Nursing Now

Today's Issues, Tomorrow's Trends

third edition

Joseph T. Catalano, RN, PhD, CCRN
Department Chair
Professor of Nursing
East Central University
Ada, Oklahoma

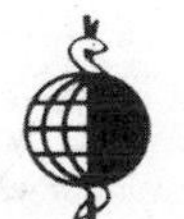
F. A. DAVIS COMPANY • Philadelphia

F. A. Davis Company
1915 Arch Street
Philadelphia, PA 19103
www.fadavis.com

Printed in the United States of America

Last digit indicates print number: 10 9 8 7 6 5 4 3

The painting used on the front cover is 'The Prophecy - Sleep Suite 2', 1955, by Stanton MacDonald-Wright, (1890-1973). Courtesy of Goldfield Galleries, 8380 Melrose Ave., Los Angeles, CA 90069, (323) 651-1122.

Acquisitions Editor: Robert G. Martone
Developmental Editors: Melanie J. Freely and Michelle Clarke
Production Editors: Nwakaego Fletcher-Perry and Arlene Chappelle
Cover Designer: Louis Forgione

As new scientific information becomes available through basic and clinical research, recommended treatments and drug therapies undergo changes. The author(s) and publisher have done everything possible to make this book accurate, up to date, and in accord with accepted standards at the time of publication. The author(s), editors, and publisher are not responsible for errors or omissions or for consequences from application of the book, and make no warranty, expressed or implied, in regard to the contents of the book. Any practice described in this book should be applied by the reader in accordance with professional standards of care used in regard to the unique circumstances that may apply in each situation. The reader is advised always to check product information (package inserts) for changes and new information regarding dose and contraindications before administering any drug. Caution is especially urged when using new or infrequently ordered drugs.

Library of Congress Cataloging-in-Publication Data

Catalano, Joseph T.
Nursing now : today's issues, tomorrow's trends / Joseph T. Catalano.–3rd. ed.
p. ; cm.
Includes bibliographical references and index.
ISBN 0-8036-1040-8 (pbk.)
1. Nursing–Vocational guidance. 2. Nursing–Practice. 3. Nursing–Social aspects.
4. Nursing–Philosophy. I. Title.
[DNLM: 1. Nursing–trends. WY 16 C357n 2003]
RT82 .C33 2003
610.73'06'9–dc21

2002031371

Dedication

To all those dedicated students with high stress levels who are the hope and future of our profession.

Preface

The dawn of a new century has brought changes no one could have dreamed of only a few short years ago. New technological advances have pushed health care into areas of genetics and bioscience that challenge the imaginations of even futuristic science fiction writers. Unimaginable acts of terror have induced a type of societal paranoia never seen before. Yet, many of the traditional challenges remain. The nursing shortage has reached panic levels in many parts of the country. The quality of health care in general remains a challenge for health-care providers. Changing management systems increase the stress on nurses.

If nothing else, the profession of nursing is finally receiving its long overdue recognition as a vital part of the health-care system. Nurses preparing to work in a changing health-care setting are faced with ever increasing demands to learn more, do more, and be more. Students entering nursing schools today come from diverse cultural, personal, and educational backgrounds. Yet, they are required to master a tremendous amount of information and learn a wide variety of skills so that they can successfully pass the licensure exam and become competent registered nurses.

As with the second edition, we have been listening to our readers. The third edition of *Nursing Now! Today's Issues, Tomorrow's Trends* incorporates many of the suggestions that have been made since its last publication. We are very excited about the revised text and believe its quality and content meet the high standards demanded by our readers.

Although the second edition had substantial content on leadership and management, it was integrated with other chapters. Because of the emphasis that is currently being placed on changing institutional organizational structures, this material was collected and emphasized in a separate unit on Leading and Managing. New chapters in this section include Chapter 12, Principles of Leadership and Management, and Chapter 14, Delegation and Supervision in Nursing.

In response to a suggestion by our readers, Chapter 2, Historical Perspectives, was added to the text. A substantial expansion of Chapter 10, NCLEX: What You Need to Know, was also made.

The book still retains its interactive format, with its journal layout, current issues boxes, and integrated questions throughout. The overall purpose of the book remains the presentation of an overview and synthesis of the important issues and trends that are basic to the development of professional nursing and affect nursing both today and into the future. Our readers tell us that the book can be used both at the beginning of the students' educational process as the basis for an "Introduction to Nursing" course and toward the end of the process as part of an "Issues and Trends" course. Nursing students remain the primary intended audience for *Nursing Now*. However, practicing nurses have reported that there is a sufficiently wide range of current issues and topics covered in enough depth to be useful for their practice.

Thinking about the future and what is required sometimes seems overwhelming. One characteristic that nurses and the nursing profession have always had and will continue to possess into the future is flexibility. The ability to adapt to changes in the health-care system while remaining focused on providing high-quality care is essential for the survival of the nursing profession. The only way that nurses will be able to effectively practice their profession in a demanding health-care system is to remain firmly rooted in those values and beliefs that have always served as their source of strength. Even more so than in the past, nurses need to look to each other for the inspiration and the strength that allow them to succeed. Professional organizations still serve as the single most powerful force for nurses, and membership in professional organizations is becoming increasingly important.

It is my belief that this book will help future nurses become familiar with the important issues and trends that affect the profession and health care. The nursing profession needs highly skilled nurses who can teach, do research, solve complicated client problems, provide high-level care, and obtain advanced degrees. The leaders of the profession will come from those students who have a clear understanding of what it means to be a professional nurse and who are willing to invest the effort in attaining their goals.

JOSEPH T. CATALANO, RN, PHD

Acknowledgments

I would like to express my thanks to all my students and colleagues who have over the years shaped my thoughts and ideas about the nursing profession. I would particularly like to acknowledge Peggy Hart, RN, PhD, a co-professor for many years, for her insights, dedication, and support. Finally, this text would never have been completed without the direction, encouragement, and support of Melanie Freely and Michelle Clarke.

Contributors

Contributors to the second edition

Tonia Aiken, RN, BSN, JD
President and CEO
Aiken Development Group
New Orleans, Louisiana

Mary Evans, RN, JD
Colorado Springs, Colorado

Deborah Finfgeld, RN, PhD
Professor of Nursing
Illinois Wesleyan University
School of Nursing
Bloomington, Illinois

Anita G. Hufft, RN, PhD
Associate Professor
East Central University
Ada, Oklahoma

Donna Gentile O'Donnell, RN, MSN
Deputy Health Commissioner (Formerly)
Health Commissioner's Office, Policy and Planning
Philadelphia, Pennsylvania

Cindy Peternelj-Taylor, RN, MSC
Associate Professor
University of Saskatchewan
Saskatoon, Saskatchewan
Canada

Nancy C. Sharts-Hopko, RN, PhD, FAAN
Professor
Villanova University
Villanova, Pennsylvania

Kathleen Mary Young, RN,C, MA
Instructor
Western Michigan University
Kalamazoo, Michigan

The author also wishes to acknowledge the contributors from the previous edition.

Contributor to the third edition

Lydia DeSantis, RN, PhD, FAAN
University of Miami
School of Nursing
Miami, Florida

Consultants

Nicole Harder, RN, MPA
Lecturer, Faculty of Nursing
University of Manitoba
Helen Glass Centre for Nursing
Winnipeg, Manitoba
Canada
(BSN program)

Deirdre A. Krause, RN, PhD, ARNP, CS
Associate Professor
Lynn University
Boca Raton, Florida
(BSN program)

Pamela H. Linkous, RN, BSN, MS
(ADN program)

Kathleen Mitchell, RN, CS, NP, MEd, DNS
Professor of Nursing
William Carey School of Nursing
O.N.O.B.T.S.
New Orleans, Louisiana
(BSN program)

Dianna Scherlin, RN, MS, CAGS
Nursing Programs Director, Department Chair, and Professor
New Hampshire Community Technical College-Claremont Nashua
Nashua, New Hampshire
(LPN, ADN, and Nursing Assistant programs)

Marshelle Thobaben, RNC, MS, PNP, PHN, FNP
Professor
Humboldt State University
Department of Nursing
Arcata, California
(BSN program)

Patty Tillman-Annear, RN, MSN
Assistant Professor, Nursing and Allied Health
Butler County Community College
Butler, Pennsylvania
(ADN program)

Contents

1

The Growth of Nursing

1

The Development of a Profession

Joseph T. Catalano

Learning Objectives

After completing this chapter, the reader will be able to:

- Define the terms *position, job, occupation*, and *profession*.
- Compare the three approaches to defining a profession.
- Analyze those traits defining a profession that nursing has attained.
- Evaluate why nursing has failed to attain some of the traits that define a profession.
- Correlate the concept of power with its important characteristics.

Since the time of Florence Nightingale, each generation of nurses, in its own way, has fostered the movement to professionalize the image of nurses and nursing. The struggle to change the status of nurses from that of female domestic servants to one of high-level health-care providers who base their protocols on scientific principles has been a primary goal of nursing's leaders for many years. Yet some people, both inside and outside of the profession of nursing, question whether the search for and attainment of professional status is worth the effort and price that must ultimately be paid.

At some levels in nursing, the question of **professionalism** takes on immense significance. However, to the busy **staff nurse**—who is trying to allocate client assignments for a shift; distribute the medications at 9 A.M. to 24 clients; and supervise two aides, a licensed practical nurse (LPN) or licensed vocational nurse (LVN), and a nursing student—the issue may not seem very significant at all.

Indeed, when nurses were first developing their identity separate from that of physicians, there was no thought about their being part of a **profession**. Over the years, however, as the scope of practice has expanded and the responsibilities have increased, nurses have increasingly begun to consider what they do as professional activities.

This chapter presents some of the current thought concerning professions and where nursing stands in relationship to these viewpoints.

Approaches to Defining a Profession

In common usage, terms such as *position*, *job*, *occupation*, *profession*, *professional*, and *professionalism* are often used interchangeably and incorrectly. The following definitions will clarify what is meant by these terms within this text.

Position: A group of tasks assigned to one individual.

Job: A group of positions that are similar in nature and level of skill that can be carried out by one or more individuals.

Occupation: A group of jobs that are similar in type of work and that are usually found throughout an industry or work environment.

Profession: A type of occupation that meets certain criteria (discussed later in this chapter) that raise it to a level above that of an occupation.

Professional: A person who belongs to and practices a profession. (The term *professional* is probably the most misused of all these terms when describing people who are clearly involved in jobs or occupations, such as a "professional truck driver," "professional football player," or even a "professional thief.")

Professionalism: The demonstration of high-level personal, ethical, and skill characteristics of a member of a profession.[1]

Experts in social science have been attempting to develop a "foolproof" approach to determine what constitutes a profession for almost 100 years, but with only minimal success. Three common models are the process approach, the power approach, and the most widely accepted trait approach.

What Do You Think?

Do you really care if nursing is a profession? How will it affect the way that you practice nursing?

Process Approach

The process approach views all occupations as points of development into a profession along a continuum ranging from position to profession.

Continuum of Professional Development:

Position ←——→ Profession

Using this approach, the question becomes not whether nursing and truck driving are professions, but where they are located along the continuum. Occupations, such as medicine, law, and the ministry, are widely accepted by the public as being closest to the professional end of the continuum.[2] Other occupations may be less clearly defined.

The major difficulty with this approach is that it lacks criteria on which to base judgments. Final determination of the status of an occupation or profession depends almost completely on public perception of the activities of that occupation. Nursing has always had a rather poor public image when it comes to being viewed as a profession.

Power Approach

The power approach uses two criteria to define a profession:

1. How much independence of practice does this occupation have?
2. How much power does this occupation control?

The concept of power is discussed later in this chapter, but in this context it refers to political power and the amount of money that the person in that occupation earns.[3]

Using this determinant, occupations such as medicine, law, and **politics** would clearly be considered professions. The members of these occupations earn high incomes, practice their skills with a great deal of independence, and exercise significant power over individuals, the public, and the political community, both individually and in organized groups. The ministry is generally perceived as having power and influence. However, most persons in this group, except for a few individuals such as television evangelists, have relatively low income levels. Nursing, of course, with its relatively poor salaries, low membership in organizations, and perceived lack of political power, would clearly not meet the power criteria for a profession.

The question that comes to mind is whether power, independence of practice, and high incomes are the only elements that determine professional status. Although those three factors confer status in our culture, other elements can be considered as significant in how a profession is viewed. For example, for many, members of the clergy have a great deal of power when they act as counselors, speakers of the truth, and community leaders.

Trait Approach

Of the many researchers and theorists who have attempted to identify the traits that define a profession, Flexner,[4] Bixler,[5] and Pavalko[6] are most widely accepted as the leaders in the field. These three social scientists have determined that the following common characteristics are important:

- High intellectual level
- High level of individual responsibility and **accountability**
- Specialized body of knowledge
- Knowledge that can be learned in institutions of higher education
- Public service and altruistic activities
- Public service valued over financial gain
- Relatively high degree of **autonomy** and independence of practice
- Need for a well-organized and strong organization representing the members of the profession and controlling the quality of practice
- A **code of ethics** that guides the members of the profession in their practice
- Strong professional identity and commitment to the development of the profession
- Demonstration of professional competency and possession of a legally recognized license

Nursing as a Profession

How does nursing compare with other professions when measured against these widely accepted professional traits? The profession of nursing meets most of the criteria but falls short in a few areas.

High Intellectual Level of Functioning

In the very early stages of the development of the practice of nursing, this criterion did not apply. Florence Nightingale raised the bar for education, and graduates of her school were considered to be highly educated compared with other women of that time. However, most of the tasks performed by these early nurses are generally considered by today's standards to be menial and routine. On the other hand, as health care has advanced and made great strides in technology, pharmacology, and all branches of the physical sciences, a high level of intellectual functioning is required for even relatively simple nursing tasks, such as taking a client's temperature or blood pressure using automated equipment. Nurses use **assessment** skills and knowledge, have the ability to reason, and make routine judgments based on clients' conditions daily. Without a doubt, professional nurses must and do function at a high intellectual level.

High Level of Individual Responsibility and Accountability

Not too long ago, a nurse was rarely, if ever, named as a **defendant** in a malpractice suit. The public, in general, did not view nurses as having enough knowledge to be held accountable for errors that were made in client care. This is not the case in the health-care system today. Nurses are often the primary, and frequently the only, defendants named when errors are made that result in injury to the client. Nurses must be accountable and demonstrate a high level of individual responsibility for the care and services that they provide.

> *As health care has advanced and made great strides in technology, pharmacology, and all branches of the physical sciences, a high level of intellectual functioning is required for even relatively simple nursing tasks, such as taking a client's temperature or blood pressure using automated equipment.*

The concept of accountability has legal, ethical, and professional implications that include accepting responsibility for actions taken to provide **client** care as well as accepting responsibility for the consequences of actions that are not performed. A nurse can no longer state that "the physician told me to do it" as a method of avoiding responsibility for his or her actions.

Specialized Body of Knowledge

Most early nursing skills practiced were based either on traditional ways of doing things or on the intuitive knowledge of the individual nurse. As nursing has developed into an identifiable, separate discipline, a specialized body of knowledge called "nursing science" was compiled through the research efforts of nurses who hold advanced educational degrees. Although this body of specialized nursing knowledge is relatively small, it forms a theoretical basis for the practice of nursing today. As more nurses obtain advanced degrees, conduct research, and develop philosophies and theories about nursing, this body of knowledge will increase in scope.

Evidence-Based Practice

In professional nursing today, there is an increasing emphasis on evidence-based practice. Almost all the currently used nursing theories address this issue in some way. Simply stated, evidence-based practice is the practice of nursing in which interventions are based on data from research that demonstrates that they are appropriate and successful. It involves a systematic process of uncovering, evaluating, and using information from research as the basis for making decisions about and providing client care. Many nursing practices and interventions of the past were performed merely because that is the way it was always done (accustomed practice) or because of deductions from physiologic or pathophysiologic information. Clients are now more sophisticated and knowledgeable about health-care issues and demand a higher level of knowledge and skill from their health-care providers.

The development of information technology has made evidenced-based practice in nursing a reality. In the past, nurses relied primarily on units within their own facilities for information about the success of treatments, decisions about health care, and outcomes for clients. Nursing education now requires nursing students to perform Web-based research for papers and projects, so that by the time of graduation, these nurses feel comfortable accessing a wide range of the most current and highest quality of information through electronic sources. Of course, one of the key limiting factors of evidence-based practice is the quality of the information on which the practice is based. Evaluating the quality of information on the Web can be difficult at times.

The first step in developing an evidenced-based practice is to identify exactly what the intervention is supposed to accomplish. Once the goal or client outcome is identified, then the nurse needs to evaluate current practices and whether or not they are achieving the client outcomes. If they are not successful, or if the

ISSUES NOW

Web Sites: Friend or Foe?

Have a paper or report to do for class? Need information on pheochromocytoma, post-traumatic stress disorder, Kawasaki's disease? No problem, look it up on the Web, right? Well, yes and no. Without any question, there is a tremendous amount of information about almost any subject available just a few mouse clicks away. But the bigger question is: how good is that information? The truth of the matter is that anyone can post almost anything on-line these days, and there are no organizations or agencies that oversee or review the information for quality, accuracy, or objectivity. So how are you supposed to know what is good and what is not? Although there is no foolproof method for determining the quality of any given Web site, there are some telltale markers that can point you in the right direction when you are rating the quality of the information you are seeking.

Marker 1: Peer Review

All major professional journals have a peer review process that requires any manuscripts submitted to be reviewed by two or three professionals who are considered experts or at least knowledgeable in the subject matter. Peer review is one of the key elements in ensuring the accuracy of the information in the manuscript. When considering a Web source, look for a clear statement of the source of the information and how that information is reviewed. If the information is from an established source, such as a recognized professional journal, then it has been peer-reviewed and has a higher degree of accuracy. Examine the format and writing style of the document. If it seems to be very choppy, or the style, tone, or person the article is written in changes throughout the article, it is an indication that it was not well edited and probably not peer-reviewed. Use the information with caution.

Marker 2: Author Credentials

The name of the author and his or her titles and credentials should be listed. Be cautious if no author or publisher is listed. Of course, anyone can use another person's name as the author, but it is relatively easy to cross-check authors' names through other databases, such as those found in libraries. Before accepting the information as gospel, it is probably worth looking up the author and seeing what other articles or books he or she has written. Another key to establishing author credentials is to establish to whom the Web site belongs. In general, personal Web pages are less likely to contain authoritative information. You can also look at the last three letters in the Web site address. The ones that end in ".gov," ".org," or ".edu" will tend to have higher quality information. Also, see whether the information has a copyright. Copyrighted information means that the person felt strongly enough about what he or she was posting to go through the effort to make sure no one else can use it as their original information.

Marker 3: Prejudice and Bias

Although there is almost always a small degree of prejudice and bias in all written material, most legitimate authors will strive to be as objective as possible. Many times if you read a document with a critical eye, you can discern obvious prejudicial viewpoints. See if the author has a vested interest in the content of the document. You can be pretty sure that an article about the effects of tobacco use on the respiratory system written by a scientist who was hired by the R. J. Reynolds Company would have a decidedly different viewpoint than an article written by a scientist who was employed by the National Health Information Center. See if contact information is provided by the author and who the sponsor or publisher of the document is. If these are not provided, be suspicious about the information.

Marker 4: Timeliness

Of course all of us want the most recent information we can find and sometimes mistakenly make the assumption that because it is on the Web, it is new. In reality, professional journals that post their partial-text or full-text articles on their Web sites usually take anywhere from 6 to 9 months to do so. If you want the absolutely most current information, the hard-copy journal texts found in the library still are your best bet. Some forms of the Web have been around for as many as 10 years now, so some of the material can be well outdated. See if you can determine when the site was last updated and how extensively the information was revised. It is also a good practice to look to other sources (Web, journals, books, etc.) to compare the material for currency. Many Web sites will have links where you can access other related information. If those links have messages such as "Page discontinued" or "Link no longer available" be extremely cautious with the information. Good links should connect you to other reliable sites.

Marker 5: Presentation

Although the old saying is that "you can't tell a book by its cover," experienced Web-surfers can often tell a lot about a Web site by its presentation. There are some that look well developed and professional, and others that look very amateurish. There is no guarantee that the slick-looking Web sites are better, but it is one factor to consider in the overall evaluation of the information you are seeking. Take a look at the graphics. They should be balanced with the text and help explain or demonstrate information in the text. If the graphics seem to be just decorative, it should raise a "red flag" about the content of the site. Some sites use a compressed format that requires special programs such as Adobe Acrobat. If you do not have access to these programs, then the information in the site is unusable. Move on to the next site.

In summary, the Internet can be a very valuable source of information about a wide variety of subjects. However, each source of information needs to be evaluated carefully. Following the five markers discussed here will place you on the path to deciding the quality of the information presented in any given Web site.

Sources: Thurmond, VA: Considering theory in assessing quality of Web-based courses. Nurse Educator 27(1):20–24, 2002.

DeBourgh, GA: Using Web technology in a clinical nursing course. Nurse Educator 26(5):227–233, 2001.

Timmons, S: Use of the Internet by patients: Not a threat to nursing, but an opportunity? Nurse Education Today 21(2):104–109, 2001.

Take a byte: Evaluating Web sites. American Nursing Student 5(1):1, 2001.

http://www.mlanet.org/resources/medspeak/topten.html

nurse feels they can be more efficient with fewer complications, then research sources need to be collected. These can be from published journal articles (either electronic or hard copy) and from presentations at research or practice conferences that often present the most current information. Then a plan should be developed to implement the new findings. This process can be applied to changing policy and procedures or developing training programs for facility staff. Research data should always be used when initiating new practices or modifying old ones.

> *Evidence-based practice is the practice of nursing in which interventions are based on data from research that demonstrates that they are appropriate and successful.*

Public Service and Altruistic Activities

Almost all major nursing theorists, when defining nursing, include a statement that refers to a goal of helping clients to adapt to illness and to achieve their highest level of functioning. The public (variously referred to as consumers, patients, clients, individuals, or humans) is the focal point of all nursing models and nursing practice. The public service function of nursing has always been recognized and acknowledged by society's willingness to continue to educate nurses in public, tax-supported institutions as well as in private schools. In addition, nursing has been viewed universally as being an altruistic profession composed of selfless individuals who place the lives and well-being of their clients above their personal safety. In the earliest days, dedicated nurses provided care for victims of deadly plagues with little regard for their own welfare. Today, nurses are found in remote and often hostile areas, providing care for the sick and dying, working 12-hour shifts, being "on call," and working rotating shifts.

Few individuals enter nursing in order to become rich and famous. It is likely that those who do so for these reasons quickly become disappointed. Although the pay scale has increased tremendously since the 1990s, nursing is, at best, a middle-income occupation. Surveys among students entering nursing programs continue to indicate that the primary reason for wishing to become a nurse is to "help others" or "make a difference" in someone's life and to have "job security." Rarely do these beginning students include "to make a lot of money" as their motivation.[7]

Well-Organized and Strong Professional Organization

Professional organizations represent the members of the profession and control the quality of professional practice. The National League for Nursing (NLN) and the American Nurses Association (ANA) are the two major national organizations that represent nursing in today's health-care system. The NLN is primarily responsible for regulating the quality of the educational programs that prepare nurses for the practice of nursing, whereas the ANA is more concerned with the quality of nursing practice in the daily health-care setting. These and other organizations are discussed in more detail in Chapter 3.

Both these organizations are well organized, but neither can be considered powerful when compared with other professional organizations, such as the American Medical Association (AMA) or the American Bar Association (ABA). One reason for their lack of strength is that fewer than 15 percent of all nurses in the United States are members of any professional organization at the national level.[3] Many nurses do belong to specialty organizations that represent a specific area of practice, but these lack sufficient political power to produce changes in health-care laws and policies at the national level.

Nurses' Code of Ethics

Nursing has several codes of ethics that are used to guide nursing practice. The ANA Code of Ethics for Nurses, the most widely used in the United States, was first published in 1971, updated in 1985, and last updated in 2001. The current ANA Code of Ethics, while maintaining the integrity found in earlier versions, is now more relevant to current health-care and nursing practices. This code of ethics is recognized by other professions as a standard with which others are compared. The nurses' code of ethics and its implications are discussed in greater detail in Chapter 7.

Competency and Professional License

Nurses must pass a national licensure examination to demonstrate that they are qualified to practice nursing. Only after passing this examination are nurses allowed to practice. The granting of a nursing **license** is a legal activity conducted by the individual state under the **regulations** contained in that state's nurse practice act.

When Nursing Falls Short of Meeting the Criteria for a Profession

Before Florence Nightingale practiced nursing, people considered it to be unnecessary, if not outright dangerous, to educate nurses through independent nursing programs in publicly supported educational institutions. As nursing has developed, particularly in the United States, the recognition of the intellectual nature of the practice, as well as the vast amount of knowledge required for the job, has led to a belief by some nursing leaders that college education for nurses is now a necessity.

Nursing is the only major discipline that does not require its members to hold at least a baccalaureate degree in order to obtain licensure. Although the number of diploma programs in nursing has decreased tremendously since 1990, associate degree programs continue to maintain high enrollment and graduate large numbers of individuals. Whether a baccalaureate degree nursing program should be the minimum requirement for entry-level nurses remains a hotly debated issue.[1,6,7,10]

Autonomy and Independence of Practice

Historically, the handmaiden or servant relationship of the nurse to the physician was widely accepted. It was based on several factors, including social norms. For example, women became nurses, whereas men became physicians; and women were subservient to men, the nature of the work being such that nurses cleaned and physicians cured. In terms of the relative levels of education of the two groups, the average nursing program lasted for 1 year, whereas physician education lasted for 6 to 8 years. Unfortunately, despite efforts to expand nursing practice into more independent areas through updated nurse practice legislation, nursing retains much of its subservient image. In reality, nursing is both an independent and interdependent discipline. Nurses in all health-care settings must work closely with physicians, hospital administrators, pharmacists, and other groups in the provision of care. In some cases, nurses in **advanced practice** roles, such as **nurse practitioners**, can and do establish their own independent practices. Actually, most state **nurse practice acts** allow nurses more independence in their practice than they realize. To be considered a true profession, nursing will need to be recognized by other disciplines as having practitioners who practice nursing independently.

Professional Identity and Development

The issue of job versus career is in question here. A job is a group of positions that are similar in nature and level of skill that can be carried out by one or more individuals. There is relatively little commitment to a job, and many individuals move from one job to another with little regard to the long-term outcomes. A career, in contrast, is usually viewed as a person's major lifework, which progresses and develops as the person grows older. Careers and professions have many of the same characteristics, including a formal education, full-time employment, requirement for lifelong learning, and a dedication to what is being achieved. Although an increasing number of nurses view nursing as their life's work, many still treat nursing more as a job.

The problem becomes circular. The reason nurses lack a strong professional identity and do not consider nursing a lifelong career is because nursing does not have full status as a profession. Until nurses are fully committed to the profession of nursing, identify with it as a profession, and are dedicated to its future development, nursing will probably not achieve professional status.

Members of the Team

The health-care delivery system employs large numbers of diagnosticians, technicians, direct care providers, administrators, and support staff (Table 1–1). It is estimated that there are more than 300 job titles used to describe health-care workers. Among these are nurses, physicians, physician assistants, social workers, physical therapists, occupational therapists, respiratory therapists, clinical psychologists, and pharmacists. All these individuals provide services that are essential to daily operation of the health-care delivery system in this country.

Of particular importance among this array of health-care workers are various types of nurses: registered nurses, licensed practical (vocational) nurses, nurse practitioners, case managers, and clinical nurse specialists. Each of these requires a different type of educational background, clinical expertise, and, sometimes, professional credentialing. In general, all nurses make valuable contributions within the health-care delivery system. There has been an increased demand for nurses who are educated to deliver care in the

Table 1–1
Other Key Health-Care Team Members

TITLE	CREDENTIAL	PRACTICE
Physician (MD)	License–Medical	Medical—limited only by specialization Some serve as primary care providers
Physician (DO)	License–Osteopath	Medical, with focus on body movement and holistic health—similar to MD Can serve as primary care providers
Physician (DC)	License–Chiropractor	Limited—focus on spinal column and nervous system Unable to prescribe medications
Physician (DPM)	License–Podiatry	Limited—foot problems Can prescribe medications, perform foot surgery
Physician Assistant	Certification–no individual license	Practice on physician's license Practice limited by medical practice act and wishes of supervising physician
Social Workers	License	Increasingly important as health care becomes more complex Resolve financial, housing, psychosocial, and employment problems; do discharge planning and assist clients in transfer between facilities. May serve in case management roles to coordinate services.
Physical Therapists	License	Focus on helping clients maintain or regain the highest level of function possible after strokes, spinal cord injury, arthritis, or residual effects of traumatic accidents. Help prevent physical decline and regain the ability to groom, eat, and walk through individualized range of motion and exercise programs. Therapy occurs in hospitals, clinics, or in the community
Respiratory Therapists	License	Strive to restore normal or as near normal pulmonary functioning as possible by conducting diagnostic tests and administering treatments that have been prescribed by a physician
Clinical Psychologists	License	Assist clients to manage mental health problems Private practice, clinics
Pharmacists	License	Distribute prescribed and over-the-counter medications, educate clients, monitor appropriate medication selections, detect interactions and untoward responses in community pharmacies and institutional settings Valuable resource for nurses

community setting and in long-term health-care settings rather than in the hospital. There has also been a need for nurse case managers who are prepared to coordinate care for vulnerable populations requiring costly services over extended periods. Nursing education programs are attempting to meet these needs by preparing individuals who can practice independently and autonomously, network, collaborate, and coordinate services. These programs also offer more clinical experiences in rehabilitation, nursing home, and community settings.

What Do You Think?

List and rate several of your recent experiences with the health-care system. In what roles did you observe registered nurses functioning?

Registered Nurses, Licensed Practical Nurses, and Unlicensed Assistive Personnel

Registered nurses (RNs) who have been educated at the associate, diploma, or baccalaureate level have traditionally been considered the cornerstone of the current health-care delivery system. In the past, most RNs worked within hospital settings and provided direct client care and nursing administration functions within these facilities. Owing to past trends in health-care funding, there were fewer hospital admissions, which temporarily decreased the demand for RNs in acute care facilities and increased the need for well-prepared nurses who could function autonomously within the community. However, current trends in population and health care have demonstrated a need for RNs in both acute care and community settings. The need still remains within institutional settings, for licensed practical nurses (LPNs) and unlicensed assistive personnel (UAP) who work under the supervision of an RN. This pattern of care is particularly evident in nursing homes and other long-term care facilities.[2]

Advanced Practice Nurses

For individuals who are unfamiliar with the health-care delivery system, it is sometimes difficult to understand the similarities and differences between nursing titles and roles. This confusion is particularly evident in the case of clinical nurse specialists (CNSs) and nurse practitioners (NPs), who are sometimes collectively referred to as advanced practice nurses (APNs). In general, NPs are prepared to provide direct client care in primary care settings, focusing on health promotion, illness prevention, early diagnosis, and treatment of common health problems. Their educational preparation varies, but in most cases individuals successfully complete a graduate nurse practitioner program and are certified by the American Nurses Credentialing Center (ANCC) or an appropriate professional nursing organization. Depending on the individual state practice act, NPs have a range of responsibility for diagnosing diseases and prescribing both treatments and medications. A growing number of states now grant NPs direct third-party reimbursement for their services without a physician.

Clinical nurse specialists usually practice in secondary or tertiary care settings and focus on care of individuals who are experiencing an acute illness or an exacerbation of a chronic condition. In general, they are prepared at the graduate level and are ANCC certified. CNSs are highly skilled practitioners who are comfortable working in high-tech environments with seriously ill individuals and their families. Because of the nature of their work, they are excellent health-care educators and physician collaborators.

Attempts have been made to combine the roles of the CNS and NP so that the best qualities of both roles are preserved. The goal of this combination is to provide high-quality care to individuals in a wide array of health-care settings who have a wide range of health problems. Advocates of this movement include the NLN, American Association of Colleges of Nursing (AACN), and the ANA. Titling for this new blended role is unconfirmed, and state legislatures may make the final decisions through their licensing laws. As such, titling, educational preparation, and practice privileges will probably vary from one state to another.

Case Managers

One argument for the blended NP/CNS role is the need for case managers who possess the expertise of both levels of preparation. Case managers coordinate services for clients with high-risk or long-term health problems who have access to the full continuum of health-care services. Case managers provide services in various settings, such as acute care facilities, rehabilitation centers, and community agencies. They also work for managed-care companies, insurance companies, and private case management agencies. Their roles vary depending on the circumstances of their employment; however, their overall goal is to coordinate the use of health-care services in the most efficient and cost-effective manner possible. Case management is the "glue" that holds health-care services together across practitioners, agencies, funding sources, locations, and time. Titling, educational preparation, and certification of nurse case managers are now available. The ANCC has developed certification eligibility criteria for nurse case managers, and an examination is available. At this time, case managers can be physicians, social workers, registered nurses, and even well-intentioned laypersons with little health-care education.

Empowerment in Nursing

One of the concerns that has plagued nurses and nursing almost from its development as a separate health-care specialty is the relatively large amount of personal responsibility shouldered by nurses combined with a relatively small amount of control over their practice. Even in the more enlightened atmosphere of today's society, with its concerns about equal opportunity, equal pay, and collegial relationships, many nurses still seem uncomfortable with the concepts of power and control in their practice. Their discomfort may arise from the belief that nursing is a helping and caring profession whose goals are separate from issues of power. Historically, nurses have never had much power, and previous attempts at gaining power and control over their practice have been met with much resistance from groups who benefit from keeping nurses powerless. Nevertheless, all nurses use power in their daily practice, even if they do not realize it. Until nurses understand the sources of their power, how to increase it, and how to use it in providing client care, they will be relegated to a subservient position in the health-care system.

The Nature of Power

The term *power* has many meanings. From the standpoint of nursing, power is probably best defined as the ability or capacity to exert influence over another person or group of persons. In other words, power is the ability to get other people to do things even when they do not want to do them. Although power in itself is neither good nor bad, it can be used to produce either good or bad results.

Power is always a two-way street. By its very definition, when power is exerted by one person, another person is affected; that is, the use of power by one person requires that another person give up some of his or her power. Individuals are always in a state of change, either increasing their power or losing some; the balance of power rarely remains static. **Empowerment** refers to the increased amount of power that an individual or group is either given or gains.

Origins of Power

If power is such an important part of nursing and the practice of nurses, where does it come from? Although there are many sources, some of them would be inappropriate or unacceptable for those in a helping and caring profession. The following list includes some of the more accessible and acceptable sources of power that nurses should consider using in their practice.[3,8,9] These sources are:

- Referent
- Expert
- Reward
- Coercive
- Legitimate
- Collective

Referent Power

The referent source of power depends on establishing and maintaining a close personal relationship with someone. In any close personal relationship, one individual often will do something he or she would really rather not do because of the relationship. This ability to be able to change the actions of another is an exercise of power. Nurses often obtain power from this source when they establish and maintain good therapeutic relationships with their clients. Clients take medications, tolerate uncomfortable treatments, and participate in demanding activities that they would clearly prefer to avoid because the nurse has a good relationship with them. Likewise, nurses who have good collegial relationships with other nurses, departments, and physicians are often able to obtain what they want from these individuals or groups in providing care to clients.

Expert Power

The expert source of power derives from the amount of knowledge, skill, or expertise that an individual or group has. This power source is exercised by the individual or group when knowledge, skills, or expertise is either used or withheld in order to influence the behavior of others. Nurses should have at least a minimal amount of this type of power because of their education and experience. It follows logically that increasing the level of nurses' education will, or should, increase this expert power. As nurses attain and remain in positions of power longer, the increased experience will also aid the use of expert power. Nurses in advanced practice roles are good examples of those who have expert power. Their additional education and experience provide these nurses with the ability to practice skills at a higher level, compared with nurses prepared at the basic education level.

Nurses access this expert source of power when they use their knowledge to teach, counsel, or motivate clients to follow a plan of care. Nurses can also use this source of power when dealing with physicians. By demonstrating their knowledge of the client's condition, recent laboratory tests, and other elements that are vital in the client's recovery, nurses demonstrate their expert power. This knowledge may increase the amount of respect that they are given by physicians.

By demonstrating their knowledge of the client's condition, recent laboratory tests, and other elements that are vital in the client's recovery, nurses demonstrate their expert power. This knowledge may increase the amount of respect that they are given by physicians.

Power of Rewards

The reward source of power depends on the ability of one person to grant another some type of reward for specific behaviors or changes in behavior. The rewards themselves can take on many different forms, including personal favors, promotions, money, expanded privileges, and eradication of punishments. Nurses, in their daily provision of care, can use this source of power to influence client behavior. For example, a nurse can give a client extra praise for completing the prescribed range-of-motion exercises. There are many aspects of the daily care of clients over which nurses have a substantial amount of reward power. This reward source of power is also the underlying principle in the process of behavior modification.

Coercive Power

The coercive source of power is the flip side of the reward source. The ability to punish, withhold rewards, and threaten punishment is the key element underlying the coercive source of power. Although nurses do have access to this source of power, it is probably one that they use minimally, if at all. Not only does the use of the coercive source of power destroy thera-

ISSUES IN PRACTICE

Kasey is an RN who has worked on the busy surgical unit of a large city hospital for the past 6 years. As one of three RNs on the unit's day shift, she often serves at the charge nurse when the assigned charge nurse has a day off. She is hard working, caring, and well organized and provides high-quality care for the often very unstable postoperative clients they receive on a daily basis.

Approximately 2 weeks ago, Kasey's mother was admitted for a high-risk surgical removal of a brain tumor that was not responding to chemotherapy or radiation therapy. The surgery did not go well, and Kasey's mother was admitted to the surgical unit after the procedure. During the past 2 weeks, she has shown a gradual but steady decline in condition and is no longer able to recognize her family, speak, or do any self-care. It is believed she will probably not live more than a week longer.

Per hospital policy, Kasey is not assigned to care for her mother; however, during her shifts, Kasey is spending more and more time with her mother, sometimes to the detriment of her assigned clients. She is also beginning to make more demands on the unit nursing staff, often overseeing their care and requesting that only certain nurses care for her mother. One of the other nurses on the unit suggested that Kasey's mother be moved to a less specialized unit. When Kasey heard about the suggestion, she became livid and loudly scolded the nurse for her insensitivity in the middle of the nurses station.

Questions for thought:

1. Is the practice of not allowing nurses to provide care for their relatives evidence-based or accustomed practice?
2. Identify the steps in making this policy evidence-based.
3. Do you think nurses should be allowed to care for relatives? Why? Why not?

peutic and personal relationships, but it can also be considered unethical and even illegal in certain situations. Threatening clients that they will get an injection if they do not take their oral medications may motivate them to take those medications, but it is generally not considered to be a good example of therapeutic communication technique.

Legitimate Power

The legitimate source of power depends on a legislative or legal act that gives the individual or organization a right to make decisions that they might not otherwise have the authority to make. Most obviously, political figures and **legislators** have this source of power. But this power can also be disseminated and delegated to others through legislative acts. In nursing, the state board of nursing has access to the legitimate source of power because of its establishment under the nurse practice act of that state. Similarly, nurses have access to the legitimate source of power when they are licensed by the state under the provisions in the nurse practice act or when they are appointed to positions within a health-care agency. Nursing decisions made about client care can come only from individuals who have a legitimate source of power to make those decisions—that is, licensed nurses.

Collective Power

The collective source of power is often used in a broader context than individual client care and is the underlying source for many other sources of power. When a large group of individuals who have similar beliefs, desires, or needs become organized, a collective source of power exists. For individuals who belong to professions, the professional organization is the focal point for this source of power. The main goal of any organization is to influence those policies that affect the members of the organization. This influence is usually in the form of political activities carried out by politicians and **lobbyists**.

Professional organizations that can deliver large numbers of votes have a powerful means of influencing politicians. The use of the collective source of power contains elements of reward, coercive, expert, and even referent sources. Each source may come into play at one time or another.

How to Increase Power in Nursing

Despite some feelings of powerlessness, nurses really do have access to some important, and rather substantial, sources of power. What can nurses, either as individuals or as a group, do in order to increase their power?

Professional Unity

Probably the first, and certainly the most important, way in which nurses can gain power in all areas is through professional unity. The most powerful groups are those that are best organized and most united. The power that a professional organization has is directly related to the size of its membership. According to the ANA, there are approximately 3 million nurses in the United States. It is not difficult to imagine the power that the ANA could have to influence legislators and legislation if all of those nurses were members of the organization rather than the 250,000 who actually do belong. This point—that nurses need to belong to their nursing national organization—cannot be emphasized too much.

Political Activities

A second way in which nurses can gain power is by becoming involved in **political action**. Although this produces discomfort in many, nurses must realize that they are affected by politics and political decisions in every phase of their daily nursing activities.

The simple truth is that if nurses do not become involved in politics and participate in important legislation that influences their practice, someone other than nurses will be making those decisions for them. Nurses need to become involved in political activities from local to national levels. The average legislator knows little about issues such as clients' rights, national health insurance, quality of nursing care, third-party reimbursement for nurses, and expanded practice roles for nurses. Yet, they make decisions about these issues almost daily. It would seem logical that more informed and better decisions could be made if nurses took an active part in the legislative process.

> *Probably the first, and certainly the most important, way in which nurses can gain power in all areas is through professional unity. The most powerful groups are those that are best organized and most united.*

Accountability and Professionalism

A third method of increasing power is by demonstrating the characteristics of accountability and professionalism. Nursing has made great strides in these two areas in recent years. Nurses, through professional organizations, have been working hard to establish standards for quality client care. More important, nurses are now concerned with demonstrating competence and delivering high-quality client care through processes such as peer review and evaluation. By accepting responsibility for the care that they provide and by setting the standards to guide that care, nurses are taking the power to govern nursing away from non-nursing groups.

Networkings

Finally, nurses can gain power through establishing a nurse support network. It is common knowledge that the "old boy" system remains alive and well in many segments of our seemingly enlightened twenty-first century society. The "old boy" system, which is found in most large organizations ranging from universities to businesses and governmental agencies, provides individuals, usually men, with the encouragement, support, and nurturing that allows them to move up quickly through the ranks in the organization to achieve high administrative positions. Nursing and nursing organizations have never had this type of system for the advancement of nurses. Part of this system of doing business involves never criticizing another "old boy" in public, even though there may be major differences of opinion in private. Presentation of a united front is extremely important in maintaining power within this system.

Part of the difficulty in establishing a nurse support network arises from the fact that nurses really have not been in high-level positions for very long. The framework for a support system for nurses is now in place; and with some commitment to the concept and activity, it can grow into a well-developed network to allow the brightest, best, and most ambitious people in the profession to achieve high-level positions.

Future Trends in the Nursing Profession

Clearly, it would be difficult to make an airtight case for nursing as a profession. Yet nursing does meet many of the criteria proposed for a profession. Although it would probably be most accurate to call nursing a developing or aspiring profession, for the purposes of this book, nursing will be referred to as a profession. Only when nurses begin to think of nursing as a profession, work toward raising the educational standards for entry level, and begin practicing independently as professionals, will the profession become a reality for nursing. The movement of any discipline from the status of occupation to one of profession is a dynamic and ongoing process with many considerations.

All the experts now predict a severe shortage of professional nurses, ranging from between 400,000 to as many a 1 million, by the year 2020. In the past, the way that nursing shortages were handled was to use a "quick-fix" method of producing more nurses in a shorter period of time by reducing the educational requirements. The current nursing education system is producing approximately 40,000 graduates from diploma and associate degree programs every year.[10] Although this number may help alleviate the nursing shortage, the more critical question to ask is whether this level of education is going to prepare nurses to meet the challenges of a rapidly changing and demanding health-care system into the twenty-first century.

As the national employment picture continues to evolve for registered nurses from bedside caregivers to coordinators of care, and financial resources become stressed, perhaps more nurses will begin to look on what they do as a lifelong commitment. Professional commitment is a complicated issue, but little doubt exists that nurses will not have increased independence of practice until they begin to demonstrate that they are professionals committed to the field of nursing.

Conclusion

Ongoing changes in the health-care system will have a major impact on how, where, and even who practices nursing. Unless nurses become involved in decisions about the direction in which health care is going, band together as a profession, and exert some of the tremendous potential power that they have, politicians, physicians, hospital administrators, and insurance companies will ultimately be shaping their future. The move toward mandated staffing ratios is one way that nurses are demonstrating their power to achieve a goal when they band together and exert power as a group.

Nursing has taken great strides forward in achieving professional status in the health-care system. Currently, many nurses accept the premise that nursing is a profession and therefore are not very concerned about furthering the process. Even as nursing has matured and evolved into a field of study with an identifiable body of knowledge, the questions and problems that have plagued this profession persist. In addition, advances in technology, management, and society have raised new questions about the nature and role of nursing in the health-care system. Only by understanding and exploring the issues of professionalism will nurses be prepared to practice effectively in the present and meet the complex challenges of the future.

ISSUES IN PRACTICE

Mandated Staffing Ratios: Creative Solution or Worsening Problem?

The nation is currently looking to California as the state moves toward approving the first laws that mandate nurse-to-client staffing ratios. Although approved in concept by the California legislature in late 1999, it took until January 2002 for specific guidelines to be developed (see following discussion). The delays in instituting the proposed ratios were caused by an ongoing controversy between nursing and consumer organizations who favor the ratios and hospital and physician organizations who strongly oppose them. If approved by the legislature, the ratios are to be phased in starting in July 2003. The proposal can still be amended following statewide hearings and a 45-day period to allow for public input.

Following in California's footsteps, a bill that would establish even stricter nurse-to-client ratios has been passed in the Florida Senate. This bill also proposes eliminating mandatory overtime for nurses involved in direct hands-on care. Predictably, the bill is opposed by the Florida Hospital Association, which argues that hospitals must be allowed to determine their own staffing needs based on client census and condition.

The slow, but inevitable move toward legislated nurse-to-client ratios is based on research that demonstrates the connection between staffing and positive or negative health-care outcomes for hospitalized clients. Nursing associations and consumer groups believe the proposal is a step toward increasing the quality of care, increasing client safety, and eventually reducing the nursing shortage by addressing one of the leading causes of attrition among nurses—burnout from poor working conditions.

Supporters of the mandated minimal staffing ratios believe that they will actually be more cost-effective for hospitals in the long run. With more nurses caring for fewer clients, clients will recover more quickly from surgeries and serious illnesses, and facilities will ultimately save money because of reduced times of stay. Similarly, the readmission rates should be reduced along with the incidence of health-care errors that increase malpractice insurance costs.

One difficulty faced was trying to determine what exactly were the optimal ratios. The current numbers were a compromise between the 1-to-10 ratio suggested by the California Healthcare Association (representing hospital administration) and the 1-to-3 ratio promoted by the California Nurses Association. Although nursing and medical literature clearly point to better outcomes when more nurses care for fewer clients, unfortunately it does not provide any hard scientific findings about what the optimal staffing ratios should be. It will likely be a trial-and-error process over many years before the magic numbers, if there are any, are determined.

However, some nursing groups feel that establishing ratios is not the entire answer to the problems in the health-care system, and in some instances may actually make problems worse. Fixed numerical ratios may not take into consideration the complexity of client care needs or the levels of education of the nursing staff. Care needs should be determined by considering all factors involved in care, including client care needs, nurses' abilities, and the priorities set by the organization. One potential problem with fixed ratios is that the hospitals may view them as staffing ceilings, rather than minimal requirements, and use the law to support inadequate staffing practices in certain situations.

Another important concern is that staffing ratios will actually accentuate the nursing shortage in the short run. States are already experiencing a significant shortage of nurses. In California, which is ranked 49 among states in nurse-to-population ratio (544 nurses per 100,000 residents), it is estimated that more than 5000 additional nurses would be needed the first day the staffing ratios go into effect. Currently, California hospitals, like many hospitals across the country, have a number of services and floors closed down because of the nursing shortage. At times, it seems that almost every hospital in even large cities like Los Angeles is on "divert" and cannot or will not accept emergency clients brought in by ambulance.

Clearly, this issue will be under discussion for many years to come. A steering committee is currently being developed for the Call to the Profession collaboration that involved more than 100 nursing organizations. Issues to be addressed by this group include staffing, mandatory overtime, nursing shortage, competitive salaries, recognition of the value of nursing, level of education and expertise, and autonomy of practice.

The nursing shortage and other nursing-related issues have not gone unnoticed by the national legislature. Congress is looking at a number of bills, including the Nurse Reinvestment Act (S 1864), the Registered Nurse and Patients Protection Act (HR 1289), and the Safe Nursing and Patient Care Act of 2001 (S 1686).

California Proposed Nurse-to-Client Ratios (April 2002)

HOSPITAL UNIT	RATIO
ICU	1:2*
Operating Room	1:1*
Neonatal ICU	1:2*
Intermediate care nursery	1:4*
Well-baby nursery	1:8*
Postpartum (multiple births never to exceed 8 per nurse)	1:8 (1:4 couplets; 1:6 mothers only)
Labor and delivery	1:2
Postanesthesia care unit (recovery room)	1:2

(Continued)

California Proposed Nurse-to-Client Ratios (April 2002)

HOSPITAL UNIT	RATIO
Emergency departments	1:4 (1:2 critical; 1:1 trauma)
Burn unit	1:2
Pediatrics	1:4
Step-down/telemetry	1:4
Specialty care (oncology)	1:5
Telemetry unit	1:5
General medical/surgical	1:6 initially 1:5 phased in
Behavioral health psychiatric units	1:6
Mixed units	1:6 initially 1:5 phased in

* These units currently have minimum nurse-to-client rations in statute and/or regulations.

Questions for thought:

1. Are you familiar with bills being proposed by the national legislature? Your state legislature? If not, obtain copies of the bills, read them, and discuss them with your class.
2. Do you know who your legislator is? Have you contacted him or her about how you feel about any proposed bills? If not, call him or her today!
3. Do you think the proposed staffing ratios are a good thing? Why or why not? How would they affect health care in your town?

Sources: Stringer, H: Agencies compromise on 1-to-6 staffing ratio. Nurse Week 14, February 4, 2002 (Special edition).

Staffing standards proposed. AACN News 19(3):1, 18, 2002.

Critical Thinking Exercises

- Distinguish between an occupation and a profession.
- Is nursing a profession? Defend your position.
- Discuss four ways in which nursing can improve its professional status.
- Name the three sources of power to which nurses have the most access. Discuss how nurses can best use these sources of power to improve nursing, nursing care, and the health-care system.

References

1. Manthey, M: Continuing the case for the baccalaureate. J Prof Nurs 18(1):7, 2002.
2. Adams, D, and Miller, BK: Professionalism in nursing behaviors of nurse practitioners. J Prof Nurs 17(4):203–210, 2001.
3. Smith, GR: Power and health care reform. J Nurs Educ 33:194–197, 1994.
4. Bellack, JP, and O'Neil, EH: Recreating nursing practice for a new century. Nursing and Health Care Perspectives 21(1):14-24, 2000.
5. Lindeman, CA: The future of nursing education. J Nurs Educ 39(1):5–12, 2000.
6. Lusk, M, and Decker, I: Moving towards a model of nursing education and practice. Nursing and Health Care Perspectives 22(2):81–84, 2001.
7. Gatxke, H, and Ransom, JE: New skills for a new age: Preparing nurses for the 21st century. Nursing Forum 36(3):18–28, 2001.
8. Fitzpatrick, ML: Prologue to Professionalism. Robert J. Brady, Bowie, MD, 1983.
9. O'Grady, ET: Health policy and politics. Nursing Economics 18(2):88–90, 2001.
10. American Nurses Association: Nursing Social Policy Statement. ANA, Washington, DC, 1999.

Bibliography

Bellack, JP, and O'Neil, EH: Recreating nursing practice for a new century. Nursing and Health Care Perspectives 21(1):14–24, 2000.

Brady, M, et al: Differentiating the 21 Pew Competencies by level of nursing education. Nursing and Health Care Perspectives 22(1):30–38, 2001.

Burke, RJ: The ripple effect: Staffing post restructuring. Nursing Management 33(2):41–43, 2002.

Freeman, LH, et al: New curriculum for a new century. Nursing Education 41(1):38–40, 2002.

Irving, JA, and Sniper, J: Preserving professional values. J Prof Nurs 18(1):5, 2002.

Kinsman, L, and James, EL: Evidence based practice needs evidence based implementation. Lippincott's Case Management 6(5):208–219, 2001.

Latter, S, et al: Nurse educational preparation for a medication education role. Nurse Education Today 21(2):143–154, 2001.

Manthey, M: Continuing the case for the baccalaureate. J Prof Nurs 18(1):7, 2002.

Narayan, MC, et al: Searching for nursing's future. Nursing Management 33(1):26–30, 2002.

O'Bryan, L, et al: Rework the workload. Nursing Management 33(3):38–40, 2002.

2

Historical Perspectives

Joseph T. Catalano

Learning Objectives

After completing this chapter, the reader will be able to:

- Explain why studying the history of health care and nursing is important to the profession of nursing.
- Name three "historical threads" found in the study of nursing history, and discuss why they are important.
- Discuss Christian influences on health care and nursing.
- Discuss the influences of the Renaissance and Reformation on health care and nursing.
- Describe the major changes in health care and nursing that occurred during and immediately after World War II.

Knowledge about the profession's past can help us understand how nursing developed and even suggest solutions to problems that face the profession today. There are several threads that run throughout the history of nursing, including society's beliefs about the causes of illness, the value placed on individual life, and the role of women in society. The wars of modern history have also had a significant impact on nursing, particularly in influencing the development of technology and guiding the direction of health care. This chapter is not a treatise on the history of health care and nursing, but presents some key historic milestones that helped to form the foundations of health and nursing care.

Origins of Nursing

Before Nursing

Current nursing practice is a relatively recent development. The major concern of most early civilizations was the survival of the group, and because illness and injury threatened this survival, many primitive health-care practices grew from processes of trial and error. In prehistoric times, women tended to care for the ill and injured. Evil spirits were thought to be the cause of illness, and the medicine men and women who practiced witchcraft were considered religious figures.

In ancient eastern civilizations, starting from about 3500 B.C., health care was intertwined with religion. Taoism emphasized balance and the driving of demons out of the ailing body. Acupuncture developed over the next several thousands of years, and medicinal herbs were used in preventive health care. In Southeast Asia, Hinduism emphasized the need for good hygiene, and written records would soon chronicle a number of surgical procedures. This was also the first culture to document medical treatment outside the home, although women were prohibited from working. The rise of Buddhism around 530 B.C. caused a surge in health care, with public hospitals and high standards for doctors and other hospital workers, and an emphasis on hygiene and prevention of disease. The development of medical knowledge was hindered to a degree by the refusal of the physicians to come in contact with blood and infectious body secretions and the prohibition against dissection of the human body.

> *The major concern of most early civilizations was the survival of the group, and because illness and injury threatened this survival, many primitive health-care practices grew from processes of trial and error.*

During the same period, the ancient Egyptians' belief that all disease was caused by evil spirits and punishing gods was changing. Health-care providers from that time showed a well-developed understanding of the basis for disease. Writings from 1500 B.C. refer to surgical procedures, the role of the midwife, bandaging, preventive care, and even birth control. Women enjoyed a higher status in Egyptian society and even worked in hospitals.[1] Physicians, however, were still men, who served in multiple roles, as surgeon, priest, architect, and politician.

The Babylonian Empire, united in 2100 B.C., was a civilization that focused on astrology. Its health-care practices included special diets, massage therapy, and rest to drive evil spirits from a body. People would go to the marketplace to seek advice on how to treat their ailments. During the height of the empire, strict guidelines governed doctors' fees and responsibility in medical practice. There is also evidence in this period of child care and treatment for some diseases, but most care still took place in the home.

By 1900 B.C., the Hebrews had formed a nation along the Mediterranean and adopted many of the health practices of their neighbors. They integrated elements of the Egyptian sanitary laws to form the Mosaic Code that, as in many other cultures, mixed religion and medicine. Caring for widows, orphans, and other strangers in need was part of daily life. Hebrews had good knowledge of anatomy and physiology, especially the circulatory systems. Physician-priests routinely performed operations such as cesarean sections (named later by the Romans), amputation, and circumcisions. They also enforced rules of purification, performed sacrifices, and conducted rituals related to food preparation.

Ancient Greece was a culture that focused on appeasing the gods, and its medical practice was no exception. The god Apollo was devoted to medicine and good health. The Greeks performed sacrifices to appease the gods and practiced abortion and infanticide in an attempt to control the population. People took hot baths at spas to improve health, but the sick and injured were cared for at clinics. Although women were held in high esteem, they were not permitted to provide any health care outside the home. Around 400 B.C., the writings of Hippocrates began to change medical practice in Greece. One of a roving group of physician-priests, Hippocrates was called "the father of medicine." His beliefs focused on harmony with the natural law instead of on appeasing the gods. He emphasized treating the whole

What Do You Think?

Is the study of history really necessary for nursing students?

Why or why not?

client—mind, body, spirit, and environment—and making diagnoses based on symptoms rather than on an isolated idea of a disease. He was also concerned with ethical standards for physicians, expressed in the now-famous Hippocratic oath.

Ancient Romans clung to superstitions and polytheism as the foundations for medical as well as religious practices. This dominant empire ruled from around 290 B.C. and absorbed useful elements of whatever culture they conquered—including the Greeks and Hebrews—into their own. They developed a quite advanced system of medicine and a pharmacology that included more than 600 medications derived from herbs and plants. Roman physicians were eventually able to distinguish between various conditions and performed many surgeries. They also did physical therapy for athletes; diagnosed symptoms of infections; identified job-related dangers of lead, mercury, and asbestos; and published medical textbooks.

The Romans' advances in creating an unlimited supply of clean water via aqueducts were critical in maintaining the good health of its citizens, as were central heating, spas and baths, and more advanced systems for sewage disposal. Because the great Roman armies were so crucial to the empire, they developed early hospitals to care for sick and injured soldiers. These were mobile and were staffed by female as well as male attendants, who performed duties that would today be thought of as nursing care: cleaning and bandaging wounds, feeding and cleaning clients, and providing comfort to the wounded and dying. In many ways, women enjoyed an equal place in society, and they provided home health care as well as midwifery.

> *The term* nurse *is thought to have originated in this period, from the Latin word* nutrire, *meaning to nourish, nurture, or suckle a child.*

Early Efforts at Nursing

The rise of Christianity, starting from 30 A.D., brought with it a strong belief in the sanctity of all human life. Christians considered practices like human sacrifice, infanticide, and abortion—which had been common in Roman society—to be murder. Following the teachings of Jesus meant that caring for the sick, poor, and disadvantaged was of primary importance, and groups of believers soon organized to offer care for those in need.

Early writings of the Christian period record women's important role in ministering to the sick and providing food and care for the poor and homeless. Wealthy Roman women who had converted to Christianity established hospital-like institutions and residences for these caregivers in their homes. The term *nurse* is thought to have originated in this period, from the Latin word *nutrire*, meaning to nourish, nurture, or suckle a child. The majority of care was still provided by a family member in the home. Most early Christian hospitals were roadside houses for the sick, poor, or destitute, who were cared for by male and female attendants alike. The attendants learned from a process of trial and error and by observing others.

The Dark Ages, from roughly 500 to 1000 A.D., were marked by widespread poverty, illness, and death. Plagues and other diseases like smallpox, leprosy, and diphtheria ravaged the known world and killed large segments of populations. Health care at this time was almost nonexistent. However, the strong beliefs of the Catholic Church, which was based in Rome, produced monasteries and convents that became centers for the care of the poor and the sick. By 500 A.D., there were several religious nursing orders in what is today England, France, and Italy. Men and women worked there and also traveled to rural areas where they were needed, combining religious rituals and home remedies as well as treatments such as bandaging, cautery, bloodletting, enemas, and leeching.

The biggest contribution to health care in this period may have been the insistence on cleanliness and hygiene, which lessened the spread of infections. Medieval nurses did not have any formal schooling but learned through apprenticeships with older monks or nuns. Eventually hospitals came to be built outside of monastery grounds. Secular orders were also established, which could provide a wider range of services to the sick because they were not limited by religious restrictions and obligations.

At the end of the Dark Ages, there were a series of holy wars and invasions, including the Crusades, which produced many sick and injured who were far from home. Military nursing orders developed to care for the soldiers, but these were made up exclusively of men who wore suits of armor to protect themselves and their hospitals against attacks. These orders, with the emblem of the red cross, were extremely well organized and dedicated, and they existed well into the Renaissance.

The military nursing orders, with the emblem of the red cross, were extremely well organized and dedicated, and they existed well into the Renaissance.

Development of the Modern Nurse

In the intellectual reawakening of the Renaissance in Europe, starting in about 1350, nursing emerged in a recognizable form, although it did not grow steadily as a profession during this period. Inventions from this time include the microscope and thermometer, but the use of more modern diagnoses and treatment was viewed with skepticism. Monastic hospitals still regarded the restoration of health as secondary to the salvation of the soul. Major political changes initiated by the Protestant Reformation in 1517 had the greatest effect on the health care of the period. In Catholic nation-states, including Italy, France, and Spain, health care remained generally unchanged from that of the Middle Ages, although the number of male nursing orders gradually decreased. By 1500, the majority of health care was provided by female religious orders.

What Do You Think?

Imagine yourself living in one of the historical periods discussed in this chapter. Given your or your family's health-care problems, how would your lives be different?

In the nation-states that broke away from the Catholic Church, such as England, Germany, and the Netherlands, health care soon degenerated to a point that was even worse than that of the Middle Ages. The role of women was reduced under Protestant leadership, and the male nurse all but disappeared. Secular nursing orders gradually took over the duties of the many substandard hospitals that had been established in metropolitan areas. The most famous of these was the Sisters of Charity, established in 1600. These orders were the first to establish a nursing hierarchy. Primary nurses were called sisters and those assisting them were called helpers and watchers. It is at this time that people began to recognize the benefit of skilled nursing care. The first nursing textbooks appeared, and the use of midwives became widespread. Although hospitals were gaining importance, most clients still received health care at home.

The Industrial Revolution (1850–1950) caused a flood of people from rural areas throughout Europe into cities, and cramped conditions caused very bad health conditions and the spread of disease and plagues. Factory owners supported some forms of health care to keep their workers on the job, and this led to an early form of community health nursing. The Sisters of Charity expanded their care to include home care. Only a few male nursing orders survived the Protestant Reformation and Industrial Revolution, and several non-Catholic nursing orders were founded, including the famous Quaker Society of Protestant Sisters of Charity, which provided care primarily for prisoners and children.

Nursing in the United States

Five hospitals existed in America before the Revolutionary War, housing the homeless, the poor, and rudimentary infirmaries. However, there were no identifiable groups of nurses for these infirmaries.[2] Health care in America at this time reflected that of the European country where the settlers had come from. Infant mortality rates were very high, ranging between 50 and 75 percent. One of the first schools of nursing was established in 1640 by the Sisters of St. Ursula in Quebec, and Spanish and French religious orders would establish hospital-based training schools in the New World over the next 100 years.

During the Revolutionary War there was no organized medical or nursing corps, but small groups of untrained volunteers cared for the wounded and sick in their homes or in churches or barns.

During the Revolutionary War, there was no organized medical or nursing corps, but small groups of untrained volunteers cared for the wounded and sick in their homes or in churches or barns. Benjamin Franklin founded Pennsylvania Hospital in 1751, which was the first U.S. hospital dedicated to treating the sick.

Between the Revolutionary and the Civil Wars, health care in the United States increased markedly with the influx of religious nursing orders from Europe. More early schools of nursing developed at this time. Despite the rapid increase in the number of hospitals, most nursing care was still given at home by family members. Hospitals were considered a last resort and still had very high mortality rates.

The Civil War caused more death and injury than any war in the history of the United States, and the demand for nurses increased dramatically. Women volunteers (as many as 6000 for the North and 1000 for the South) began to follow the armies to the battlefield to provide basic nursing care, although many of them were untrained. Navy Nurses, the American Red Cross, and the Army Nurse Corps all date from this period. Large numbers of women came out of their homes to work in the hospitals, and a number of African-American volunteers in the North paved the way for others to enter the health-care field in the future.

Technological developments in the nineteenth century included medications such as morphine and codeine for pain and quinine to treat malaria. The arrival of 30 million immigrants in this century meant that the need for health care increased accordingly. Hospitals sprang up, and many instituted their own schools of nursing. Still, home care was the preferred type of nursing.

At the beginning of World War I, there were only about 400 nurses in the Army Nurse Corps, but by 1917 that number swelled to 21,000. Because many hospitals were recruiting untrained women to provide basic care, a committee on nursing was formed to establish standards, and eventually the Red Cross began a training program for nurse's aides. This was supported by physicians, but opposed by many nursing leaders, who were concerned that it relegated nursing to "women's work," which would be seen as something anyone could do with minimal training. Because nurse's aides were a cheap source of labor, they began to replace more trained nurses in hospitals. Unfortunately this also resulted in a lower quality of care.

After the war, a segment of the nursing profession began to focus intensely on improving the educational standards of nursing care. At this time, 90 percent of nursing care was still given at home, but nurses began to practice in industry and in branches of government outside of the military. The standards of nursing care were low, and external quality controls were nonexistent. The Great Depression took its toll on health care and nursing, as jobs became scarce and many nursing schools closed. At this time, the federal government became one of the largest employers of nurses. The newly organized Joint Committee on Nursing recommended that jobs should go to more qualified nurses and that the work day be reduced from 12 to 8 hours, although these measures were not widely implemented. During this period, hospitals became the primary source of health care, supported by hospital insurance programs. As the size of hospitals increased, more nursing jobs became available.

World War II produced another nursing shortage, and in response, Congress passed the Bolton Nurse Training Act, which shortened hospital-based training programs from 36 to 30 months. The new Cadet Nurse Corps established minimum educational standards for nursing programs and forbade discrimination on the basis of race, creed, or sex.[2] Many schools revised and improved their curriculums to meet these new standards. To encourage more nurses to enter the military, the U.S. government granted women full commissioned status and gave them the same pay as men with the same rank. By the end of the war, African-American and male nurses were also admitted to the armed services.

> *The Civil War caused more death and injury than any war in the history of the United States, and the demand for nurses increased dramatically.*

The advancements in health care made during World War II required that nurses receive more highly specialized education to meet clients' unique needs. After the war, many nurses left the profession to raise families, and the spaces were filled by graduates of new programs, which trained licensed practical nurses (LPNs) and licensed vocational nurses (LVNs) in just 1 year. At this time, the concept of team nursing came to be widely accepted, although it removed the registered nurses (RNs) from direct client care, requiring them to serve as team leaders.

Technical nursing programs, which granted associate degrees (associate degree nurse [ADN]) at 2-year community colleges, were developed to help with the nursing shortage. With the baby boom, the need for nurses continued to grow, and what had been a quick-fix solution began to take a stronger hold. By the mid-1960s, ADNs outnumbered the nurses with baccalaureate degrees (BSNs) and the technical LPNs. ADNs also won the right to take the same licensing examinations as RN graduates from diploma and BSN programs. Still, as the health-care system became increasingly complicated, some nursing leaders questioned whether 1- or 2-year LPN and ADN programs were adequate to meet the needs of the profession. Slowly the number of BSN programs and graduate-level programs began to increase.

The Mobile Army Surgical Hospital (MASH) units that had been developed during the Korean War were replaced during the Vietnam War with Medical Unit, Self-Contained Transportable (MUST) hospitals, which were staffed by nurses as well as physicians. Some 5000 nurses served in this war, and for the first time graduates of 2-year ADN programs were commissioned into the armed services. Several Navy nurses were injured in the line of duty, and one army nurse was killed. Only recently have the efforts of these and other women who served been recognized at the Vietnam Women's War Memorial in Washington, dedicated in 1993.

Nursing Leaders

The nursing profession as it is practiced today owes a great deal to a number of outstanding nurses who had a vision for the future. The few discussed here are representative of the great drive and dedication of the many individuals who created change and influenced the development of the nursing profession, even to this day.

ISSUES NOW

Health and Human Services Report Released

A recent sampling of registered nurses (RNs) across the nation was performed by the Department of Health and Human Services (HHS). The data generated by HHS are considered the most comprehensive statistical resource on the nation's RN population. Key points of the data collected include:

1. The average age of RNs continues to increase to the current high of 45 years.
2. The rate of younger nurses entering the profession continues to decline.
3. The rate of nurses entering the workforce between 1996 and 2000 was down by more than 10% from the previous 4 years.
4. The number of practicing licensed RNs had increased to approximately 2,697,000—up 137,666 nurses from the previous 4 years.
5. The number of practicing licensed RNs employed in nursing stands at 81.7%.
6. Approximately 12.3% of RNs report being of one or more racial or ethnic minority. U.S. population minority rate now stands at 30%.
7. The number of men entering the nursing profession increased slightly from 5.4% to 5.9%.
8. The number of nurses working in the acute care setting increased from 1,270,870 to 1,300,323.
9. The majority of the nation's nursing homes (90%) are understaffed to a point where they are unable to provide safe basic care.

To help address the nation's growing need for RNs, the administration's budget for the year 2003 proposes a total of $15 million—an increase of 50% over the previous year's allotment. Most of the money is earmarked for the Nursing Education Loan Repayment Program and should support loans for 800 new nursing students. The program also is directed to repaying a substantial portion of the educational loans of nurses who agree to work for 2 years in designated public or nonprofit health-care facilities with an identified shortage of nurses.

HHS is also offering grants and contracts totaling more than $27.4 million to increase the number of qualified nurses and the quality of nursing services nationally. About half the money is designated for nursing scholarships to increase the number of registered nurses; the other half will be used to improve the quality of health-care services in communities nationwide.

Source: www.dhhs.gov/ Contact: webmaster@os.dhss.gov

Florence Nightingale (1820–1910)

Universally regarded as the founder of modern nursing, Florence Nightingale dedicated her long life to improving health care and nursing standards. Raised in England, Nightingale was considered highly educated for her time. Through travels with her family, she became aware of the substandard health care in many countries in Europe. In 1851, she attended a 3-month nurses training program at the church-run hospital in Kaiserwerth, Germany. She was impressed with the program but came to believe that this brief training was insufficient. She later ran a private nursing home and realized that the only way to improve health care was to educate women to be reliable, high-quality nurses.

Plans to develop a school of nursing in England were interrupted in 1854 by a cholera epidemic. Nightingale volunteered her services and learned a great deal about how to prevent the spread of disease. When the Crimean War broke out that same year, she got permission to take a group of 37 volunteer nurses into the battlefield. British medical officers initially refused their assistance, but as conditions worsened they were admitted to the hospital. After just 6 months of the nurses' cleaning and bandaging wounds, cooking, and cleaning the wards, the mortality rate dropped from 42 to 2 percent.[3] Nightingale expanded her reform to include supplies, a military post office, convalescent camps for long-term recovery, and residences for soldiers' families. She also began to help with the care given at the front lines. At the height of her work in the war, she supervised some 125 nurses in several large hospitals, and her accomplishments were recognized by the Queen of England with an Order of Merit, the highest award given to English civilians.

What Do You Think?

What would current nursing practice and nursing education be like without the influences of Florence Nightingale?

This war experience strengthened Nightingale's convictions that nursing education required major reform. Believing that nursing schools should be run by nurses and be independent of hospitals and physicians, she advocated a program of at least 1 year that included basic biological science, techniques to improve nursing care, and supervised practice. She regarded nursing as a lifelong endeavor and felt that nurses should be in direct contact with clients rather than doing menial jobs such as cooking and cleaning. She worked tirelessly for the reform of health care and nursing and was appointed to many related committees and commissions. A prolific writer, she wrote extensively about improving hospital conditions, sanitation, nursing education, and health care in general.

Her famous Nightingale Training School for Nurses opened in 1860 and began to train nurses who were in great demand throughout Europe and the United States. At this school, she advocated health maintenance and the concept that nursing was both an art and a science. She taught that each person should be treated as an individual and that nurses should meet the needs of clients, not the demands of physicians. The school flourished, although it faced strong opposition from physicians who felt that nurses were already overtrained. Many early graduates of her school went on to become important nursing leaders. Nightingale's ideas were somewhat diluted during the first half of the twentieth century, but they have since resurfaced and are now evaluated in the light of a rapidly changing health-care system.

Isabel Adams Hampton Robb (1860–1910)

Hampton Robb started out as a teacher in her home city of Ontario, Canada, but in 1881 she went to New York City to train to be a nurse. After graduation, she moved to Rome and became a superintendent of a hospital there. She had always focused on the academic rather than the clinical side of nursing, but in Italy her conviction grew that nurses needed a solid theoretical education—a belief that was not well accepted by the medical community of the time. From that point on, she dedicated her life to raising the standards of nursing education in the United States, first as director of the Illinois Training School for Nurses, a school that was unique for its time in that it was university-based and emphasized academic learning. She later headed the new Johns Hopkins Training School for Nurses and would implement her ideas there as well.

Hampton Robb brought together leaders from key nursing schools to form the American Society of Superintendents of Training Schools for Nurses, and she served as its chairman. The group was the precursor to the National League for Nursing, which was dedicated to improving the standards for nursing education. In 1896, Hampton Robb became the first president of a group for staff nurses in active practice, called the Nurses Associated Alumnae of the United States and Canada, which would later become the American Nurses Association (ANA), dedicated to the improvement of clinical practice. She later helped develop the *American Journal of Nursing*, the first professional journal dedicated to the improvement of nursing, which is still the official journal of the ANA.

Lillian Wald (1867–1940)

Wald was raised in Ohio and graduated from the New York Hospital School of Nursing in 1901. After working as a hospital nurse, she entered medical school, but encounters with New York's poor and sick caused her to change direction. She instead opened the Henry Street Settlement, a storefront health clinic in one of the poorest sections of the city, which organized nurses to make home visits, focusing on sanitary conditions and children's health. Wald became a dedicated social reformer, an efficient fundraiser, and an eloquent speaker. Although women still did not have the right to vote, her political influence was felt worldwide.

> **What Do You Think?**
>
> Who is your favorite historical nursing leader? What are some of that person's characteristics that attracted you? Are there any current nurses or nurse educators who provide you with a role model? What are some of that person's characteristics that attract you?

Under Wald's auspices, Columbia University developed courses to prepare nurses for careers in public health. She also advocated wellness education, which the medical community did not value at the time. The Metropolitan Life Insurance Company saw the value in her beliefs, however, and asked her to organize its nursing branch. She is also credited with founding the American Red Cross's Town and Country Nursing Service and with initiating the concept of school nursing. In 1912, she founded and became the first president of the National Organization of Public Health Nursing. Many child health and wellness programs in use today are based on her efforts. Current proposals for health-care reform often include her ideas about public health nursing, independent clinics, and health maintenance.

Lavinia Lloyd Dock (1858–1956)

Dock left her home in Pennsylvania to attend New York's Bellevue Training School for Nurses in 1885. She noticed that many of her fellow students struggled to learn about all the medications that were becoming available, and she would later write the first medication textbook for nurses. She worked alongside Lillian Wald at the Henry Street Settlement and Isabel Hampton Robb at Johns Hopkins Hospital. Like Wald, Dock believed that poverty and squalor contributed to poor health, and she dedicated herself to social reform to address these problems. However, she soon learned that she was limited in her influence because she was a woman, and she spent most of her career dedicated to the pursuit of equal rights. For 20 years she lobbied legislators at all levels about women's right to vote, believing that this was the only way to influence social reform and health care. An excellent example of the diverse ways that nurses can help achieve higher quality health care, she is considered one of the most influential leaders in the early twentieth century.

Annie W. Goodrich (1866–1954)

Goodrich was active at Lillian Wald's Henry Street Settlement in New York after receiving her nursing degree. She was known as an outstanding nursing educator and ran a number of nursing schools in New York; and in 1910, she was appointed a state inspector of nursing schools, a position that up to that time had been held only by physicians. After the U.S. Army asked her to survey its hospital nursing departments, Goodrich proposed that it organize its own nursing school. The school opened later that year, with her as its dean, and this school would serve as the model for others established at Army hospitals during World War I.

To respond to the need for nurses in the war, Goodrich also established a nursing training program at Vassar College, and after the war other colleges and universities slowly began to develop their own nursing programs. She had demonstrated that learning theoretical information in a classroom was just as important in training highly skilled nurses as clinical practice. When the war was over, Goodrich returned to the Henry Street Settlement and then became a nursing educator, eventually serving as dean at the Yale University School of Nursing. Her many writings about nursing education and her experiences with military nursing have been a great contribution to the nursing profession.[4]

Conclusion

Many of the problems and difficulties with today's health-care system, and those of nursing in particular, are based in the historical development of the profession. Knowledge of these historic roots can help us understand why the profession of nursing is the way it is and even suggest solutions to problems that may seem unsolvable. For example, nursing today appears to be a profession with a high level of responsibility but a low level of power. How did this situation develop? What can be done about it? A great deal of confusion exists about the education of nurses, unlike the situation in other health-care professions. Why does nursing have this problem, and how can this confusion be addressed? Those who belong to the nursing profession have a responsibility not only to learn about how these and other conditions developed, but also to relate that knowledge to nursing's possibility for growth in the future.

ISSUES IN PRACTICE

Case Study

Clara, who is 108 years old, is admitted through the hospital emergency room (ER) for nonspecific complaints of chest pain and dizziness. This is the third time that she has come to the hospital with this complaint in the last month. Although previous examinations and tests have shown no acute disease process, the ER physician thought that because of her age and long history of coronary artery disease, Clara should be monitored and evaluated more closely. Clara has no private insurance, but she is covered under Medicare, Parts A and B, with supplemental coverage from a small insurance company in her state.

Despite her age, Clara is mentally alert and competent. She lives by herself in a small apartment and manages basic daily care, including shopping and cleaning, with only minimal assistance from friends. She has no living family members, except for a few aging cousins in a distant state. She is taking several medications at home: diltiazem (Cardizem) for her heart problems, ranitidine (Zantac) for a hiatal hernia, and papaverine (Pavabid) to increase her general circulation.

After a complete physical examination, including several laboratory tests and an electrocardiogram (ECG), she is scheduled for a cardiac catheterization. A significant block is seen in one of the major coronary arteries, and the physicians decide to perform an angioplasty on the artery. She is admitted to the intensive care unit (ICU) after the procedure, where she also receives 2 units of blood because she is anemic. She recovers without incident and is discharged 5 days after her admission. The total cost for her hospitalization, including tests and angioplasty, is more than $15,000.

Clara is not a typical client for her age group. Many medical experts would categorize the treatment given her as overtreatment because of the current emphasis on quality of life, death with dignity, and the futility of treating the hopelessly ill. Yet, as people in the United States continue to age, it is more likely that Clara will become the norm rather than the exception. Many issues—ethical, financial, and others—surround this case.

Critical Thinking Questions

1. As a general rule, should a complicated and expensive procedure, such as an angioplasty, always be approved for a 108-year-old client? If not, what should be the exceptions?
2. From a historical perspective, how would a client with Clara's health-care problems be treated in the Roman Empire? The Middle Ages? The United States in the 1800s? The United States in the 1950s?

3. The state where Clara lives has a severe budget shortfall, and substantial cuts in Medicaid benefits have taken place. The entire budget for immunizations of the state's children is only $10,000. What would you do as administrator of the state's Medicaid program if faced with the option of immunizing the children or paying for Clara's angioplasty?
4. The elderly, through the various entitlement programs, consume a large proportion of the national budget. This cost is borne mainly by young and middle-aged workers through their taxes. Is it fair that the young be required to carry the burden for the care of the old?
5. Is the government ever justified in rationing health care and/or limiting access to health care?

References

1. Jenson, DM: History and Trends in Professional Nursing. CV Mosby, St. Louis, 1959.
2. Kalisch, PA, and Kalisch, BJ: The Advance of American Nursing. JB Lippincott, Philadelphia, 1995.
3. Woodham-Smith, C: Florence Nightingale. McGraw-Hill, New York, 1957.
4. Mason, DJ: Policy and Politics for Nurses. WB Saunders, Philadelphia, 1993.

Bibliography

Cristy, T: The first fifty years. Am J Nurs 9(9):1778–1784, 1971.

Cristy, T: Portrait of a leader: Lavinia Lloyd Dock. Nurs Outlook 17(6):72–75, 1969.

Cristy, T: Portrait of a leader: M. Adelaide Nutting. Nurs Outlook 17(l):20–24, 1969.

Cristy, T: Portrait of a leader: Isabel Hampton Robb. Nurs Outlook 17(3):26–29, 1969.

Cristy, T: Portrait of a leader: Isabel Maitland Stewart. Nurs Outlook 17(10):44–48, 1969.

Jamieson, EM, et al: Trends in Nursing History. WB Saunders, Philadelphia, 1968.

Murphy-Ende, K: Advanced practice nursing: Reflections on the past, issues for the future. Oncol Nurs Forum 29(1):26–33, 2002.

Scribner, CJ: Analysis of historical trends in nursing education: Is there application to the current environment? Seminars in Perioperative Nursing 10(2):63–66, 2001.

Selanders, LC: Florence Nightingale: Perseverance, power, possibilities. Maryland Nurse 4(3):1–2, 2001.

Smoyak, SA: Florence Nightingale, insane nurse. J Psychosoc Nurs Ment Health Serv 39(10):6–8, 2001.

3

The Evolution of Licensure, Certification, and Nursing Organizations

Joseph T. Catalano

Learning Objectives

After completing this chapter, the reader will be able to:

- Identify the purposes and needs for nurse licensure.
- Distinguish between permissive and mandatory licensure.
- Explain why institutional licensure is unacceptable in today's health-care system.
- Evaluate the importance of nurse practice acts.
- Analyze the significance of professional certification.

Almost from the inception of nursing, societal needs and expectations have been the driving forces behind the establishment of the standards that guide the profession. In the early days of nursing when health care was relatively primitive and society's expectations of nurses were low, there was little demand for regulations or controls over and within the profession. However, as technology and health care have advanced and become more complex, there has been a corresponding increase in societal expectations for nurses. All nurses now accept **licensure** and **certification** examinations as a given in today's health-care system. But where did these examinations come from? And what do they mean to the profession? This chapter explores the answers to these questions.

Rather than looking on the advent of sophisticated telecommunications, growing information technologies, redesigned health-care organizations, and increasing **health-care consumer** demands with fear and trepidation, nurses should consider this as an exciting time of growth and opportunity. In today's health-care system, nurses have an almost unlimited number of ways to provide new and creative nursing care for clients in all settings. As society's needs and expectations change, so will the regulations and standards that help define nursing practice. Through their professional nursing organizations, nurses can help shape health-care regulations that establish the most freedom to provide effective care while maintaining the goal of protection of the public. It is likely that in the future state boards of nursing will look much different, just as the profession of nursing will differ from that of its past.

The Development of Nurse Practice Acts

A nurse practice act is state legislation regulating the practice of nurses that protects the public and makes nurses accountable for their actions. Nurse practice acts establish state boards of nursing (SBNs) and define specific SBN powers regarding the practice of nursing within the state. Rules and regulations written by the SBNs become **statutory laws** under the powers delegated by the state **legislature**.

Although nurse practice acts differ from one state to another, the SBNs have many powers in common. All SBNs have the power to grant licenses, to accredit nursing programs, to establish standards for nursing schools, and to write specific regulations for nurses and nursing in general in that state. Of particular importance is the SBN's power to deny or revoke nurse licenses (Box 3–1). Other functions of nurse practice acts include defining nursing and the scope of practice, ruling on who can use the titles registered nurse (RN) and licensed practical nurse/licensed vocational nurse (LPN/LVN), setting up an application procedure for licensure in the state, determining fees for licensure, establishing requirements for renewal of licensure, and determining responsibility for any regulations governing expanded practice for nurses in that particular state.

> *Rather than looking on the advent of sophisticated telecommunications, growing information technologies, redesigned health-care organizations, and increasing health-care consumer demands with fear and trepidation, nurses should consider this as an exciting time of growth and opportunity.*

The Need for Licensure

Imagine what the quality of health care would be if anyone could walk into a hospital, claim to know how to care for clients, and be given a job as a nurse. This situation might sound impossible in today's health-care system, but not too long ago it was the norm rather than the exception.

Throughout the last half of the nineteenth century and the first half of the twentieth century, rapid growth in health-care technology led to the increasing use of hospitals as the primary source of health care. Individuals who were qualified to provide this care, however, were in short supply. There were wide variations both in the abilities of those who claimed to be nurses and in the quality of the care that they provided. Paradoxically, nursing leaders who had always advocated some type of **credentialing** for nurses to ensure competency found that their attempts to initiate registration or licensure met with strong opposition from physician groups, hospital administrators, and practicing nurses themselves.[1]

Early Attempts at Licensure

Although the idea of registering nurses had been in existence for some time, Florence Nightingale was the first to establish a formal register for graduates of her nursing school. In the United States and Canada, there was widespread recognition of the need for some type of credentialing of nurses as far back as the middle 1800s. The first organized attempt to establish a credentialing system was initiated in 1896 by the Nurses Associated Alumnae of the United States and Canada (later to become the American Nurses Association). As with other early attempts at

Box 3–1

Reasons the State Boards of Nursing May Revoke a Nursing License

- Conviction for a serious crime
- Demonstration of gross negligence or unethical conduct in the practice of nursing
- Failure to renew a nursing license while still continuing to practice nursing
- Use of illegal drugs or alcohol during the provision of care for clients, or use that carries over and affects client's care
- Willful violation of the state's nurse practice act

Box 3–2

Key Points in the New York State Licensure Bill (1904)

- Established minimum educational standards
- Established the minimum length of basic nursing programs at 2 years
- Required all nursing schools to be registered with the state board of regents (who oversee all higher education)
- Established a state board of nursing (SBN) with five nurses as members
- Formulated rules for the examination of nurses
- Formulated regulations for nurses that, if violated, could lead to the revocation of licensure

Source: Hirsh, IL: Statement on nursing's scope describes how two levels of nurses practice. American Nurse 20:13, 1988.

licensure, it was met with resistance and eventually failed.[2]

Several nursing leaders, including Lillian Wald, Annie Goodrich, and Isabel Stewart, recognized the inconsistent quality of nursing care and the need for licensure to protect the public. In 1901, after an extensive and lengthy campaign to educate the public, physicians, hospital administrators, and nurses themselves about the need for licensure, the International Council of Nurses passed a resolution that required each state to establish a licensure and examination procedure for nurses. It took 3 years before the state of New York, through the New York Nurses Association, developed a licensure bill that passed the legislature (Box 3–2).

Other states that followed New York's lead were North Carolina, New Jersey, and Virginia. Although these states had bills that were weaker than New York's nurse practice act, passage of such legislation was considered a major accomplishment for several reasons. Women did not even have the right to vote in general elections at the time these bills were passed. In addition, few requirements and regulations for licensure existed during this period in the history of the United States, even for the medical profession.

The Importance of Licensure Examinations

The thought of having to take an examination that can determine whether or not one can practice nursing can make even the best student anxious. Adding to the tension is the fact that the examination is given outside of the academic setting, by computer, and is created by individuals other than the students' teachers. (See Chapter 10 for a detailed discussion of NCLEX-RN, CAT.)

Some type of objective method, however, to prove that the individual is qualified to practice nursing safety is necessary to protect the public from unqualified practitioners. Early attempts at creating licensure examinations for nurses were met with resistance. Although all states had some form of licensure examination by 1923, the format and length of the examinations varied widely. Some states required both written and practical examinations to demonstrate safety of practice; others added an oral examination.

Although licensure was and is a state-controlled activity, the major nursing organizations in the United States eventually realized that in order to have some consistency of quality across the country, a single examination that all nurses needed to pass should be devised. The American Nurses Association (ANA) Council of State Boards of Nursing was organized in 1945 to oversee development of a uniform examination for nurses that could be used by all state boards of nursing. The National League for Nursing Testing Division developed such a test, which was implemented in 1950. Originally the test was simply called the State Board Examination, but it was renamed the National Council Licensure Examination (NCLEX) in 1987. In 1994, the computerized version of the examination was implemented—the National Council Licensure Examination Computerized Adaptive Testing, for Registered Nurses (NCLEX-RN, CAT).

Licensure for nurses has undergone a major change. States are currently in the process of implementing the Mutual Recognition Model for Nursing Licensure, which will allow nurses licensed in one state to practice nursing in other states that belong to their regional agreement. The eventual goal is to have a "universal" nursing license that will allow nurses to practice in all states without having to become relicensed each time they cross a state border.

Registration versus Licensure

The terms *registration* and *licensure* are often used interchangeably, although they are not synonymous. They serve a similar purpose, but some technical differences exist.

Registration

Registration is the listing, or registering, of names of individuals on an official roster who have met certain pre-established criteria. Before universal licensure by the states, any health-care institution that wanted to know whether a person applying for a position had met the standards for that position by graduating from a school of nursing or by passing an examination could call the school and see whether the applicant's name appeared on the official roster or register, hence the origin of the term *registered nurse*. With the advent of state board examinations, an institution merely has to call the SBN to find out whether the individual is registered or licensed.

Licensure

Licensure is an activity conducted by the state through the enforcement powers of its regulatory boards to protect the public's health, safety, and welfare by establishing professional standards. Licensure for nurses, as for other professionals who deal with the public, is necessary to ensure that everyone who claims to be a nurse can function at a minimal level of competency and safety. There are several different types of licensure.

Permissive Licensure

Permissive licensure allows individuals to practice nursing as long as they do not use the letters "RN" after their names. Basically, permissive licensure protects the "registered nurse" designation but not the practice of nursing itself. Under a permissive licensure law, anyone could carry out the functions of an RN, regardless of their level of education, without having to pass an examination indicating competency. Health-care administrators seem to support the concept of permissive licensure because it allows them to employ less-educated and lower-paid employees rather than the more highly paid RNs. However, they also recognize that the quality of care decreases when the education level of health-care providers is lower. Although most early licensure laws were permissive, all states now have mandatory licensure.

Mandatory Licensure

Mandatory licensure requires anyone who wishes to practice nursing to pass a **licensure examination** and become registered by the SBN. Because different levels of nursing practice exist, different levels of licensure are necessary. At the technical level, the individual must take and pass the LPN/LVN examination; at the professional level, the individual must take and pass the RN examination. Mandatory licensure forced SBNs to distinguish between the activities that nurses at different levels could legally perform. The scope of practice defines the boundaries for each of the levels: advanced practice nurse (APN), RN, and LPN/LVN. As more levels of nursing education (e.g., the associate degree in nursing [ADN]) have been added, however, lines dividing the different scopes of practice have become blurred. In the current health-care system, it is not unusual to find LPNs/LVNs performing activities that are generally considered professional.

A particularly confusing element in today's health-care system is the use of unlicensed individuals to provide health care. The advent of certified nurse's assistants (CNAs) and unlicensed assistive personnel (UAP) has led to widespread use of such individuals in all health-care settings. Although they must be supervised by an RN or LPN/LVN, these individuals are sometimes illegally assigned nursing tasks much more advanced than their levels of training. (See Chapter 14 for a more detailed discussion of delegation.) Despite the fact that permissive licensure is no longer legal, CNAs and UAP appear to fall under an unofficial type of permissive licensure.

Institutional Licensure

Although universally rejected by every major nursing organization, **institutional licensure** has become a reality for many other types of health-care workers, such as respiratory therapists and physical therapists. In some state legislatures, bills have been introduced to allow **foreign graduate nurses** and nurses who are licensed in foreign countries to work in specific institutions without taking the U.S. licensure examination. Up to this point, these bills have been stopped by the state nursing organizations before they could become law. Institutional licensure has been proposed periodically over the years as an alternative to governmental licensure.

The idea behind institutional licensure is that the individual health-care institution will be permitted to determine which individuals are qualified to practice nursing within general guidelines established by an outside board. Although this type of licensure appeals to hospitals and nursing homes because it would allow them to hire individuals with less education at a reduced cost, it has some serious difficulties associated with it.

Probably the most critical problem is the lack of any external control to determine a minimal level of competency. The designations of RN and LPN/LVN would be virtually meaningless under institutional licensure. These nurses would not be under the control of a state **licensing board** and thus would not be held to the same **standards of practice** as other nurses who were licensed by the states. A second problem is that nurses who wished to move to a new place of employment would have to undergo whatever licensure procedure the new institution had established before being allowed to work there. Currently, nurses who move from one state to another can obtain **licensure by endorsement** by having the state recognize their nursing license from the original state of licensure. This process is generally referred to as **reciprocity**.

Certification

At first glance, not much difference may be seen between certification and licensure. Strictly defined, licensure can actually be considered a type of legal certification. In the more widely accepted use of the term, however, certification is a granting of credentials to indicate that an individual has achieved a level of ability higher than the minimal level of competency indicated by licensure.[3] As technology increases and the health-care environment becomes more complex and demanding, nurses are finding a need to increase their knowledge and skill levels beyond the essentials taught in their basic nursing courses. Certification acknowledges the attainment of increased knowledge and skills and provides nurses with a means to validate their own self-worth and competence.

Some certification also carries with it a legal status, like licensure; but in many cases, certification merely indicates a specific professional status. The public, employers, and even nurses themselves have difficulty understanding what certification means. Another element that adds confusion to the understanding of the process of certification is that a large number of groups can offer certification. These are usually professional specialty groups like the National Association of Pediatric Nurse Associates and Practitioners (NAPNAP) and the American Association of Critical-Care Nurses (AACN), but they can also be national organizations like the National League for Nursing (NLN) or the ANA.

Individual Certification

The most common type of certification is called individual certification. When a nurse has demonstrated that he or she has attained a certain level of ability above and beyond the basic level required for licensure in a defined area of practice, that nurse can become certified. Usually some type of written and practical examination is required to demonstrate this advanced level of skill. The American Nurses Credentialing Center (ANCC) offers certifications in more than 40 areas that are widely recognized. Almost all nurses with individual certification are required to maintain their skills and competencies through continuing education and a specified number of continuing education units (CEUs). Recertification may be achieved through CEUs or retaking of the certification examination.

Organizational Certification

Organizational certification is the certification of a group or health-care institution by some external agency. It is usually referred to as accreditation and indicates that the institution has met standards established by either the government or by a nongovernmental agency. Often the ability of the institution to collect money from insurance companies or the federal government depends on whether or not the institution is certified by a recognized agency. Most hospitals are accredited by the Joint Commission on Accreditation of Healthcare Organizations (JCAHO) as a minimum level of accreditation.

Advanced Practice

Some state governments may either award or recognize certification granted to nurses in areas of advanced practice. In these cases, the certification becomes a legal requirement for practice at the APN level. Depending on the individual state's nurse practice act, nurses thus certified fall under regulations in the state's practice act that control the type of activities nurses may legally carry out when they perform advanced roles. For example, many states recognize the position of nurse **midwife** as an advanced practice role for nurses. In these states, a nurse midwife is allowed to practice those skills allowed under the nurse practice act of that state after obtaining certification. Generally nurse midwives are allowed to conduct prenatal examinations, do prenatal teaching, and deliver babies vaginally in

ISSUES NOW

Mutual Recognition Model of Nursing Licensure Continues to Expand

The Delegate Assembly of the National Council of State Boards of Nursing continues the process of expanding the mutual recognition model of nursing licensure that allows nurses licensed in one state to practice in other states without the necessity of seeking additional licensure. As of July 1, 2001, the number of states that officially belonged to the Interstate Nurse Licensure Compact had risen to 13. The newest members were Mississippi, Idaho, and Maine. Other compact states are Arkansas, Delaware, Iowa, Maryland, Nebraska, North Carolina, South Dakota, Texas, Utah, and Wisconsin. The number continues to grow as Arizona and North Dakota implement the compact in 2002 and 2003, and Illinois, Virginia, Georgia, and New Jersey are writing laws to open their states to honor nurse licenses from other compact states.

Although the number of states participating has increased, several issues continue to plague long-range plans to implement the compact nationwide. A primary hurdle preventing many states from joining the compact is concerns about disciplinary actions from the state of practice to the state of residence. It may be difficulty to track offenses and discipline nurses when they are practicing in states that have not issued their licenses. The question becomes: Who is responsible for the disciplinary action? The state where the license was issued or the state where the violation takes place? It seems likely that the state of residence would not be inclined to enthusiastically pursue disciplinary action against a nurse who committed a violation in another state because of the cost involved in investigating violations across state lines. In an attempt to deal with this question, the compact agreement allows states to restrict or revoke a nurse's privilege within its borders, regardless of where the license was issued. In addition, the state where the license was issued is permitted to take action against a nurse's license even if a violation takes place in another compact state.

Some states actually view the compact as a way to enhance the ability to track information about nurses with disciplinary problems. When states belong to the compact, the usual rules on sharing confidential information between state boards no longer hold. Any state belonging to the compact can share complete discipline information freely with any other state that belongs to the compact. This coordinated licensure information system between states includes all licensing information and disciplinary history of each nurse and serves as an additional measure in the protection of the public from unsafe practitioners.

The other major hurdle revolves around financial concerns. Currently, nurses who do not belong to compact states, but are employed in several different states, must pay the licensure fees for each state where they are employed. If the nurse is employed in compact states, he or she only pays the fee from the state of residence and then can work in any state within the compact without paying additional licensure fees. The total loss can be substantial. In a state the size of Virginia, it is estimated that the loss from license fees from out-of-state nurses would be in the range of $250,000 per year. In order to compensate for this loss of revenue, the state boards of nursing of some compact state have raised licensure fees substantially. Then the question becomes, is it fair to subsidize a small percentage of a state's nurses who work in other states by increasing the fees for all nurses in the state?

An important restriction on practicing across state lines arises when nurses change residence from a compact state to a nonparticipating state. The nurse can retain a valid license for the former state of residence; however, he or she will lose interstate privileges to practice in compact states. Likewise, nurses who obtain second licenses in compact states but do not live in those states do not have multistate licensure privileges.

It will most likely be many years before all the wrinkles in the compact plan are ironed out. Some states that are interested in the compact are taking a wait-and-see approach before making the commitment. They want to be sure that it is going to work. Other states, particularly those that have strong labor unions, will oppose the compact plan if it allows nurses to work in states where they are not required to join unions and pay union dues. In addition to the convenience and savings that multistate licensure offers for nurses who practice in two or more states, it provides a method of monitoring that is lacking in the current noncompact system. It is the first step in creating a national register for nurses and their licensure histories. Protection of the public is always the major concern. Although all the particular policies have not been formulated at this time, the proposed system would likely be similar to what is currently being used by nurses in the military, who can practice anywhere in the United States as long as they have a valid license from one state.

The movement toward a national licensure has been stimulated by several trends and developing issues in health care. These include the trend of nurses to increase their practice across state lines, the use of new technologies in numerous settings often located in different states, and the need by employers for quick approval for practice. Major issues that influence the movement include the demand by health-care consumers for qualified practitioners without regard to state boundaries, efficient and cost-effective use of limited registration and management resources for licensure, and questionable compliance with state requirements for licensure.

This movement is seen by many as an historic turning point in nursing that will affect every nurse in the United States. Mutual recognition will usher in a new and innovative method of regulation of nursing licensure and nursing practice, again demonstrating the nursing profession's creative leadership in health care.

Source: McPeck, P: Cross-country nursing: Multistate licensure allows RNs greater flexibility but raises cost, legal and practical questions. Nurse Week 14(18):25–26, 2001.

What Do You Think?

Should permissive licensure be re-established because it will help to reduce the cost of health care? Why? Why not?

uncomplicated pregnancies. They are not usually allowed to perform cesarean sections.

An independent certification center was proposed in 1978 to establish uniform criteria and standards and to oversee all certification activities. Although it would eliminate much of the current confusion about certification and would help with the legal recognition of advanced practice nurses, this proposal has not yet been acted upon because of opposition from physician and health-care administration groups.

Unfortunately, there is no uniformity among states in the recognition of certification of advanced practice nurses. Some states recognize almost all certifications and have provisions in their nurse practice acts to help guide these practices. Other states have very little legal recognition of certification levels and thus few guidelines for practice. This confusion may result from so many organizations offering certification in different areas. In some advanced practice areas, like nurse practitioners, two or more organizations may offer certification for the same title. The certification standards vary from organization to organization, and the method of determining certification may also be different.

It is expected that advanced practice nurses will play a larger role in the rapidly evolving health-care system of the future. What that role will be depends on how well governmental organizations and the public understand the contributions practitioners can make as **primary care** providers. Without a uniform definition of this specialty, such nurses will not be utilized to their full potential.

Licensure and certification are both methods of granting credentials to demonstrate that an individual is qualified to provide safe care to the public. Without proof of competency, the profession of nursing would become chaotic, disorganized, and even dangerous. It is important for nurses to keep a watchful eye on pending legislation and practices that health-care institutions are initiating. Many of these proposals and practices are covert ways of reintroducing permissive and institutional licensure.

Nursing Organizations and Their Importance

The establishment of a professional organization is one of the most important defining characteristics of a profession. Many professions have a single major professional organization to which most of its members belong and several specialized suborganizations that members may also join. Professions with just one major organization generally have a great deal of political power.

Nurses need and use power in every aspect of their professional lives, ranging from supervising nonlicensed personnel to negotiating with the administration for increased independence of practice. Clearly, an individual nurse probably does not have much power; but for nurses as a group, the potential is increased exponentially by the organization. The dedication to high-quality nursing standards and improved methods of practice by the major nursing organizations has led to improved care and increased benefits to the public as a whole.

> *Clearly, an individual nurse probably does not have much power; but for nurses as a group, the potential is increased exponentially by the organization.*

National nursing organizations need the participation and membership of all nurses in order to claim that they are truly representative of the profession. A large membership allows the organization to speak with one voice when making its values about health-care issues known to politicians, physicians' groups, and the public in general.

The National League for Nursing

Purposes

The primary purpose of the National League for Nursing (NLN) is to maintain and improve the standards of nursing education. The NLN is also a strong force in community health nursing, occupational health nursing, and nursing service activities. Its bylaws state that its purpose is to foster the development and improvement of hospital, industrial, public health, and other organized nursing services and of nursing education through the coordinated action of nurses, allied professional groups, citizens, agencies, and schools so that the nursing needs of the people will be met.

Membership

Although membership is open to individual nurses, the primary membership in the NLN comes in the form of agency membership, usually through schools of nursing. One of the major functions of this organization, through the National League for Nursing Accrediting Commission (NLNAC), is to accredit schools of nursing through a self-study process. The schools are given a set of criteria or **essentials for accreditation** and are then required to evaluate their programs against these criteria. After the evaluation report is written and sent to the NLNAC, site representatives visit the school to verify the information in the report and see whether the school has met the criteria. If the school meets the evaluation criteria, it is accredited for up to 8 years. NLNAC accreditation of a school of nursing indicates that the school meets national standards. In some work settings, it is a requirement that a nurse be a graduate of an NLNAC-accredited school of nursing before the nurse can be hired or accepted into many master's level nursing programs.

Other services and activities that the NLN carries out include testing, evaluating new graduate nurses, supplying career information and continuing education workshops and conferences for all levels of nursing, publishing a wide range of literature and videotapes covering current issues in health care, and compiling statistics about nursing, nurses, and nursing education.

American Association of Colleges of Nursing

Purposes

The American Association of Colleges of Nursing (AACN) was established to help colleges with schools of nursing work together to improve the standards for higher education for professional nursing. The AACN, through the Commission on Collegiate Nursing Education (CCNE), has developed standards for the **accreditation** of baccalaureate schools of nursing and is poised to become a major accreditation agency, competing with the NLNAC. The AACN has developed and published a set of guidelines for the education of professional nursing students that is widely used as the theoretical basis for baccalaureate curricula.

> *The American Association of Colleges of Nursing (AACN) was established to help colleges with schools of nursing work together to improve the standards for higher education for professional nursing.*

Membership

Only deans and directors of programs that offer baccalaureate or higher degrees in nursing with an upper-division nursing major are permitted membership.

American Nurses Association

Purposes

The American Nurses Association (ANA) grew out of a concern for the quality of nursing practice and the care that nurses were providing. The major purposes for the existence of the ANA, as stated in its bylaws, include improvement of the standards of health and the access to health-care services for everyone, improvement and maintenance of high standards for nursing practice, and promotion of the professional growth and development of all nurses, including economic issues, working conditions, and independence of practice.[4]

Membership

Membership in the ANA is limited to 52 constituents: 50 state organizations and Washington, DC, and Puerto Rico. An individual joins a state organization and through the state organization indirectly is a member of ANA. Certain discounts in membership are offered for new members and new graduate nurses. Various levels of membership are available for nurses who work part-time or those who are retired. The ANA makes every effort to encourage individual nurses to join the organization. Unfortunately, most nurses do not belong to this potentially powerful, politically active, and very influential organization.

Each state has the opportunity to determine what is needed from each member to run the state association; the amount of the dues that is sent to ANA is predetermined. Although dues are not inexpensive (they change a little from year to year, but are about $200 per year), the ANA offers various plans for payment, such as three equal payments over the course of a year or monthly payroll deductions. Because of the efforts of the ANA, nurses' salaries have risen to a point where this sum is affordable.

Other Services

When nurses pursue advanced education and levels of practice, as many are doing today, the ANA ANCC is essential for testing and certification of many of these practice levels. Although other organizations offer advanced practice certification, without the ANCC, there would be even less standardization for and less recognition of these practitioners by the public, physicians, or lawmakers.

Another important issue that the ANA has been involved in is the entry-level education requirement for professional nurses. The ANA has supported the baccalaureate degree as the minimum educational requirement for nurses for the last 25 years. The ANA is in the forefront of the debate over **entry into practice**, which has continued into the twenty-first century.

Additional functions carried out by the ANA include the establishment and continual updating of standards of nursing practice. These standards are the yardstick against which nurses are measured and held accountable by courts of **law**. The ANA also established the official code of ethics that guides professional practice.

Many of the political and economic activities of the ANA are carried out in the halls of legislatures and offices of legislators. The ANA Political Action Committee (PAC) is one of the most powerful in Washington, DC. (See Chapter 18 for more detailed discussion.) Such activities have a profound effect on the role that nurses play and will continue to play in health care well into the twenty-first century. Successful PAC activities require money and the power of a large, unified membership. The ANA-PAC seeks to influence legislation about nurses, nursing, and health care in general. It has been and will be a strong voice in the formulation of current national health-care reform.

Another important function of the ANA is economic. In many states, the ANA is the official **bargaining agent** for nurses in the negotiation of **contracts** with hospitals, nursing homes, and other health-care agencies that employ nurses. However, **collective bargaining** is done on a state-to-state basis—some states are **collective bargaining units** and others are not. (See Chapter 15 for more detailed discussion.) Professional organizations represent professional groups better than a labor union that has little knowledge of professional activities or needs.

The National Student Nurses' Association

Purposes

The National Student Nurses' Association (NSNA) is an independent legal corporation established in 1953 to represent the needs of nursing students. Working closely with the ANA, which offers services, an official publication, and close communication, the NSNA consists of state chapters that represent student nurses in those particular states.

The main purpose of the NSNA is to help maintain high standards of education in schools of nursing, with the ultimate goal of educating high-quality nurses who will provide excellent health care. Students' ideas, concerns, and needs are extremely important to nursing educators. Most nursing programs have committees in which students are asked to participate, including curriculum development and evaluation techniques. It is important that students belong to these committees and actively participate in the committees' activities.

Membership

Membership consists of all nursing students in registered nurse programs. Students can join at the local, state, or national level, or at all levels if desired. Dues are low, with a discount for the first year's membership.

Other Services

Additionally, the NSNA is concerned with developing and providing workshops, seminars, and conferences that deal with current issues in nursing and health care, with a wide range of subjects, from ethical and legal concerns to recent developments in pharmacology, test-taking skills, and professional growth. Student nurses who belong to the NSNA and who take an active part in its functions are much more likely to join the ANA after they graduate. Professional identity and professional behavior are learned. By beginning the process during the formal school years, student nurses develop professional attitudes and behaviors that they will continue for the rest of their lives.

Many benefits exist for student nurses who belong to the NSNA. A number of scholarships are available through this organization to members of the NSNA. Members receive the official publication of the organization, *Imprint*, and the *NSNA News*, keeping the student nurse current on recent developments in health care and nursing. The student member also has political representation on issues that may affect the student now or in the future. Some of these issues include educational standards for practice, standards of professional practice, and health insurance. The NSNA is also concerned with the difficulty that many nursing students from minority groups experience in the educational process. The Breakthrough project is an attempt by the NSNA to help such students enter the profession of nursing.

Student nurses who join the NSNA experience firsthand the operation, activities, and benefits of a professional organization. In schools with active memberships, the NSNA can be a very exciting and useful organization for students. Many NSNA chapters are involved in community activities that provide services at a local level and allow the student to practice "real" nursing. These services include providing community health screening programs for hypertension, lead poisoning, vision, hearing, and birth defects; setting up information and education programs; giving immunizations; and working with groups concerned with drug abuse, child abuse, drunk driving, and teen pregnancy. All nursing students should be encouraged to belong to this organization.

In response to the nursing shortage, the Oklahoma Nursing Student Association (ONSA) initiated a program in which the members of the association gave presentations to grade school and junior high school level students about the nursing profession. These are groups that are not usually targeted by college recruitment, although research has shown that recruitment among high school level students is largely nonproductive. Most individuals, by the time they reach high school, have made up their minds about the direction of their careers. The ONSA is funding its recruitment activities by obtaining donations from regional hospitals and other heath-care facilities that are experiencing the nursing shortage firsthand.

The International Council of Nurses

Membership in the International Council of Nurses (ICN) consists of national nursing organizations, and it serves as the international organization for professional nursing. The ANA is one member among 104 nursing associations around the world. Each member nation sends delegates and participates in the international convention held every 4 years. The quadrennial conventions or congresses are open to all nurses and delegates from all nations.

The goal of the ICN is to improve health and nursing care throughout the world. The ICN coordinates its efforts with the United Nations and other international organizations when appropriate in the pursuit of its goal.

Some issues that have been the focus of concern by the ICN are social and economic welfare of nurses, the changing role of nurses in the present health-care environment, the challenges being faced by the various national nursing organizations, and how government and politics affect the nursing profession and health care. Overseeing the ICN is the Council of National Representatives. This body meets every 2 years and serves as the governing organization. ICN headquarters is located in Geneva, Switzerland.

Sigma Theta Tau

Sigma Theta Tau is an honorary organization that was established in colleges and universities to recognize those individuals who have demonstrated leadership or made important contributions to professional nursing. It is international, and candidates are selected from among senior nursing students or graduate or practicing nurses.

The organization has its headquarters in Indianapolis, where it has a large library open to members to use for scholarly activities and research. It also boasts the first on-line nursing journal, which can be accessed by any nurse with a computer anywhere in the world. Local chapters of Sigma Theta Tau collect and distribute funds to nurses who are conducting nursing research. The organization also holds educational conferences and recognizes those who have made contributions to nursing.

Grassroots Organizations

A growing trend in contemporary nursing has been the formation of grassroots nursing organizations. In reality, all nursing organizations start as the grassroots efforts of local nursing groups who are trying to solve a particular problem. Over time, these small grassroots organizations become more structured, larger, and eventually become national or international when they spread to other areas across the country or around the world. Unfortunately, the large organizations tend to lose sight of the fundamental issues they were originally formed to solve, or they are unable to deal effectively with local problems.

Grassroots organizations usually have relatively small memberships; are localized to a town, city, or sometimes a state; and attempt to solve a problem or deal with an issue that the members feel is not being adequately handled by a large national organization. They may be created as a completely new and separate organization, or they may break away from a larger, established group. Because all the members of the grassroots organizations are passionately concerned about only one or two issues at a time that affect them directly, they tend to work hard to effect change and can bring a great deal of concentrated power to bear upon those, such as legislators, who make the decisions about the issues.

A number of techniques that are often frowned upon by the more established organizations are used by grassroots groups to attain their goals. In addition to the traditional techniques of writing letters, sending e-mail, and calling legislators, grassroots groups actively seek media attention, march on capitol buildings and state houses, introduce resolutions, and testify before committee hearings. Their success varies from issue to issue and location to location.

Two examples of successful grassroots efforts are found in California and Pennsylvania. The California Nurses Association decided to break away from the ANA because it was not addressing some key state issues such as length of hospital stays, reduction in professional nursing staffs, and the preoccupation with profit of **managed care**. The grassroots group in Pennsylvania formed a completely new organization, the Nurses of Pennsylvania (NPA), and focused their energies on the trend to replace licensed registered nurses with unlicensed technicians, sometimes called "downskilling."

Special-Interest Organizations

The historical origins of special-interest organizations in nursing are even older than those of the main national organizations. For example, the Red Cross, established in 1864, is one of the oldest special-interest organizations that nurses have been involved with. Like the Red Cross, most specialty organizations in nursing were founded when a group of nurses with similar concerns sought professional and individual support. These organizations usually start out small and informal, then increase in size, structure, and membership over a number of years. There were relatively few of these organizations until 1965, when an explosion in specialty organizations in nursing took place. During the next 20 years, almost 100 new organizations were formed, with the associated effect of diminishing membership levels in the ANA.

Specialty organizations are usually organized according to clinical practice area. Organizations exist for almost every clinical specialty and subspecialty known in nursing, such as obstetrics/gynecology, critical care, operating room, emergency room, and occupational health, as well as less known areas such as flight nurses, urology, and cosmetic surgery. Another focal area for these organizations is education and ethics. Organizations such as the American Association of Colleges of Nursing and the Western Interstate Commission for Higher Education fall into this category. Often organizations focus on the common **ethnic group**, cultural, or religious backgrounds of nurses. The National Association of Hispanic Nurses and the National Black Nurses Association represent this type of specialty organization.

Although many of these organizations promote the personal and professional growth of their membership, they also carry out many other activities. Particularly important among these activities is establishing the standards of practice for the particular specialty area. Much as the ANA establishes overall standards of practice for nursing in general, the specialty organizations establish standards for their particular clinical areas. Providing educational services for their members is another important activity of specialty organizations. Conferences, workshops, and seminars in the clinical area represented are important venues for nurses to keep current on new developments and to maintain high standards of practice.

How many of these specialty nursing organizations are there? No one really knows. Many such organizations are informal and run by volunteers. Organizations are continually being formed, and others are being disbanded. Should

ISSUES IN PRACTICE

Juanita R., an RN at a large, inner-city hospital, has been working on her off-hours as a volunteer in a storefront clinic to treat the indigent and underserved population of that part of the city. The clinic clientele is primarily Mexican-American, as are the majority of the 20 nurses working at the clinic. Because all the nurses, including a family nurse practitioner, volunteer their time and receive no pay, the small private grant that Juanita had managed to secure was adequate to cover the cost for rental of the building, basic supplies for the clinic, and a few medications. However, the grant is about to run out and is nonrenewable.

Juanita first tried to obtain money from the hospital to keep the clinic going, but she was told that the hospital was having its own financial problems because of managed care demands and could not spare any money. At a staff meeting of the nurses from the clinic, the nurses decided to band together and form a grass-roots organization called the Store-Front Clinic Nurses in order to focus their efforts on obtaining funds to keep the clinic open. They printed and passed out flyers, called local and city politicians, encouraged the patrons of the clinic to talk to people they knew, and even called the local television station for an interview about their plight.

Although most of the nurses' effort went unrewarded, a large pharmaceutical company became aware of their plight and wanted to provide a sizable financial stipend to the clinic, in addition to supplying free medications, for a period of at least 5 years. In addition to their philanthropic interests, the pharmaceutical company also wanted to gather long-term data about a newly developed antihypertensive medication. The company would provide the medication free to the clients at the clinic, the majority of whom had some degree of hypertension, and all the nurses would have to do is take and record the clients' blood pressure readings and complete "reported side effects" forms on each client. Client identifier codes, rather than names, would be used to maintain confidentiality. Juanita, as the group's coordinator, would be responsible for coordinating and preserving the data.

Although Juanita saw it as an answer to her prayers, she was concerned about the medication project. The pharmaceutical company said that no research consent forms were needed because the medication had already been through clinical trials and had received approval by the Food and Drug Administration. Juanita called another meeting of her nurses to discuss the issue. Without the grant, the clinic would close, but if they accepted the grant, they would have to participate in a medication research project that made Juanita feel uncomfortable.

1. What are the main issues in this case study?
2. What ethical principles are being violated? What is the ethical dilemma that Juanita is facing?
3. Are there any other solutions to this problem?

What Do You Think?

What type of power does the individual nurse have? Cite examples of individual nurses who have used their power to effect changes in health care and nursing?

nurses belong to these organizations? The answer is yes, but only after they belong to the ANA. Many of the larger specialty organizations have recognized this fact and have established close ties with the ANA. The ANA, in its turn, is well aware of the membership bleed-off from the specialty organizations and has initiated efforts to become more involved in the specialty nursing areas.

Before nurses join a specialty organization, they should determine whether its purposes are at odds with those of the ANA. Many of the large specialty organizations have their own lobbyists in both state and national legislatures. Because the legislators really do not know the differences between the various nursing organizations, they can easily become confused over health-care issues if they are receiving pressure from two nursing groups representing opposing sides of the same issue. At this point, legislators may simply surmise that nurses really do not know what they want and vote on an important issue without regard to nurses and nursing.

Conclusion

Nursing, in its journey toward professionalism, has been propelled and shaped by its nursing organizations, which were the main vehicles for the development of educational and practice standards, initiation of licensure, promotion of advanced practice, and general improvement in the level of care nurses provided. From their beginnings, nursing organizations have served as channels of communication between nurses, consumers of health care, and other health-care professionals. In many cases, the nursing organizations have served as a focus of power for the profession to influence those important health policies that affect the whole nation. That continued unity is essential for the survival of nursing.

The tendency toward specialization has led to an ever-increasing number of nursing organizations, however, each focusing on a particular practice field within the profession. This trend has diluted the unity and ultimately lessened the power that nursing as a profession can exert in health-care issues. Although it is important to recognize the complexity of today's health-care system and the pluralism inherent in nursing, unity of opinion on major issues is essential if nursing is to have any influence on the future of the profession. The challenge for nurses in the future is to use the diversity in the profession as a positive force and to unite as a group on important issues. Awareness of earlier development of nursing organizations provides a perspective for the current situation and can act as a framework for planning the future.

Critical Thinking Exercises

- Develop a strategy for increasing the membership in the ANA.
- A labor union is attempting to organize the nurses at your hospital. Is it better for the professional nursing organization to represent the nurses? Why?
- A new graduate nurse is working in the intensive care unit (ICU) of a large hospital. She wants to join a nursing organization but only has a limited amount of money to spend. Her coworkers in the ICU want her to join the AACN, but she would also like to join the ANA. Basing her decision on economic and professional issues, which organization should she join?
- Compare and contrast certification and licensure. Should certification be legally recognized? Justify your answer.

References

1. Kleinpell, RM: Two-tiered certification model debuts. Nursing Spectrum 13A(1):19, 2001.
2. McDonald, T: Professional issues: Nurses at work creating nursing futures. Lamp 58(11):29–30, 2001.
3. Mills, AC, and McSweeny, M: Nurse practitioners and physician assistants revisited. J Prof Nurs 18(1):36–46, 2002.
4. American Nurses Association: Nursing's Social Policy Statement. ANA, Washington, DC, 1995.

Bibliography

Adams, D, and Miller, BK: Professionalism in nursing behaviors of nurse practitioners. J Prof Nurs 17(4):203–210, 2001.

Barkley, TW, et al: Practice issues: Credentialing, perscriptive authority, and liability. Nurse Practitioner Forum 2001 12(2):106–114, 2001.

Garnero, T: On solving the nursing shortage. Nurse Week (Special Edition) Feb 4, 2002, p 11.

Glassford, B: Certification connection: Recognizing certification as an effective tool. AACN News 18(11):11, 2001.

Humphery, K: A guide to specialty certification. Dimensions of Critical Care Nursing 20(5):41–42, 2001.

Kleinpell, RM: Evolving nursing practice prompts changes to licensure exam. Nursing Spectrum 14(4):5, 2001.

Martin, SA: Network to promote advanced practice mentoring relationships. AACN News 19(3):5, 2002.

McPeck, P: Cross-country nursing: Multistate licensure allows RNs greater flexibility but raises cost, legal and practical questions. Nurse Week 14(18):25–26, 2001.

O'Neale, M, and Kurtz, S: Certification: Perspectives on competency assurance. Seminars in Perioperative Nursing 10(2):88–92, 2001.

Richards, JM: License endorsement applications require research. RN2001 64(7):32–33, 2001.

4

Theories and Models of Nursing

Joseph T. Catalano

Learning Objectives

After completing this chapter, the reader will be able to:

- Explain why theories and models are important to the profession of nursing.
- Analyze the four key concepts found in nursing theories and models.
- Interrelate systems theory as an important element in understanding nursing theories or models.
- Evaluate how the four parts of all systems interact.
- Synthesize three nursing theories, identifying how the different nursing theorists define the key concepts in their theories.

For many nurses, and for most nursing students, the terms *theory* and *model* evoke images of textbooks filled with abstract, obscure words and convoluted sentences. The visceral response is often "Why is this important? I want to take care of real people!" The simple answer is: Understanding and using nursing theories or models will help you to be a better nurse and provide better care to real people.

Differences Between Theory and Model

Although the terms *theory* and *model* are not synonymous, in nursing practice they are often used interchangeably. Strictly speaking, a theory refers to a speculative statement involving some element of reality that has not been proved. For example, the theory of relativity has never been proved, although the results have often been observed. The nursing profession tends to use the term *theory* when attempting to explain apparent relationships between observed behaviors and their effects on a client's health. In this nursing context, the goal of a theory is to describe and explain a particular nursing action in order to make a **hypothesis** or predict its effect on a client's outcome, such as improved health or recovery from illness. For example, the action of turning an unresponsive client from side to side every 2 hours should help prevent skin breakdown and improve respiratory function.

A model, on the other hand, is a hypothetical representation of something that exists in reality. The purpose of a model is to attempt to explain a complex reality in a systematic and organized manner.

What Do You Think?

Do you consider yourself to be healthy? What factors make you healthy? What factors are indicators of illness?

For example, a hospital organizational chart is a model that attempts to demonstrate the interrelationships of the various levels of the hospital's administration.[1]

Although a model tends to be more concrete than a theory, they both help explain and direct nursing actions. This ability, using a systematic and structured approach, is one of the key elements that raises nursing from a task-oriented job to the level of a real profession. With the use of a **conceptual model**, nurses can provide intelligent and thoughtful answers to the question "What do nurses do?" Consider this scenario:

> Mr. X had surgery for intestinal cancer 4 days ago. He has a colostomy and needs to learn how to take care of it at home because he is going to be discharged from the hospital in 2 days. When the nurses attempt to teach him colostomy care, he looks away, makes sarcastic personal comments about the nurses, and generally displays a belligerent and hostile attitude.

Without an understanding of the underlying dynamics involved, the nurse's reactions to this client's behavior might be to become sarcastic and scold the client about his behavior or simply to minimize the amount of contact with him.[1] This type of response will not improve Mr. X's health status. If the nurses knew, however, and understood the dynamics of the grief theory, they would realize that Mr. X was probably in the anger stage of the grief process. This understanding would direct the nurse to allow, or even to encourage, Mr. X to express his anger and **aggressiveness** without condemnation, and to help him deal with his feelings in a constructive manner. Once Mr. X gets past the anger stage, he can move on to taking a more active part in his care and thus improve his health status. The **client goals** would then be achieved.

If a researcher were to stop 10 people at random on the street and ask the question, "What do nurses do?", he or she would likely get 10 different answers. But the confusion about nurses' activities extends far beyond the public at large. What if the researcher asked 10 hospital administrators, 10 physicians, or even 10 nurses the same question? It could be anticipated that the answers would vary almost as much as the answers from laypeople. In an attempt to identify what exactly it is that nurses do, McCloskey and Bulechek, two nurse researchers at the University of Iowa, have been conducting a research project since 1990 to develop a **taxonomy** of the **interventions** that nurses use in their practice (Box 4–1). This research has been called Nursing Interventions Classification (NIC), the Iowa Interventions Project, or simply the Iowa Project.[2-5]

The first results, published in 1994, categorized and ranked 336 interventions that nurses use when they provide care to clients. A follow-up study was conducted about 2 years after the original and published in 1996. This study categorized and ranked 433 interventions used by nurses. McCloskey and Bulechek[6] also investigated what nursing interventions were commonly used by nurses in specialty settings. Forty specialty areas responded, and the researchers were able to develop a table that lists what core skills are used by each organization. This type of research helps identify the important contributions made by nursing to the health and well-being of clients. It also demonstrates the complex and demanding nature of the nursing profession. Although additional research has been conducted into this topic, the findings of McCloskey and Bulechek[4-6] continue to be considered the standard for all subsequent studies.

Key Concepts Common to Nursing Models

Although nursing models vary in terminology and approach to health care, there are four **concepts** that are common to almost all of them: client or patient (individual or collective), health,

Box 4–1

At first glance, it would seem that everybody knows that nurses take care of clients. But what constitutes care? A study conducted by the faculty of the University of Iowa, called the Nursing Interventions Classification (NIC) or simply the Iowa Project, has identified 336 tasks or interventions that nurses are responsible for in their care of patients. Not all nurses carry out all 336 of these tasks all the time, but during an average career, a nurse would likely be involved in the majority of these tasks. Although this project was undertaken in the mid-1990s, it remains as the benchmark study. Since the original study, several additional studies have been conducted that reaffirm the findings of the Iowa Project, and several researchers have undertaken projects to use the data generated by the Iowa Project in actual client care situations.

This project is an excellent example of how a nursing theory led to a research project that developed information that can be used by nurses in their daily practice. Based on the belief that nursing interventions are specific actions that a nurse can perform to bring about the resolution of a potential or actual health-care problem, the NIC attempted to identify and classify nursing interventions. It also attempted to rank those interventions according to the number of times a nurse was likely to perform one during a working day. The goal of the project was to develop a nursing information system that could be incorporated into the current information systems of all clinical facilities. By using the NIC system, hospital administrators, physicians, nurses, and even the public should be better able to recognize and evaluate the multiple interventions that nurses are responsible for in their daily work.

It is a generally acknowledged fact that nurses, as the largest single group of health-care providers, are essential to the welfare and care of most clients. Yet, in an age of health-care reform, nurses are finding it increasingly difficult to delineate the specific contributions they make to health care. And if nurses themselves are unable to define the care they provide, how are the reformers, politicians, and the public going to be able to identify the unique contribution made by nursing?

Unfortunately, many of the contributions that nurses make to health care are currently invisible because there is no method of classification for them in computerized database systems now in use. Commonly used nursing interventions such as active listening, emotional support, touch, skin surveillance, or even family support cannot be measured and quantified by most current information systems.

The large number of different interventions used daily by nurses demonstrates the complex and demanding nature of the profession. The breadth and depth of knowledge and skills demanded of nurses on a daily basis is much greater than is found in many other health-care professions. One study found that nurses working in general medical/surgical units during a 6-month period were likely to care for 500 clients with more than 600 individual diagnoses (many clients have multiple diagnoses). These researchers also found that the physical demands of the work were actually less difficult and tiring than dealing with the emotional and technical demands of handling the huge amounts of information generated by the care given.

Sources: McCloskey, JC, and Grace, CK: Current Issues in Nursing, ed. 5. Mosby–Year Book, St. Louis, 1997.

Bulechek, GM, et al: Nursing interventions used in nursing practice. Am J Nurs 94(10):59–61, 1994.

O'Connor, NA, et al: Documenting patterns of nursing interventions using cluster analysis. Journal of Nursing Measurement 9(1):73–90, 2001.

Determining cost of nursing interventions: A beginning… Iowa Intervention Project. Nursing Economics 19(4):146–160, 2001.

environment, and nursing. Each nursing model has its own specific definition of these terms, but the underlying definitions of the concepts are similar.

Client

The concept of client (or patient) is central to all nursing models, because it is the client who is the primary recipient of nursing care. Although the term *client* is usually used to refer to a single individual, it can also refer to small groups or to a large collective of individuals (for community health nurses, the community is the client).

The concept of client has changed over the years as the knowledge and understanding of human nature developed and increased. A client constitutes more than a person who simply needs **restorative care** and comes to a health-care facility with a **disease** to be cured. Clients are now seen as complex entities affected by various interrelating factors, such as the mind and body, the individual and the **environment**, and the person and the person's family. When nurses talk about clients, the term *biopsychosocial* is often used to express the complex relationship between the body, mind, and environment.

Nursing models tend to be holistic; they are concerned with curing disease and restoring a client's health, but they also focus on prevention of disease and maintenance of health. A healthy person is just as important to many nursing models as the person with a disease.

A client, in many of the nursing models, does not have to have an illness in order to be the central element of the model (this explains the current preference of using the term *client* over the term *patient*). This is also one of the clearest distinctions between medical models and nursing models. Medical models tend to be restrictive and are almost exclusively devoted to curing diseases and to restoring health. Nursing models tend to be **holistic**; they are concerned with curing disease and restoring a client's health, but they also focus on prevention of disease and maintenance of health. A healthy person is just as important to many nursing models as the person with a disease.

Health

Like the concept of client, the concept of health has undergone much development and change over the years as knowledge has increased. Originally thought of as an absence of disease, a more current realistic view is that of health as a continuum, ranging from a completely healthy state where there is no disease to a completely unhealthy state, which results in death. At any given time in their lives, everyone is located somewhere along the health continuum and may move closer to one side or the other depending on circumstances and health status.[7]

Health is difficult to define because it varies so much from one individual to another. For example, a 22-year-old bodybuilder who has no chronic diseases perceives health differently than an 85-year-old who has diabetes, congestive heart failure, and vision problems. The perception of health also varies from one culture to another and at different historical periods within the same culture. In some past cultures, a sign of health was pure white skin, whereas in the modern American culture, a dark bronze suntan has been more desirable as a sign of health—although there is an increasing recognition of the harmful effects of ultraviolet light on the skin.

Environment

The concept of environment is another element in most current nursing models. Nursing models often broaden the concept of environment from the simple physical environment to include elements such as living conditions, public sanitation, and air and water quality. Factors such as interpersonal relationships and social interactions are also included.

Some internal environmental factors that affect health include the personal psychological processes, religious beliefs, sexual orientation, personality, and emotional responses. It has long been known that individuals who are highly self-motivated and internally goal directed (i.e., type A personality) tend to develop ulcers and have myocardial infarctions at a higher rate than the general population. Medical models, which are primarily illness oriented, although acknowledging this factor, may not consider it to be treatable. Nursing models that consider personality as one of the environmental factors that affect health are more likely to attempt to modify the individual's behavior (internal environment) to decrease the risk of disease.

Like the other key concepts found in nursing models, the concept of environment is used so that it is consistent within a particular model's overall context. Nursing models try to show how various aspects of environment interrelate and how they affect the client's health status. In addition, nursing models treat environment as an active element in the overall health-care system and assert that positive alterations in the environment will improve the client's health status.

Nursing

The culminating concept in all the various nursing models is nursing itself. After consideration of what it means to be a client, what it means to be healthy, and how the environment influences the client's health status either positively or negatively, the concept of nursing delineates the function and role nurses have in their relationship with clients. Historically, the profession of nursing has been interested in providing basic physical care (i.e., hygiene, activity, nourishment), psychological support, and relief of discomfort for clients. But modern nursing, although still including these basic elements of client care, has expanded into areas of health care that were only imagined a generation ago.

> **What Do You Think?**
>
> How do you define nursing? What activities are important for the nurse to carry out?

In the modern nurse-client relationship, the client is no longer the passive recipient of nursing care. The relationship has been expanded to include clients as key partners in curing and in the health maintenance process. In conjunction with the nurse, clients set goals for care and recovery, take an active part in achieving those goals, and help in evaluating whether or not those actions have achieved the goals.[8]

Because of the broadened understanding of environment, several nursing models include manipulation of environmental elements that affect health as an important part of the nurse's role. The environment may be directly altered by the nurse with little or no input from the client, or the client may be taught by the nurse to alter the environment in ways that will contribute to curing disease, increasing comfort, or improving the client's health status.[9]

To analyze and understand any nursing model, it is important to look for these four key concepts: client, health, environment, and nursing. These concepts should be clearly defined, closely interrelated, and mutually supportive. Depending on the particular nursing model, one element may be emphasized more than another. The resultant role and function of the nurse depend on which element is given greater emphasis.

General Systems Theory

A widely accepted method for conceptualizing and understanding the world and what is in it is derived from a systems viewpoint. Generally understood as an organized unit with a set of components that interact and affect each other, a system acts as a whole because of the interdependence of its parts.[10] As a result, when part of the system malfunctions or fails, it interrupts the function of the whole system rather than affecting merely one part. Humans, plants, cars, governments, the health-care system, the profession of nursing, and almost anything that exists can be viewed as a system. The terminology and principles of systems theory pervade U.S. society.

Although general systems theory in its pure form is rarely, if ever, used as a nursing model, its process and much of its terminology underlie many nursing models. Elements of general systems theory in one form or another have found their way into many textbooks and much of the professional literature. General systems theory often acts as the unacknowledged **conceptual framework** for many educational programs. An understanding of the mechanisms and terminology of general systems theory is helpful in providing an orientation to understanding nursing models.

General systems theory, sometimes referred to simply as **systems theory**, is an outgrowth of an innate intellectual process. The human mind has difficulty comprehending large, complex entities as a single unit. As a result, the mind automatically divides that entity into smaller, more manageable fragments and then examines each fragment separately. This is similar to the process of deductive reasoning, in which a single complex thought or theory is broken down into smaller, interrelated pieces. All scientific disciplines, from physics to biology and social sciences (e.g., sociology and psychology), use this method of analysis.

Systems theory, however, takes the process a step further. After analyzing or breaking down the entity, systems theory attempts to put it back together by showing how the parts work individually and together within the system. This interrelationship of the parts makes the system function as a unit. And often, particularly when the system involves biologic or sociologic entities, the system that results is greater than the sum of its parts. For example, a human can be considered to be a complex, biosocial system. Humans are made up of a large number of smaller systems such as the endocrine system, neurologic system, gastrointestinal system, urinary system, and so forth. Although each of these systems is important, in and of themselves they do not make a human. Many animals have the same systems, yet the human is more than the animal and more than the sum of the systems.

Although the early roots of general systems theory can be traced as far back as the 1930s, von Bertalanffy is usually credited with the formal development and publication of general systems theory around 1950.[11] His major achievement was to standardize the definitions of the terms used in systems theory and make the concept useful to a wide range of disciplines. Systems theory is so widely applicable because it reflects the reality that underlies the basic human thought processes.

Very simply, a system is defined as a set of interacting parts. The parts that compose a system may be similar or they may vary a great deal from each other, but they all have the common function of making the system work well to achieve its overall purpose. A school is a good example of how the dynamics and interrelatedness of a system work. A school as a system consists of a large number of units including buildings, administrators, teachers, students, and various other individuals (e.g., counselors, financial aid personnel, bookkeepers, and maintenance persons). Each of these individuals has a unique job but also contributes to the overall goal of the school, which is to provide an education for the students and also to further the development of knowledge through research.

All systems consist of four key parts: the system itself (i.e., whether an open system or a closed system); input and output; throughput; and a feedback loop.

Open and Closed Systems

A system is categorized as being either open or closed. In reality, very few systems are completely open or completely closed. Rather, they are usually a combination of both open and closed systems.

Open systems are those in which relatively free movement of information, matter, and **energy** into and out of the system exists. In a completely open system, there would be no restrictions on what moves in and out of the system, thus making its boundaries difficult to identify. Most systems have some control on the movement of information, energy, and matter around them. This control is maintained through the semipermeable nature of their boundaries, which allows some things in and keeps some things out as well as allowing some out while keeping others in. This control on input and output leads to the dynamic equilibrium found in most well-functioning systems.

Theoretically, a **closed system** prevents any movement into and out of the system. In this case, the system would be totally static and unchanging. Probably no absolutely closed systems exist in the real world, although there are systems that may tend to be closed to outside elements. A stone, for example, considered as a system, seems to be very nearly a perfectly closed system. It does not take anything in or put anything out. It does not change very much over long periods. In reality, though, it is affected by a number of elements in nature. It absorbs moisture when it is damp, freezes when cold, and becomes hot in the summer. Over long periods, these factors may cause the stone to crack, break down, and eventually become topsoil.

Systems that nurses deal with frequently are relatively open. Primarily, the client can be categorized as a highly open system that requires certain input elements and has output elements also. Other systems that nurses commonly work with (e.g., hospital administrators and physicians) are generally considered to be open systems, although their degree of openness may vary widely.

Input and Output

The processes by which a system interacts with elements in its environment are called input and output. **Input** is defined as any type of information, energy, or material that enters the system from the environment through its boundaries. Conversely, **output** is defined as any information, energy, or material that leaves the system and enters the environment through the system's boundaries. The **end product** of a system is a type of output that is not reusable as input. Open systems require relatively large amounts of input and output.

Throughput

A third term sometimes used in relationship to the system's dynamic exchange with the environment is *throughput*. **Throughput** is a process that allows the input to be changed so that it is useful to the system. For example, most automobiles operate on some form of liquid fossil fuel (input) such as gasoline or diesel fuel. However, going to the gas station and pouring liquid fuel on the roof of the car will not produce the effects desired when most people buy fuel for their cars. But if the fuel is put into the gas tank, it can be transformed by the carburetor or fuel injection system into a fine mist, which when mixed with air and ignited by a spark plug burns rapidly to produce the force necessary to propel the car. Without this internal process (throughput) found in the car, liquid fuel is not a useful form of energy.

Feedback Loop

The fourth key element of a system is the feedback loop. The **feedback** loop allows the system to monitor its internal functioning so that it can either restrict or increase its input and its output and maintain the highest level of functioning.

Two basic types of feedback exist. Positive feedback leads to change within the system, with the goal of improving the system. Students in the classroom, for example, receive feedback from the teacher in several ways; it may be in the form of direct verbal statements such as "good work on this assignment" or feedback by examination and homework grades. Feedback is considered positive if it produces a change in a student's behavior, such as motivating him or her to study more, spending more time on assignments, or preparing more thoroughly for class.

Negative feedback maintains stability; that is, it does not produce change. Negative feedback is not necessarily bad for a system. Rather, when a system has reached its peak level of functioning, negative feedback helps it maintain that level. For example, an athlete who has reached his or her peak level of performance through long hours of practice knows what type of practice is required to stay at that level of ability. Negative feedback—in the form of optimal times in the case of runners or number of pounds lifted in the case of weightlifters—indicates that no changes in practice patterns are required.

> *Positive feedback leads to change within the system, with the goal of improving the system.*

The feedback loop is an important element in systems theory. It makes the process circular and links the various elements of the system together. Without a feedback loop, it is virtually impossible for the system to have any meaningful control over its input and output.

Feedback loops are used at all levels in a hospital. Nurses get feedback about the care that they provide both from clients and from their supervisors. The hospital administration gets feedback from clients and accrediting agencies. Physicians get feedback from clients, nurses, and the hospital administration. Systems theory is present, if sometimes unseen, in almost all health-care settings. Professional nurses need to be able to understand and identify the components of systems theory when they are encountered to improve their nursing practice and quality of care.

Major Nursing Theories and Models

At least 15 published nursing models (or theories) have been used to direct nursing education and nursing care.[12] The six nursing models discussed here (Table 4–1) have been selected because they are the most widely accepted and are good examples of how the concepts of client, health, environment, and nursing are used to explain and guide nursing actions. Discussion of these theories is not intended to be exhaustive, but rather to provide an overview of the main concepts of the **nurse theorist**. It is important to understand the terms used in the theories as defined by their authors and to see the interrelationship between the elements in each theory as well as the similarities and differences among the various different models.

The Roy Adaptation Model

As developed by Sister Callista Roy, the Roy Adaptation Model of nursing is very closely related to systems theory.[13] The main **goal** of this model is to allow the client to reach his or her highest level of functioning through **adaptation**.

Client

The central element in the Roy Adaptation Model is man (a generic term referring to humans in general, or the client in particular, collectively or individually). Man is viewed as a dynamic entity with both input and output. As derived from the context of the four modes in the Roy Adaptation Model, the client is defined as a biopsychosocial being who is affected by various stimuli and displays behaviors to help adapt to the stimuli. Because the client is constantly being affected by stimuli, adaptation is a continual process.[13]

Input are called stimuli and include internal stimuli that arise from within the client's environment as well as stimuli coming from external

Table 4–1

Comparison of Selected Nursing Models

NURSING THEORY	CLIENT	HEALTH	ENVIRONMENT	NURSING
Roy Adaptation Model	Man—as a dynamic system with input and output	A continuum—the ability to adapt successfully to illness	Both internal and external stimuli that affect behaviors	Multistep process that helps the client adapt and reach the highest level of functioning
Orem Self-Care Model	Humans—biologic, psychological social beings with the ability for self-care	Ability to live life to the fullest through self-care	The medium through which the client moves	Helping the client achieve health through assistance in self-care activities
King Model of Goal Attainment	Person—exchanges energy and information with the environment to meet needs	Dynamic process to achieve the highest level of functioning	Personal, interpersonal, and social systems and the external physical world	Dynamic process to identify and meet the health-care needs of the person
Watson Model of Human Caring	Individual—has needs, grows, and develops to reach a state of inner harmony	Dynamic state of growth and development leading to full potential as a human being	Those factors the client must overcome to achieve health	Science of caring that helps clients reach their greatest potential
Johnson Behavioral System Model	Person—a behavioral system that is an organized and integrated whole composed of seven subsystems	A balanced and steady state within the behavioral system of the client	All those internal and external elements that affect client behavior	Activities that manipulate the environment and help clients achieve the balanced state of health
Neuman Health-Care Systems Model	An open system that constantly interacts with internal and external environment	Relatively stable internal functioning of the individual in a high state of wellness (stability)	Internal and external stressors that produce change in the client	Identifies boundary disruption and helps clients in activities to restore stability

environmental factors such as physical surroundings, family, and society. The output in the Roy Adaptation Model is the behavior that the client demonstrates as a result of stimuli that are affecting him or her.

Output, or behavior, is a very important element in the Roy Adaptation Model, because it provides the **baseline data** about the client that the nurse obtains through assessment techniques. In this model, the output (behavior) is always modified by the client's internal attempts to adapt to the input, or stimuli. Roy has identified four internal adaptational activities that clients use and has called them the four adaptation modes:

1. The physiologic mode (using internal physiologic process)
2. The self-concept mode (developed throughout life by experience)
3. The role function mode (dependent on the client's relative place in society)
4. The interdependence mode (indicating how the client relates to others)

Health

In the Roy Adaptation Model, the concept of health is defined as the location of the client along a continuum between perfect health and complete illness. Health, in this model, is rarely an absolute. Rather, "a person's ability to adapt to stimuli, such as injury, disease, or even psychological stress, determines the level of that person's health status."[13] For example, a client who was in an automobile accident, had a broken neck, and was paralyzed but who eventually went back to college, obtained a law degree, and became a practicing lawyer would, in the Roy Adaptation Model, be considered to have a high degree of health because of the ability to adapt to the stimuli imposed.

Environment

The Roy Adaptation Model's definition of environment is synonymous with the concept of stimuli. The environment consists of all those factors that influence the client's behavior, either internally or externally. This model categorizes these environmental elements, or stimuli, into three groups: (1) focal, (2) contextual, and (3) residual.

Focal stimuli are environmental factors that most directly affect the client's behavior and require most of his or her attention. Contextual stimuli form the general physical, social, and psychological environment from which the client emerges. Residual stimuli are factors in the client's past, such as personality characteristics, past experiences, religious beliefs, and social norms that have an indirect effect on the client's health status. Residual stimuli are often very difficult to identify because they may remain hidden in the person's past memory or may be an integral part of the client's personality.

Nursing

In the Roy Adaptation Model, nursing becomes a multistep process, similar to the **nursing process**, to aid and support the client in the attempt to adapt to stimuli in one or more of the four adaptive modes. To determine what type of help is required to promote adaptation, the nurse must first assess the client. The primary **nursing assessments** are of the client's behavior (output). Basically, the nurse should try to determine whether the client's behavior is adaptive or maladaptive in each of the four adaptational modes previously defined. Some first-level assessments of the pneumonia client might include a temperature of 104°F, a cough productive of thick green sputum, chest pain on inspiration, and signs of weakness or physical debility, such as the inability to bring in wood for the fireplace or to visit friends.

A second-level assessment should also be made to determine what type of stimuli (input) are affecting the client's health-care status. In the case of the client with pneumonia, this might include a culture and sensitivity of the sputum to identify the invasive bacteria, assessment of the client's clothes to determine whether they were adequate for the weather outside, and an investigation to find out whether any neighbors could help the client when he or she is discharged from the hospital.

After performing the assessment, the nurse analyzes the data and arranges them in such a way so as to be able to make a statement about the client's adaptive or maladaptive behaviors, that is, identifies the problem. In current terminology, this identification of the problem is called a **nursing diagnosis**.

After the problem has been identified, goals for optimal adaptation are established. Ideally, these goals should be a collaborative effort between the nurse and the client. A determination of the actions that need to be taken to achieve the goals is the next step in the process. The focus should be on manipulation of the stimuli to promote optimal adaptation. Finally, an evaluation is made of the whole process to evaluate whether the goals have been met. If the goals have not been met, the nurse must then determine why, not how, the activities should be modified to achieve the goals.[11]

The Orem Self-Care Model

Dorothea E. Orem's model of nursing is based on the belief that health care is each individual's own responsibility. The model is aimed at helping clients direct and carry out activities that either help maintain or improve their health.[14]

Client

As with most other nursing models, the central element of the Orem model is the client, who is a biologic, psychological, and social being with the capacity for self-care. Self-care is defined as the practice of activities that individuals initiate and perform on their own behalf to maintain life, health, and well-being. Self-care is a requirement both for maintenance of life and for optimal functioning.

Health

In the Orem Self-Care Model, health is defined as the person's ability to live fully within a particular physical, biologic, and social environment, achieving a higher level of functioning that distinguishes the person from lower life forms. Quality of life is an extremely important element in this model of nursing. A person who is healthy is living life to the fullest and has the capacity to maintain that life through self-care. An unhealthy person is an individual who has a self-care deficit. This deficit is indicated by the inability to carry out one or more of the key health-care activities. These activities have been categorized into six groups:

> *The primary goal of nursing in the Orem model is to help the client conduct self-care activities in such a way as to reach the highest level of human functioning.*

- Air, water, and food
- Excretion of waste
- Activity and rest
- Solitude and social interactions
- Hazards to life and well-being
- Being normal mentally under universal self-care. This group of unhealthy individuals also includes adults with diseases and injuries, young and dependent children, the elderly, and the disabled.

Universal Self-Care

In the Orem model, self-care is a two-part concept. The first type of self-care is called universal self-care and includes those elements commonly found in everyday life that support and encourage normal human growth, development, and functioning. Persons who are healthy, according to the Orem model, carry out the activities listed in order to maintain a state of health. To some degree, all these elements are necessary activities in maintaining health through self-care.[15]

The second type of self-care comes into play when the individual is unable to conduct one or more of the six self-care activities. This second type of self-care is called health deviation self-care. Health deviation self-care includes those activities carried out by individuals who have diseases, injuries, physiologic or psychological stress, or other health-care concerns. Activities such as seeking health care at an emergency room or clinic, entering a drug **rehabilitation** unit, joining a health club or weight control program, or going to a physician's office fall into this category.

Environment

Environment, in the self-care model, is the medium through which clients move as they conduct their daily activities. Although less emphasized in this model, the environment is generally viewed as a negative factor on a person's health status because many environmental factors detract from the ability to provide self-care. Environment includes social interactions with others, situations that must be resolved, and those physical elements that affect health.

Nursing

The primary goal of nursing in the Orem model is to help the client conduct self-care activities in such a way as to reach the highest level of human functioning. Because there is a range of levels of self-care ability, three distinct levels, or systems, of nursing care are delineated, based on the individual's ability to undertake self-care activities. As clients become less able to care for themselves, their nursing care needs increase.

A person who is able to carry out few or no self-care activities falls into the wholly compensated nursing care category in which the nurse must provide for most or all of the client's self-care needs. Examples of clients who require this level of care include comatose and ventilator-dependent clients in an intensive care unit, clients in surgery and the immediate recovery period, women in the labor and delivery phases of childbirth, and clients with emotional and psychological problems so severe as to render them unable to conduct normal activities of daily living.

Clients in the partially compensatory category of nursing care can meet some to most of their own self-care needs, but still have certain self-care deficits that require nursing intervention. The nurse's role becomes one of identifying these needs and carrying out activities to meet them until the client reaches a state of health and is able to meet the needs personally. Examples of this level of nursing care include the postoperative client who can feed himself and do basic activities of daily living (ADLs) but is unable to care for his or her catheter and dressings, or a client with newly diagnosed diabetes who has not yet learned the technique of self-administered insulin injections.

Clients who are able to meet all of their basic self-care needs require very little or no nursing interventions. These clients are recipients of the supportive developmental category of nursing care, in which the nurse's main functions are to teach the client how to maintain or improve health and to offer guidance in self-care activities and provide emotional support and encouragement. Also, the nurse may adjust the environment to support the client's growth and development toward self-care or may identify community resources to help in the self-care process.[15] Conducting prenatal classes, arranging for discharge planning, providing child screening programs through a community health agency, and organizing aerobic exercise classes for post-coronary clients all are nursing actions that belong in the supportive developmental category of care.

Nursing care is carried out through a three-step process in the Orem model. Step 1 determines whether nursing care is needed. This step includes a basic assessment of the client and identification of self-care problems and needs. Step 2 determines the appropriate nursing care system category and plans nursing care according to that category. Step 3 provides the indicated nursing care or actions to meet the client's self-care needs.

What Do You Think?

Based on your experiences with the health-care system, write your own definition of client (patient). What factors led you to this definition?

Five Methods

In the Orem model, step 3—the provision of nursing care (**implementation** phase)—is carried out by helping the client through one or a combination of five nursing methods:[12]

- Acting for or doing for another person
- Guiding another person

- Supporting another person (physically or psychologically)
- Providing an environment that promotes personal development
- Teaching another person

The King Model of Goal Attainment

The current widely accepted practice of establishing health-care goals for clients, and directing client care to meet these goals, has its origins in the King Model of Goal Attainment developed by Imogene M. King. It is also called the King Intervention Model.[16]

The King model also noted that nursing must function in all three system levels found in the environment: personal, interactional, and social. The primary function of nursing is at the personal systems level, whereby care of the individual is the main focus. However, nurses can effectively provide care at the interactional systems level, at which they deal with small- to moderate-sized groups in activities such as group therapy and in health promotion classes. Finally, nurses can provide care at the social systems level through activities such as programs in community health. In addition, the role of nursing at the social systems level can be expanded to include involvement in policy decisions that have an effect on the health-care system as a whole.

Client

As in other nursing models, the focal point of care in the King model is the person or client. The client is viewed as an open system that exchanges energy and information with the environment, a personal system with physical, emotional, and intellectual needs that change and grow during the course of life. Because these needs cannot be met completely by the client alone, interpersonal systems are developed through interactions with others depending on the client's perceptions of reality, communications with others, and transactions to reduce stress and tension in the environment.

Environment

Environment is an important concept in the King model and encompasses a number of interrelated elements. The personal and interpersonal systems or groups are central to King's conception of environment. They are formed at various levels according to internal goals established by the client.

Personal Systems. At the most basic level are the personal systems, where an interchange takes place between two individuals who share similar goals. An example of such a personal system is a client-nurse relationship.

Interpersonal Systems. At the intermediate level are the interpersonal systems that involve relatively small groups of individuals who share like goals, for example, a formal weight-loss program in which the members have the common goal of losing weight. Human interactions, communications, role delineation, and stress reduction are essential factors at this level.

Social Systems. At the highest level are social systems, which include the large, relatively homogeneous elements of society. The health-care system, government, and society in general are some important social systems. These social systems have as their common goals organization, authority, power, status, and decision. Although the client may not be in direct interaction with the social systems, these systems are important because the personal and interpersonal systems necessarily function within larger social systems. Evoking the principle of nonsummativity,* whenever one part of an open system is changed, all the other parts of the system feel the

*Nonsummativity is the degree of interrelatedness among the systems parts. The higher the degree of nonsummativity, the greater the interdependence of parts.

effect. For example, a decision made at the governmental level to reduce **Medicare** or **Medicaid** payments may affect when and how often a client can use health-care services such as doctor's office visits, group therapy, or emergency room care.

The King model also includes the external physical environment that affects a person's health and well-being. As the person moves through the world, the physical setting interacts with the personal system to either improve or degrade the client's health-care status.

Health

Viewed as a dynamic process that involves a range of human life experiences, health exists in people when they can achieve their highest level of functioning. Health is the primary goal of the client in the King model. It is achieved by continually adjusting to environmental **stressors**, maximizing the use of available resources, and setting and achieving goals for one's role in life. Anything that disrupts or interferes with people's ability to function normally in their chosen roles is considered to be a state of illness.

Nursing

The King model considers nursing to be a dynamic process and a type of personal system based on interactions between the nurse and the client. During these interactions, the nurse and the client jointly evaluate and identify the health-care needs, set goals for fulfillment of the needs, and consider actions to take in achieving those goals. Nursing is a multifaceted process that includes a range of activities such as the promotion and maintenance of health through education, the restoration of health through care of the sick and injured, and preparation for death through care of the dying.[11]

The process of nursing in the King model includes five key elements considered central to all human interactions:

- Action
- Reaction
- Interaction
- Transaction
- Feedback

The Watson Model of Human Caring

Although the concept of caring has always been an important, if somewhat obscure, element in the practice of nursing, the Watson Model of Human Caring defines caring in a detailed and systematic manner. In the development of her model, Jean Watson used a philosophical approach rather than the systems theory approach seen in many other nursing models. Her main concern in the development of this model is to balance the impersonal aspects of nursing care that are found in the technological and scientific aspects of practice with the personal and interpersonal elements of care that grow from a humanistic belief in life. Watson is also one of the very few theorists who openly recognizes the client's and family's spirituality and spiritual beliefs as an essential element of health.[17]

Watson is also one of the very few theorists who openly recognizes the client's and family's spirituality and spiritual beliefs as an essential element of health.

Client

The concept of client or person in the Watson model is not well developed as separate from the concept of nursing. The individuality of the client is a key concern. The Watson model views

ISSUES NOW

Looking to the Future—The Pew Commission Final Report

Projected estimates of the nursing shortage based on data collected by the U.S. Bureau of the Census Current Population Survey, Division of Nursing, the Pew Commission, and the Buerhaus and Staiger data collection agency in 1998 are now considered woefully inadequate. Current projections of the nursing shortage range from 400,000 to as many as 1,000,000 by the year 2010. The Pew Commission's final report addressed the competencies that nurses in the future will need:

Twenty-one Competencies for the Twenty-first Century

1. Embrace a personal ethic of social responsibility and service.
2. Exhibit ethical behavior in all professional activities.
3. Provide evidence-based, clinically competent care.
4. Incorporate the multiple determinants of health in clinical care.
5. Apply knowledge of the new sciences.
6. Demonstrate critical thinking, reflection, and problem-solving skills.
7. Understand the role of primary care.
8. Rigorously practice preventive health care.
9. Integrate population-based care and services into practice.
10. Improve access to health care for those with unmet health needs.
11. Practice relationship-centered care with individuals and families.
12. Provide culturally sensitive care to a diverse society.
13. Partner with communities in health-care decisions.
14. Use communication and information technology effectively and appropriately.
15. Work in interdisciplinary teams.
16. Ensure care that balances individual, professional, system, and social needs.
17. Practice leadership.
18. Take responsibility for quality of care and health outcomes at all levels.
19. Contribute to continuous improvement of the health-care system.
20. Advocate for public policy that promotes and protects the health of the public.
21. Continue to learn and help others to learn.

The Pew Commission also went on to identify five key areas for professional education:

1. Change professional training to meet the demands of the new health-care system.

2. Ensure that the health professions workforce reflects the diversity of the nation's population.
3. Require interdisciplinary competence in all health professionals.
4. Continue to move education into ambulatory practice.
5. Encourage public service of all health professional students and graduates.

The changes that will occur over the next decade may threaten some health-care professionals, but they will also open up a vista of opportunities for those willing to look into the future creatively. Nursing has to recognize that it will grow only to the extent that it is able to contribute to the needs of an evolving health-care system. These needs will change with time. The Pew Report, although broad in scope, provides the nursing profession a blueprint for dealing with these changes as they occur. It is a call to action that nurses and the nursing profession need to hear.

Sources: Critical Challenges: Revitalizing the Health Professions for the 21st Century. Pew Health Professions Commission, San Francisco, 1995.

Bellack, JP, and O'Neil, EH: Recreating nursing practice for a new century: Recommendations of the Pew Health Professions Commission's Final Report. Nursing and Health Care Perspectives 21(1):14–21, 2000.

Brady, M, et al: A Proposed framework for differentiating the 21 Pew Competencies by level of nursing education. Nursing and Health Care Perspectives 22(1):30–36, 2001.

Pontious, M: Where have all the nurses gone? The Oklahoma Nurse 47(1):1, 18, 2002.

More than one million new nurses needed by 2010. The American Nurse 34(1):5, 2002.

the client as someone who has needs, who grows and develops throughout life, and who eventually reaches a state of internal harmony. The client is also seen as a gestalt, or whole, who has value because of inherent goodness and capacity to develop. This gestalt, or holistic, view of the human being is a recurring theme in the Watson model; it emphasizes that the total person is more important to nursing care than the individual injury or disease process that produced the need for care.

Environment

Environment in the Watson model is a concept that is also closely intertwined with the concept of nursing. Viewed primarily as a negative element in the health-care process, the environment consists of those factors that the client must overcome to achieve a state of health. The environment can be both external physical and social elements and internal psychological reactions that affect health.

Health

To be healthy according to the Watson model, the individual must be in a dynamic state of growth and development that leads to reaching full potential as a human. As with other nursing models, health is viewed as a continuum along which a person at any point may tend more toward health or more toward illness. Illness, in the Watson model, is the client's inability to integrate life experiences and the failure to achieve full potential or inner harmony. In this model, the state of illness is not necessarily synonymous with the disease process. If the person reacts to the disease process in such a way as to find meaning, then that response is considered to be healthy. A failure to find meaning in the disease experience leads to a state of illness.

Nursing

Watson makes a clear distinction between the science of nursing and the practice of curing (medicine).[12] She defined nursing as the science of caring in which the primary goal is to assist the client reach the greatest level of personal potential. The practice of curing involves the conduct of activities that have the goal of treatment and elimination of disease.

The process of nursing in the Watson model is based on the systematic use of the scientific problem-solving method for decision making. In order to best understand nursing as a science of caring, the nurse should hold certain beliefs and be able to initiate certain caring activities.

Values. Basic to the beliefs necessary for the successful practice of nursing in the Watson model is the formation of a humanistic altruistic system of values based on the tenet that all people are inherently valuable because they are human. In addition, the nurse should have a strong sense of faith and hope in people and their condition because of the human potential for development.

Caring. A number of activities are important when practicing nursing according to Watson's caring way. These activities include establishing a relationship of help and trust between the nurse and the client; encouraging the client to express both positive and negative feelings with acceptance; manipulating the environment to make it more supportive, protective, or corrective for the client with any type of disease process; and assisting in whatever way deemed appropriate to meet the basic human needs of the client.

The Johnson Behavioral System Model

By integrating systems theory with behavioral theory, Dorothy E. Johnson has developed a model of nursing that considers client behavior to be the key to preventing illness, and also to restoring health when illness occurs. Johnson holds that human behavior is really a type of system in itself that is influenced by input factors from the environment and has output that in its turn affects the environment.[12]

Client

Drawing directly on the terminology of systems theory, the Johnson model describes the person, or client, as a behavioral system that is an organized and integrated whole. The whole is greater than the sum of its parts because of the integration and functioning of its **subsystems.** In the Johnson model, the client as a behavioral system is composed of seven distinct behavioral subsystems. In turn, each of these seven behavioral subsystems contains four structural elements that guide and shape the subsystem.

Security. The first behavioral subsystem is the attachment or affiliate subsystem, which has security as its driving force. The type of activity that this subsystem undertakes is, for the most part, inclusion in social functions, and the behavior that is observed from this subsystem is social interactions.

Dependency. The second behavioral subsystem is the dependency subsystem and has as its initiating force the goal of assisting or helping others. The primary type of activity involved is nurturing and promoting self-image. The observable behaviors that are a result of this activity include approval, attention, and physical assistance of the person.

Taking In. The third behavioral subsystem is called the ingestive subsystem and has as its driving force the meeting of the body's basic physiologic needs of food and nutrient intake. Correspondingly, its primary activity is seeking and eating food, which manifests itself in the behavior of eating.

Eliminative Behavior. The fourth behavioral subsystem is the eliminative; its goal is removal of waste products from the system. Its primary activity is means of elimination, which is observed as the behavior of expelling waste products.

Sexual Behavior. The fifth behavioral subsystem is sexual behavior and is found in the Johnson model's description of the person. The sexual subsystem has gratification and procreation of the species as its goals. It involves the complex activities of identifying gender roles, sexual development, and actual biologic sexual activity. It manifests itself in courting and mating behaviors.

Self-Protection. The sixth behavioral subsystem is called the aggressive subsystem, and its driving force is the goal of self-preservation. All the actions that individuals undertake to protect themselves from harm, either internal or external, derive from this subsystem and are shown in actions toward others and the environment in general.

Achievement. The seventh, and final, behavioral subsystem is identified as achievement. Achievement has as its driving force the broad goal of exploration and manipulation of the environment. Gaining mastery and control over the environment is the primary activity of this subsystem; it can be demonstrated externally when the individual shows that learning has occurred and higher-level accomplishments are being produced.[18]

As with all open systems, the behavioral system that makes up the person seeks to maintain a dynamic balance by regulating input and output. This regulation process takes the form of adapting to the environment and responding to others. However, the Johnson model sees human behavior as being goal directed, which leads the person to constant growth and development beyond the maintenance of a mere steady state.

Health

A state of health exists, according to the Johnson model, when balance and steady state exist within the behavioral systems of the client. Under normal circumstances, the human system has enough inherent flexibility to maintain this balance without external intervention. At times, however, the system's balance may be disturbed to such a degree by physical disease, injury, or emotional crisis as to require external assistance. This out-of-balance state is the state of illness.

Environment

In the Johnson model, the environment is defined as all those internal and external elements that have an affect on the behavioral system. These environmental elements include obvious external factors, such as air temperature and relative humidity; sociologic factors, such as family, neighborhood, and society in general; and the internal environment, such as bodily processes, psychological states, religious beliefs, and political orientation. All seven behavioral subsystems of the client are involved with his or her relationship to the environment through the regulation of input and output. The client is continually interacting with the environment in the attempt to remain healthy by maintaining an internal dynamic balance.

Nursing

In the Johnson model, nursing is an activity that helps the individual achieve and maintain an optimal level of behavior (state of health) through the manipulation and regulation of the environment.[11] Nursing has functions in both health and illness. Nursing interventions to either maintain or regain health involve four activities in the regulation of the environment:

- Restricting harmful environmental factors
- Defending the client from negative environmental influences
- Inhibiting adverse elements from occurring
- Facilitating positive internal environmental factors in the recovery process

As a professional, the nurse in the Johnson model provides direct services to the client. By interacting with, and sometimes intervening in, the multiple subsystems that are found in the client's environment, the nurse acts as an external regulatory force. The goal of nursing is to promote the highest level of functioning and development in the client at all times. Nursing actions include helping the client act in a socially acceptable manner, monitoring and aiding with biologic processes necessary for maintenance of a dynamic balance, demonstrating support for medical care and treatment during illness, and taking actions to prevent illness from recurring. In this model, nursing makes its own unique contribution to the health and well-being of individuals and provides a service that is complementary to that provided by other health-care professionals.

The Neuman Health-Care Systems Model

As envisioned by Betty Neuman, the Health-Care Systems Model focuses on the individual and his or her environment and is applicable to a variety of health-care disciplines apart from nursing. Drawing from systems theory, the Neuman model also includes elements from stress theory with an overall holistic view of humanity and health care.[19]

Client

In this model, the client is viewed as an open system that interacts constantly with internal and external environments through the system's boundaries. The client-system's boundaries are called lines of defense and resistance in the Neuman model and may be represented graphically as a series of concentric circles that surround the basic core of the individual. The goal of these boundaries is to keep the basic core system stable by controlling system input and output.

Neuman classifies these defensive boundaries according to their various functions. The internal lines of resistance are the boundaries that are closest to the basic core and thus protect the basic internal structure of the system. The normal lines of defense are outside the internal lines of resistance; they protect the system from common, everyday environmental stressors. The flexible line of defense surrounds the normal line of defense and protects it from extreme environmental stressors. The general goal of all these protective boundaries is to maintain the internal stability of the client.

Health

Health, then, in the Neuman model is defined as the relatively stable internal functioning of the client. Optimal health exists when the client is maintained in a high state of wellness or stability. As in other nursing models, health is not considered an absolute state, but rather a continuum that reflects the client's internal stability while moving from wellness to illness and back. It takes a considerable amount of physical and psychological energy to maintain the stability of the person who is in good health.

The opposite of a healthy state, illness exists when the client's core structure becomes unstable through the effects of environmental factors that overwhelm and defeat the lines of defense and resistance. These environmental factors, whether internal or external, are called stressors in this model.

Environment

The environment is composed of internal or external forces or stressors that produce change or response in the client. Stressors may be helpful or harmful, strong or weak.

Stressors are also classified according to their relationship to the basic core of the client-system. Stressors that are completely outside the basic core are termed extrapersonal stressors and are either physical in nature, such as atmospheric temperature, or sociologic, such as living in either a rural or an urban setting.

Interpersonal stressors arise from interactions with other human beings. Marital relationships, career expectations, or friendships are included in this group of interpersonal stressors. Those stressors that occur within the client are called intrapersonal and include involuntary physiologic responses, psychological reactions, and internal thought processes.

Nursing

The nurse's role in the Neuman model is to identify at what level or in which boundary a disruption in the client's internal stability has taken place, and then to aid the client in activities that strengthen or restore the integrity of that particular boundary. The Neuman model expands the concept of client from the individual to include families, small groups, the community, or even society in general.

> *Although the search for the perfect nursing model continues, the emphasis in recent years has shifted from developing new theories to the application of existing theories to nursing practice.*

Nursing's main concern in this model is either to identify stressors that will disrupt a defensive boundary in the future (prevention) or to identify a stressor that has already disrupted a defensive boundary, thereby producing present instability (illness).[19] The Neuman model is based on the nursing process, and identifies three levels of intervention: primary, secondary, and tertiary.

A **primary intervention** has as its main goal the prevention of possible symptoms that could be caused by environmental stressors. Teaching clients about stress management, giving immunizations, or encouraging aerobic exercises to prevent heart disease are examples of primary interventions. A **secondary intervention** is aimed at treating symptoms that have already been produced by stressors. Many of the actions that nurses perform in the hospital or clinic (e.g., giving pain medications or teaching a client with cardiac disease about the benefits of a low-sodium diet) fall into this secondary intervention category. **Tertiary care** actions seek to restore the client's system to an optimal state of balance by adapting to negative environmental stressors. Teaching a client how to care for a colostomy at home after discharge from the hospital is an example of nursing activities at the tertiary level.

Trends for the Future in Nursing Theory

Although the search for the perfect nursing model continues, the emphasis in recent years has shifted from developing new theories to the application of existing theories to nursing practice. Also, the new theorists seem to be more interested in expanding existing nursing theories by including such concepts as cultural diversity, spirituality, family, and social change rather than starting all over again from the beginning. A good example of this trend is the cultural meaning–centered theory that was published by Mendyka and Bloom.[20] This theory expands the King model by adding a cultural perspective.

One of the more recent of the established nursing theories is the Man-Living-Health Model proposed by Parse. Although her original work started in 1981, a more developed form of her theory was published in 1987.[21–23] Parse's theory stresses the elements of experience, personal **values**, and lifestyle choices in the maintenance of health.

In this theory, the client can be any person or family who is concerned with the quality of their life situation. The client is viewed as an open, whole being who is influenced by past and present life experiences. The ability to make free choices is essential in this theory. The client, through choices that are made, interacts with the environment to influence health either positively or negatively.

Health, for Parse, is an ongoing process. By making free choices, the client's health status is continually unfolding. In addition, health is determined by lived experiences, synthesis of values, and the way the client lives.[24]

Therefore, the main role of nursing in the Parse model is to guide clients in finding and understanding the meaning of their lives. Once the client chooses a healthy life situation, then the nurse can further increase the quality of the client's life and improve his or her health status. The ability to change the client's health-related values is an important skill for nurses to master in this model.

Parse never really defines the concept of environment in relationship to her theory. Specifically, it seems to be any health-related setting, but it can also be expanded to include past and present experiences.

As with any developing science, nursing will continue to change and respond to the dynamic trends of society. Older nursing models will either be replaced by new ones or modified to include developing concepts. Indeed, one of the hallmarks of a sound nursing theory or model is its flexibility and ability to adapt to new discoveries. The increasing number of **independent nurse practitioners** and other advanced practice nurses are testing nursing theories as they have never been tested before. The theories that are flexible, realistic, and usable in actual practice will survive and remain as the pillars of professional nursing.[24] Others that are too theoretical or rigid will fall by the wayside and become mere footnotes in nursing texts.

Conclusion

As nursing takes its rightful place among the other helping professions, nursing theory will take on additional importance. Nursing theory and models are the systematic conceptualizations of nursing practice and how it fits into the health-care system. Nursing theories help describe, explain, predict, and control nursing activities to achieve the goals of client care. By understanding and using nursing theory, nurses will be better able to incorporate theoretical information into their practice to provide new ways of approaching nursing care and improving nursing practice.

The development of nursing theory and models indicates a maturing of the profession. As the knowledge associated with the profession increases, becomes unique, more complex, and better organized, the general body of nursing science knowledge also increases. Only when nursing has a well-developed body of specialized knowledge will it be fully recognized as a separate scientific discipline and a true profession.

Critical Thinking Exercises

Mrs. McCann, an 88-year-old woman, has been a resident of St. Martin's Village, a lifetime care community, since her husband died 8 years ago. Her health status is fair. She has adult-onset diabetes controlled by oral medication and a scar from a tumor behind her left ear that was removed surgically. The wound from this tumor removal has never healed completely, and it has continuously oozed a serous fluid requiring a dressing. At St. Martin's Village, Mrs. McCann has her own apartment, which she maintains with minimal assistance, receives one hot meal each day in a common dining room, and has access to a full range of services such as a beauty shop, recreational facilities, and a chapel. She is generally happy in this setting. She has no immediate family nearby, and the cost of the facility was covered by a large, one-time gift from her now deceased husband. Recently, she has become much weaker and has had difficulty walking, attending activities including meals, and changing the dressing on her ear. The nurse at St. Martin's Village is sent to evaluate this client.

- Select two nursing models and apply the principles of the model to this case study. Make sure that you include the concepts of client, health, environment, and nursing.

References

1. Algase, DL, et al: Nursing theory across curricula. J Prof Nurs 17(5):248–255, 2002.
2. Bulechek, GM, et al: Nursing interventions used in nursing practice. Am J Nurs 94(10):61, 1994.
3. Rice, B: CIC work in year 2: Data gathering, analysis, and work force modeling. Colleagues in Caring Newsletter, October 1997, pp. 3–4.
4. Titler, MG, et al: Use of the nursing interventions classification by critical care nurses. Critical Care Nurse 16(4):38–54, 1996.
5. Felton, G, et al: How Does the NLNAC support the Pew Health Commission competencies? Nursing and Health Care Perspectives 21(1):53, 2000.
6. McCloskey, JC, et al: Nursing interventions core to specialty practice. Nurs Outlook 46(3):67–76, 1998.
7. Mitchell, PR, and Grippando, GM: Nursing Perspectives and Issues. Delmar, Albany, NY, 1993.
8. McCann-Flynn, JB, and Heffron, PB: Nursing: From Concept to Practice. Robert J. Brady, Bowie, MD, 1984.
9. Riehl-Sisca, JP: Conceptual Models for Nursing Practice. Appleton & Lange, E. Norwalk, CT, 1989.
10. Putt, A: General Systems Theory Applied to Nursing. Little, Brown, Boston, 1978.
11. Stevens, BJ: Nursing Theory: Analysis, Application, Evaluation. Little, Brown, Boston, 1984.
12. Fawcett, J: Analysis and Evaluation of Conceptual Models of Nursing. FA Davis, Philadelphia, 1989.
13. Roy, C, and Andrews, HA: The Roy Adaptation Model: The Definitive Statement. Appleton & Lange, E. Norwalk, CT, 1991.
14. Orem, DE: Nursing: Concepts of Practice. Mosby–Year Book, St. Louis, 1991.
15. Leininger, MM (ed): Cultural Care Diversity and Universality: A Theory of Nursing. National League for Nursing, New York, 1992.
16. King, IM: King's theory of goal attainment. Nursing Science Quarterly 5:19–25, 1992.
17. Watson, J: Nursing: Human Science and Human Care: A Theory of Nursing. Appleton-Century-Crofts, E. Norwalk, CT, 1985.
18. Schaefer, KM, and Pond, JB: Levine's Conservation Model: A Framework for Nursing Practice. FA Davis, Philadelphia, 1991.
19. Neuman, B: The Neuman Systems Model. Appleton & Lange, E. Norwalk, CT, 1989.
20. Davidson, AW: Research issues. Person-environment mutual process: Studying and facilitating healthy environments from a nursing science perspective. Nursing Science Quarterly 14(2):101–108, 2001.
21. Parse, RR: Man-Living-Health: Theory of Nursing. Wiley, Philadelphia, 1987.
22. Parse, RR: The lived experience of contentment: A study of the Parse Research Method. Nursing Science Quarterly 14(4):330–338, 2001.
23. Fawcett, J: Scholarly dialogue. The nurse theorists: 21st-century update—Rosemarie Rizzo Parse. Nursing Science Quarterly 14(2):126–131, 2001.
24. Gaudine, AP: Demonstrating theory in practice: Examples of the McGill Model of Nursing. Journal of Continuing Education in Nursing 32(2):77–85, 2001.

Bibliography

Algase, DL, et al: Nursing theory across curricula. J Prof Nurs 17(5):248–255, 2002.

Brewer, C, and Kovner, CT: Is there another nursing shortage? What the data tell us. Nurs Outlook 49(1):20–26, 2001.

Coffey-Love, JG: Said another way. The nursing shortage: What is your role? Nursing Forum 36(2):29–35, 2001.

Determining cost of nursing interventions: Iowa Intervention Project. Nursing Economics 19(4):146–160, 2001.

More than one million new nurses needed by 2010. The American Nurse 34(1):5, 2002.

Narayan, MC, et al: Searching for nursing's future? Nursing Management 33(1):26–30, 2002.

Nightingale, F: Notes on Nursing: What It Is and What It Is Not. Harrison, London, 1859 (Reprinted by JB Lippincott, Philadelphia, 1966).

Nursing shortage puts patients at risk and creates liability problems. Health Care Risk Management 23(6):61–65, 2002.

O'Connor, NA, et al: Documenting patterns of nursing interventions using cluster analysis. J Nurs Meas 9(1):73–90, 2001.

Pontious, JM: Where have all the nurses gone? The Oklahoma Nurse 47(1):1, 18, 2002.

5

The Process of Educating Nurses

Joseph T. Catalano

Learning Objectives

After completing this chapter, the reader will be able to:

- Compare the major differences between the diploma, associate degree nursing, and bachelor of science in nursing educational programs.
- Discuss at least three types of advanced nursing degrees.
- Distinguish between the different types of doctoral degrees available to nurses.
- Explain the concept of advanced practice for nurses.

Unlike many other professions, nursing has several related, but unique, educational pathways that lead to licensure and professional status. Indeed, the current system of nursing education creates a great deal of confusion about nursing, not only among the public, but even among nurses themselves. Perhaps the belief that "a nurse is a nurse is a nurse is a nurse" developed from the fact that even though registered nurses may be prepared in educational programs that vary in length, orientation, and content, the graduates all take the same licensing examination, and, superficially, all seem to be able to provide the same level of care. The licensure examination measures knowledge at the minimal level of safe practice. The workplace has not provided pay differences to distinguish levels of education despite studies showing performance differences.

Paradigm Shifting

The millennium has become the metaphor for the difficult challenges and extraordinary opportunities facing nursing. Current and future trends in health care are being driven by a number of powerful societal forces that are producing an inevitable reshaping of health-care delivery. Traditionally somewhat insulated from the forces of change, nursing education has been forced to recognize that graduates need to be prepared with knowledge and skills that are in tune with a rapidly evolving health-care system. The most powerful of these forces of change are:

Box 5–1

Johnson & Johnson Promotes Nursing

The "Discover Nursing" ad campaign was initiated by the Johnson & Johnson Company in response to the nursing shortage. The goal is to bring more people into nursing. Working with nursing leaders and other concerned health-care organizations, the ad campaign is running a series of high-quality and catchy television commercials that feature nurses, both women and men, speaking about their work, its effect on society, and the rewards of a career in nursing.

A second element of the campaign is an associated Web site (www.discovernursing.com). The site has several sections that include answers to the question of "Why Nursing?"; details on the nursing market, benefits, and salaries; and nursing specialties. Under the "How?" section of the site, there is information concerning nursing basics, a nursing program search with links to nursing programs across the country, a scholarship search program, and information about additional funds for nursing education.

The site also has profiles of nurses who share their stories of why they became nurses and the elements of their careers that they find most rewarding.

Johnson & Johnson has committed $25 million to this campaign for the television ads, maintenance of the Web site, and scholarship money for nursing students. The campaign should run for several more years and is an excellent example of how private industry, with the encouragement of the nursing profession, can work together with nurses to benefit the health-care system.

- The movement toward a market-driven health-care economy
- The wider use of capitated managed care for financing coverage
- The increasing age and diversity of the U.S. population
- A woeful shortage of registered nurses
- The rapid leaps forward in health care and information technology

What Do You Think?

Does an individual prepared in a technical course of study have enough knowledge to be a provider of professional nursing care in today's more complex health-care system? Do you think that the American Nurses Association (ANA) position statement on nursing education advocates a valid position? If yes, what can be done to bring nursing education into line with it?

According to the Department of Health and Human Services, Division of Nursing, in a report based on a survey conducted in 2001, slightly less that 60 percent of registered nurses remained employed in hospitals, about the same as in 1998, and down from 66 percent in 1992.[1] The remainder were employed in a wide variety of settings, including private practice, public health agencies, home health care, primary nursing school–operated nursing centers, **ambulatory care centers**, insurance and managed care companies, education, and health-care research. There is also an ever-growing group of **emerging health occupations** that have not yet been officially recognized by professional organizations.

The Pew Report

The Pew Health Professions Commission Report, sometimes referred to as the Pew

Report, was a major study of health care and nursing education that also reinforces the belief that there is a need for reform in nursing education.[2,3] Its 21 recommendations for all schools preparing health-care professionals are comprehensive and include:

- Expanding the scientific basis of the programs
- Promoting interdisciplinary education
- Developing cultural sensitivity
- Establishing new alliances with managed care companies and government
- Increasing the use of computer technology and interactive software

The Pew Report also recommended a differentiated practice structure to simplify and consolidate the titles that are used for the different practitioner levels so that there is just one title for each level.

As more and more health care shifts to ambulatory and community-based settings, nursing educators need to re-evaluate whether the graduates of their programs are adequately prepared to meet the demands posed by these areas of care and whether their own educational and skill preparation is sufficient.

> *Perhaps the belief that "a nurse is a nurse is a nurse is a nurse" developed from the fact that even though registered nurses may be prepared in educational programs that vary in length, orientation, and content, the graduates all take the same licensing examination, and, superficially, all seem to be able to provide the same level of care.*

Nurses of the Future

Nurses of the future will need to practice with self-reliance, independence, and flexibility. They will be required to have well-developed decision-making skills based on critical thinking ability, a working knowledge of community resources, and computer and technical competencies. And just as important, they will need to deliver high-quality client education and care while working within the constraints of a managed care system with tight cost control measures.

Will nursing education ever be able to prepare a graduate who fulfills all the qualities required of nurses of the future? Nursing education responds with a "yes," but only with curricular changes that provide graduates with the tools to continue to learn as they advance in their careers.

Hospital-based acute care nursing practice will always have an important place in any health-care system. Highly skilled, acute care nurses will always find a place to practice. It is generally accepted that the older population requires more health care of all types—acute, chronic, and community based. Although the current system had experienced a decrease in the utilization of acute care beds, a gradual reverse in this trend is beginning as the "baby boomers" become the senior citizens who require more care for acute problems.

Paradigm shifting in nursing education does not need to be an either/or proposition. It is sometimes felt that nursing education is either acute care focused or it is community focused. Nursing education needs to combine the two so that the graduate can practice with competence in either or both settings. The skills are similar; however, the emphasis may be different. Although some hospital skills are being done by non-nurses at a cheaper cost, nursing education must still teach such important skills as critical thinking, therapeutic relationship, **primary care** and **case management**, as well as how to be comfortable with a consumer-driven health-care system.

Critical thinking has been a buzzword in nursing education for the past several years. It is generally recognized as the ability to use basic core knowledge and decision-making skills in deciding and resolving situations where there is a

ISSUES NOW

Ten Health-Care Trends to Watch

Nursing students and nurse educators alike need to remain in tune with the unprecedented transformations that are and will be taking place in health-care delivery and professional nursing. These trends have a number of driving forces, including technological advancements, financial restructuring, shifts in social structure, and consumer demands.

Ten trends that will affect health care

1. **Changing Demographics and Increasing Cultural Diversity.** Increasing numbers of minority groups as well as an aging population is a trend that will have a major effect on health care for many years to come. It is projected that by the year 2020, more than 20 percent of the population will be 65 and older, with those older than 85 constituting the most rapidly increasing segment of the population. Other projections indicate that by the year 2050, the white population of the United States will no longer be the majority.
2. **Explosion of Technology.** Telehealth, telemedicine, nanotechnology, electronic medical records, and health-oriented Internet databases all are a common part of today's health-care system that were unheard of even a few short years ago. Nurses of the twenty-first century will not only need the basic computer skills that many children currently master by the time they reach high school, but will also need to have a high degree of technological sophistication.
3. **Economic and Social Globalization.** Although globalization may seem to many nurses to be an abstract concept concerning events that happen "out there," events such as those of 9/11 have a way of bringing the reality home in a very dramatic way. Information technology and communications, international travel and commerce, multinational corporations, and political changes everywhere all contribute to the trend to globalization.
4. **Better Educated Consumers, the Genome Project, Alternative Health-Care Practices, and Palliative Care.** Clients in today's health-care system are consumers who want to actively participate in the planning of the care they are to receive. Through the Internet, clients now have access to information that was formerly available only to health-care practitioners. A better-educated consumer is more likely to be interested in health promotion and maintenance, resulting in a greater interest in alternative health-care practices.

   Only recently have new settings for and types of care—such as hospice, pain management, support groups, bereavement counseling, and spiritual practices—been advocated as valid parts of total client care. Nurses need to not only understand and feel comfortable when providing care to clients who use these settings, but actually be prepared for an active role in the provision of care.

5. **Increasing Complex Health Care and Shift to Population-Based Care.** Although more and more health care is being provided outside the traditional hospital setting, clients who are admitted to hospitals are much more seriously ill than in the past. Currently, there is a ratio of one critical care or specialty unit care bed to each general care bed in hospitals across the country. This means that fully half of the clients admitted to the hospital are in need of high-level, complex health care such as is provided in critical care units.
6. **Managed Health Care and Out-of-Control Health-Care Costs.** Over the last decade, managed care has become a reality of life. Despite the promise for flexible financing, prevention of illness, and promotion of health when first started, managed care still remains an illness-based, fee-for-service system with all the problems associated with that process.

   Health-care costs now approach 15 percent of the gross national product (GNP). There are more than 40 million Americans who have no health insurance. Cost concerns will continue to influence almost every aspect of nursing practice, from staffing, work assignments, and use of unlicensed personnel to increased out-of-pocket cost of health-care services and medications not covered by insurance.
7. **Governmental Health-Care Regulations and Policies.** Complex and sometimes contradictory health-care regulations from both the federal and state levels add to the confusion found in nursing practice. It is imperative that nurses belong to their professional nursing organization and participate actively in political activities to move the health-care system in a direction that is more nurse and client friendly.
8. **Collaborative Practice.** Health care has been a team effort for many years. As the health-care system becomes more complex in the future, and clients have increasingly more complex health-care problems, the need for collaborative practice will only increase.
9. **Nursing Shortage.** Over the years, there have been cycles of nursing shortages coupled with nursing surpluses; however, current projections are for a very deep nursing shortage that will last well into the twenty-first century. Despite the problems produced by the shortage, there are opportunities too. There has already been an upward trend in salaries, and many facilities are offering more flexibility in working hours. Nurses are also finding new opportunities for advancement, interesting work settings, increased demand for advanced practice nurses (APNs), and careers in case management.
10. **Advances in Nursing Research.** One of the key characteristics of a profession is the development of a unique body of knowledge through research. The growing body of research provides a scientific basis for client care practices. As nursing research advances in the future, client outcomes will improve, the health of communities will be promoted, and the most vulnerable of the population will be protected.

Sources: Lindeman, CA: The future of nursing. Nurs Educ 39(1):5–12, 2000.
Heller, BR, et al: 10 Trends to watch. Nursing and Health Care Perspectives 21(1):9–14, 2001.

relatively small amount of data and a high degree of risk and ambiguity. Although it has not always been called critical thinking, nursing has long been concerned with the ability to make good judgments and decisions about client care. (See Chapter 6 for a fuller discussion of critical thinking.) At a fundamental level, the nursing process is a type of critical thinking. Unfortunately, in the health-care system of the future, a nurse's critical thinking skills must go far beyond those of the basic nursing process. Nursing education will need to prepare students for more advanced critical thinking by exposing them to real-life situations that require the use of creativity, intuition, analysis, and deductive and inductive reasoning. These situations are introduced in the classroom as case studies and are reinforced in the clinical setting through guided experiences and mentoring.

Therapeutic relationship skills have been long stressed by mental health nursing faculty as a key element in the treatment of psychiatric problems. In reality, therapeutic relationship skills are essential for all nurses to fulfill their roles as health-care providers and healers. Although these skills are currently being taught in a limited and focused way in most schools of nursing, they need to be expanded to involve directed services and relationship-centered nursing care.

Relationship-centered nursing care is client focused and revolves around the client's trust in, value of, and understanding of the nurse's skills and role in the healing process. The client must be able to feel comfortable with the nurse and share his or her understanding of both illness and health. Currently, in many licensed practical nurse/licensed vocational nurse (LPN/LVN) programs and schools offering the associate degree in nursing, clinical experiences consist of one-time, 8-hour provision of care for an acute or chronically ill client. Little time is spent in follow-up care. However, many bachelor of nursing science (BSN) programs and some associate degree nursing (ADN) programs have expanded clinical experiences to include **discharge planning** and follow-up home health care experiences. To meet the demands of the future health-care system, all nursing education programs must be able to develop learning experiences for students that involve care for selected individuals or families over extended periods of time, perhaps ranging from several weeks to several semesters.

Care management is a general term that refers to a method of coordinating care either with an individual client or on a system-wide basis. **Case management**, a new entity in a health-care system driven by the urge for cost-effective care, usually is associated with coordinating care for an individual client as he or she moves from one level to another through the health-care system. Case management is now a certified specialty. Almost all the proposals for revisions in the health-care system include the **case manager** as an important element in the overall management of care. Currently, case managers do not have to be registered nurses. Many individuals with degrees in social work and human resources as well as registered nurses are serving in the capacity of case managers. Perhaps the ideal situation would be to function as a **health-care team**, with both a registered nurse and a social worker coordinating all aspects of the client's care.

As case managers, nurses are responsible for developing **clinical pathways** and also for directing and guiding the overall health care of a specific group of clients. Case management includes not only overseeing the clients' care while they are in the hospital but also following clients through their rehabilitation at home, long-term follow-up, health-care practices, and developmental stages.

The knowledge and thinking required by an effective case manager go far beyond what is currently required of new graduates. Nurses must be able to understand not only the immediate disease process but also the long-term outcomes and factors that influence the disease. Case managers must also practice health-focused nursing and primary levels of intervention. Decisions will need to be made about care from a broad **database** as well as an understanding of the client's abilities, knowledge level, and even financial status.

Nursing education will be severely challenged to provide experiences to prepare students for this role. Students must be allowed to experience the authority, accountability, and responsibility of guiding a client's health care over an extended period. It might be beneficial to combine the learning experiences mentioned earlier in establishing the therapeutic relationship with the managed care experience.

A consumer-driven health-care system is at one and the same time the nurse's dream and nightmare. Many widely used nursing models or theories claim to be client centered, which translates into being consumer driven. Yet, when these models are put into practice, the care given is more provider driven than anything else. A client/consumer-driven health-care system means that the care given is defined by the consumer and the outcomes are also determined by the consumer. The nurse must be able to accept the authority of the group or community as a determinant of health care. The nurse's role becomes one of a partner in guiding, implementing, and overseeing ways to deliver requested health care for a given community.

Many nursing programs, particularly baccalaureate programs, include a course in community health and home-health-care nursing. A requirement of these courses is often to have the students perform a community survey in which they determine the needs of the community as they perceive them. Currently, many of these courses have been modified so that the students learn from the community what the community perceives to be their own needs.

Paradigm shifting is never easy. Major paradigm shifts in thinking and acting are even more difficult. Nursing education is currently dealing with a huge paradigm shift. How educators are meeting these challenges will, to a large extent, shape the future of professional nursing.

ANA Position Paper on Education for Nurses

After evaluating the changes that occurred in the health-care system during the 1950s and studying the projected educational needs for nurses, the American Nurses Association (ANA) published a paper in 1965 that took a stand on an issue that was, and still is, highly controversial. Although written almost 40 years ago, this document is still relevant to many of the issues in nursing education today.

For full appreciation of the significance of this paper, it must be examined from a historical perspective. The overall purpose of the ANA has always been to ensure high-quality nursing care to the public by fostering high standards of nursing practice. In addition, the ANA was concerned with furthering the professional and educational advancement of nurses as well as protecting the occupational welfare of nurses. To achieve these goals, the ANA took responsibility for establishing the scope of practice for nurses and for guaranteeing the competence of those who claim the title of nurse.

> *The overall purpose of the ANA has always been to ensure high-quality nursing care to the public by fostering high standards of nursing practice.*

After World War II, there was an explosion of scientific and technological knowledge used in health care. The educational level of the population was also increasing, thus resulting in greater public demand for higher-quality health care. In re-evaluating the nature and scope of nursing practice, and the type and level of quality of education needed to meet these new demands, the ANA reached the conclusions that are presented in its position paper.

Since 1965, the ANA has upheld the belief that baccalaureate education should be the basic level of preparation for professional nurses. Specifically, the ANA concluded that:

> *The education for all those who are licensed to practice nursing should take place in institutions of higher education; minimum preparation for beginning professional nursing practice at the present time should be the baccalaureate degree education in nursing; minimum preparation for beginning technical nursing practice at the present time should be associate degree education; education for assistants in the health care service occupations should be short, intensive pre-service programs in vocational education institutions rather than on the job training.*[4]

There were several assumptions on which the ANA based this position paper:

- Nursing is a helping profession and, as such, provides services that contribute to the health and well-being of people.
- Nursing is of vital significance to the individual receiving services; it meets needs that cannot be met by the person, the family, or other persons in the community.
- The demand for the services of nurses will continue to increase.
- The professional practitioner is responsible for the nature and quality of all nursing care that clients receive.
- The services of professional practitioners of nursing will continue to be supplemented and complemented by the services of nurse practitioners who will be licensed.
- Education for those in the health-care professions must increase in depth and breadth as scientific knowledge expands.
- The health care of the public, in the amount and to the extent needed and demanded, requires the services of large numbers of health occupation workers, in addition to those licensed as nurses, to function as assistants to nurses. These workers are presently designated nurses' aides, orderlies, assistants, and attendants.
- The professional association must concern itself with the nature of nursing practice, the methods for improving nursing practice, and standards for membership in the professional association.[4]

The rationale for taking such a strong stand on the future of nursing education derived from recognition by the profession of its heritage, its immediate problems, the emerging social issues and trends, the nature of nursing practice, and the extent to which nurses could realistically enact changes for continued professional progress. The ANA drew on Florence Nightingale's vision of nursing and nursing education, which emphasized the value of education for the development of the profession. It was important to Nightingale that schools of nursing be independent of hospitals and that they have a strong theoretical component on which to base clinical practice.

By recognizing the increasing complexity of society, the ANA realized that nursing was not only becoming more specialized but was also moving toward greater interdependence with other groups in society. One of these key groups was the U.S. federal government. As the government began increasing aid for nursing education, educational facilities expanded, providing greater opportunities for professional advancement. Larger numbers of students with more varied backgrounds were recruited into the profession, requiring greater flexibility in nursing education programs to accommodate their needs. Schools of nursing were, at the same time, also hard-pressed to meet the attendant demands of science and technology that were changing the traditional role of nurses. In addition to expanding roles for nurses, greater consumer awareness and expectations were placing new demands on the abilities of nurses.

Even in 1965, the ANA recognized that nurses were required to master a very large and extremely complex body of knowledge. In addition, nurses were being called up increasingly to make critical and independent decisions about client care.

Effects of the ANA Paper

The implications of this paper were far-reaching and highly controversial. The ANA paper affected many different elements of society and the health-care industry.

Hospitals recognized that they would no longer retain their traditional role of preparing nurses for practice. Even though pressure to move nursing education from hospital-based diploma schools to institutions of higher education had been building for some time, in the mid-1960s, a full 75 percent of the graduating nurses were from hospital-based diploma programs.[5]

Colleges and universities were hard pressed to develop undergraduate and graduate curricula quickly for increasing numbers of nursing majors. The relatively few baccalaureate programs in existence at the time were generally small and found it difficult to expand their programs rapidly. It also became evident that a clear distinction between technical and professional programs needed to be made.

To this day, the ANA remains firmly committed to its stand that all nursing education should be housed in institutions of higher learning. Nearly 40 years after this statement was made, the profession of nursing is still trying to reach a consensus on the issue of basic educational preparation for entry into practice.

Hospitals recognized that they would no longer retain their traditional role of preparing nurses for practice.

A similar resolution was again proposed by the ANA in 1985, but it also met strong opposition and was never enacted. In 1996, the American Association of Colleges of Nursing (AACN) presented its own position paper emphasizing the belief that the baccalaureate degree should be the minimal requirement for entry into the nursing profession. The discussion has continued into the twenty-first century with little hope for resolution. The most influential reasons why these proposals have not been adopted are economic, not conceptual.

Continuing discussion and efforts to bring about collaborative agreement on nursing education is a goal that the profession must work toward. Only after the issue of basic entry-level education for professional nursing is resolved, and when nurses, like all other professionals, obtain their knowledge from recognized schools of higher education, will nursing as a profession be able to resolve its other important problems. Advancement of clinical practice, preparation for advanced practice roles, and increased body of nursing knowledge all depend on baccalaureate entry-level education for professional nurses.

Diploma Schools

The Nightingale School of Nursing was a diploma school in the strict use of the term. When nurses graduated from this school they were given a certificate or diploma noting their graduation, but no academic degree. The first graduates from the Nightingale School soon began to establish their own schools of nursing based on the Nightingale model and adhered to her philosophy of nursing education. These were also diploma schools. After an initial period of uncertainty and trepidation, both physicians and hospital administrators began to recognize that when the quality of nurses was improved, so too was the overall quality of the care provided by their hospitals. They also understood that these types of schools that were closely associated with hospitals could provide a source of free, or inexpensive, labor in the form of nursing students. Diploma schools sprang up throughout Europe so that, in time, each hospital had its own school of nursing. Many of Nightingale's principles and concerns about nursing education were abandoned during this period of growth.

In the United States, developments in nursing education, as with health care in general, lagged behind those in Europe. It was not until the mid-1870s that the first school of nursing was established in the United States. This was a diploma school that was attached to the New England Hospital for Women.[6] As in Europe, the idea of diploma schools quickly caught on, and within 10 years almost every large hospital in the United States had its own diploma school of nursing. These schools had very little in common with the Nightingale School of Nursing. There was no uniformity in curriculum, length of program, or requirements. To guarantee adequate enrollment, candidates were again being recruited from the lowest levels of society.

The hospitals used the student nurses as a major source of free labor for their facilities. There was little or no classroom or theoretical study. The students learned exclusively by hands-on experience during their 12- to 14-hour, 7-days-a-week work shifts. Most of the students were young, single women recruited just after they graduated from high school. The students were confined to dormitories on the hospital property. The dormitories were monitored closely by a housemother who enforced the rigorous rules of behavior covering all aspects of the students' lives and dismissed students for even minor infractions of the rules. The early diploma schools of nursing were organized and administered on a model that was similar to the strictest of the religious orders.

> *In 1952, the National League for Nursing (NLN) assumed accrediting responsibilities for all schools of nursing.*

The nurses who graduated from these schools were proficient in basic nursing skills and could assume positions in the hospital where they were trained or in home nursing, where they worked on a case-by-case basis without any additional orientation or education. Because of the 24-hour-a-day, 7-day-a-week socialization process administered by these schools, diploma graduate nurses tended to be very submissive to authority and willing to carry out any duty to please the physician, administrator, or head nurse. Before the advent of licensure examinations and standardization of practice, nurses from diploma schools were often limited to employment in their own training institutions or in the home-health-care setting.

Diploma schools of nursing remained relatively unchanged in the United States until 1949 when the National Nursing Accrediting Service, working under the guidance of the National League for Nursing Education, became the licensing body for all schools of nursing that voluntarily sought accreditation. The first formal accreditation of nursing schools occurred in the early 1950s. In 1952, the National League for Nursing (NLN) assumed accrediting responsibilities for all schools of nursing.[7] Accreditation by the National League for Nursing Accrediting Commission (NLNAC) has always been and remains a voluntary undertaking.

In order to be accredited by the NLN, schools of nursing had to meet specific **outcome criteria** and teach specific content in their curricula. Many of the diploma schools of nursing could not or would not comply with these criteria and eventually closed. Some of the requirements for the schools that did choose to comply with the NLN included:

- Implementing a 3-year course of study meeting the criteria established by the state board of nursing using only faculty with baccalaureate or higher degrees in nursing
- Developing a unique philosophy and demonstrating how that philosophy was implemented through learning objectives, course objectives, and outcome criteria
- Showing an adequate pass rate on the State Board or National Council Licensure Examination (NCLEX)

One of the key factors that all state boards of nursing were concerned about was that the school be able to demonstrate that the students were not being used as unpaid hospital personnel while they were in their education and training programs. When students could no longer be used as free labor, diploma nursing schools went from being virtually free to the hospital to being very expensive. Not only did they still have to pay for the room and board of the students, but they also now had to hire and pay additional staff because the students could no longer be included in the overall staff numbers. Even more diploma schools closed because of the financial burdens to the hospitals. The schools that stayed open began increasing their tuition rates to the point that they were as expensive as programs granting academic degrees.

During the 1960s and 1970s, many diploma schools became associated with universities and converted their curricula into degree-granting programs. According to the 2001–2002 statistics published by the NLN, there are only 115 accredited diploma programs still functioning. They are of universal high quality and meet all the standards necessary for NLN accreditation. The main emphasis remains on preparing nurses who are highly competent in the technical nursing skills through extensive hands-on practice in the clinical setting, but elements of leadership, humanities, and general sciences are also included in the classroom setting.[8]

Associate Degree Nursing

The **associate degree nursing (ADN) program** was developed by Mildred Montague as a short-

Box 5–2

Students' Thoughts About Their Programs

PROGRAM	PROS	CONS
Diploma Usually a 3-year program Located in a hospital sometimes in conjunction with a community college Prepares nurses for the staff positions in hospitals and other inpatient facilities	"The diploma school in my area is very inexpensive." "I know from high school that I am the type of stuent who needs a lot of one-on-one time. I heard the hospital schools offer that." "We have lots of clinical time. I'm quite comfortable on the hospital floor now."	"I sometimes feel that other nurses look down on us—like we are part of a dinosaur-age system." "It's hard to work during school because you spend so much time at clinical." "It's like we're living in a fishbowl because we spend so much time around other students.
Associate Degree (AD) Usually a 2-year program Usually located in a community college Prepares nurses for staff positions in hospitals and other inpatient facilities	"Convenience—the community college I attend is 10 minutes walk from my front door." "I already have a promise of a job when I graduate, and they will pay 100% of my BSN courses. It's like getting 4 years of education for the price of 2."	"I'm afraid I won't be able to get a job anyplace but a nursing home." "Now I have to go back to school to get my BSN. Ugh! Sometimes I wonder if it would have been easier to do it all at once."
Bachelor of Science in Nursing (BSN) Usually a 4- to 5-year program Located in colleges and universities Prepares nurses for positions in both inpatient and community settings	"It's easier to compete for a job—there are a million AD programs in my city and not that many places to work." "I'm ready to start graduate school anytime. Anytime I get the courage that is!"	"I'm in debt up to my ears!" "I'm a sophomore and getting tired of theory classes. I just want to see a patient."

Source: Dunham, KS: How to Survive and Maybe Even Love Nursing School. FA Davis, Philadelphia, 2001, with permission.

term solution to the nursing shortage experienced after World War II.[9] Originally designed to prepare students for technical nursing practice, the 2-year ADN programs were offered through community colleges with an emphasis on developing the skills necessary to provide high-quality bedside care in less time than BSN programs. A successful pilot program for ADNs was conducted by Montague at Teachers' College in Columbia University in New York City in 1952 to prepare technical nurses who could assist professional nurses. It demonstrated that community college–based programs could attract large numbers of students, prove cost effective, and produce skillful technical nurses in half the time required for BSN programs.[10]

Early on, there was some heated debate concerning licensure and titling for this group of nurses. The technical orientation of the curriculum was, and is, very similar to that found in programs that prepare LPNs, but the location of the programs in the community college setting and the increased theoretical orientation seemed to elevate these programs to a higher educational plane. It was finally decided that the ADN graduates should take the registered nurse (RN) licensure examination rather than the LPN/LVN examination.

The emphasis on technical skills of the ADN programs met a need in the health-care system of the 1960s and 1970s. By the early 1980s, there were more than 800 ADN programs across the United States; as of 2002, the number was close to 900, with more than 63,000 students attending.[11] Graduates from these programs soon exceeded the number of graduates from all the BSN and LPN/LVN programs combined.

Although it is possible to complete the requirements for an ADN in 2 academic years, most programs actually take at least 3 years to complete for a new student who has no prior college credit.[11] ADN graduates have a proven track record for providing safe bedside care for clients from the first day they are hired. They function well as team members and, after a period of orientation, can assume responsibility for the care of clients who are more acutely ill.

Baccalaureate Education

The development of schools of nursing in the university and college setting was a gradual process that extended over several decades. Only a few collegiate nursing programs were established during the years when the diploma programs were expanding. Some of these early collegiate programs were a hybrid mixture of college-level classes and diploma school clinical experiences that still granted only a diploma rather than an academic degree. Early attempts at college-level nursing programs sometimes took the form of "pre-nursing" courses over a 1- or 2-year period that prepared students to enter upper division schools of nursing. Generally acclaimed as the first university program to be completely conducted in the higher education setting, the University of Minnesota School of Nursing was opened in 1909. In 1923, the Yale School of Nursing began accepting students; it is considered the first autonomous college of nursing in the United States.

The number of university-based nursing programs gradually increased over the years, and by the beginning of World War II there were 76 programs granting baccalaureate degrees in nursing. These programs tended to specialize in preparing nurses for public health nursing, teaching, administration, and supervisory positions in hospitals. Although all these programs included a clinical component, the emphasis was more on theoretical knowledge, development of decision-making skills, and leadership. Universities in general enjoyed rapid growth immediately after World War II, and higher education nursing programs expanded along with the universities. Many military nurses prepared by the Cadet Nurse Corps during World War II went back to school under the G.I. Bill to complete their baccalaureate degrees.

During this rapid growth period, these **baccalaureate degree nursing programs** were plagued with problems similar to those found in the diploma programs during their own rapid expansion period. Primarily, the lack of uniformity in content, curriculum, and even length of programs was problematic. It was difficult to find qualified faculty because most of the nurses up to this time had received their education in diploma programs. No doctorate degrees existed in nursing; few nurses had master's degrees; and only a smattering of nurses had baccalaureate degrees. During the late 1940s and early 1950s, awareness began to develop that there was a need to stratify nursing education programs into technical levels and professional levels. It became apparent that all health-care professionals should have, at minimum, a baccalaureate degree.[12]

The NLN began to develop strict criteria for the accreditation of baccalaureate nursing programs. These criteria included courses in general education, general sciences, humanities, and language as well as specific nursing courses. They required a certain number of hours to be spent in the clinical setting practicing nursing skills, a faculty prepared at the master's degree level, and the availability of laboratory and library facilities for the students. Faculty-to-student ratios were limited, particularly in the clinical setting, and outcome criteria were required for the students.[13]

Although all university-level baccalaureate degrees in nursing have the same number of required credit hours and educational requirements for baccalaureate degrees, there are three avenues for attaining this degree. The BSN degree fulfills the criteria to be known as a professional degree. It meets the overall requirements for a college baccalaureate degree (124 credit hours, 65 hours of nursing major, and most of the general education requirements), but does not meet all the general education requirements for an academic bachelor of science (BS) degree. Although this degree is usually obtained in a traditional college setting, it can also be obtained through an **external degree** program where the student has to meet the criteria for the BSN.

The second approach is found in programs that offer a bachelor of science degree with a major in nursing (BS Nursing). This degree is the full academic college degree and guarantees that the person holding it has met all of the general education, science, and major subject requirements. According to statistics published by the NLN for academic year 2001–2002, there were more than 530 accredited programs offering baccalaureate degrees in nursing.

A third avenue that may be pursued is sometimes called the career ladder program (see section on Ladder Programs).

Practical/Vocational Nursing

The practical/vocational nurse, in one form or another, has been a part of the health-care system in the United States for more than 100 years. Although the earliest formal schools of practical/vocational nursing were started around 1890, informal training programs for this level of nursing probably existed well before that time—for example, in the Young Women's Christian Association (YWCA), particularly in New York City. These programs took uneducated girls who had migrated from rural areas and farms to the cities in search of employment and taught them a useful trade with which they could support themselves. With no regulation or accreditation for the early practical/vocational nurse programs, there were wide variations in the quality, length, and focus of what was being taught. Generally, the students were taught to provide home care, similar to that given by private duty nurses, for clients ranging from newborns to the elderly and invalids.

The number of **practical/vocational nursing programs** gradually increased over the next 50 years. Graduates of these 3-month programs were beginning to find employment in hospitals and nursing homes as well as in areas of private duty. During the nurse shortage after World War I, many hospitals found that these relatively undereducated nurses, after receiving on-the-job training in the hospital, could function at a fairly high level of skill, and at a much reduced cost. The word got around, and soon the number of these unlicensed nurses grew.

By the late 1930s, the ANA saw the need to regulate the quality of the practical/vocational nursing programs in order to protect public safety. It was not until 1938 that the state of New York took seriously the ANA's recommendation for compulsory licensure for practical/vocational nurses and enacted the first law requiring such licensure. In 1960, all practical/vocational nurses were required to pass a licensure examination before they could practice. These nurses are now referred to as licensed practical nurses (LPNs). In Texas and California, these nurses are called licensed vocational nurses (LVNs).

Although education for LPNs and LVNs varies slightly from one state to another, there are some common characteristics. Most of the programs are from 9 to 12 months and are measured in clock hours rather than academic hours. They are often offered in hospitals, high schools, vocational schools, or trade schools, although some programs are conducted in community colleges or even in universities. Orientation of the curricula in these programs is highly technical and emphasizes the learning of skills in the setting of a hospital or nursing home with less emphasis on theoretical knowledge. As a **technician**, it is much more important for practical/vocational nurses to learn how to do something than why it is being done.

> *A ladder program allows nurses to upgrade their education and move from one educational level to another with relative ease and without loss of credits from previous education.*

The stated scope of practice for the practical/vocational nurse involves providing care for clients in hospitals, nursing homes, or the home setting for those who have stable conditions. LPNs/LVNs are to be under the supervision of an RN or a licensed physician. However, in the real world, LPNs/LVNs are often required to provide care well outside of their scope of practice, often functioning in leadership roles or providing care in acute settings with highly unstable clients. LPNs/ LVNs are often hired when there are shortages of RNs to fill the gaps in client care. Many associate degree RN programs have developed a ladder curriculum whereby an LPN/LVN can go back to school for a shorter period, often receiving credit for years of experience, complete the program in 1 year, and then take the RN licensure examination.

Ladder Programs

Career ladder, educational ladder, **articulation**, or educational mobility programs have become increasingly popular as a result of an interest in **upward mobility**, educational articulation, and **career mobility**. A ladder program allows nurses to upgrade their education and move from one educational level to another with relative ease and without loss of credits from previous education. Each ladder program is developed according to the philosophy of the particular nursing school, may use any one of a number of curricular patterns, uses one of several means of **advanced placement**, or granting credit for previous education, and must meet NLNAC accreditation standards. Ladder programs take several different forms. Some ladder programs provide a **competency-based education** that allows the students to proceed at their own pace as long as they fulfill required educational outcomes. Ladder programs have become increasingly popular as colleges move toward Web-based courses and programs.

The LPN/LVN-to-ADN ladder allows individuals who have been licensed as LPNs/LVNs to take a minimal number of courses in an associate degree program to obtain their ADN and then take the NCLEX-RN, CAT to become licensed as registered nurses. Programs vary widely as to how many credits they will accept from the LPN/LVN programs and how many courses the students take to complete the degree. Some of the requirements for number of hours are out of the control of the nursing programs, because they have been established as general education requirements of the college or are state regents requirements. These programs are highly compatible because of the similarity of curricula and the technical orientation of both types of programs.

There are also LPN/LVN-to-BSN ladder programs that either allow licensed LPNs/LVNs to challenge out of a number of courses or grant them credit for nursing courses based on previous experience and demonstrated competency. Students who enter these types of ladder programs usually spend more time in school than those in the LPN/ LVN-to-ADN programs. In addition to meeting the requirements of the BSN, they also have to meet the general education requirements for a baccalaureate degree and complete 124 hours of college-level courses.

Nursing education has seen a marked increase in the number of ADN-to-BSN and diploma-to-BSN ladder programs sometimes called **two plus two (2+2) programs**. These programs admit individuals who are already licensed as registered nurses but who have either a diploma or associate degree. These programs may take several different forms. Upper division baccalaureate programs work exclusively with ADN-RNs, have no generic students, and are designed exclusively to meet the educational needs of students who are already RNs. Other programs accept ADN or diploma graduates as students, in addition to generic students. These schools often have separate programs for ADN or diploma RNs that allow them to take examinations to prove educational knowledge and nursing proficiency (**challenge examinations**) in specific classes, thus granting credit for their nursing experience. The RNs then take advanced-level nursing courses such as Community Health/Home Health Care, Leadership, and Critical Care, which are not commonly found in diploma or ADN programs. In either case, on completion of the degree requirements, these nurses are granted a baccalaureate degree. Some of these programs have an **open curriculum** that allows students to enter and leave the program freely. There are 418 such programs accredited by the NLNAC.[11]

A growing trend in educational ladder programs is the ADN-to-MSN programs. Schools that offer this type of ladder must have an MSN program in place. The ADN students who enter these programs are given credit for prior classes and work experience and take both undergraduate and graduate level courses, receiving a BSN along the way to obtaining the MSN. These programs vary a great deal from school to school and may require from three to five semesters of classes. Often they are offered on a part-time basis, with many evening and weekend classes or Web-based classes to meet the needs of working students.

Another type of educational ladder program that is less common is the nurse practitioner (NP)-to-MSN program. These programs admit nurse practitioners who graduated from programs that allowed the student to become certified but did not include enough credit hours for a master's degree. Again, the students are granted credit for past classes and work experience and often are allowed to challenge a certain number of core courses. Then they take the remaining required courses and are granted an MSN at graduation.

Master's and Doctoral Level Education

The baccalaureate degree is considered a generalist degree that exposes a student to a wide range of subjects during the 4 years spent in college. The master's degree, on the other hand, is a specialist's degree.[14] Students who pursue a master's degree concentrate their study in one particular subject area and become expert in that given area.

Master's degree nursing programs have been in existence almost from the time baccalaureate level nursing programs were started. These early master's degree in nursing programs were designed for students who had baccalaureate degrees in other majors, such as biology, who wanted to become nurses. After completion of an additional 36 to 42 credit hours in nursing courses only, these students were awarded the MSN, and could then take the licensure examination for registered nurses.

Today, most master's degree in nursing programs are restricted to registered nurses who have the baccalaureate degree. Many of these programs require at least 1 year of clinical practice after the BSN and require an additional 36 to 46 college credit hours. Most students who enter master's degree programs attend classes on a part-time basis while they are working and may take up to 5 years to complete the requirements. Many universities have recognized this trend and have tailored their programs to meet the needs of these part-time students; universities now offer courses over the Internet, by distance education in the evening, on weekends, or 1-day-a-week programs. There are 296 accredited master's degree programs in the United States.[11]

There are a number of available areas of study for those pursuing master's degrees in nursing. Some of the more popular areas include nursing administration, community health, psychiatric mental health, adult health, maternal-child health, gerontology, rehabilitation care, nursing education, and some more advanced areas of practice, such as anesthesiology, pediatric nurse practitioner (PNP), family nurse practitioner, geriatric nurse practitioner (GNP), and obstetric-gynecology nurse practitioner.[15] Most of these programs require the student to pass a comprehensive written or oral examination, and some courses require the student to write an extensive research thesis before graduation.

There are two basic types of master's degrees in nursing. The master's of science in nursing (MSN) is the professional degree, and the master's of science with a major in nursing degree (MS Nursing) is the formal academic degree.[16] In practice, however, little differentiation is made between the two. Almost all master's programs accredited by the NLNAC require the applicant to have at least a 3.0 grade point average (GPA) and to demonstrate academic proficiency by achieving a satisfactory score on the Graduate Record Examination (GRE) or the Miller's Analogy Test before admission. The GRE is also used to recommend remedial coursework needed to correct deficiencies before the master's program is undertaken.

In the evolution of the various levels of education, the baccalaureate degree is a generalist's degree, the master's degree is a specialist's degree, and the doctoral degree is a generalist's degree, although at a much higher academic level than that of the baccalaureate degree. Actually, the major purpose of early doctoral degrees was to prepare the individual to conduct advanced research in a particular area of interest.

Currently there is a wide range of available doctoral degrees for nurses. The doctor of philosophy (PhD) degree is the most accepted academic degree and is designed to prepare individuals to conduct research. The doctor of education (EdD) degree is considered to be a professional degree, although in many programs there is little difference between the courses of study taken by the EdD and PhD candidates. In other programs, the PhD focuses primarily on research, whereas the EdD focuses more on administration in the educational setting. The classes and research credits differ somewhat between the two degrees.

Since the 1970s, other doctoral programs for nurses have been developed that stress the clinical rather than academic nature of nursing.[17] These include the doctor of nursing science (DNSc) and the doctor of science in nursing (DSN), which is a clinically oriented nursing degree. The doctor of nursing (DN or ND) degree is for the person with a BS or MS in a field other than nursing who wants to pursue nursing as a career. It is a generalist's degree at a basic level of education. In addition, for nurses who wish to pursue a career in higher education, the doctor of nursing education (DNEd) degree is available.

Despite the wide range of doctoral degrees in nursing, there are relatively few programs across

What Do You Think?

Have you ever been to an advanced practice nurse for care? How would you rate the quality of that care? If you have not been to an advanced practice nurse, would you consider going to one for care? Why or why not?

the United States that offer these degrees. Many nurses who seek them may obtain them in fields such as higher education, psychology, college teaching, and adult education. Fewer than 2 percent of nurses hold doctoral degrees.

The requirements for doctoral education are similar, even though the specific degrees being sought are different. The student must have attained a master's degree and must have achieved a satisfactory score on the GRE. Often there is an admission interview and preprogram examination that must be passed before the candidate can be formally admitted to the program. Doctoral programs are at least 60 college credit hours in length, require many statistics and research courses, and often have a residency requirement. Before the doctoral degree can be granted, the student must successfully complete both oral and written comprehensive examinations, as well as write a doctoral dissertation explaining the conduct of a major research project.

Some individuals pursuing doctoral degrees do so on a part-time basis while they are working full-time, whereas others attend classes full-time while working full-time, often completing the program in 3 to 4 years. Many programs require that the individual complete all the requirements within a 10-year time period. Although this may seem a like a long time, it is not unusual for the dissertation process itself to take 2 to 3 years.

Nurses with master's or doctoral degrees are regarded as leaders in the profession of nursing. Many of the larger hospitals in the United States require their unit managers and supervisors to have master's degrees and their directors of nursing or vice presidents of nursing to have doctorates. Of course, in baccalaureate programs, the minimal requirement for teaching is the master's degree, and the doctorate is preferred. Nurses with these advanced degrees provide direction and leadership for the profession through their publications, research, and theory development. As health-care delivery becomes more complicated, larger numbers of nurses with advanced degrees will be required.

Education for Advanced Practice

Advanced practice is one of those often misused terms in nursing that adds to the public's confusion about educational levels of those in the profession. It is sometimes referred to as **expanded role** or practice. Nurses who obtain certification are allowed to practice at a higher and more independent level depending on the nurse practice act of their individual state. Advanced practitioners diagnose illnesses, prescribe medications, conduct physical examinations, and refer clients to specialists for more intensive follow-up care. These nurses practice nursing under their own licenses as **independent practitioners** but often work closely with a physician so that they can quickly refer clients who have medical problems that lie outside their scope of practice.

The nurse practitioner levels of nursing are most widely accepted as advanced practice areas for nursing. These include the pediatric nurse practitioner (PNP), the neonatal nurse practitioner (NNP), the geriatric nurse practitioner (GNP), the obstetrics-gynecology nurse practitioner, the family nurse practitioner (FNP), the rehabilitation nurse practitioner (RNP), the psychiatric nurse practitioner, and the nurse midwife. The certified registered nurse anesthetist (CRNA) and nurse midwife are the oldest of the advanced practice specialties for nurses and are already well accepted in the medical community. Other advanced practice nurses experience varying levels of acceptance from physicians, although the public in general likes the care they receive from advanced practice nurses. All states now have granted some type of **prescriptive authority** to nurse practitioners.

In the past, nurses with baccalaureate degrees (or even associate degrees in California as late as the 1990s) could attend highly concentrated courses of study for 1 to 2 years and become increasingly proficient in a particular specialty area without, however, obtaining an MSN. They could then take the certification examination and become certified as nurse practitioners. Currently, most nurse practitioner programs are

ISSUES NOW

Physicians' Attitudes Changing Slowly

Although slow to evolve, physicians' attitudes toward nurse practitioners have made a 180-degree turnaround in the past few years. As managed care stresses and seeks more economical methods of delivering cost-effective primary care, nurse practitioners have experienced an increase in demand for their services. The shift of care from hospital-based to community-based services has many physicians looking at nurse practitioners from a new perspective.

Physicians are beginning to recognize that modern health care is a team process involving physicians, nurses, dietitians, social workers, and nurse practitioners. Not only do nurse practitioners expand the physicians' practice by allowing for increased numbers of clients to be treated, they also offer a unique aspect to the care. The additional time that nurse practitioners spend with clients, coupled with their traditional nurse orientation toward caring, produces an atmosphere in clinics, physicians' offices, and health-care facilities where clients perceive that they are important and the focus of the care.

The National Advisory Council on Nurse Education and Practice estimates that the United States had only 20,000 certified nurse practitioners of all types in 1993. The Council projects that by the year 2020, the United States will require almost 100,000 nurse practitioners to meet the primary health-care needs of a predominantly managed care system.

Schools of nursing are responding to this trend by increasing the number of master's level nurse practitioner programs. All nurse practitioner programs are reporting full classes. Many nurses who have been practicing for several years view the move to nurse practitioner as a method to advance in nursing without moving to an administrative or desk job far away from direct client care. Also, many nurses who were classified as clinical specialists recognized the uncertainty of this position and began entering nurse practitioner programs.

Managed health-care institutions are beginning to recognize that nurse practitioners excel at health promotion and management of clients' with chronic and disabling diseases. When nurse practitioners keep clients healthier and out of the hospital, the managed systems can keep their costs lower. Relatively simple practices routinely performed by nurse practitioners, like calling clients to see whether they are taking their blood pressure medications, drawing blood samples to monitor clients conditions, or simply listening attentively to client complaints, add a humanistic touch to the cold world of medical treatment. Clients tend to be more willing to follow health-care teaching if they feel the health-care provider is really interested in them as a person.

Across the nation, more and more physicians are beginning to use or considering using nurse practitioners in their practice. They recognize that the key to success in a managed health-care world is to keep clients as healthy as possible. Nurse practitioners are particularly well suited to provide wellness and health maintenance care because of both their education and their orientation toward caring.

Sources: Job security, better pay spur nurses to better training. St. Louis Post Dispatch, August 25, 1997, 10BP–13BP.

Spross, JA, and Heaney, CA: Shaping advanced nursing practice in the new millennium. Oncology Nursing 16(1):12–24, 2000.

Oberle, K, and Allen, M: The nature of advanced practice nursing. Nurs Outlook 49(3):148–153, 2001.

Adams, D, and Miller, BK: Professionalism in nursing behaviors of nurse practitioners. Prof Nurs 17(4):203–210, 2001.

offered in major universities, requiring students to complete the master's degree before allowing them to take the certification examination.

One level of nursing that falls under the umbrella of advanced practice is the **nurse specialist**, or **clinical nurse specialist** (CNS). Although there are only a few schools that offer specific clinical nurse specialists curricula, more often these nurses are self-classified as clinical nurse specialists after completing a master's degree, or some additional education, in a particular clinical area. However, in a few states, such as Ohio, the clinical nurse specialist designation requires a master's degree and a special licensing examination. CNSs are usually hired by hospitals and often function as in-service educators for the hospital.

In 1988, an amendment to the New York Nurse Practice Act established a separate scope of practice and title protection for nurse practitioners (NPs). Subsequent to the NP amendment, there has been some confusion regarding which of the advanced nursing practice categories are included within the scope of practice, particularly by clinical nurse specialists, nurse midwives, and certified nurse anesthetists. This confusion, especially in psychiatric mental health nursing and nurse anesthesia, is related to the legal interpretations of the NP amendment. The resultant debate about this issue has led to a clearer definition and understanding of the term advanced practice nurse.

The career opportunities for advanced practice nurses are numerous.[18] Many nurse practitioners work for county health departments, rural clinics, and on Native-American reservations; others work in hospitals, with physicians in private practice, and in rehabilitation centers. They have even established their own independent clinics. They provide primary health-care services in areas where there is a lack of primary care physicians. Although many of these areas are traditionally rural, today inner-city areas also often have need for this type of health care.

In addition, a common element of several proposed national health-care plans is the requirement that a client seeking entry into the health-care system be evaluated by a primary health-care practitioner before referral to any specialized health-care practitioner. Although the family practice physician, or general practitioner, would be the most common primary health-care provider to evaluate the client, the nurse practitioner could also function in this role. If any of these proposed health-care plans are adopted on a national level, the demand for nurse practitioners will increase tremendously.

Conclusion

In today's rapidly changing health-care environment, there is an ever-increasing need for health-care professionals who are educated to practice at the highest levels.[1] It is imperative that the schools that will be educating future nurses be responsive to the changes, challenges, and demands of an ever more sophisticated and technologically advanced health-care system. Nursing education is an important part of a much larger network of health-care systems, including the service and practice sector, government and regulatory agencies, and licensing and credentialing institutions. All of these interact with each other and together form what is called the health-care system.

The nursing profession has, over the years, developed a number of different types of education programs in an attempt to meet the demands of a growing health-care system. Some of the programs that were developed for specific needs that no longer exist should be examined for their usefulness and viability in today's advanced health-care atmosphere. Perhaps their resources could be rechanneled to programs that are more in tune with current needs. Students should carefully evaluate programs that they might enter and decide which one best meets their care goals. Meanwhile, nursing education continues to develop innovative approaches to help nurses meet the demands for more education, more technical skills, and more leadership ability. The ladder programs are a good example. By recognizing the dynamic state of nursing education, and implementing changes that respond to or even anticipate changes in the health-care system, the nursing profession will continue as one of the pillars of the health-care system.

Educators in nursing have begun to recognize that it is impossible to teach nursing students everything they need to know in the short time allowed for formal education. The demands of the changing health-care system will make that goal even more difficult. However, it may not be necessary to teach nursing students everything. It is more important to teach these students the thinking, decision-making, and management skills that will allow them to adjust to an ever-changing and developing health-care system.

Critical Thinking Exercises

- Discuss why the current educational system for nurses leads to confusion over the role and scope of practice for nurses.
- The literature reports that there will be a nursing shortage well into the twenty-first century. What aspects of health-care reform are likely to produce changes in nursing education? Identify possible changes that may occur in nursing education because of the projected nursing shortage. Will these changes be beneficial or harmful to the profession of nursing?
- What historical factors had an important influence on the development of nursing education as it is currently conducted in the United States?
- What should the minimum level of education be for the professional nurse—ADN, BSN, or MSN? Defend your position.

References

1. Freeman, LH, et al: New Curriculum for a new century. Nursing Education 41(1):38–40, 2002.
2. Bellack, JP, and O'Neil, EH: Recreating nursing practice for A new century: Recommendations and implications of the Pew Health Professions Commission's Final Report. Nursing and Health Care Perspectives 21(1):14–21, 2002.
3. de Tornyay, R: Critical challenges for nurse educators. J Nurs Educ 35(4):146–147, 1996.
4. American Nurses Association: Position Paper on Education. ANA, Kansas City, MO, 1965.
5. Fitzpatrick, ML: Prologue to Professionalism. Robert J. Brady, Bowie, MD, 1983.
6. Jamieson, EM, et al: Trends in Nursing History. WB Saunders, Philadelphia, 1968.
7. Hegner, BR, and Caldwell, E: Nursing Assistant: A Nursing Process Approach, ed. 6. Delmar Publishers, Albany, NY, 1995.
8. National League for Nursing: Trends in Education, 2002. Available at: www.nln.org.
9. Ketefian, S: Moving beyond traditional boundaries. J Prof Nurs 9:25–31, 1993.
10. Calhoun, J: The Nightingale pledge: A commitment that survives the passage of time. Nursing & Health Care 14:130–136, 1993.
11. National League for Nursing: Statistics on Education, 2002. Available at: www.nln.org.
12. Manthey, M: Continuing the case for the baccalaureate. J Prof Nurs 18(1):7, 2002.
13. Felton, G, et al: How does NLNAC support the Pew Health Commission Competencies? Nursing and Health Care Perspectives 21(1):53, 2000.
14. Forni, PR: Nursing's diverse master's programs: The state of the art. Nursing & Health Care 8:770–775, 1987.
15. Lipman, TH, and Deatrick, JA: Enhancing specialist preparation for the next century. J Nurs Educ 33:53–58, 1994.
16. Kalisch, PA, and Kalisch, BJ: The Advance of American Nursing, ed. 3. JB Lippincott, Philadelphia, 1995.
17. American Association of Colleges of Nursing: Indicators of quality in doctoral programs in nursing. J Prof Nurs 3:72–74, 1987.
18. Lynch, MP, et al: Advanced practice issues: Results of the ONS Advanced Practice Nursing Survey. Oncol Nurs Forum, 28(10):1521–1530, 2001.

Bibliography

Brady, M, et al: A Proposed framework for differentiating the 21 Pew Competencies by level of nursing education. Nursing and Health Care Perspectives 22(1):30–35, 2002.

Brewer, C, and Kovner, CT: Is there another nursing shortage? What the data tell us. Nurs Outlook 49(1):20–26, 2001.

Clark, L, and Thornam, C: Using educational technology to teach cultural assessment. Nursing Education 41(3):117–120, 2002.

Coffey-Love, M: Said another way: The nursing shortage: What is your role? Nursing Forum 36(2):29–35, 2001.

Fondiller, SH: The advancement of baccalaureate and graduate nursing education 1952–1972. Nursing and Health Care Perspectives 21(1):10–13, 2002.

Freeman, LH, et al: New curriculum for a new century. Nursing Education 41(1):38–40, 2002.

Gatzke, H, and Ransom, JE: New skills for a new age: Preparing nurses for the 21st century. Nursing Forum 36(3):13–17, 2001.

Good, DM, and Schubert, CR: Faculty practice: How it enhances teaching. J Nurs Educ 40(9):397–403, 2001.

Kotecki, CN: Baccalaureate nursing students' communication process in the clinical setting. Nursing Education 41(2):61–68, 2002.

Sandelowski, M: Visible humans, vanishing bodies and virtual nursing. ANS 24(3):58–70, 2002.

6

Critical Thinking

Joseph T. Catalano

Learning Objectives

After completing this chapter, the reader will be able to:

- Demonstrate logical, rational, and creative critical thinking.
- Describe the steps of the critical thinking process in resolving a client care issue.
- Apply critical thinking to client care.
- List five characteristics of critical thinking.

One of the most important responsibilities that nurses have is to make correct and safe decisions in a variety of client care situations. The decisions made by nurses affect the health status, recovery time, and even the life or death of a client. For example, the critical care nurse must decide when to give certain medications based on changes in the client's condition. The emergency room nurse must decide which client is treated first based on the extent of his or her injuries. The hospital staff nurse must decide what PRN medication to give for which set of symptoms. The home health nurse must decide when to call the physician about a change in a client's condition.

The process by which these decisions are made involves the use of critical thinking. Critical thinking is based on reason and reflection, knowledge and instinct derived from experience. It has also been defined as "the art of thinking about thinking." It is both an attitude about and an approach to solving problems. Critical thinking helps nurses make decisions about problems for which there are no simple solutions. Often nurses have to make these decisions with less than complete information.

Although critical thinking has always been used by nurses to some degree and is recognized as important in the provision of care, its status increased greatly when the National League for Nursing Accrediting Commission (NLNAC) designated critical thinking as one of its mandatory outcome objectives in 1992. Since then, schools of nursing have been challenged to demonstrate where and how they teach and measure critical thinking in the curriculum. It is fairly easy to claim, "Yes, we teach our students how to think critically," but much more difficult to accurately define what critical thinking actually is and then demonstrate that the graduates of the program have attained and can use the skill.

A definition is a short statement that identifies and distinguishes something from all other things so that it can be recognized. Generally, things that are easy to define have one or a few definitions. Things that are more difficult to define tend to have many definitions that may or may not overlap. It would seem that critical thinking falls into the latter category. There are at least 10 different definitions for critical thinking that have been developed over the years by the various experts in the subject. Perhaps a better approach to recognizing and developing critical thinking is to look at the characteristics that seem to be common to most of the definitions.

> *Jumping to conclusions often produces poor decisions and negative results.*

Characteristics of Critical Thinking

Critical Thinking Is Creative

Nurses who think creatively explore new ideas and alternative ways of solving client care problems. Creative thinkers are able to bring together bits of knowledge or information that may initially seem unrelated and formulate them into a plan that leads to effective decision making and solves the problem by finding connections between the thoughts and concepts. This process is similar to the linear approach used in the nursing process. All the situational variables must be considered, and decision making becomes more complex as the number of variables increases.

Example of Creative Thinking

In a small hospital, a policy was instituted that required all post–cesarean delivery clients to be monitored in the recovery room just like all other postoperative clients. Because the operating room (OR) nurses were on call for the recovery room, they thought that they were being required to do more work with no additional staff. The circulating and scrub obstetric (OB) nurses could go home after the delivery. The OR nurses became very resentful of the extra call for the post-delivery clients and often called in sick the day after they were required to attend a post-cesarean client. This practice left the OR short staffed during the day and led to increased tension and frequent unfriendly confrontations between the OR and the OB nurses.

The nurse managers of the OB and OR units resolved the problem by instituting a policy of "cross-training" with the OR and OB nurses. OB nurses were taught how to monitor the recovery of postoperative clients and were rotated through recovery for 1 week every 2 months to keep these skills current. The OR nurses were taught how to assist at cesarean deliveries and were rotated through the OB unit for 1 week every 2 months. This system kept the staffing levels constant and allowed the OB nurses to assist with the post–cesarean delivery clients. Although not everyone was happy with the practice, it did reduce the resentment levels between the two units and gave the nurses a better appreciation of the other nurses' responsibilities.

> **What Do You Think?**
>
> Identify two situations that you have been involved with that required critical thinking. How did you resolve these situations? What elements of critical thinking did you use?

Critical Thinking Is Logical, Rational, and Reflective

Although the critical thinking process is often expanded beyond fundamental logical thinking, it must always be based on rationales and facts rather than emotions or egocentric impulses. Intuition can play a part in critical thinking when it is recognized as a rational thought process that brings together and processes a number of factors at the subconscious level rather than a simple "gut feeling." If at all possible, critical thinkers must take the time to collect as much data as they can and examine them under the light of reason before making a decision or taking an action. Decisions must at times be made on a limited amount of information in situations where there is a high degree of risk and ambiguity. In these situations, the nurse's past experiences resolving similar situations as well as intuition can help. However, in most cases, merely jumping to conclusions often produces poor decisions and negative results. Logical reasoning is often divided into deductive and inductive reasoning.

Example of Deductive Reasoning

Deductive logic or reasoning is a process whereby the individual proceeds from the general to the particular. The conclusions reached by deductive reasoning based on a valid argument are certain and true.

Either John Smith or George Jones is to be given a dose of IV penicillin before surgery.
There was no order for IV penicillin for John Smith before surgery.
Therefore, George Jones is to be given IV penicillin before surgery.

The conclusion is valid. The rationale is that all of the information in the conclusion is found in the premises; therefore, the conclusion must logically follow if the premises are true.

Example of Inductive Reasoning

Inductive logic or reasoning involves proceeding from the particular to the general. The conclusions reached by inductive reasoning are probable or contingent. Inductive reasoning is more frequently used in health-care situations than deductive reasoning because of the wide range of variables involved in client care.

Mr. Jones has bacterial lobar pneumonia.
Antibiotics are usually used to treat this disease.
Therefore, Mr. Jones should be given an antibiotic.

The conclusion is valid. The rationale is that the conclusion is uncertain because the use of the word "usually" in the premise leaves room for alternative conclusions.

Keep in mind that all critical thinking, including both inductive and deductive reasoning, is open to fallacies. A fallacy is generally defined as an error in reasoning that leads to a conclusion that does not follow from its premises.[1] Some arguments are valid, sound, or cogent, whereas others are false, illogical, and invalid. The most common type of fallacy seen in nursing is the non sequitur, a fallacy in which the conclusion does not follow from the arguments or premise. For example, a 72-year-old male client who had a colon resection and colostomy 12 days ago and who is being prepared for discharge expresses fear about returning to his one-room apartment in the inner city. He also has a heart murmur. On these two factors alone, a nursing diagnosis of "severe dependency needs" is formulated. Another common example of this fallacy is often seen when there are staffing shortages. It is not unusual for nursing supervisors to say to a staff nurse, "We need you to work this extra shift because everyone else called in. I know you take classes in the evening, but the clients always come first. Therefore, if you don't work, you might as well start looking for employment elsewhere." This situation also adds the element of irrelevant appeal to force.

People commit fallacies for various reasons. In some cases, individuals have such a strong ideological commitment to a religious, economic, or political belief that they refuse to listen to any ideas or opinions that contradict what they believe. Basically, their minds are closed to any alternative conclusions, thus they stick to their own conclusions regardless of the reasoning process. Some individuals have difficulty acknowledging that they have made a mistake and will refuse to see the lack of logic in their reasoning and conclusions. Still others must "win" at all cost and will subvert the critical thinking process and logic by abuse, twisting the other person's words, and using personal attacks. Being able to recognize conclusions that are valid or invalid is an important part of critical thinking.

For practice, analyze each of the following arguments, decide whether they are inductive or deductive, note whether they are valid or invalid, and give a rationale for the decision.

1. The largest city in a country is usually the capital of the country.
   New York City is the largest city in the United States.
   Therefore, New York City is the capital of the United States.
   Type of reasoning ____________
   Conclusion valid? Yes No
   Rationale: ____________
2. All nurses are women.
   Pat is a nurse.
   Therefore, Pat is a woman.
   Type of reasoning ____________
   Conclusion valid? Yes No
   Rationale: ____________
3. Nora is a premature infant who weighs 1 pound.
   Nora has two congenital abnormalities: myelomeningocele and ventricular septal defect.
   Premature infants with congenital abnormalities usually die within 2 weeks of birth.
   Therefore, Nora will die within the next 2 weeks.
   Type of reasoning ____________
   Conclusion valid? Yes No
   Rationale: ____________
4. In prison, criminals perform hard labor.
   Tom is a prisoner performing hard labor.
   Therefore, Tom is a criminal.
   Type of reasoning ____________
   Conclusion valid? Yes No
   Rationale: ____________
5. 96% of nurses are women.
   Terry is a nurse.
   Therefore, Terry is probably a woman.
   Type of reasoning ____________
   Conclusion valid? Yes No
   Rationale: ____________
6. Mary is staggering around the room.
   Mary was just at a cocktail party.
   Therefore, Mary drank too much alcohol.
   Type of reasoning ____________
   Conclusion valid? Yes No
   Rationale: ____________
7. Almost every identified carcinogen causes cancer in animals.
   Humans are animals.
   Therefore, almost every identified carcinogen causes cancer in humans.
   Type of reasoning ____________
   Conclusion valid? Yes No
   Rationale: ____________
8. O.J. owns a pair of Bruno Magli shoes.
   Footprints from Bruno Magli shoes were found at the crime scene.
   Therefore, O.J. committed the crime.
   Type of reasoning ____________
   Conclusion valid? Yes No
   Rationale: ____________
9. Ada, Betty, and Clara are the staff nurse, the head nurse, and the supervisor (but not necessarily in that order).
   Ada was beaten by the head nurse in a bridge game.
   Betty is the supervisor's neighbor.
   Betty is unbeatable at bridge when playing the other two nurses.
   Clara wants to become a head nurse or supervisor.

a. Who is the head nurse? ________
b. Who is the supervisor? ________
c. Who is the staff nurse? ________
Type of reasoning ________
Rationale: ________

10. Smith, Jones, and Brown are a surgeon, a scrub nurse, and an OR tech (but not necessarily in that order).
The OR tech, who is an only child, earns the least amount of money.
Brown, who married Smith's sister, earns more than the scrub nurse.
Who is the surgeon? ________
Who is the scrub nurse? ________
Who is the scrub tech? ________
Type of reasoning ________
Rationale: ________

Keep in mind that these exercises are simplified examples of inductive and deductive reasoning and are presented as an introduction to logical reasoning. However, using simple reasoning processes alone in client care decisions can lead to serious fallacies and error in judgment. All the other characteristics of critical thinking discussed here must be included for sound clinical decision making.

> *Nurses who think critically are not easily influenced by others with strong opinions.*

Critical Thinking Is Independent

Nurses who think critically are not easily influenced by others with strong opinions. They demonstrate their autonomy by thinking for themselves and not passively succumbing to peer pressure or the belief system of the majority.

Example of Independent Thinking

An 82-year-old woman was brought into the emergency room (ER) by her family with complaints of "difficulty urinating." During the initial assessment, the RN noted that the client had +2 edema of her ankles and feet, congested lung sounds, and shortness of breath. The ER physician ordered a Foley catheter, urinalysis, and a consultation with a urologist for the urinary complaint. The RN pointed out the client's history of congestive heart failure (CHF) and current symptoms and also the fact that only 10 mL of urine was obtained when the catheter was inserted. The ER physician insisted that the problem was urinary and refused to discuss the client's condition any more.

While waiting for the urinalysis results, the client became increasingly short of breath and restless. The RN called for a chest x-ray and measurement of arterial blood gases (ABGs). The chest x-ray showed that 75 percent of the client's lung fields were filled with fluid, and the ABGs showed respiratory acidosis with hypoxia. The nurse asked the physician to order furosemide (Lasix) for the client based on these findings. The physician became angry, accused the nurse of practicing medicine, and refused to write the order. The nurse then called the client's attending physician, who decided to admit the client to the hospital and begin treatment with IV furosemide for the obvious CHF.

Critical Thinking Challenges Rituals and Assumptions About Client Care

A healthy, constructive questioning of long-used health-care practices prevents the nurse from the mindless provision of rote care. Improvement and advance in health-care practices occur only when nurses understand the rationale behind the practices, then accept or reject them based on evidence that they either do or do not work as intended.

Example of Challenging Rituals and Assumptions

A newly hired nurse was beginning her first shift on the obstetric (OB) unit when a 28-year-old client in her sixth month of pregnancy was admitted with abdominal cramps and vaginal bleeding. A spontaneous abortion was suspected. Another nurse who had worked on the OB unit for 10 years knew the client and her family. She told the newly hired nurse to call the client's sister (her number was on the chart), even though the client had not requested it. The newly hired nurse felt uncomfortable making the call and refused on the grounds that it was a violation of client **confidentiality**. The experienced nurse became angry at the refusal and berated the new nurse with the statement, "We've been notifying the families of our clients for years and you're not going to change that practice."

The next day, the newly hired nurse had a conference with the OB unit nurse manager and arranged for several in-service presentations on the right to privacy.

> *In order to use effective critical thinking, biases and stereotypes must be identified and eliminated.*

Critical Thinking Is Free of Bias and Prejudice

Biases are unjustified personal opinions. When a bias, as well as **stereotype**, is taken as fact, it becomes a prejudice. A belief is not true just because it has been in existence for a long period of time or because many people believe it. In order to use effective critical thinking, biases and stereotypes must be identified and eliminated.

Analyzing and viewing a situation from all points of view before arriving at a conclusion prevents the nurse from making one-sided decisions. It also helps determine bias or prejudice on the part of physicians, nurses, and even clients and the backlash effect that it may produce on other decision makers.

Recognition of bias does not always eliminate it, but helps the decision-maker compensate for it when making the final decision.

Example of Bias and Prejudice-Free Thinking

A homosexual, HIV-positive client with full-blown symptoms of AIDS is admitted to a medical/surgical unit for care. The nurse assigned to care for the client has very strong religious beliefs about homosexuality. She believes that her obligation as a nurse requires her to care for this client despite his diagnosis and sexual preference, yet she also believes that caring for this client would tacitly condone his sexual preferences and lifestyle. She tries to place herself in the client's situation and recognizes that an ill client deserves quality care without consideration of his beliefs or background.

Critical Thinking Is Action Oriented

The goal of critical thinking in health care should always be the resolution of a problem or a method to improve client care. Critical thinking is used at all levels of the health-care system and is essential to the formulation and evaluation of policies and procedures, use of effective communication, and resolution of management and personnel conflicts.

Example of Action-Oriented Critical Thinking

A physician with a reputation for striking fear in the hearts of the nurses in the medical/surgical unit was in a particularly bad mood one day. After making his rounds, the physician criticized the care that the nurses were giving to his clients loudly and publicly in the nurses' station and proceeded to announce numerous mistakes that the nurses had made over the past year. The unit manager took the physician aside and told him that if he was having problems with the nurses on the unit, he should follow correct channels to file complaints and not make a scene in the nurses' station where many of the clients could hear him.

The physician became even more irate and stormed out of the unit directly to the office of the director of nursing (DON). He told the DON that he was filing an official **complaint** against the unit manager for unprofessional behavior, disrespect for a physician, and failure to follow medical orders. The DON told him that she would investigate the complaint and take appropriate action.

After talking with all the nurses on the medical/surgical unit and nurses on other units, as well as a number of physicians, it was discovered that the physician who filed the complaint was well known for his **capricious** and obnoxious behavior toward nurses. He was referred to the hospital medical board, reprimanded for his behavior toward the nurses, and required to drop the complaint about the manager of the medical/surgical unit. In addition, a special meeting was called for all the physicians practicing in the hospital to discuss the problem and to better understand what was involved regarding professional behavior.

Critical Thinking Skills

Although there are different approaches to developing critical thinking, certain concepts are common to the skill. Some individuals seem to have an innate ability to master these concepts, whereas others have difficulty with them. As with most skills, practice and repetition increase efficiency and the ability to make safe decisions in complex nursing situations where there are multiple variables that affect the client's health status.

Identify the Problem

The saying "It's hard to know when you have arrived if you don't know where you are going" applies particularly well to critical thinking. If the underlying problem has not been identified, then it is almost impossible to develop a plan to solve it. One way to identify the underlying problem is to try to restate the issue as a declarative statement. For example, a public health nurse may identify that "sexually transmitted diseases (STDs) among teenagers in our society are increasing at a rapid rate."

Gather Pertinent Data

It sometimes happens that when trying to apply critical thinking to the resolution of a problem, there is only a small amount of information that relates to the situation. On the other hand, in our information-oriented society, there may be an overabundance of data. It becomes necessary for the nurse to sort through the data, use the data that relate to the problem, and reject the data that are extraneous and perhaps misleading. In the previous example of STDs in teenagers, the Internet can provide copious data, including general population statistics, racial and ethnic breakdowns, STD incidents by region, the most common STDs, treatment regimens, and even projections for the future.

Rational analysis and consideration of the data may produce a re-examination and refocusing of the problem. For example, after examining the

What Do You Think?

What five values are most important to you? How do these influence the way you act? What happens when these values conflict?

abundance of information about teenage STD, the community health nurses may decide to focus their emphasis on dealing with the problem in their community rather than the entire state.

Identify and Challenge Assumptions, Beliefs, Ideas, and Issues

Developing a contextual awareness requires primarily the use of deductive reasoning. Contextual awareness is a very broad concept that is not merely limited to values but also includes everything that may have an affect on the client, such as physical symptoms and environment. Everyone, including nurses, has feelings and beliefs about all issues. Some of these beliefs are personal; some are cultural; some are stated overtly, whereas others remain deeply rooted but hidden in the unconscious. In any case, these beliefs influence how situations are perceived and what decisions are made.

In order to make solid decisions based on critical thinking, nurses must examine their own philosophy, beliefs, and value systems. **Values clarification** is an important element in critical thinking. At some point in the nurse's career, preferably in the early stages, he or she should make a list of all the things they consider as valuable (Box 6–1). It should also be recognized that values are not static and that values will be added or deleted or will change in priority with time.

In addition, nurses must examine their own philosophy of nursing and health care as it relates to that of the agency for which they are working. Then, they need to compare how societal values relate to their own personal philosophy and that of the agency. Do societal values reflect or contradict the philosophy? How do the standards of care, the nurse practice act of the state, facility

Box 6–1

Personal Values

Listed below are a number of values that almost everyone has. Circle the ones that you feel are important to you, adding additional values as necessary. Then rank the values according to priority.

family 1 4
education 3
career
honesty 5
good health 2
respect
leisure time
nonjudgmental attitude
cooperative work relationships
professional integrity
competency
empathy
flexibility
trust 7
teamwork
dependability 6
punctuality
accountability
self-determination
independence
veracity
justice
commitment
____
____
____
____

protocols, and even the code of ethics affect the care being provided?

Challenging assumptions and rituals of care requires use of inductive reasoning. The nurse needs to ask whether there are any assumptions about the care provided; what they are; how they affect care; and whether any of these assumptions can be challenged.

In much the same way, rituals about care should also be identified and challenged. What are the rituals that are done routinely without much thought? Are they beneficial, or can they be changed or eliminated?

The community health nurse, for example, may have the philosophy that an STD among teenagers represents a dangerous and serious threat to the health of the community. On the other hand, the community may have an underlying philosophy that teenage STD is to be expected and is only one of the rites of passage that must be experienced. Where such a major difference in philosophy exists, it would be extremely difficult for the nurse to implement any action that would resolve the problem.

Some assumptions that could be challenged might revolve around the cause of the problem. An increase in STDs among teenagers may be caused by (1) a lack of sexual education in school, (2) a lack of morals in our society, or (3) an atmosphere of permissiveness and egocentrism that is projected in the media.

A nurse using critical thinking will often be able to identify more than one solution to a problem.

One health department philosophy about teenagers that may need to be challenged might be that all teenagers are rebellious, uncooperative, and promiscuous, when in reality, many teenagers work well with others, are highly productive, and have high moral standards.

Nurses also need to learn and evaluate the value systems of those with whom they are working. Even though they may not agree with those values, it is important to recognize them and work with them when attempting to affect health. For example, when teaching a group of high-school students about STDs, it would be essential to know what their attitudes toward sex and health were. In all likelihood, these attitudes would be different from those of the nurse. An education program organized around only the nurse's belief and value system would be doomed to failure. Presenting the information from a viewpoint of the students would help them better understand and perhaps be more willing to accept it.

Imagine and Explore Alternatives Creatively

Once the nurse has identified the problem and explored the assumptions and rituals, he or she needs to consider the possible alternatives to care delivery. However, the nurse does not need to do this alone.

The information can be obtained from a variety of sources, such as written reports, surveys, and published articles. Information may also be obtained from others informally, such as in discussions with individuals who work in the field or have dealt with a similar problem before, or via feedback from the clients who are receiving the care. No matter what the source of information, it needs to be evaluated critically for accuracy, consistency, cause and effect, and biases.

A nurse using critical thinking will often be able to identify more than one solution to a problem. For example, possible solutions to the teenage STD problem may include providing condoms for all high-school students, performing tubal ligations on sexually active girls, or establishing strict nighttime curfews.

Although all these solutions may be effective, the nurse would have to evaluate the cause-and-effect relationship, value, and consequences of each of these courses of action. A nurse who is a critical thinker would consider each one of these before implementing a course of action.

Critical Thinking in Decision Making

Although critical thinking is used in all aspects of decision making, it is particularly important in the nursing process. It is important to remember that although the nursing process and critical thinking are interrelated and interdependent, they are not identical.

As a way of looking at the world, critical thinking allows the nurse to consider new ideas and then evaluate those ideas in light of accepted information as well as client and personal value systems. Nurses are constantly making decisions in both their professional and personal lives. By viewing critical thinking as a purposeful mental activity in which ideas are evaluated and decisions reached, nurses will be able to make ethical, creative, rational, and independent decisions related to client care.

Critical thinking, when applied to the nursing process, makes it a powerful client problem-solving tool. Critical thinking expands the usual linear nursing process into a gestalt that allows the nurse to sort through the multiple variables that are often encountered in client care. Effective use of critical thinking within the nursing process is evident when the nurse successfully applies knowledge from other disciplines in the resolution of client problems, deals with stressful environments, and creatively resolves unique nursing care problems.

Conclusion

Nurses practicing in today's health-care system are required to master many skills. Critical thinking underlies many of these skills. By examining assumptions, beliefs, propositions, and meanings, nurses are able to make sound and valid decisions about client care. Critical thinking both underlies and expands the nursing process in the practical provision of nursing care. When students and nurses master critical thinking concepts and skills, they open their perspectives on client care. An important transformation occurs when students are taught how to think rather than what to think.

The profession of nursing is in an active state of change, continually developing new theories, redefining its practice, and adapting to changing public policy and social mandates. Nurses who use critical thinking in making nursing judgments tend to consider the client's human rights and be effective client advocates. These nurses will also be able to adapt the rules of the nursing process to meet a wide range of client needs.

Critical Thinking Exercises

Use the steps in the nursing process to provide a plan of care, including at least two nursing diagnoses, for the following client situation:

> Mr. Y. is 49 years old and has been complaining of chest pain starting in the center of his chest and radiating to his left arm and hand for 2 hours. He is having trouble breathing, is very pale, and has cool and moist skin. His pulse is 134 beats per minute and irregular; his blood pressure is 92/50 mm Hg; and his respiratory rate is 24 breaths per minute. He is very anxious and expresses concern about having to leave his job as an accountant because of these symptoms. He is diagnosed as having an acute anterior myocardial infarction and is admitted to the intensive care unit.

- What key assessment does the nurse need to identify as essential to this client's problem?
- What problems does this client have that a nurse can treat independently? Write nursing diagnoses for these problems.
- What can be accomplished in the nursing treatment of this client's problems (goals)?
- What type of activities can the nurse undertake to achieve the goals (intervention)?
- What does the nurse need to look for to see whether the interventions have worked (evaluation)?

References

1. Strasser, JA: Critical thinking: Health and the capacity for building health. DNA Reporter 26(1):10–12, 2001.

Bibliography

Alfaro-LeFevre, R: Applying Nursing Process: A Step by Step Guide, ed. 4. JB Lippincott, Philadelphia, 1998.

Beeken, JE, et al: Teaching critical thinking skills in undergraduate nursing students. Nurse Educator 22(3):37–39, 1997.

Benner, P: From Novice to Expert. Addison-Wesley, Menlo Park, CA, 1984.

Chau, JPC, et al: Effects of using videotaped vignettes on enhancing students' critical thinking ability in a baccalaureate nursing programme. J Adv Nurs 36(1):112–119, 2001.

Cioffi, J: Clinical simulations: Development and validation. Nurse Education Today 21(6):477–486, 2001.

Daily, WM: The development of an alternative method in the assessment of critical thinking as an outcome of nursing education. J Adv Nurs 36(1):120–130, 2001.

Doenges, ME, et al: Application of Nursing Process and Nursing Diagnosis: An Interactive Text for Diagnostic Reasoning. FA Davis, Philadelphia, 1995.

Farrell, M: Planning for critical outcomes. J Nurs Educ 35:278–281, 1996.

Fetter, MS: Transforming clinical practice to foster critical thinking habits of the mind. Dean's Notes 22(5):1–3, 2001.

Green, CJ: Critical Thinking in Nursing. Prentice Hall, Upper Saddle River, NJ, 2000.

Hunt, R: Community-based nursing: Philosophy or setting? Am J Nurs 98(10):44–49, 1998.

Maslow, AH: Motivation and Personality. Harper & Row, New York, 1971.

Mill, JE, et al: Critical theory: Critical methodology to disciplinary foundations in nursing. Canadian Journal of Nursing Research 33(2):109–127, 2001.

Mogale, NM: Problem-based case study to enhance critical thinking in nursing students. Durationis: South African Journal of Nursing 24(3):27–35, 2001.

Myrick, F, and Yonge, OJ: Creating a climate for critical thinking in the preceptorship experience. Nurse Education Today 21(6):461–467, 2001.

Nicoll, LH: Nurses' Guide to the Internet, ed. 2. JB Lippincott, Philadelphia, 1998.

Nicoteri, JA: Critical thinking skills. Am J Nurs 98(10):62–68, 1998.

Pesult, DJ: Clinical judgement: Foreground and background. J Prof Nurs 17(5):215, 2001.

Proctor, H, et al: In the nursing interest: Reading and thinking critically in the new millennium. Contemporary Nurse 9(3/4):201–204, 2000.

Redding, DA: The development of critical thinking among students in baccalaureate nursing education. Holistic Nursing Practice 15(4):57–64, 2001.

Shell, R: Perceived barriers to teaching for critical thinking by BSN nursing faculty. Nursing and Health Care Perspectives 22(6):286–291, 2001.

Stewart, M: Health care community faces the year 2000. American Nurse 29(6):24, 1997.

Sullivan, TJ: Collaboration: A Health Care Imperative. McGraw-Hill, New York, 1998.

Taylor, C: Clinical problem solving in nursing. J Adv Nurs 31(4):847–849, 2000.

Thurmond, VA: The holism in critical thinking: A concept analysis. Journal of Holistic Nursing 19(4):375–389, 2001.

Van Eerden, K: Using critical thinking vignettes to evaluate student learning. Nursing and Health Care Perspectives 22(5):231–234, 2001

Winningham, ML, and Preusser, BA: Critical Thinking in Medical-Surgical Settings. Mosby, St. Louis, 2001.

2

Making the Transition to Professional

7

Ethics in Nursing

Joseph T. Catalano

Learning Objectives

After completing this chapter, the reader will be able to:

- Discuss and analyze the difference between law and ethics.
- Define the key terms used in ethics.
- Discuss the important ethical concepts.
- Distinguish between the two most commonly used systems of ethical decision making.
- Apply the steps in the ethical decision-making process.

Nurses who practice in today's health-care system soon realize that making ethical decisions is a common part of daily nursing care. However, experience shows that in the full curricula of many schools of nursing, the teaching of ethical principles and ethical decision making gets less attention than the topics of nursing skills, pathophysiology, and nursing care plans. As health-care technology continues to advance into the twenty-first century, it will become more and more difficult for nurses to make these ethical decisions. Many nurses thus feel the need to be better prepared to understand and deal with the complex ethical problems that keep evolving as they attempt to provide care for their clients.

Ethical decision making is a skill that can be learned. The ability to make sensible ethical decisions is based on an understanding of underlying ethical principles, ethical theories or systems, a decision-making model, and the profession's Code of Ethics. This skill, like others, involves mastery of the theoretical material and practice of the skill itself. This chapter presents the basic information required to understand ethics, the code of ethics, and ethical decision making. It also highlights some of the important bioethical issues that confront nurses in the current health-care system.

Important Definitions

In Western cultures, the study of ethics is a specialized area of philosophy, the origins of which can be traced to ancient Greece. In fact, certain ethical principles articulated by Hippocrates still serve as the basis of many of the current debates. Like most specialized areas of study, ethics has its own language and uses terminology in precise ways. The following are some key terms that are encountered in studies of health-care ethics.

Values

Values are ideals or concepts that give meaning to the individual's life. Values are derived most commonly from societal norms, religion, and family orientation and serve as the framework for making decisions and taking action in daily life. A person's values tend to change as his or her life situations change, as the person grows older, and as he or she encounters situations that cause value conflicts. For example, prior to the 1950s, pregnancy outside of marriage was unacceptable, and unmarried women who were pregnant were shunned and generally separated from society. Today, it is much more accepted, and it is not uncommon to see pregnant high-school students attending classes.

Values are usually not written down; however, at some time in their professional careers, it may be important for nurses to make a list of their values. This value clarification process requires that the nurse assess, evaluate, and then determine a set of personal values and prioritize them. This will help the nurse make decisions when confronted with situations in which the client's values differ from the nurse's own values.

Value conflicts that often occur in daily life can force an individual to select a higher priority value over a lower priority one. For example, a nurse who values both her career and her family may be forced to decide between going to work and staying home with a sick child.

> *A moral person is generally someone who responds to another person in need by providing care and who maintains a level of responsibility in all relationships.*

What Do You Think?

What type of value conflicts have you experienced in the past week? How did you resolve them? Were you satisfied with the resolution, or did it make you feel uncomfortable?

Morals

Morals are the fundamental standards of right and wrong that an individual learns and internalizes, usually in the early stages of childhood development. An individual's moral orientation is often based on religious beliefs, although societal influence plays an important part in this development. The word *moral* comes from the Latin word **mores**, which means customs or values. Moral behavior is often manifested as behavior in accordance with a group's norms, customs, or traditions. A moral person is generally someone who responds to another person in need by providing care and who maintains a level of responsibility in all relationships.[1] In many situations in which moral convictions differ, it is difficult to find a rational basis for proving one side right over the other. For example, animal rights activists believe that killing animals for sport, their fur, or even food is morally wrong. Most hunters do not even think of the killing of animals as a moral issue at all.

Laws

Laws can generally be defined as rules of social conduct made by humans to protect society, and these laws are based on concerns about fairness and justice. The goals of laws are to preserve the species and promote peaceful and productive interactions between individuals or groups of individuals by preventing the actions of one citizen from infringing on the rights of another. Two important aspects of laws are that they are enforceable through some type of police force and that they should be applied equally to all persons.

Ethics

Ethics are declarations of what is right or wrong and of what ought to be. Ethics are usually presented as systems of value behaviors and beliefs; they serve the purpose of governing conduct to ensure the protection of an individual's rights. Ethics exist on several levels, ranging from the individual or a small group to the society as a whole. The concept of ethics is closely associated with the concept of morals in both their development and purposes. In one sense, ethics can be considered a system of morals for a particular group. There are usually no systems of enforcement for those who violate ethical principles.

A **code of ethics** is a written list of a profession's values and standards of conduct. The code of ethics provides a framework for decision making for the profession and should be oriented toward the daily decisions made by members of the profession.

An **ethical dilemma** is a situation that requires an individual to make a choice between two equally unfavorable alternatives. When ethical dilemmas are reduced to their elemental aspects, conflicts of one individual's rights with those of another, or one individual's obligations with the rights of another, or a combination of one group's obligations and rights conflicting with those of another group usually form the basis of the dilemma. By the very nature of an ethical dilemma, there can be no simple correct solution, and the final decision must often be defended against those who disagree with it. For example, a client went to surgery for a laparoscopic biopsy of an abdominal mass. After the laparoscope was inserted, the physician noted that the mass had metastasized to the liver, pancreas, and colon, and even before the results of the tissue biopsy returned from the laboratory, the physician diagnosed metastatic cancer with a poor prognosis. When the client was returned to his room, the physician told the nurses about the diagnosis but warned them that under no circumstances were they to tell the client about the cancer. When the client awoke, the first question that he asked the nurses was "Do I have cancer?" This posed an ethical dilemma for the nurses. If they were to tell the client the truth, they would violate the principle of fidelity to the physician. If they lied to the client, they would violate the principle of veracity.

Key Concepts in Ethics

In addition to the terminology used in the study and practice of ethics, several important principles often underlie ethical dilemmas. These principles include autonomy, justice, fidelity, beneficence, nonmaleficence, veracity, standard of best interest, and obligations.

Autonomy

Autonomy is the right of self-determination, independence, and freedom. Autonomy refers to the client's right to make health-care decisions for himself or herself, even if the health-care provider does not agree with those decisions.

Autonomy, as with most rights, is not absolute, and under certain conditions, limitations can be imposed on it. Generally these limitations occur when one individual's autonomy interferes with another individual's rights, health, or well-being. For example, a client generally can use his or her right to autonomy by refusing any or all treatments. In the case of contagious diseases (e.g., tuberculosis [TB]) that affect society, however, the individual can be forced by the health-care and legal systems to take medications to cure the disease. The individual can also be forced into isolation to prevent the disease from spreading. Consider the following situation:

> June, who is the 28-year-old mother of two children, is brought into the emergency

department after a tonic-clonic-type seizure at a shopping mall. June is known to the emergency room (ER) nurses because she has been treated several times for seizures because she did not take her antiseizure medications. She states that the medications make her feel "dopey" and tired all the time and she hates the way that they make her feel.

Recently, June has started to drive one of her children and four other children to school in the neighborhood car pool 1 day a week. She also drives 62 miles one way on the interstate highway twice a week to visit her aging mother in a nursing home in a different city. The nurse who takes care of June this day in the ER knows that the state licensing laws require that an individual with uncontrolled seizures must report the fact to the Department of Motor Vehicles and is usually ineligible for a driver's license. When the nurse mentions that she is going to have to report the seizure, June begs her not to report it. She would have no means of taking her children to school or visiting her mother. She assures the nurse that she will take her medication no matter how it makes her feel.

Justice

Justice is the obligation to be fair to all people. The concept is often expanded to what is called **distributive justice**, which states that individuals have the right to be treated equally regardless of race, sex, marital status, medical diagnosis, social standing, economic level, or religious belief. The principle of justice underlies the first statement in the American Nurses Association (ANA) Code of Ethics for Nurses:

> *The nurse provides services with respect for human dignity and the uniqueness of the client unrestricted by considerations of social or economic status, personal attributes, or the nature of health problems.*[2]

Distributive justice sometimes includes ideas such as equal access to health care for all. As with other rights, limits can be placed on justice when it interferes with the rights of others. For example, a middle-aged homeless man who was diagnosed with type I, insulin-dependent diabetes mellitus demanded that Medicaid pay for a pancreas transplant. His health record showed that he refused to follow the prescribed diabetic regimen, drank large quantities of wine, and rarely took his insulin. The transplant would cost $48,000, which is the total cost of immunizing all the children in the state for 1 year.

Fidelity

Fidelity is the obligation of an individual to be faithful to commitments made to himself or herself and also to others. In health care, fidelity includes the professional's faithfulness or loyalty to agreements and responsibilities accepted as part of the practice of the profession. Fidelity is the main support for the concept of accountability, although conflicts in fidelity might arise from obligations owed to different individuals or groups.

For example, a nurse who was just finishing a very busy and tiring 12-hour shift may experience a conflict of fidelity when she is asked by a supervisor to work an additional shift because of the hospital's being short-staffed. The nurse has to weigh her fidelity to herself against fidelity to the employing institution and against the fidelity to the profession and clients to do the best job possible, particularly if she felt that her fatigue would interfere with the performance of those obligations.

What Do You Think?

Identify a situation in which a law is or may be unethical. Which system has higher authority? How do you resolve the conflict?

Beneficence

Beneficence, one of the oldest requirements for health-care providers, views the primary goal of

ISSUES IN PRACTICE

A Question of Distributive Justice

Jessica B. was diagnosed with acute lymphocytic leukemia at age 4. She is now 7 years old and has been treated with chemotherapy for the past 3 years with varying degrees of success. She is currently in a state of relapse, and a bone marrow transplant seems to be the only treatment that might improve her condition and save her life. Her father is a day laborer who has no health insurance, so Jessica's health care is being paid for mainly by the Medicaid system of her small state in the Southwest.

The current cost of a bone marrow transplant at the state's central teaching hospital is $1.5 million, representing about half of the state's entire annual Medicaid budget. Although bone marrow transplants are an accepted treatment for leukemia, this therapy offers only a slim chance for a total cure of the disease. The procedure is risky, and there is a chance that it may cause death. The procedure will involve several months of post-transplant treatment and recovery in an intensive care unit far away from the family's home and will require the child to take costly antirejection medications for many years.

The family understands the risks and benefits. They ask the nurse caring for Jessica what they should do. How should the nurse respond? Does the nurse have any obligations toward the Medicaid system as a whole?

health care as doing good for clients under their care. In general, the term *good* includes more than providing technically competent care for clients. Good care requires that the health-care provider take a holistic approach to the client, including the client's beliefs, feelings, and wishes as well as those of the client's family and significant others. The difficulty in implementing the principle of beneficence is in determining what exactly is good for another and who can best make the decision about this good.

Consider the case of the man involved in an automobile accident who ran into a metal fence pole. The pole passed through his abdomen. Even after 6 hours of surgery, the surgeon was unable to repair all the damage. The man was not expected to live for more than 12 hours. When the man came back from surgery, he had a nasogastric tube inserted, thus the physician ordered that the client should have nothing by mouth (NPO) to prevent depletion of electrolytes. Although the man was somewhat confused when he awoke postoperatively, he begged the nurse for a drink of water. He had a fever of 105.7°F. The nurse believed the physician's orders to be absolute, thus she repeatedly refused the client water. He began to yell loudly that he needed a drink of water, but the nurse still refused his requests. At one point, the nurse caught the man attempting to drink water from the icepacks that were being used to lower his fever. This continued for the full 8-hour shift until the man died.

Nonmaleficence

Nonmaleficence is the requirement that health-care providers do no harm to their clients, either intentionally or unintentionally. In a sense, it is the opposite side of the concept of beneficence, and it is difficult to speak of one term without referring to the other. In current health-care practice, the principle of nonmaleficence is often violated in the short term to produce a greater good in the long-term treatment of the client. For example, a client may undergo painful and debilitating surgery to remove a cancerous growth in order to prolong his life.

By extension, the principle of nonmaleficence also requires that health-care providers protect those from harm who cannot protect themselves. This protection from harm is particularly evident in groups such as children, the mentally incompetent, the unconscious, and those who are too weak or debilitated to protect themselves. In fact, very strict regulations have developed around situations involving child abuse and the health-care provider's obligation to report suspected child abuse. (This issue is discussed in more detail in Chapter 8.)

Veracity

Veracity is the principle of truthfulness. It requires the health-care provider to tell the truth and not to deceive or mislead clients intentionally. As with other rights and obligations, limitations to this principle exist. The primary limitation is when telling the client the truth would seriously harm (principle of nonmaleficence) the client's ability to recover or would produce greater illness. Health-care providers often feel uncomfortable giving a client bad news, and they tend to avoid answering these questions truthfully. An uncomfortable feeling is not a good enough reason to avoid telling clients the truth about their diagnosis, treatments, or prognosis. Clients have a right to know this information.

One common situation in which veracity is violated is in the use of placebo medications. At some point during their careers, most health-care providers will observe the placebo effect among some clients. Sometimes when a client is given a gel capsule filled with sugar powder and it seems to relieve the pain, this has the same effect as giving the person a narcotic, but without the side effects or potential for addiction. Of course, if the client was told that it was just a sugar pill (veracity), it would not have the same effect. How should nurses feel about this practice?

ISSUES IN PRACTICE

The nurse is caring for a critically ill client after a radical neck surgery in the surgical ICU. The client is connected to a ventilator and is on a sedation protocol with continuous IV infusion of midazolam HCl (Versed), a powerful sedative that requires constant monitoring and titration to maintain the required level of sedation. During the night shift, the nurse discovers that the medication bag is almost empty and the pharmacy, which is closed, did not send up another bag. She looks the medication up in a drug guide and proceeds to mix the drip herself. The night charge nurse was busy supervising a cardiac arrest situation out of the ICU and was unavailable to double-check how the medication was mixed.

Inadvertently, the nurse had mixed a double-strength dose of the medication. Thirty minutes after she hung the new drip, the client's blood pressure was 44/20. The client required a saline bolus and a dopamine drip to stabilize the blood pressure. The family was notified that the client had "taken a turn for the worse" and that they should come to the hospital immediately. In backtracking for the cause of the hypotension, the nurse realizes that she had mixed the sedative double-strength and reduces the rate by half.

When the family arrives, the client's blood pressure has started to return to normal. They ask the nurse what happened and why their mother was on the new IV medication. Should the family be told about the error? Who should tell them? The nurse? The physician? What approach should be used?

Source: McNutty, J: Disclosure of medical errors: An ethical dilemma. AACN News 19(3):4, 2002.

Another issue that has come into the public eye in recent months is medical errors. Some studies indicate that the incidence of medical errors in the current health-care system is extremely high and accounts for as many as 44,000 deaths per year. Nurses are often involved in these incidents. What is the nurses ethical obligation to reveal this information? Some believe that if there is no injury to clients, then the error needs not be revealed.

Consider the following case study from the view point of veracity:

> Tisha S., a senior nursing student, was acting as the team leader during her final clinical experience. Jamie D., a close friend of Tisha's, was one of three junior nursing students in Tisha's team that day. Because of some personal problems, Jamie had been late and unprepared for several clinical experiences. She was informed by her instructor that she might fail unless she showed marked improvement during clinical training.
>
> Claire, B., a 64-year-old woman with diabetes and possible renal failure, was one of Jamie's clients. Mrs. B. was having a 24-hour urine test to help determine her renal function. After the test was completed later that afternoon, she was to be discharged and treated through the renal clinic. Jamie understood the principles of the 24-hour urine test and realized that all the urine for the full 24 hours needed to be saved. But she became busy caring for another client and accidentally threw away the last specimen before the test ended. She took the specimen container to the laboratory anyway.
>
> At the end of the shift, when Jamie was giving her report to Tisha, she confided that she had thrown away the last urine specimen but begged Tisha not to tell the instructor. This mistake would mean that the test would have to be started over again, and Mrs. B. would have to spend an extra day in the hospital. Out of friendship, Tisha agreed not to tell the instructor, rationalizing that they had got almost all the urine and she was going to be treated for renal failure anyway. When the instructor asked Tisha for her final report for the day, she specifically asked if there had been any problems with the 24-hour urine test. What would be the consequences of telling the truth and of not telling the truth?

Standard of Best Interest

Standard of best interest describes a type of decision made about a client's health care when the client is unable to make the informed decision regarding his or her own care. The standard of best interest is based on what health-care providers and the family decide is best for that individual. It is very important to consider the individual client's expressed wishes, either formally in a written declaration (e.g., a living will) or informally in conversation with family members. Individuals can also legally designate a specific person to make health-care decisions for them in case they become unable to make decisions for themselves. The designated person then has what is called durable power of attorney for health care (DPOAHC). The Omnibus Budget Reconciliation Act (OBRA) of 1990 made it mandatory for all health-care facilities, such as hospitals, nursing homes, and home-health-care agencies, to provide information to clients about the living will and DPOAHC.

The standard of best interest should be based on the principle of beneficence. Unfortunately, when clients are unable to make decisions for themselves and no DPOAHC has been designated, the resolution of the dilemma can be a unilateral decision made by health-care providers. The making of a unilateral decision by health-care providers that disregards the client's wishes implies that the providers alone know what is best for the client; this is called paternalism.

Obligations

Obligations are demands made on an individual, a profession, a society, or a government to fulfill and honor the rights of others. Obligations are often divided into two categories.

Legal Obligations

Legal obligations are those that have become formal statements of law and are enforceable under the law. For instance, a nurse has a legal obligation to provide safe and adequate care for clients assigned to him or her.

Moral Obligations

Moral obligations are those based on moral or ethical principles but are not enforceable under the law. In most states, no legal obligation exists for a nurse on a vacation trip to stop and help an automobile accident victim.

> *The making of a unilateral decision by health-care providers that disregards the client's wishes implies that the providers alone know what is best for the client; this is called paternalism.*

Rights

Rights are generally defined as something owed to an individual according to just claims, legal guarantees, or moral and ethical principles. Although the term *right* is frequently used in both the legal and ethical systems, its meaning is often blurred in daily usage. Individuals sometimes mistakenly claim things as rights that are really privileges, concessions, or freedoms. Several classification systems exist in which different types of rights are delineated. The following three types of rights include the range of definitions.

Welfare Rights

Welfare rights (also called **legal rights**) are based on a legal entitlement to some good or benefit. These rights are guaranteed by laws (e.g., the **Bill of Rights** of the U.S. Constitution), and violation of such rights can be punished under the legal system. For example, citizens of the United States have a right to equal access to housing regardless of race, sexual preference, or religion.

Ethical Rights

Ethical rights (also called **moral rights**) are based on a moral or ethical principle. Ethical rights usually do not need to have the power of law in order to be enforced. Ethical rights are, in reality, often privileges allotted to certain individuals or groups of individuals. Over time, popular acceptance of ethical rights can give them the force of a legal right. An example of an ethical right in the United States is the belief in universal access to health care. In the United States, it is really a long-standing privilege, whereas in many other industrialized countries, such as Canada, Germany, Japan, and England, universal health care is a legal right.

Option Rights

Option rights are rights that are based on a fundamental belief in the dignity and freedom of humans. These are **basic human rights** that are particularly evident in free and democratic countries such as the United States and much less evident in totalitarian and restrictive societies such as Iraq. Option rights give individuals freedom of choice and the right to live their lives as they choose, but within a given set of prescribed boundaries. For example, people may wear whatever clothes they choose, as long as they wear some type of clothing.

Ethics Committees

Physicians, nurses, and other staff members often encounter ethical conflicts that they are unable to resolve on their own. In these cases, the interdisciplinary ethics committee can help the health-care provider resolve the dilemma. An increasing number of health-care facilities, particularly hospitals, have instituted ethics committees that make their consultation services available to health-care providers.

The people who belong to the ethics committee vary somewhat from one institution to another, but almost all include a physician, a member of administration, an RN, a clergy person, a philosopher with a background in ethics, a lawyer, and a person from the community. Members of ethics committees should not have any personal agenda that they are promoting and should be able to make decisions without prejudice on the basis of the situation and ethical principles.

Depending on the institution, the scope of the ethics committee's duties can range widely, from very limited activity with infrequent meetings on an ad hoc basis to active promotion of ethical thinking and decision making through educational programs. Other common functions of ethics committees include making evaluations of institutional policies in the light of ethical considerations, making recommendations about complex ethical issues, and providing education programs for medical and nursing schools as well as the community. It is extremely important that nurses participate in these committees and that the ethical concerns of the nurses are recognized and addressed.

Ethical Systems

An ethical situation exists every time a nurse interacts with a client in a health-care setting. Nurses are continually making ethical decisions in their daily practice, whether or not they recognize it. These are called normative decisions. **Normative ethics** deal with questions and dilemmas that require a choice of actions when there is a conflict of rights or obligations between the nurse and the client, the nurse and the client's family, or the nurse and the physician. In resolving these ethical questions, these nurses often use just one ethical system, or they may use a combination of several ethical systems.

The two systems that are most directly concerned with ethical decision making in the health-care professions are utilitarianism and deontology. Both apply to **bioethical issues**, the ethics of life (or, in some cases, death). *Bioethics* and *bioethical issues* are terms that are in common use. These terms have become synonymous with health-care ethics and encompass not only questions concerning life and death but also questions of quality of life, life-sustaining and life-altering technologies, and biologic science in general. It is in the context of bioethics that the following discussion of these two systems of ethics is undertaken.

Utilitarianism

Ethical Precepts

Utilitarianism (also called **teleology**, consequentialism, or situation ethics) is referred to as the ethical system of utility. As a system of normative ethics, utilitarianism defines good as happiness or pleasure. It is associated with two underlying principles: "The greatest good for the greatest number," and "The end justifies the means." Because of these two principles, utilitarianism is sometimes subdivided into act utilitarianism and rule utilitarianism. According to rule utilitarianism, the individual draws on past experiences to formulate internal rules that are useful in determining the greatest good. With act utilitarianism, the particular situation in which a nurse finds himself or herself determines the rightness or wrongness of a particular act. In practice, the true follower of utilitarianism does not believe in the validity of any system of rules because the rules can change depending on the circumstances surrounding whatever decision needs to be made.

Situation ethics is probably the most publicized form of act utilitarianism. Joseph Fletcher, one of the best-known proponents of act utilitarianism, outlines a method of ethical thinking in which the situation itself determines whether the act is morally right or wrong. Fletcher views acts as good to the extent that they promote happiness and bad to the degree that they promote unhappiness. Happiness is defined as the happiness of the greatest number of people, yet the happiness of each person is to have equal weight. Abortion, for example, is considered ethical in this system in a situation where an unwed mother on welfare with four other children becomes pregnant with her fifth child. The greatest good and the greatest amount of happiness are produced by aborting this unwanted child.

Because utilitarianism is based on the concept that moral rules should not be arbitrary but should rather serve a purpose, ethical decisions derived from a utilitarian framework weigh the effect of alternative actions that influence the overall welfare of present and future populations. As such, this system is oriented toward the good of the population in general and also toward the individual in the sense that the individual participates in that population.

Advantages

The major advantage of the utilitarian system of ethical decision making is that many individuals find it easy to use in most situations. Utilitarianism is built around an individual's needs for happiness in which the individual has an immediate and vested interest. Another advantage is that utilitarianism fits well into a society that otherwise shuns rules and regulations. A follower of utilitarianism can justify many decisions based on the happiness principle. Also, its utility orientation fits well into Western society's belief in the work ethic and a behavioristic approach to education, philosophy, and life.

The follower of utilitarianism will support a general prohibition against lying and deceiving because ultimately the results of telling the truth will lead to greater happiness than the results of lying. Yet truth telling is not an absolute requirement to the follower of utilitarianism. If telling the truth will produce widespread unhappiness for a great number of people and future generations, then it would be ethically better to tell a lie that will yield more happiness than to tell a truth that will lead to greater unhappiness. Although such behavior might appear to be unethical at first glance, the strict follower of act utilitarianism would have little difficulty in arriving at this decision as a logical conclusion of utilitarian ethical thinking.

Disadvantages

Some serious limitations exist when using utilitarianism as a system of health-care ethics or bioethics. An immediate question is whether happiness refers to the average happiness of all or the total happiness of a few. Because individual happiness is also important, one must consider how to make decisions when the individual's happiness is in conflict with that of the larger group. More fundamental is the question of what constitutes happiness. Similarly, what constitutes the greatest good for the greatest number? Who determines what is good in the first place? Is it society in general, the government, governmental policy, or the individual? In health-care delivery and the formulation of health-care policy, the general guiding principle often seems to be the greatest good for the greatest number. Yet where do minority groups fit into this system?

Also, the tenet that the ends justify the means has been consistently rejected as a rationale for justifying actions. It is generally unacceptable to allow any type of action as long as the final goal or purpose is good. The Nazis in the 1930s and 1940s used this aphorism to justify many actions that may be viewed by others to be considerably less than good.

The other difficulty in determining what is good lies in the attempt to quantify such concepts as good, harm, benefits, and greatest. This problem becomes especially acute when dealing with health-care issues that involve individuals' lives. For example, an elderly family member has been sick for a long time, and that course of illness has placed great financial hardship on the family. It would be ethical under utilitarianism to allow this client to die or even to euthanize her to relieve the financial stress created by her illness.

Utilitarianism as an ethical system in the health-care decision-making process requires use of an additional principle of distributive justice as an ultimate guiding point. Unfortunately, whenever an unchanging principle is combined with this system, it negates the basic concept of pure utilitarianism. Pure utilitarianism, although easy to use as a decision-making system, does not work well as an ethical system for decision making in health care because of its arbitrary, self-centered nature. In the everyday delivery of health care, utilitarianism is often combined with other types of ethical decision making in the resolution of ethical dilemmas.

Deontology

Ethical Precepts

Deontology is a system of ethical decision making based on moral rules and unchanging principles. This system is also termed the formalistic system, the principle system of ethics, or duty-based ethics. A follower of a pure form of the deontological system of ethical decision making believes in the ethical absoluteness of principles regardless of the consequences of the decision. Strict adherence to an ethical theory, in which the moral rightness or wrongness of human actions is considered separately from the consequences, is based on a fundamental principle called the categorical imperative. It is not the results of the act that make it right or wrong, but the principles by reason of which the act is carried out. These fundamental principles are ultimately unchanging and absolute and derived from the universal values that underlie all major religions. Focusing on a concern for right and wrong in the moral sense is the basic premise of the system. Its goal is the survival of the species and social cooperation.

Rule deontology is based on the belief that standards exist for the ethical choices and judgments made by individuals. These standards are fixed and do not change when the situation changes. Although the number of standards or rules is potentially unlimited, in reality—and particularly in dealing with bioethical issues—many of these principles can be grouped together into a few general principles. These principles can also be arranged into a type of hierarchy of rules and include such maxims as the following: People should always be treated as ends and never as means; human life has value; one is always to tell the truth; above all in health care, do no harm; humans have a right to self-determination; and all people are of equal value. These principles echo such fundamental documents as the Bill of Rights and the American Hospital Association's Patient's Bill of Rights.

Advantages

The deontological system is useful in making ethical decisions in health care because it holds that an ethical judgment based on principles will be the same in a variety of given similar situations regardless of the time, location, or particular individuals involved. In addition, deontological terminology and concepts are similar to the terms and concepts used by the legal system. The legal system emphasizes rights, duties, principles, and rules. Significant differences, however, exist between the two. Legal rights and duties are enforceable under the law, whereas ethical rights and duties are usually not. In general, ethical systems are much wider and more inclusive than the system of laws that they underlie. It is difficult to have an ethical perspective on law without having it lead to an interest in making laws that govern health care and nursing practice.

Disadvantages

The deontological system of ethical decision making is not free from imperfection. Some of the more troubling questions include the following: What do you do when the basic guiding principles conflict with each other? What is the source of the principles? Is there ever a situation where an exception to the rule will apply? Although various approaches have been proposed to circumvent these limitations, it may be difficult for nurses to resolve situations in which duties and obligations conflict, particularly when the consequences of following a rule end in harm or hurt being done to a client. In reality, there are probably few pure followers of deontology, because most people will consider the consequences of their actions in the decision making process.

Application of Ethical Theories

Ethical theories do not provide recipes for resolution of ethical dilemmas. Instead, they provide a framework for decision making that the nurse can apply to a particular ethical situation.

At times, ethical theories may seem too abstract or general to be of much use to specific ethical situations. Without them, however, ethical decisions may often be made without reasoning or forethought and may be based on personal emotions. Most nurses in attempting to make ethical decisions combine the two theories presented here.

Nursing Code of Ethics

A code of ethics is generally defined as the ethical principles that govern a particular profession. Codes of ethics are presented as general statements and thus do not give specific answers to every possible ethical dilemma that might arise. These codes do, however, offer guidance to the individual practitioner in making decisions.

Ideally, codes of ethics should be reviewed periodically to reflect necessary changes in the profession and society as a whole. Although codes of ethics are not judicially enforceable as laws, consistent violations of the code of ethics by a professional in any field may indicate an unwillingness to act in a professional manner and will often result in disciplinary actions ranging from reprimands and fines to suspension of licensure.

Although similar, there are several different codes of ethics that nurses may adopt. In the United States, the American Nurses Association (ANA) Code of Ethics is the generally accepted code. After several years of work, the ANA revised the Code of Ethics in 2001 to be more reflective of the health-care challenges in the new century (Box 7–1). There is also a Canadian Nurses Association Code of Ethics.

The ANA Code of Ethics has been acknowledged by other health-care professions as one of the most complete. It is sometimes used as the benchmark against which other codes of ethics are measured. Yet, a careful reading of this code of ethics reveals only a set of clearly stated principles that the nurse must apply to actual clinical situations. For example, the nurse involved in resuscitation will find no specific mention of **no-code orders** in the ANA Code of Ethics. Rather, the nurse must be able to apply general statements such as "The nurse . . . practices with compassion and respect for the inherent dignity, worth and uniqueness of every individual, unrestricted by considerations of social or economic status, personal attributes or the nature of health care problems" and "The nurse is responsible and accountable for individual nursing practice and determines the appropriate delegation of tasks consistent with the nurse's obligation to provide optimum patient care" to the particular situation.

The revised Code of Ethics restates and reinforces the basic values and commitments that have been and remain essential to the profession of nursing. Traditional ethical principles such as

Box 7–1

The American Nurses Association Code of Ethics

1. The nurse in all professional relationships practices with compassion and respect for the inherent dignity, worth, and uniqueness of every individual, unrestricted by considerations of social or economic status, personal attributes or the nature of health problems.
2. The nurse's primary commitment is to the patient, whether an individual, family, group or community.
3. The nurse promotes, advocates for, and strives to protect the health, safety, and rights of the patient.
4. The nurse is responsible and accountable for individual nursing practice and determines the appropriate delegation of tasks consistent with the nurse's obligation to provide optimum patient care.
5. The nurse owes the same duties to self as to others including the responsibility to preserve integrity and safety, to maintain competence, and to continue personal and professional growth.
6. The nurse participates in establishing, maintaining, and improving health care environments and conditions of employment conducive to the provision of quality health care and consistent with the values of the profession through individual and collective action.
7. The nurse participates in the advancement of the profession through contributions to practice, education, administration, and knowledge development.
8. The nurse collaborates with other health professionals and the public in promoting community, national, and international efforts to meet health needs.
9. The profession of nursing, as represented by associations and their members, is responsible for articulating nursing values, for maintaining the integrity of the profession and its practice, and for shaping social policy.

Source: Code for Nurses with Interpretive Statements, 2001; p.1.

American Nurses Publishing, American Nurses Foundation/American Nurses Association, 600 Maryland Avenue, SW, Suite 100W, Washington, DC 20024-2571, with permission.

veracity, justice, beneficence, and autonomy are re-emphasized. The nurse is still expected to practice with cooperation, wisdom, compassion, honesty, courage, and respect for the client's privacy. However, the revised code, in response to current health-care practices, defines new boundaries of duty and loyalty. Ethical challenges such as cost containment, delegation, and information technology require nurses to look at health care from new perspectives.

The revised code supports nurses in their attempts to upgrade their employment conditions and environment through measures such as collective bargaining. The revised code addresses and supports nurses who are involved in whistle-blowing when dealing with health-care team members who may be chemically impaired or otherwise incompetent in practice. It also supports nurses in their right to refuse to practice in treatments that violate the nurse's beliefs. The revised code also expands nursing duties beyond individual nurse-client interactions. It recognizes that professional nurses now work in multiple practice areas and are responsible for developing and using the knowledge used in these expanded areas through research and collaborative practice. The 2001 Code for Nurses is an important document that nurses need to be familiar with, both to help ensure ethical practice and to shape an improved future for the profession of nursing.

Decision-Making Process

Nurses, by definition, are problem solvers, and one of the important tools that nurses use is the nursing process. The nursing process is a systematic step-by-step approach to resolving problems that deal with a client's health and well-being.

Although nurses deal with problems related to the physical or psychological needs of clients, many feel inadequate when dealing with ethical problems associated with client care. Nurses in any health-care setting can, however, develop the decision-making skills necessary to make sound ethical decisions if they learn and practice using an ethical decision-making process.

An ethical decision-making process provides a method for the nurse to answer key questions about ethical dilemmas and to organize his or her thinking in a more logical and sequential manner. Although there are several ethical decision-making models, the problem-solving method presented here is based on the nursing process. It should be a relatively easy transition for the nurse to move from the nursing process used in the resolution of a client's physical problems to the ethical decision-making process for the resolution of problems with ethical ramifications.

The chief goal of the ethical decision-making process is to determine right and wrong in situations where clear demarcations are not readily apparent. This process presupposes that the nurse making the decision knows that a system of ethics exists, knows the content of that ethical system, and knows that the system applies to similar ethical decision-making problems despite multiple variables. In addition to identifying his or her own values, the nurse also needs an understanding of the possible ethical systems that may be used in making decisions about ethical dilemmas.

What Do You Think?

Think of a time when you were faced with an ethical dilemma. How did you resolve it? Did you use a decision-making process? If you did not use the decision-making process, would you have come to the same solution to the problem?

The following ethical decision-making process is presented as a tool for resolving ethical dilemmas (Fig. 7–1).

Step 1: Collect, Analyze, and Interpret the Data

Obtain as much information as possible concerning the particular ethical dilemma. Unfortunately, such information is sometimes very limited. Among the issues important to know are the client's wishes, the client's family's wishes, the extent of the physical or emotional problems causing the dilemma, the physician's beliefs about health care, and the nurse's own orientation to issues concerning life and death.

Many nurses, for example, face the question of whether or not to initiate resuscitation efforts when a terminally ill client is admitted to the hospital. Physicians often leave instructions for the nursing staff indicating that the nurses really should not resuscitate the client but should, instead, merely go through the motions to make the family feel better, which is sometimes referred to as a **slow-code order**. The nurse's dilemma is whether to make a serious attempt to revive the client or to let the client die quietly.

Important information that will help the nurse to make the decision might include:

- The mental competency of the client to make a no-resuscitation decision
- The client's desires
- The family's feelings
- Whether the physician previously sought input from the client and the family
- Whether there is a living will or DPOAHC

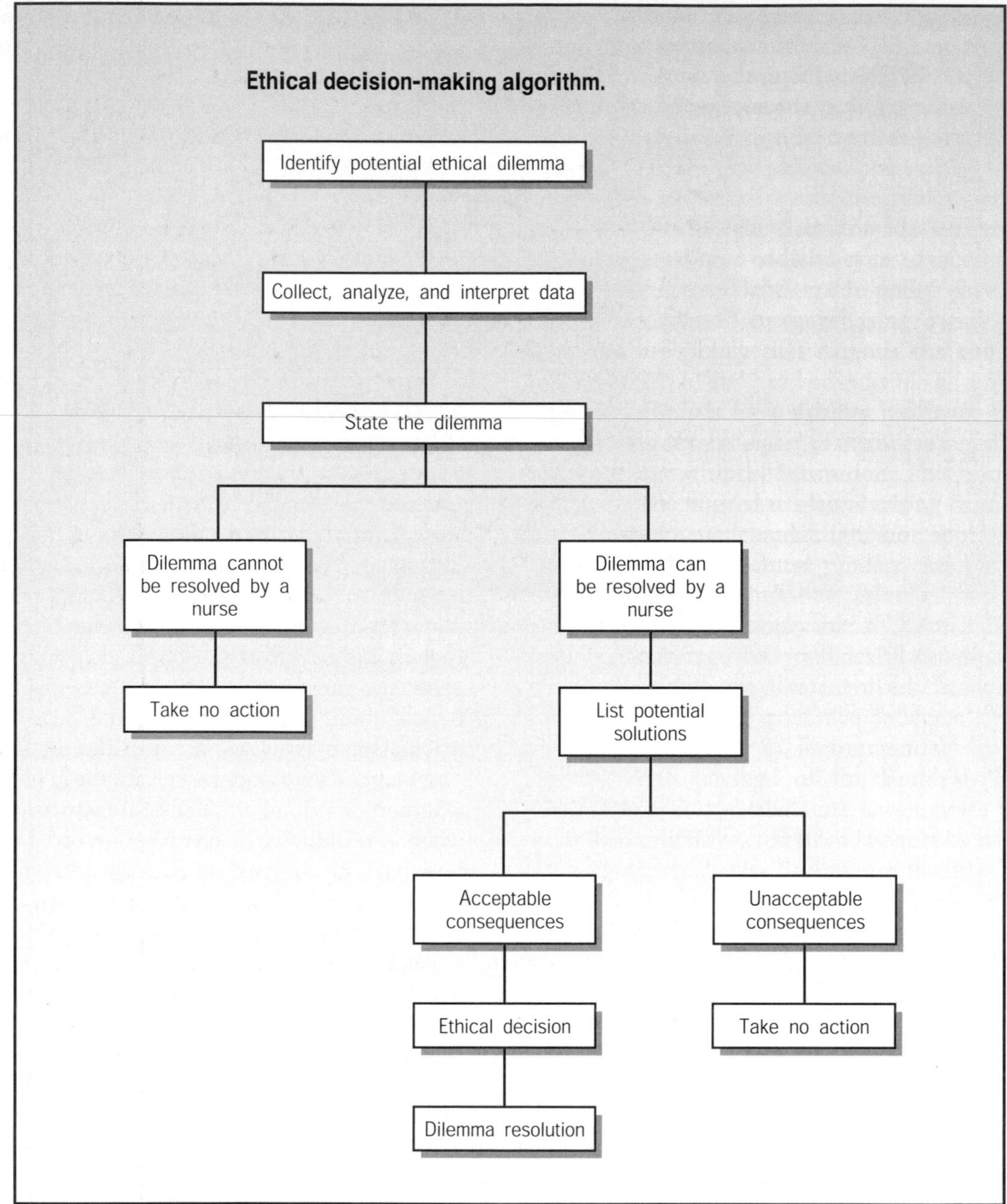

Figure 7–1. Ethical decision-making algorithm. (Adapted from Catalano, JT: Ethical decision making in the critical care patient. Crit Care Nurs Clin North Am 9(1):45–52, 1997.)

Many institutions have policies concerning no-resuscitation orders, and it is wise to consider these during data collection. After collecting information, the nurse needs to bring the pieces of information together in a manner that will give the clearest and sharpest focus to the dilemma.

Step 2: State the Dilemma

After collecting and analyzing as much information as is available, the nurse then needs to state the dilemma as clearly as possible. In this step, it is important to identify whether the problem is one that directly involves the nurse or is one that can be resolved only by the client, the client's family, the physician, or the DPOAHC.

Recognizing the key aspects of the dilemma helps focus attention on the important ethical principles. Most of the time, the dilemma can be reduced to a few statements that encompass the key ethical issues. Such ethical issues often involve a question of conflicting rights, obligations, or basic ethical principles.

In the case of a no-resuscitation order, the statement of the dilemma might be: "The client's right to death with dignity versus the nurse's obligation to preserve life and do no harm." In general, the principle that the competent client's wishes must be followed is unequivocal. If the client has become unresponsive before expressing his or her wishes, then the family members' input must be given serious consideration. Additional questions can arise if the family's wishes conflict with those of the client.

Step 3: Consider the Choices of Action

After stating the dilemma as clearly as possible, the next step is to attempt to list, without consideration of their consequences, all possible courses of action that can be taken to resolve the dilemma. This brainstorming activity in which all possible courses of action are considered may require input from outside sources such as colleagues, supervisors, or even experts in the ethical field. The consequences of the different actions are considered later in this chapter.

Some possible courses of action for the nurse in the resuscitation scenario might include the following:

- Resuscitating the client to the nurse's fullest capabilities despite what the physician has requested
- Not resuscitating the client at all
- Only going through the motions without any real attempt to revive the client
- Seeking another assignment so as to avoid dealing with the situation
- Reporting the problem to a supervisor
- Attempting to clarify the question with the client
- Attempting to clarify the question with the family
- Confronting the physician about the question
- Consulting the institution's ethics committee

For nurses who are unsure about which issues can be referred to the ethics committee, the facility's policy and procedure manual can give direction.

Step 4: Analyze the Advantages and Disadvantages of Each Course of Action

Some of the courses of action developed during the previous step are more realistic than others. The identification of these actions becomes readily evident during this step in the decision-making process, when the advantages and the disadvantages of each action are considered in detail. Along with each option, the consequences of taking each course of action must be thoroughly evaluated.

Consider whether initiating discussion might anger the physician or cause distrust of the nurse involved. Both these responses may reinforce the attitude of submission to the physician, and either could make continuing to practice nursing at that institution difficult. The same result might occur if the nurse successfully resuscitates a client despite orders to the contrary. Failure to resuscitate the client has the potential to produce a lawsuit unless a clear order for no resuscitation has been given. Presenting the situation to a supervisor may, if the supervisor supports the physician, cause the nurse to be considered a troublemaker and thus have a negative effect on future evaluations. The same process could be applied to the other courses of action.

When considering the advantages and disadvantages, the nurse should be able to narrow the realistic choices of action. Other relevant issues need to be examined when weighing the choices of action. A major factor would be choosing the appropriate code of ethics. The ANA Code of Ethics should be part of many client-care decisions affected by ethical dilemmas.

Step 5: Make the Decision and Act on It

The most difficult part of the process is actually making the decision, following through with action, and then living with the consequences. Decisions are often made with no follow-through, because nurses are fearful of the consequences of their decisions. By their nature, ethical dilemmas produce differences of opinion and not everyone will be pleased with the decision.

In the attempt to solve any ethical dilemma, there will always be a question of the correct course of action. The client's wishes almost always supersede independent decisions on the part of health-care professionals. A collaborative decision made by the client, physician, nurses, and family about resuscitation is the ideal situation and tends to produce fewer complications in the long-term resolution of such questions.

Conclusion

Ethical dilemmas, by definition, are difficult to resolve. Rarely will a nurse find ethical dilemmas covered in policy, procedure, and protocol manuals; but nurses can develop the skills necessary to make appropriate ethical decisions. The key to developing these skills is the recognition and frequent use of an ethical decision-making model and application of the appropriate ethical theories to the dilemma. As an orderly approach in solving the often disorderly aspects of ethical questions encountered in nursing practice, the decision-making model presented in this chapter can be applied to almost every type of ethical dilemma. Although each situation is different, ethical decision making based on ethical theory can provide a potent tool for resolving dilemmas found in client-care situations.

Critical Thinking Exercises

1. Compare and contrast ethics with laws by delineating the purposes, scopes, and methods of enforcement of each.
2. Distinguish between the two types of obligations.
3. Compare the three categories of rights.
4. Analyze the following ethical dilemma case study using the ethical decision-making process:

- What are the important data in relation to this situation?
- State the ethical dilemma in a clear, simple statement.
- What are the choices of action and how do they relate to specific ethical principles?
- What are the consequences of these actions?
- What decision can be made?

Bill L., a veteran emergency room (ER) nurse, called the resident physician about a client just admitted to the ER after a fall from a ladder. The client, a 52-year-old man, had been fixing his roof when the accident occurred. He had suffered a minor head injury, a twisted ankle, and a badly bruised arm. He also had a long history of asthma and heavy smoking. Not long after his admission to the ER, the client became cyanotic, dyspneic, and semiconscious. By the time the resident physician arrived, the nurse had prepared the client for endotracheal intubation and had already notified the personnel in the medical intensive care unit (MICU) that they would be receiving this client.

After a hasty evaluation of the client, the resident decided to perform an emergency tracheostomy before transporting the client to the MICU. While performing the tracheostomy, the physician severed a major blood vessel and the client hemorrhaged profusely. After several tense minutes, the endotracheal tube was inserted, and the client was quickly transported to the MICU. The client remained cyanotic and had great difficulty breathing. Shortly after leaving the ER, the nurse realized that the oxygen tank that the client had been connected to was empty. The client never regained consciousness and died 3 days after admission. His death was due to respiratory failure and not to the injuries sustained in the fall.

When the client's wife came to the unit to collect the deceased's belongings, the nurse was torn between telling her about the mistakes that were made in the treatment of her husband and remaining silent. What are the key ethical principles involved in this situation? Are there any statements in the ANA Code of Ethics that may help resolve this dilemma? What would be the consequences of informing the client's wife of the truth? What are the consequences of not informing her?

References

1. Esterhuizen, P, and Kooyuman, A: Empowering moral decision making in nurses. Nurse Education Today 21(8):640–647, 2001.
2. Spangler, C: New Code of Ethics for Nurses. Maryland Nurse 3(3):31, 2001.

Bibliography

Aston, S: Ethics of intensive care admission: Using a decision analysis model. Nursing in Critical Care 6(2):71–75, 2001.

Austin, W: Nursing ethics in an era of globalization. ANS Adv Nurs Sci 24(2):32–46, 2001.

Bjarnascon, D, and Lehman, C: Ethical issues from critical care to rehabilitation: A challenge for specialty nurses. Crit Care Clin North Am 13(3):341–347, 2001.

Chinn, PL: Nursing and ethics: The maturing of a discipline. ANS Adv Nurs Sci 24(2):32–36, 2001.

Elliott, AC: Health care ethics: Cultural relativity of autonomy. Journal of Transcultural Nursing 12(4):326–330, 2001.

Engelhardt, HT, and Cherry, MJ: Allocating Scarce Resources. Georgetown University Press, Baltimore, 2002.

Geyer, N: Ethics and law. Nursing Update 25(7):20, 2001.

Gregory Dawes, BS: Establishing ethical practices and eliminating the "gray." AORN J 74(4):456, 458, 2001.

Irving, JA, and Sniper, J: Preserving professional ethics. J Prof Nurs 18(1):5, 2002.

Kinsella, L: Truth telling in patient care. Nursing 2001 31(12):52–55, 2001.

McNulty, J: Disclosure of medical errors: An ethical dilemma. AACN News 19(3):4, 2002.

8

Bioethical Issues

Joseph T. Catalano

Learning Objectives

After completing this chapter, the reader will be able to:

- Discuss the key ethical principles involved in:
  - Abortion
  - Genetic research
  - Fetal tissue research
  - Organ transplantation
  - Use of scarce resources
  - Assisted suicide
  - Acquired immunodeficiency syndrome (AIDS)
  - Children
- Discuss the nurse's role in these ethical dilemmas.
- Analyze and make a thoughtful ethical decision in a complex situation.

In the recent history of nursing, numerous biomedical and ethical dilemmas have arisen. Historically, nurses have been concerned with moral responsibility and ethical decision making. The nursing code of ethics and its frequent revisions demonstrate the profession's concern with providing ethical health care. The earliest codes of ethics made obedience to the physician the nurse's primary responsibility. The present code of ethics recognizes that the primary responsibility of the nurse is the client's well-being. This change in emphasis reflects the profession's increased self-awareness, independence, and growing accountability for its actions. Unfortunately, this new attitude has also heralded an era of increased tension, self-doubt, and ethical confusion. By examining the issues and identifying the key moral and ethical conflicts, nurses will be able to accept their moral responsibilities and make good ethical decisions.

In the course of their careers, nurses are likely to face ethical dilemmas. Although a complete analysis of every issue is beyond the scope of this book, some of the more common situations and their important ethical features are presented as examples of ways to analyze such dilemmas and to make informed decisions. The resolution of ethical dilemmas is never an easy task, and it is likely that someone may disagree with the decision.

Abortion

Few issues evoke as strong an emotional reaction as abortion. Because of its religious, ethical, social, and legal implications, the abortion issue touches everyone in one way or another. There seems

What Do You Think?

Do you support or reject elective abortion? On what ethical principles do you base your belief? What advice would you give to a pregnant teenager who wanted to have an abortion?

to be very little "middle ground." People are either strongly in favor of abortion or oppose it completely.

Elective abortion is the voluntary termination of a pregnancy before 24 weeks of gestation. An elective abortion may be either therapeutic or self-selected. Strictly speaking, a therapeutic abortion would be one performed in consultation with and on the recommendation of a physician or psychiatrist, based on the conclusion that the mother's health or psychological state would be damaged without the abortion. Self-selected abortions are those performed solely on the mother's own decision, without consultation with a physician or psychiatrist, usually for economic or convenience reasons. In the case of *Roe v. Wade* in 1973, the Supreme Court changed the legal status of elective abortion in the United States, but the ethical basis and moral status of this decision remain controversial.

A careful reading of the court's decision in *Roe v. Wade* reveals that the justices made no decision about the ethics or morality of elective abortion. Rather, the court said that, according to the U.S. Constitution, all people have a right to determine what they can do with their bodies (i.e., the right to self-determination) and that such a right includes termination of a pregnancy.

The fundamental issues at the heart of the abortion debate center on the right of freedom of choice, which the court recognized, and the question of when life begins. Those who argue against abortion believe that life begins at the moment of conception and therefore hold that abortion is an act of killing. Proponents of abortion argue that the fetus is not really human until it reaches the point of development when it can live outside the mother's body (i.e., the age of viability). From a deontological standpoint, abortion represents a basic conflict of rights.

On one hand, a woman's rights to privacy, self-determination, and freedom of choice are at issue. In the United States, these rights are fiercely held and are considered to be issues of public policy and **constitutional law**. Indeed, these rights form the basis of the *Roe v. Wade* decision.

The conflicting right from the antiabortion side of the dilemma is the fetus's right to life. In most Western civilizations, particularly those that are based on Judeo-Christian beliefs, the casual and intentional taking of a human life is strongly prohibited. Life is the most basic good, because without it there can be no other rights. In general, the right to life is considered to be the most profound of the rights and is absolute in most situations.

When one is attempting to resolve the ethics and morality of abortion, these two conflicting rights need to be weighed against each other. Nurses are often placed in situations where they must help clients make decisions about abortion. Just as frequently, they are asked to participate in the procedure itself. In practice, ethical issues are always affected by the health-care provider's moral values. In the dilemma over abortion, nurses must analyze their own values and perceptions of their roles in order to make the best decisions. As a client **advocate**, should a nurse be for or against abortion? How can a nurse avoid influencing the woman's decision about abortion? Can a nurse ethically and legally refuse to assist at abortions? Ought the client's reason for wanting an abortion or her stage of pregnancy (first or second trimester, or later, requiring a partial-birth procedure) have any influence on the nurse's decision? These questions are not easily answered, but understanding the underlying principles involved in the issue may help to defuse some of the emotional impact that often surrounds this topic. As in all complicated ethical dilemmas, the nurse needs to remember that the client must receive competent, high-quality care regardless of the nurse's own personal values or moral beliefs.

Genetics and Genetic Research

The ability to alter genetic material in such a way as to produce organisms that differ greatly from their original form is now a reality. Scientific and popular literature is filled with reports of new ways to identify and change the genetic material of all types of living creatures. Currently, genetically altered bacteria (e.g., *Escherichia coli*) are used to produce various medications, including a purer form of insulin. Genetically altered corn is now growing in very hot, dry places and is resistant to most insects. Abnormal genes that indicate individuals who are at risk for various types of cancer, Alzheimer's disease, Parkinson's disease, and Down syndrome have been identified.

In the twentieth century, society became so accustomed to the idea that science should be allowed to do whatever it is capable of doing that very few questions have been asked about the ethics of genetic engineering and research. As with most scientific research and techniques, the techniques of genetic engineering are ethically neutral. Procedures such as refining recombinant DNA, gene therapy, altering germ cells, and cloning other cells, in themselves, are neither good nor bad. The potential for misuse of these procedures is so great, however, that it may permanently alter or even destroy the human race.

> *In the twentieth century, society became so accustomed to the idea that science should be allowed to do whatever it is capable of doing that very few questions have been asked about the ethics of genetic engineering and research.*

Several ethical issues need to be considered when genetic engineering and research are being conducted, including those involving the safety of genetic research, the legality and morality of genetic screening, and the proper use of genetic information. Recently proposed laws attempt to regulate genetic research to prevent the production of a supervirus or superbacteria that could exterminate the entire human population.[1]

With current technology, it is possible to detect genetic patterns in newborn infants that are linked to breast and colon cancer, heart disease, Huntington's disease, and Parkinson's disease. The advantage to insurance companies, which could screen individuals as early as infancy for costly and potentially lethal diseases later in life, is obvious: These individuals could be excluded from health and life insurance coverage, thus saving the insurance companies a great deal of money. Although this practice would most likely be unethical, the concept of mandatory genetic screening is not unrealistic. Because it requires just one blood sample from a person at some point during that person's life, it is possible that this type of screening could even be done without the individual's knowledge or consent.

Informed consent is permission granted by a person based on full knowledge of the risks and benefits of what is being done. The basic question is: Do parents violate the right of informed consent if they give permission to have gene testing performed on their newborn and have the results released to an insurance company? Do insurance companies violate informed consent if they somehow obtain the information without the knowledge of the client. (Informed consent is discussed in detail in Chapter 9.)

Similarly, confidentiality is at great risk of being violated by genetic screening. The confidentiality, trust, and fidelity that exist between the health-care provider and the client have been the basis of the therapeutic relationship. Information obtained through genetic screening can be used to benefit clients and to prepare them for

What Do You Think?

Do you support genetic research? What restrictions, if any, would you place on this type of research? Are these restrictions plausible or enforceable?

future problems, or it can be released to insurance companies to give them grounds for refusal of coverage. In some cases, individuals may be denied employment based on the results of genetic testing. In this time of the information superhighway and vast computerized databases, very little of a client's health history remains confidential.[2]

An important ethical implication for nurses is the emotional impact that genetic information may have on the client. Knowledge of the possible long-term outcome of one's health, particularly if that knowledge is negative, may cause a client **anxiety**, or the person may become depressed or suicidal. Nurses must further hone their teaching and counseling skills to assist clients in dealing with implications of this type of information.

Obstetric nurses have been involved with genetic screening procedures for years. Some of the most important information obtained from amniocentesis deals with the genetic composition of the fetus. It is important that the mother understand the procedure and the type of information it may yield and also that she gives informed consent for this procedure.

A strict ethical obligation exists for nurses to refuse to participate in mandatory, involuntary screening programs as well as a strict prohibition about revealing genetic test results to unauthorized individuals. Forcing clients to be tested who are strongly opposed to finding out information about their genetic status is clearly a breach of those clients' right to self-determination. However, much as the current practice of routine screening for diseases such as tuberculosis, hepatitis, and blood lead levels promotes the general health of the population, so does the screening for genetic diseases. Clients who are strongly opposed to such genetic screening must be allowed the option to refuse it to maintain their right to self-determination.

Now that the human genome has been decoded, a whole new world of possibilities—both positive and negative—have been opened for health-care providers. The impact of the Human Genome Project, cloning research, and other related genetic procedures is on a par with the discovery of bacteria and antibiotics. The potential for the cure of almost all known diseases, ranging from viral infections to cancer to the regeneration of spinal cord nerves, is now possible. On the other side, there is the potential for the development of superviruses that could potentially wipe out the population of the earth. Nurses need to watch each development very closely and call their legal representatives when they believe science is moving into dangerous areas.[3]

Use of Fetal Tissue

Fetal tissue research has been conducted since at least the early 1990s. Traditional fetal tissue research has been generally limited to taking living cells from an aborted fetus and transplanting them into people who have chronic or severe diseases. The procedure has been found to be helpful to a limited extent in the treatment of Alzheimer's disease and Parkinson's disease.

During 1997 to 2000, the Human Genome Project has added a new twist to this research. Rather than using tissue from aborted fetuses, scientists are now growing their own fetal tissue in the laboratory through **artificial insemination** and in vitro fertilization procedures. These test-tube fetuses are then dissected. Various fetal tissues are used for genetic and other types of research. The legal system has become aware of abuses of these procedures and has proposed legislation to control their use, including limiting the age of in vitro fetuses to 6 weeks. After 6 weeks, such fetuses will have to be destroyed.

Stem cell research is a closely related issue. Stem cells are the very early cells present in the developing fetus that have not yet begun to differentiate; that is, all the cells are identical and contain all the genetic material needed to reproduce an identical individual. Stem cells can be separated and then placed in an environment where they will form more stem cells; or the genetic material from the stem cell can be removed and replaced; or the genetic material can be removed, manipulated, and then replaced. Administrative decisions have allowed stem cell research on a limited basis.

Like stem cells, fetal tissue is highly desirable for research and transplantation because it lacks some of the genetic material that makes more mature tissues and organs more likely to cause rejection in the host. These fetal tissues are also in a rapid growth mode and naturally develop more quickly than do tissues from other sources. Scientists involved in this research see fetal tissue as one of the most important means of curing diseases.

Yet, even a superficial consideration of these procedures necessarily raises many important ethical issues. Basic to the ethics of this type of research is the source of the research material. In the past, most of the material came from elective abortions. Because of the immaturity and lack of differentiation of cells during the first trimester of pregnancy, however, the best fetal tissue comes from fetuses aborted during the second trimester. Most scientists agree that second-trimester fetuses have well-developed nervous, cardiovascular, gastrointestinal, and renal systems and are capable of feeling pain. Even though fetal tissue research has not led to an increase in abortions, the potential for abuse is tremendous.

It is also not definite whether the fetal tissue research scientists are paying others for these aborted fetuses. If payment is being made for aborted fetuses, it would seem to violate both the laws that prevent payment for organs used in transplantation and the moral respect for humanity. Questions also arise concerning who is giving permission for the use of fetuses in transplantation procedures. Does anyone really own them?

Another important ethical issue concerns the use of in vitro fertilization as a source for fetal tissue. Many religious groups question the morality of the procedure itself. Even if in vitro fertilization is considered ethical for procedures such as surrogate motherhood, is it ethical to create fetuses that are going to be used only for research and transplantation? From whom are the ova and sperm coming? Have the people from whom these have been obtained given permission for such use of their tissues? What about the rights of a fetus who was created in a test tube without ever having a hope of a normal life?

The 1988 directive, which was extended indefinitely in 1990, to prevent the Department of Health and Human Services from using federal money for fetal tissue research, was amended in 2001 to allow this type of research on a very limited basis with federal funding. Local biomedical ethical panels can make decisions about this type of research. Many of these panels, which consist mainly of research scientists, have ruled in favor of continuing research.

Nurses may have an important role to play in issues involving fetal tissue research. Although they will not likely be involved directly in research itself, nurses are often employed in facilities where elective abortions are performed. Nurses employed in such places must become aware of the issues involved in abortion. They also should know where the aborted fetuses are taken and how they are disposed of. Nurses should also remain informed about developing procedures and techniques regarding fetal tissue research; they should support legal and ethical efforts to control its abuses.

Organ Transplantation

Despite widespread public and medical acceptance of organ transplantation as a highly beneficial procedure, ethical questions still remain. Whenever a human organ is transplanted, many people are involved, including the donor, the donor's family, medical and nursing personnel, and the recipient and his or her family. Society in general could also be added to this group, because of the high cost of organ transplantation, which is usually paid from tax money directly or indirectly in the form of increased insurance premiums. Each one of these persons or groups has rights that may conflict with the rights of others.

Currently, the two primary sources for organ and tissue donations are living related donors and

cadaver donors. Most institutions that perform transplants or organizations that are involved in obtaining organs and tissues have developed elaborate procedures to help deal with the ethical and legal issues involved in transplantation. Despite these efforts, some ethical uncertainties remain whenever the issue of organ transplantation is raised. One particularly sensitive issue is exemplified when a child donates an organ, for example, a kidney transplant for a sibling, a procedure that poses some risk. Although parents are usually required to give consent for medical procedures for their children, by legal definition, a child younger than 18 years of age cannot give informed consent to such a procedure. It can be argued, however, that ethically the donor child, as a participant, should have input in making such a decision. At what age can a child have a say in the decision? Can a child be forced, for example, to donate a kidney even if he or she refuses? (See the discussion of children's ethics later in this chapter.)

One situation that illustrates this dilemma is that of a teenage girl who developed leukemia. The only way to save her life was to find a bone marrow donor who matched her genetic type. When no donor could be found, the parents decided to have another baby in the hope that the bone marrow of the second child would match that of the first child. After the baby was born, it was found that the bone marrow did indeed match, and when the child was old enough to donate safely, the bone marrow was taken and transplanted into the older child.

Despite the best efforts of the medical and legal community to establish criteria for death, some ethical questions still linger about what constitutes death. Because organs such as the heart, lungs, and liver need to come from a donor whose heart is still beating, some clinicians fear that there will be a tendency for physicians to declare that a person is dead before death actually occurs. The most widely accepted criterion for death is **brain death**. Some researchers, however, question whether the death of the brain actually means that a person ceases to exist as a human. Are there some other criteria that ought to be examined in conjunction with brain death?

One of the most difficult ethical issues involved in organ transplantation is the selection of recipients. Because fewer organs are available than the numerous people who need them, the potential ethical dilemmas are great. The **Uniform Anatomical Gift Act** was passed to increase the supply of organs for donation and attempt to reduce some of the confusion over organ donation. The national organ recipient list attempts to list and rank all people who need organs in a nondiscriminatory manner. Some important criteria for ranking include need, length of time on the list, potential for survival, prior organ transplantation, value to the community, and tissue compatibility.

Nurses can be, and often are, involved in some aspect of the organ donation process. Many states have passed laws that require the health-care workers to ask the family members of potential organ donors whether they have ever thought about their dead or dying loved one being used for organ donation (Box 8–1). Many nurses, particularly nurses who work in critical care units, provide care for clients who may potentially become organ donors. Nurses in operating rooms may help in the actual surgical procedures that remove organs from a cadaver and transplant them into a recipient's body. Other nurses provide the postoperative care for clients who have received a transplanted organ. Home-health-care nurses give the follow-up care to such clients at home.

Nurses working with organ transplantation need to be sensitive to the potential for manipulation. Most people who are seeking organ transplantations are desperately ill or near death. They and their families can be very easily manipulated or can themselves become very manipulative. On the other side, the families of potential organ donors are usually distraught about the sudden and traumatic loss of a loved one. They too are vulnerable to psychological manipulation. Because of the emotionally fragile state present in the family of a trauma victim, they are vulnerable to guilt and grief. Health-care providers should avoid appealing to these

Box 8–1

Organ Donation

Seven Questions That Families Often Ask About Organ Donation and How You Should Answer Them

Many families refuse to donate a loved one's organs simply because they do not fully understand organ donation. By being prepared to address their concerns, you can help them make a decision they are comfortable with.

Here are the most common questions families ask about organ donation. Review them along with the answers so that you are prepared the next time that you need to counsel a family on this sensitive issue.

1. *Whose consent is needed to allow organ donation?*
   Consent must come from the patient's legal next of kin, even if the patient has a signed donor card or an organ donation sticker on his or her driver's license.
2. *How can you ask us to make this decision at such a tragic time?*
   "I know that this is a very stressful time for you, but I need to ask that you think about organ donation. Is it what your loved one would have wanted?"
   "I understand that you may not be able to say yes right now, and that's okay. However, if you decide to donate, we need to know as soon as possible so that any tissues or organs may be removed in time to help another person."
3. *What does brain death mean?*
   Brain death is an irreversible condition that occurs when blood no longer flows to the brain and the brain tissue dies. Although the brain is dead, other organs and tissues can function if supported by artificial means. A doctor will pronounce brain death only after everything possible has been done for your loved one and there is no chance of survival.
4. *Is the body disfigured when the organs are removed?*
   Surgeons use as few incisions as possible to recover the donated organs or tissues. Donation shouldn't interfere with an open casket funeral, if that's what you have planned.
5. *Will we be charged for donation costs?*
   No. All costs related to removal of the organs are covered by the donor program. However, you'll still be responsible for the funeral, burial arrangements, and related costs.
6. *How are recipients chosen?*
   Recipients are chosen from the United Network of Organ Sharing, a national computer registry. They're selected according to degree of need, how long they've been on the waiting list, and certain medical criteria, such as blood type compatibility, tissue matching, and body size.
7. *We're not sure if our religion allows organ donation. What should we do?*
   Many religions support organ donation; but if you're concerned, speak with your religious leader.

Teresa M. Odell, RN
Coordinator, Nursing Staff Education
Cobb Hospital and Medical Center
Kennesaw, GA

Source: Odell, TM: Organ donation. What families need to know. Nursing 94 December 1994, p. 321, with permission.

emotions when obtaining permission to harvest organs for transplantation.

As a general rule, neither the donor nor his or her family should play any part in the selection of a recipient. Nurses need to avoid making statements or giving nonverbal indications of their approval or disapproval of potential recipients.

Use of Scarce Resources in Prolonging Life

In these days of restructuring and downsizing, money for health care is in short supply. It is recognized that most public money allocated for health care is spent during the last year of life for many elderly clients. Expensive procedures, therapies, technologies, and care are provided to terminally ill individuals to extend their lives by a few days or even a few hours. It is not unusual to spend as much as $5000 a day on a client receiving care in an intensive care unit.

The traditional belief has been that life should be preserved at all cost and by any means available. Health-care providers feel uncomfortable when cost considerations are mentioned regarding treatments for terminally ill clients. Yet, in the context of current problems in society, such considerations are both economic and ethical realities. The necessity of conserving resources has forced society, through governmental action, to face this issue. All the currently proposed health-care plans take into consideration some type of cost-control measures related to restricting payment for client care. In addition, the **hospice care** movement and a growing number of physicians and other health-care professionals support **palliative** care for the terminally ill that provides pain relief and comfort measures but does not try to prolong the person's life.

In reality, the current health-care system is already rationing care to some degree. Many people who are not covered by health-care insurance do not seek health care. Groups such as the poor, who are covered by massive governmental programs, shy away from seeking health care because of the numerous restrictions placed on it. Individuals who are covered by insurance often have restrictions placed on them by the insurance companies.

A highly controversial procedure is tube feedings. It is a relatively simple procedure that is used in all areas of health care, from feeding premature infants in the neonatal intensive care unit to maintaining the elderly postoperative client at home under the supervision of home-health-care staff. Additionally, it is a way of maintaining nutrition and hydration, two of the most basic needs of life. Nurses who work with terminally ill clients often believe that once a feeding tube has been inserted, it cannot be removed for any reason because that would constitute active euthanasia, or mercy killing. But is that belief justified in all circumstances? Consider the following scenario:

> Her large family—consisting of her husband of many years, three sons, and two daughters—were very upset. Mrs. Ada Floral, 82 years old, had just suffered a massive stroke that rendered her unresponsive. Although she was breathing on her own, she had no voluntary movements and seemed to be completely paralyzed. Magnetic resonance imaging (MRI) showed a large area of bleeding around the midbrain and brain stem. Her pupils were constricted and unresponsive. The physician explained that the prognosis was extremely grave, and the likelihood of Mrs. Floral's survival was minimal.
>
> However, the family members all agreed that "everything" should be done, so the physician reluctantly initiated aggressive medical therapy with IV glucocorticoids, osmotic diuretics, antihypertensives, and physical therapy. After a week, there was no change. The family wondered whether Mrs. Floral might be "starving to death" and asked the physician to have a feeding tube inserted and feedings started.
>
> One month later, the still unresponsive Mrs. Floral is being cared for at home by her family with the supervision of the local hospice/home-health-care program. She is off all IV medications; however, she is receiving

some medications, a commercially prepared feeding, and water through the feeding tube. Some of the family members are beginning to question whether they did the right thing by insisting that everything be done and wish to remove the feeding tube so that Mrs. Floral could die a peaceful and dignified death, rather than just hanging on for months. Other family members feel that if they give permission for the tube's removal, they would be killing their mother and could not live with the guilt.

The hospice nurse in charge of the case had discussed the issue with the family. She too believes that once a feeding tube has been placed, it should not be removed, even if all the family agrees on its removal. She feels that it's not an issue a family can "just change their minds about." Although she is in frequent contact with Mrs. Floral's physician, she has not mentioned that the family is thinking about removing the feeding tube in fear that the physician might agree.

Is the hospice nurse correct in her belief about the removal of the feeding tube? When do tube feedings stop being beneficial to clients? Is there a right to death with dignity? What ethical rationales could be used for removal of the feeding tube in this case?

The use of public funds for health care is an ethical issue that revolves around the principle of distributive justice. In this context, distributive justice requires that all citizens have equal access to all types of health care, regardless of their income levels, race, sex, religious beliefs, or diagnosis. Many complex issues are involved in this dilemma.

These issues go far beyond the questions of who gets what type of care and where and how the care takes place. Some type of **universal health-care coverage** is likely to be mandated for all Americans sometime in the future. Is it fair that some individuals (taxpayers) pay for the health care of others? Should individuals who contribute to their own poor state of health by smoking, drinking, taking illicit drugs, or overeating be provided with the same type of care as those who do not put themselves at risk? And who is going to make the decisions about who gets expensive treatment such as organ transplantations, experimental medications, placement in intensive care units, or life-extending technologies?

The use of criteria such as age, potential for a high-quality life, and availability of resources for determining who receives life-extending technologies is gaining wider acceptance. But is this a valid ethical position? Nurses are often involved in situations in which terminally ill clients are brought to the hospital for end-of-life care. Nurses need to play an active role in helping to formulate policies concerning the issues that they face daily.

The Right to Die

The right-to-die issue is an extension of the right to self-determination issue discussed in Chapter 9. It also overlaps with the dilemma of **euthanasia** and assisted suicide. Health-care providers often become involved in the decision-making process when clients are irreversibly comatose, vegetative, or suffering from a terminal disease. The choices that the families of such clients often face are death or the extension of life using painful and expensive treatments.

One of the difficulties in resolving right-to-die issues is understanding the terminology used. Often a client who has a living will states that he or she wants no extraordinary treatments if he or she should become comatose or unable to make decisions involving health care. But what actually constitutes extraordinary treatments? A general definition of ordinary treatments includes any medications, procedures, surgeries, or technologies that offer the client some hope of benefit without causing excessive pain or suffering.[4] Using this definition, extraordinary treatments (sometimes called heroic measures) become those treatments, medications, surgeries, and technologies that offer little hope for curing or improving the client's condition. Although these general definitions provide some guidelines for making decisions about ordinary and extraordinary treatments, discerning the nature of the specific modalities remains difficult. For example, a ventilator is a machine that assists a client's breathing. In intensive care units (ICUs), it is a common mode of treatment for many types of clients, including postoperative clients, clients with cardiac and respiratory diseases, and victims of trauma. Does its widespread and frequent use make the ventilator an ordinary mode of treatment? Many would say yes, whereas others would say it is still extraordinary because of its invasive nature and complicated technology.

Another issue often included in the right-to-die debate is that of codes and "do-not-resuscitate" (DNR or no code) orders. Cardiopulmonary resuscitation (CPR) is widely taught to both health-care providers and the general public. It is often used to treat clients who have suffered heart attacks and have gone into cardiac arrest as well as clients suffering from electrical shock, drowning, and traumatic injuries. In the hospital setting, the nursing staff is obligated to perform CPR on all clients who do not have a specific DNR order. This leads to situations in which terminally ill clients may be subjected to CPR efforts several times before they die.[5]

Advance directives, in the form of a living will or durable power of attorney, can and should specify which extraordinary procedures, surgeries, medications, or treatments can or cannot be used.

Advance Directives

As an issue of self-determination, it is essential that the client's wishes about health care be followed. All client communication to the nurse about desires for future care should be documented. If at all possible, the client should be encouraged to designate an individual to act as a moral surrogate, a designated decision maker, should the client become unable to make his or her own decisions. The expressed desires about future medical care are known as advance directives. They are the best means to guarantee that a client's wishes will be honored.

Advance directives, in the form of a living will or durable power of attorney, can and should specify which extraordinary procedures, surgeries, medications, or treatments can or cannot be used. These directives are often in the form of formal documents that need to be witnessed by two individuals who are not related to the client (Box 8–2). As useful as advance directives are in helping the client decide on future care, clients often are unable to anticipate all the possible types of treatments used. For example, an elderly client with a long history of cardiovascular disease specified in his living will that he did not want CPR performed and did not want a ventilator. When his heart developed a potentially lethal dysrhythmia that rendered him unresponsive, his physician made the decision to cardiovert* the client using the electric cardioverter because this mode of treatment was not specifically forbidden by the client's living will. Strictly speaking, the physician did not violate the letter of the living will, but did he violate its spirit?

Advance directives, which include living wills, are now a required part of the health care of all clients. The Omnibus Budget Reconciliation Act of 1990 requires that all hospitals, nursing-care facilities, home-health-care agencies, and caregivers ask clients about advance directives and provide information concerning living wills and durable power of attorney (DPOA) to help clients make informed health-care decisions. However, the federal law mandates only the requirements and not the directives to implement the law. The actual implementation of the

*Cardioverting is a procedure in which electrical shock is used to change the heart rhythm from ventricular tachycardia or other rhythms to normal sinus rhythms.

ISSUES IN PRACTICE

In the current health-care environment, nurses may encounter elderly clients who function independently at home and have not officially or legally been declared incompetent, but whose behavior might indicate that they are unable to make rational decisions about their care. Consider the following situation:

A 74-year-old client, Buster Mack, had been a long-haul truck driver for most of his life and was still driving his big rig into his 60s. He had been in relatively good health until 5 years ago, when he was diagnosed with lung cancer. A lobectomy was performed at that time, and he was treated with follow-up radiation and chemotherapy, but the cancer had slowly metastasized to the bone. His current hospitalization was due to a syncopal episode witnessed by a neighbor in the front yard of Mr. Mack's home, where he lives by himself.

During the admission assessment, the nurse observed that Mr. Mack had trouble focusing on the questions, and often the answers were unrelated to the question, or in the form of long rambling accounts of something that happened many years ago. Although he knew he was in some hospital (he could not remember the name), he had no idea where it was or what the date was. His demeanor was cooperative and pleasant, and he laughed easily when the nurse joked with him. He could not remember whether he had any family left living, although the name and address of a son in a distant city were listed on the old records.

Mr. Mack signed all the admission papers and consent forms placed in front of him for a number of neurologic tests. His physician was fearful that the cancer might have spread to his brain, and wanted to do a magnetic resonance imaging (MRI) test, spinal tap, and brain scan. The MRI and brain scan showed a small tumor in an area of the brain where it could be removed rather easily. Mr. Mack's physician in consultation with a neurosurgeon, felt that an immediate craniotomy with removal of the tumor was required. After explaining the procedure to Mr. Mack, the physicians placed the consent to operate form on his overbed table and gave him a pen. He promptly signed it, and gave it back.

Later on that day during her shift assessment, the nurse checked on Mr. Mack. The neighbor who had found him unconscious was visiting at the time. When the nurse asked Mr. Mack whether he was ready for the surgery scheduled for the next morning, he had a blank look on his face. On further questioning, the nurse concluded that Mr. Mack had no idea about what was going to happen to him the next day. The neighbor, who helped Mr. Mack with his bills and other paper work at home, stated: "He'll pretty much sign anything that you put in front of him." At this point the nurse felt that Mr. Mack was incapable of making an informed decision about the craniotomy.

The nurse called both the primary physician and the neurosurgeon about her observations. She was told bluntly that the consent had been signed and that they were going to operate on Mr. Mack the next day for his own good. If she wanted what was best for the client, she would just drop the issue.

Should the nurse just drop the issue? Is there anything she could do to resolve the problem? What ethical principles are involved with this situation?

Box 8–2

Checklist for Evaluating a Patient's Living Will Document

1. Statement of intention states the document was written freely when the patient was competent.
2. Statement of when the document goes into effect. This is usually when the patient is no longer able to make decisions for himself or herself.
3. A section specifies general health-care measure to be excluded from care.
4. Open section for specific measures (ventilators, pacemakers, etc.) and any other specific instructions concerning care.
5. Proxy statement (sometimes called durable power of attorney), which is optional but a strong addition. Allows another person to make decisions in situations that may not have been anticipated in the living will. (Check your state law concerning details of proxy selection.)
6. Substitute proxy. This section is optional. Specifies who can make decisions, if first choice proxy is not available.
7. Legal statement that the proxy(s) may make decisions.
8. Witness selection statement. Many states require that witnesses not be related nor members of the health-care team.
9. Signature and date. Must be signed and dated by the patient. Some states have very specific regulations concerning how long the will is valid. It may range from a few months to 5 years.
10. Legal signatures of witnesses are required.
11. Notary seal, if required by state law. State laws differ on notary seal requirement. It is usually required if a proxy is selected.

law is left to the individual states. Because of the vagueness of the law, a great deal of confusion exists, particularly with regards to living wills.

Nurses play an important role in ensuring that clients understand the implications of their choices pertaining to decisions that may prolong their lives during medical emergency. Because of their "frontline" position as caregivers within the health-care system, nurses must understand this role, specifically as it pertains to living wills.

Ethical Difficulties of Living Wills

Although a living will seems to be a simple solution to a complex care situation, there are some ethical difficulties inherent in their use that nurses need to know about. Primary among these ethical difficulties is the question of the person's level of knowledge of potential and future health-care problems at the time the will was formulated. Because living wills are often formulated long before they are to be used, there may later be serious questions about how informed the person was about the disease states and treatment modalities that might later affect care. If there is any indication that the person did not understand the full implications of future therapies or potential medical problems, then the validity of the living will is in question.

A second ethical difficulty for nurses encompasses the principles of beneficence and nonmaleficence. The principle of beneficence states that a health-care professional's primary duty is to benefit or do good for the client. The principle of nonmaleficence states that the client should be protected from harm by health-care providers. It is sometimes difficult to determine whether the primary duty is to produce benefit or prevent harm. Generally, most health-care providers think that the duty to avoid harming the client outweighs the concerns for providing benefit. When evaluated from the beneficence and nonmaleficence viewpoints, living wills seem to violate the principle of providing benefit to the client. This perception makes many health-care providers ethically uncomfortable. In some situations, the implementation of a living will might actually involve the termination of some modes of treatments already in use. Termination seems to constitute actual harm to the client. In either case, respecting a living will might often appear to health-care providers to be a violation of their duty to help clients and preserve life. Nurses, as well as other health-care providers, often experience a sense of frustration when they are not allowed to use all the skills they have learned to preserve life.

A third difficulty nurses and other health-care workers may have with living wills is their formulation and legal enforcement. In general, the language used in the standard living will document is broad and vague. Living wills are often not specific enough to include all the forms of treatments that are possible for the many types of illnesses that might render a person incompetent to make decisions. Health-care providers may have little direction as to the care they are to give if the circumstances at the time the living will is to be honored are significantly different from the declared wishes of client.

Furthermore, unless the particular state has enacted into law a special type of living will called a natural death act, the living will has no mechanism of legal enforcement. Also, when a client travels from one state to another, the legal effect of the living will may be in question. Does the non-resident state have an obligation to honor it?

In some states, a living will is considered only advisory and the physician has the right to comply with the living will or treat the client as the physician deems most appropriate. There is no protection for nurses or other health-care practitioners against criminal or civil liability in the execution of living wills in states without a natural death act. Once a valid living will exists, it only becomes effective when the person who formulated it meets the qualifications for the natural death act. In most states, the individual must be diagnosed as having a terminal condition where the continuation of treatment and life support would only prolong the client's dying process. But there is no clear consensus on the definition of "terminal condition."

Despite all these difficulties, living wills are still a good way for a client to make health-care wishes known to health-care providers. Documents that are specific about treatment modalities, are written in a "legal" format, and signed by two or more witnesses tend to be treated with an increased level of respect by health-care providers (Fig. 8–1).

Nurses can help clients plan ahead for their care should they become unable to make decisions for themselves. Although the nurse should not make the decisions for the client, the nurse can provide important information about the various treatment modalities that the client is considering. The nurse can also help clients clarify their wishes and guide them through the process in formulating an advance directive.

INSTRUCTIONS

PENNSYLVANIA DECLARATION

PRINT YOUR NAME

I, ______________________________, being of sound mind, willfully and voluntarily make this declaration to be followed if I become incompetent. This declaration reflects my firm and settled commitment to refuse life-sustaining treatment under the circumstances indicated below.

I direct my attending physician to withhold or withdraw life-sustaining treatment that serves only to prolong the process of my dying, if I should be in a terminal condition or in a state of permanent unconsciousness.

I direct that treatment be limited to measures to keep me comfortable and to relieve pain, including any pain that might occur by withholding or withdrawing life-sustaining treatment.

CHECK THE OPTIONS WHICH REFLECT YOUR WISHES

In addition, if I am in the condition described above, I feel especially strongly about the following forms of treatment:

I ( ) do ( ) do not want cardiac resuscitation.
I ( ) do ( ) do not want mechanical respiration.
I ( ) do ( ) do not want tube feeding or any other artificial or invasive form of nutrition (food) or hydration (water).
I ( ) do ( ) do not want blood or blood products.
I ( ) do ( ) do not want any form of surgery or invasive diagnostic tests.
I ( ) do ( ) do not want kidney dialysis.
I ( ) do ( ) do not want antibiotics.

I realize that if I do not specifically indicate my preference regarding any of the forms of treatment listed above, I may receive that form of treatment.

ADD PERSONAL INSTRUCTIONS (IF ANY)

Other instructions:

Figure 8–1. Sample advance directive. Because the laws on advance directives vary widely from state to state, there is no standard advance directive whose language conforms exactly with all states' laws. (Reprinted with permission of Partnership for Caring, formerly Choice in Dying, 200 Varick Street, New York. For more information visit www.partnershipforcaring.org.)

PENNSYLVANIA DECLARATION — PAGE 2 OF 2

APPOINTING A SURROGATE

Surrogate decisionmaking:

I ( ) do ( ) do not want to designate another person as my surrogate to make medical treatment decisions for me if I should be incompetent and in a terminal condition or in a state of permanent unconsciousness.

PRINT THE NAME, ADDRESS AND PHONE NUMBER OF YOUR SURROGATE

Name: ______________________________

Address: ______________________________

Phone: ______________________________

Name and address of substitute surrogate (if surrogate designated above is unable to serve):

PRINT THE NAME, ADDRESS AND PHONE NUMBER OF YOUR ALTERNATE SURROGATE

Name: ______________________________

Address: ______________________________

Phone: ______________________________

PRINT THE DATE

I made this declaration on the ____________ day of ________________.
(day) *(month, year)*

SIGN THE DOCUMENT AND PRINT YOUR ADDRESS

Declarant's signature: ______________________________

Declarant's address: ______________________________

WITNESSING PROCEDURE

YOUR TWO WITNESSES MUST SIGN AND PRINT THEIR ADDRESSES

The declarant, or the person on behalf of and at the direction of the declarant, knowingly and voluntarily signed this writing by signature or mark in my presence.

Witness's signature: ______________________________

Witness's address: ______________________________

Witness's signature: ______________________________

Witness's address: ______________________________

Courtesy of **Partnership for Caring, Inc.** 6/96
1620 Eye Street, NW, Suite 202, Washington, DC 20006 800-989-9455

Euthanasia and Assisted Suicide

The term *euthanasia* generally means killing or refusing to treat a client to allow a painless or peaceful death. A distinction is often made between passive and active euthanasia. Passive euthanasia usually refers to the practice of allowing an individual to die without any extraordinary intervention. Under this umbrella definition, practices such as DNR orders, living wills, and withdrawal of ventilators or other life support are usually included. **Active euthanasia**, on the other hand, usually describes the practice of hastening an individual's death through some act or procedure. This practice is also sometimes referred to as mercy killing and takes many forms ranging from use of large amounts of pain medication for terminal cancer clients to use of poison, gun, or knife to end a person's life.

Assisted suicide—brought to public attention by Dr. Jack Kevorkian, a Michigan physician who has publicly practiced it for many years—can be considered a type of active euthanasia or mercy killing. The central issue that has been publicized by Dr. Kevorkian is whether it is ever ethically permissible for health-care personnel to assist in taking a life. In most states the practice is illegal. The definition of homicide—bringing about a person's death or assisting in doing so—seems to fit the act of assisted suicide. In the past, there has been a great deal of hesitation on the part of the legal system to prosecute persons who are involved in assisted suicide or juries to convict physicians who participate in the activity.

> *The fundamental ethical issue in these situations is the right to self-determination.*

In the fall of 1998, Dr. Kevorkian raised the legal and ethical stakes. On a nationally broadcast network news show, "60 Minutes," he not only admitted to administering a lethal medication to a client without the client's assistance, but he also made and played a videotape that showed the whole episode. The client, who had Lou Gehrig's disease (amyotrophic lateral sclerosis), had requested that Dr. Kevorkian kill him. The client had signed a **consent** form and release and was even given an extra 2 weeks to "think about it." The client waited only for 3 days before making his final request for the lethal medication. Under Michigan law, Dr. Kevorkian could have been charged with **manslaughter** or even first-degree murder. Dr. Kevorkian admitted that his **motivation** for the act was to be tried under these laws as a test case for active euthanasia. He was arrested 2 weeks later on a charge of first-degree murder; however, he felt very strongly that a jury would not convict him. The trial verdict was guilt of second-degree murder, and he is currently serving a term of 25 years to life in prison. This verdict reinforced the belief of most health-care professionals that mercy killing or assisted suicide is always ethically wrong.

The unfortunate fallout from Dr. Kevorkian's conviction is that many physicians have become even more reluctant to write DNR orders or comply with clients' and/or families' wishes to allow clients to be removed from life support. Clearly they do not understand the distinctions between active and passive euthanasia.

The fundamental ethical issue in these situations is the right to self-determination. In almost every other health-care situation, a client who is mentally competent can make decisions about what care to accept and what care to refuse. Yet, when it comes to the termination of life, this right becomes controversial. Supporters of the practice of assisted suicide believe that the right to self-determination remains intact, even with regard to the decision to end one's life. It is the last act of a very sick individual to control his or her own fate. Many believe that medical personnel should be allowed to assist these clients in this procedure, just as they are allowed to assist clients in other medical and nursing procedures.

Those who oppose assisted suicide find these arguments unconvincing. Legally, ethically, and morally, suicide in U.S. society has never been an accepted practice. Health-care staff go to great lengths to prevent suicidal clients from injuring themselves. In addition, it would seem that individuals in the terminal stages of a disease, who are overwhelmed by pain and depressed by the thought of prolonged suffering, might not be able to think clearly enough to give informed consent for assisted suicide. Also, because the termination of life is final, it does not allow for spontaneous cures or for the development of new treatments or medications.

Nonmaleficence is the term that describes the obligation to do no harm to clients. Whether assisting in or causing the death of a client is a violation of this principle is most likely to be an issue that will continue to be debated for some time. Several states have passed laws permitting assisted suicide, but these states have very strict guidelines. The American Nurses Association (ANA) and other nurses' organizations oppose assisted suicide as a policy and believe that nurses who participate in it are violating the code of ethics.

After almost a decade of decline, the number of human immunodeficiency virus (HIV) and acquired immunodeficiency syndrome (AIDS) cases has started to rise again in the United States.

Human Immunodeficiency Virus and Acquired Immunodeficiency Syndrome

After almost a decade of decline, the number of human immunodeficiency virus (HIV) and acquired immunodeficiency syndrome (AIDS) cases has started to rise again in the United States. In some parts of Africa, it is estimated that as much as 60 percent of the population is infected with the virus. HIV and AIDS have evoked strong emotions both in the public and in the medical community. Nurses, who for years held strongly to the ethical principle that all clients regardless of race, sex, religion, age, or disease process should be cared for equally, are questioning their obligation to take care of clients who have AIDS.

Several ethical issues underlie the AIDS controversy. One of the most important is the right to privacy. Although there is a general requirement to report infection with HIV/AIDS to the Centers for Disease Control and Prevention (CDC), many states have strict laws regarding the confidentiality of the diagnosis. Unauthorized revelation of the diagnosis of HIV/AIDS brings the possibility of a lawsuit against the health-care provider or institution. However, the right to privacy is not absolute. Diseases such as tuberculosis, gonorrhea, syphilis, and hepatitis, which are highly contagious and sometimes fatal, must be reported to public health officials. If the right to privacy can be violated when the public welfare is at stake, does AIDS represent this type of threat? Is it unjust to ask health-care providers to care for clients with this disease without knowing that the client has it? Is it just to violate a client's privacy when the disease carries with it a potential for social stigma and isolation? Does the client have a right to know that a health-care provider is infected with HIV/AIDS?

Another important ethical issue is the right to care. Can a nurse refuse to care for a client with AIDS? Obviously, a fundamental right of a client is to receive care, and a fundamental obligation of a nurse is to provide care. The first statement of the ANA Code of Ethics for Nurses is that a nurse must provide care unrestricted by any considerations. Surely, though, there are some exceptions, for example if the nurse is pregnant, or is receiving chemotherapy, or has had other immunity problems. In most situations, however, the nurse is obligated to provide the best nursing care possible for all clients, including those with AIDS.

What about the tremendous cost involved in treating individuals who have AIDS? Studies estimate that the medical cost of treating a client with AIDS from the time of diagnosis to the time of death is approximately $900,000.[4] In the face of this crisis, governmental agencies, which bear the brunt of paying for AIDS treatment, will have to make some difficult decisions concerning this issue. With more than 2 million people already infected with this disease, the cost to society is astronomical.

Nurses have the obligation to care for all clients, including those with AIDS, but ought physicians, hospitals, or governmental agencies also be held to this same precept? Should our society regard health care as a right or a privilege?

Ethics Involving Children

Although children are universally acknowledged as the hope of the future, many children remain poorly fed, clothed, housed, and educated and are in dire need of all types of health care, even in affluent countries such as the United States. In the past few years, there has been a marked increase in the reporting of incidents of child neglect and abuse by parents.

Our society generally acknowledges the tremendous decision-making power that parents have on behalf of their children; however, there are limits to how parents may decide to act. These limits are sometimes obvious, such as in cases of physical abuse and cruelty to children; however, they may also be less conspicuous, such as in the cases of neglect or decisions about withholding medical care for religious reasons. Health-care professionals often find themselves trying to make decisions about the appropriateness of a parent's actions toward a child.

The legal and ethical factors surrounding the decisions that health-care providers must make about child health issues are complicated and sometimes contradictory, ranging from laws about reporting suspected abuse to obtaining permission for treatment. This section focuses on child abuse and the ethical issues that it creates for nurses and also the issues of informed consent as it pertains to children.

Issues involving children have always been an important consideration in our society. Whereas the political attention seems to focus on education, drug and alcohol abuse, and child health-care issues, ethical concerns in **pediatrics** are never forgotten and often serve as the unspoken basis for the more visible issues.

Child health ethical issues are numerous and diverse, ranging from mass screening for diseases to withholding permission for treatment.

Child Abuse

Case Study

Emily, who is 8 months old, is brought to the hospital by her 17-year-old unemployed mother, who stated that the baby refused to eat at home and vomited a lot. Emily was very small for her age and was below the growth curve for weight. She was also neurologically introverted and showed little interest in her surroundings. She slept a great deal of time. She was admitted to the hospital with a diagnosis of Nonorganic Failure to Thrive. During her stay in the hospital, Emily ate well and gained a significant amount of weight. Her neurologic status also improved. One nurse suspected that this was a case of neglect (a form of child abuse) and suggested to the physician that child protective services be notified to evaluate the case. The physician resisted because there was not enough evidence to make a definitive case and thought that it was unfair to the parents to make such a claim. The other nurses felt that by reporting the case they would lose the trust of the mother and cause her to avoid health care for Emily in the future. They also cited a case in which nurses and the hospital were sued when they reported a teenage mother for neglect; the accusation later proved to be false.

Emily was sent home after 3 weeks but was re-admitted 1 month later with the same complaints of poor feeding. She had lost weight since her discharge from the hospital, and she was again neurologically withdrawn. The physician still refused to notify child protective services because of the lack of hard evidence. He thought that an investigation and possible removal of the child from the home was too extreme based on the data available. The nurse still believed that the mother should be reported based on suspicions that could be substantiated legally.

Ethical Principles Relating to Child Abuse

There is a general legal requirement in most states that suspected child abuse must be reported by health-care providers as well as by anyone who suspects that child abuse has occurred. Abuse is more obvious when the child has physical injuries that do not fit the medical history or are atypical for the age group. However, in cases of neglect, the evidence may be very minimal or even nonexistent. Often nurses and physicians who specialize in the care of children rely on their experience in making decisions about reporting or not reporting suspected abuse.

> *A conflicting ethical principle that is sometimes forgotten in the reporting of suspected child abuse is the family's right to privacy and self-determination.*

Decisions about reporting suspected child abuse or neglect rest on the underlying ethical principles of beneficence and protection of the best interests of the child. It is always difficult to decide how far ranging these concerns for "best interest" should be. Physicians tend to focus on solving the immediate problem. Nurses hold a more holistic viewpoint and tend to see the child in relationship to his or her environment as well as the environment of the parents. Nurses also tend to think of themselves as saviors, protecting the unfortunate or disadvantaged from a malignant social system and often making value judgments about the lifestyles of others from their middle-class vantage point.

A conflicting ethical principle that is sometimes forgotten in the reporting of suspected child abuse is the family's right to privacy and self-determination. It is an equally fundamental right that Emily's parents be allowed to live their lives according to their own values, free from intrusions. However, when the child is a client in the hospital, beneficence usually outweighs fidelity and veracity.

Resolution of the Dilemma

How is the nurse going to resolve this dilemma? Should she report the case and go against the physician's decision? Should she just agree with the physician and defer to his greater experience and better judgment? Should she submit the problem to the hospital ethics committee? Are there any other possible options for action in this case?

It is likely that the physician was correct in his decision about this case, although his ethical reasoning may leave something to be desired. Legally, it is unlikely that there would be sufficient proof to remove the infant from the mother because home monitoring could achieve the same results. Therefore, how can the ethical obligations for the best interest of the child be met?

One very plausible solution is to monitor the child closely through frequent follow-up either at the physician's office or at the local health department. In addition, a follow-up and home evaluation could be arranged through a home-health-care agency, which could also make available other community resources to help in Emily's care. If the infant continued to fail to gain weight, or if it was later determined that Emily's mother was indeed unable to care adequately for her, the case could then be referred to child protective services.

The role of the nurse who cares for the very young or abused child is one of client advocate. These children need help and protection, and at times, for their very survival, must be taken out of an abusive home setting. Nurses need to be aware of and use all the assets available in these situations, including the police, child protective services, welfare, and home-health-care agencies.

Informed Consent and Children

Case Study

Peter, one of a pair of 7-year-old identical twins, developed a severe bilateral glomerulonephritis after a strep throat infection. The renal involvement was so severe that it did not respond to any medical treatment, and both of his kidneys had to be removed. Paul, Peter's identical twin, was evaluated for kidney donation and, as expected, matched on all six antigens as well as blood type and size. Paul seemed to understand what had happened to his brother and agreed to donate one of his kidneys to keep his brother alive.

However, the children's parents were having some trouble agreeing on whether Paul should donate a kidney to Peter. The twins' mother felt that the donation and transplant should be permitted because it would indeed help keep Peter alive and would also make Paul feel like he was an important part of the process. She argued that if Peter ever did die, Paul would be overcome with guilt knowing that he could have saved his brother but did not. The twins' father was not as certain about the transplant procedure. He thought that Paul was too young to make a truly free decision of that type and that he did not really understand the serious nature of a kidney removal operation. He thought that Paul, because he was so young, might have been unduly influenced by subtle, yet powerful pressures from his family. No one had directly told Paul that he *must* donate one of his kidneys, yet the fact that his brother's survival may well depend on his decision could have had a major effect on his willingness to donate. Because Peter was being maintained on dialysis and seemed to be doing fairly well, the twins' father thought that he should be put on the transplant list to see whether a suitable nonrelated donor could be found.

The nurses on the unit where Peter was being cared for were equally divided about whether the transplant should be performed. At various times during Peter's lengthy stay in the hospital, they had all been asked by the parents, usually one parent at a time, whether or not they should go ahead with the transplant.

Case Study Analysis

The question, as related to the case study, is: "Does a 7-year-old child have sufficient rational decision-making ability to decide to donate a kidney to his brother?" If, after assessing the child carefully, the answer is "yes," then under the rights-in-trust doctrine, the right to self-determination can be turned over to the child and he can make his own decision. If the answer is "no," then the child should not be permitted to donate the kidney.

But there are other ethical principles that can be brought to bear on this decision. From a utilitarian viewpoint, the child should be allowed to donate the kidney, because it would provide the greatest good or happiness for the greatest number of people. Similarly, love-based ethics, or the Golden Rule system of ethical decision making, would also support the donation on the grounds that Paul identifies closely with his brother and appears to understand the issues involved in donation. However, from an egoistic or beneficent viewpoint, because the transplant has little benefit for the donor and will surely cause pain and place him at risk for postoperative complications, the operation should not be permitted.

As with many ethical dilemmas, there is no perfect answer to this situation. The best that can be done is to ensure that the parents and children have as much of the necessary information as possible and support their decisions.

By recognizing the rights of children as individuals, their importance to society is also recognized. However, parents and health-care professionals also have the duty to nurture, support, and guide children as they grow into adolescence and adulthood. Nurses who work with children are challenged to support the independence of the child by encouraging the child to be responsible for and participate in his or her own health care.

Ethical Principles Regarding Children

One important difference between adults and children that always needs to be included in ethical decisions about child health issues is that children are dependents. As dependents, they generally are not attributed the right to self-determination that is fundamental to adult decision making. Whenever there is an ethical dilemma involving child health-care issues, a three-way relationship develops involving the child, the health-care professional, and the parents. Generally, the parents have the primary role in deciding health-care issues for their underaged, dependent children based on what they consider to be in the child's best interests.

Current routine child health practices reinforce this principle. Young children are given immunizations and medications, have blood drawn for tests, and even have operations such as tonsillectomies or myringotomies, all without asking for their permission. This exemption to the principle of self-determination in children is based on the belief that young children do not yet have the capacity to make fully rational decisions. Yet, the final expectation for children is that at some point in their lives they develop the capacity to make informed, correct decisions. The primary questions then become: When do they develop this capacity for rational decision making? and How should they be treated until they develop this capacity?

What Do You Think?

If you were the nurse, what would you suggest to the twins' parents? What ethical issues would be involved in your suggestions?

The legal system has fixed the age for rational decision making at age 18. Children who are younger than 18 years of age, with a few exceptions, require the permission of the parent for any and all medical procedures. Children older than 18 years of age can make their own decisions about health care. The difficulty with "fixing" an age is that it is arbitrary and does not reflect the reality of the individual child's development. From experience it can be observed that many children who are 9 or 10 years old exhibit rather advanced and "adult-like" decision-making skills, whereas other children who may be 18 or 19 years of age display a marked lack of this ability.

The more serious question, however, is how should underaged children be treated? One solution is to deny, because of their age, that they have rights and then treat them as being incompetent by bringing to bear paternalistic, "best interest" interventions. Another approach is to say that they do have the same rights as adults except that these rights are temporarily suspended until the child is sufficiently mature to exercise them. This is called rights-in-trust, and the rights are turned over to the child at the appropriate time. The question then becomes, when is the appropriate time?

One approach is to turn over all the rights to the child at the same time, for example, when he or she reaches 18 years of age. Another approach is to gradually release individual rights as the child grows older and is prepared to exercise them. In either case, appropriate adults, including nurses, have the role of safeguarding the child's rights and act as guardians, protectors, and advocates of the children under their care.

Box 8–3

Determining the Greatest Good

Sherry is an RN who works for a rehabilitation center that deals mainly with developmentally delayed children. For several years, Sherry has been following the case of Margie N., who is now 8 years old and has Down syndrome and moderate retardation. Margie has made steady, if slow, progress in achieving basic motor and cognitive skills but still requires close supervision of all activities and care for all basic hygiene needs. Margie is still not advanced enough to participate in group activities at the center's day clinic.

Mrs. N., Margie's mother, a 42-year-old widow, has been providing a high level of care for Margie at home as well as meeting the child's demands for love and attention. Recently, Mrs. N. has been diagnosed with systemic lupus erythematosus (SLE), which has displayed as its primary symptoms severe joint pain and stiffness. During the past several months, Mrs. N. has been finding it increasingly difficult to care for Margie because of the progressive nature of the SLE.

Mrs. N. is trying to make a decision about long-term care for Margie. She trusts Sherry's judgment completely and often relies on the information and teaching given by the nurse to make changes in Margie's care. Sherry is uncertain about what advice she should give. She recognizes that the high level of care and comfort provided by Mrs. N. have been an essential part in the advances Margie has made up to this point, but she also recognizes that Mrs. N. may soon reach a point at which that care can no longer be provided. It seems that to do what is good for Mrs. N. (i.e., placing Margie in an institution) would be harmful to Margie, whereas doing what is good for Margie (i.e., leaving her at home) would be harmful to Mrs. N. What is the best course of action in this situation? Are there any alternative solutions to this dilemma?

Conclusion

Ethical issues are a factor in the daily practice of all nurses. Any time that a nurse comes in contact with a client, a potential ethical situation exists. In today's world, with rapidly advancing technology and unusual health-care situations, ethical dilemmas are proliferating. Nurses can be prepared to deal with most of these dilemmas if they keep current with the issues and are able to follow a systematic process for making ethical decisions. At some point, difficult decisions must be made, and we should not avoid making them. One of the worst elements of ethical decision making is that it is very unlikely that everyone involved in the dilemma will be happy with the decision. However, if the decision is made after the situation has been analyzed and if it is based on sound ethical principles, it can usually be defended.

ISSUES IN PRACTICE

Analyze the following case study using the ethical decision-making process:

Ms. Sally Jones, RN, a public health nurse for a rural health department, was preparing to visit Mr. Weems, a 58-year-old client who was recently diagnosed with chronic bronchitis and emphysema. Mr. Weems was unemployed as a result of a farming accident and had been previously diagnosed with hypertension and extreme obesity. Ms. Jones was making this visit to see why Mr. Weems had missed his last appointment at the clinic and whether he was taking his prescribed antibiotics and antihypertensive medications.

As Ms. Jones pulled up in the driveway of his house, she noticed Mr. Weems sitting on the front porch smoking a cigarette. She felt a surge of anger, which she quickly suppressed, as she wondered why she spent so much of her limited time teaching him about the health consequences of smoking.

During the visit, Ms. Jones determined that Mr. Weems had stopped taking both his antihypertensive and antibiotic medications and rarely took his expectorants and bronchodilators. He coughed continuously, had a blood pressure of 196/122, and had severely congested lung sounds. Mr. Weems listened politely as Ms. Jones re-explained the need to stop smoking and the importance of taking his medications as prescribed. She also scheduled another appointment at the clinic in 1 week for follow-up.

As she drove away to her next visit, Ms. Jones wondered about the ethical responsibilities of nurses who must provide care for clients who do not seem to care about their own health. Mr. Weems took little responsibility for his health, refused to even try to stop smoking or lose weight, and did not take his medications. She wondered whether there was a limit to the amount of nursing care a noncompliant client should expect from a community health agency. She reflected that the time spent with Mr. Weems would have been spent much more productively screening children at a local grade school or working with mothers of newborn infants.

Critical Thinking Exercises

- What data are important in relation to this situation?
- State the ethical dilemma in a clear, simple statement.
- What are the choices of action and how do they relate to specific ethical principles?
- What are the consequences of these actions?
- What decisions can be made?

References

1. Recchia, B: Human biological materials in research: Ethical issues. ANS Adv Nurs Sci 24(2):32–46, 2002.
2. Williams, JK: Impact of genome research on children and their families. Journal of Child and Family Nursing 4(4):239–245, 2001.
3. Heller, BR, et al: 10 Trends to watch. Nursing and Health Care Perspectives 24(1):9–14, 2002.
4. Menzel, L: Is it worth it? Balancing the benefit of extended life with the cost of suffering during critical illness. Critical Care Nurse 18(4):67–73, 1998.
5. Austin, W: Nursing ethics in an era of globalization. ANS Adv Nurs Sci 24(2):1–18, 2002.

Bibliography

Beidler, SM, and Dickey, SB: Children's competence to participate in healthcare decisions. JONA's Healthcare Law, Ethics, and Regulation 3(3):80–87, 2001.

Bjarnascon, D, and Lehman, C: Ethical issues from critical care to rehabilitation: A challenge for specialty nurses. Crit Care Clin North Am 13(3):341–347, 2001.

Bower, J: Clinical ethics: Do not resuscitate orders in the OR. SSM 7(5):51–56, 2001.

Clark, CM: Rationing scarce life-sustaining resources on the basis of age. J Adv Nurs 35(5):799–804, 2001.

Drake, C: Informed consent? A child's right to autonomy. Journal of Child Health Care 5(3):101–104, 2001.

Elliott, AC: Health care ethics: Cultural relativity of autonomy. Journal of Transcultural Nursing 12(4):326–330, 2001.

Engelhardt, HT, and Cherry, MJ: Allocating Scarce Resources. Georgetown University Press, Baltimore, 2002.

Esterhuizen, P, and Kooyuman, A: Empowering moral decision making in nurses. Nurse Education Today 21(8):640–647, 2001.

Farcus, N, et al: Expanding the comfort zone of ethical decision making in nursing practice. Inside Case Management 8(9):5–7, 2001.

Jenkins, J: Ethical implications of genetic information. Online Journal of Issues in Nursing Feb 9, 2001.

9

Nursing Law and Liability

Mary Evans and Tonia Aiken

Learning Objectives

After completing this chapter, the reader will be able to:

- Distinguish between statutory law and common law.
- Differentiate civil law from criminal law.
- Explain the legal principles involved in:

  Unintentional torts
  Intentional torts
  Quasi-intentional torts
  Informed consent
  Do-not-resuscitate (DNR) orders

- Describe the trial process.
- List methods to prevent litigation.
- Identify the elements in delegation.

For many nurses, the mere mention of the word lawsuit provokes a high level of anxiety. At first glance, the legal system often seems to be a large and confusing entity whose intricacies are designed to entrap the uninitiated. Many nurses feel that even a minor error in client care will lead to huge settlements against them and loss of their nursing license. In reality, even though the number of lawsuits against nurses has been increasing since the early 1990s, the number of nurses who are actually sued remains relatively small.

It is important to remember that the legal system is just one element in the totality of the health-care system. Laws are rules to help protect people and to keep society functioning. The ultimate goal of all laws is to promote peaceful and productive interactions between and among the people of that society.

An understanding of basic legal principles will augment the quality of care that the nurse delivers. In our litigious society, it is important to comprehend how the law affects the profession of nursing and the individual nurse's daily practice.

Sources of Law

There are two major sources for laws in the United States—statutory law and common law (Box 9–1). The majority of the laws that govern nursing are state-level statutory laws because licensure is a function of the state's authority.

Box 9–1

Division and Types of Law

I. Statutory Law
- A. Criminal Law
  1. Misdemeanor
  2. Felony
- B. Civil Law
  1. Tort Law
     a. Unintentional tort
     b. Intentional tort
     c. Quasi-intentional tort
  2. Contract Law
  3. Treaty Law
  4. Tax Law
  5. Other

II. Common Law
- A. Criminal Law
  1. Misdemeanor
  2. Felony
- B. Civil Law
  1. Tort Law
     a. Unintentional tort
     b. Intentional tort
     c. Quasi-intentional tort
  2. Contract Law
  3. Treaty Law
  4. Tax Law
  5. Other

Statutory Law

Statutory law consists of laws written and enacted by the U.S. Congress, the state legislatures, and other governmental entities such as cities, counties, or townships. Legislated laws enacted by the U.S. Congress are called federal **statutes**. State-drafted laws are called state statutes. Individual cities and municipalities have legislative bodies that draft **ordinances**, codes, and regulations at their respective levels.

The laws that govern the profession of nursing are statutory laws. Most of these laws are written at the state level, because licensure is a responsibility of the individual states. These laws include the nurse practice act, which establishes the state board of nursing, individual licensure procedures, and schedule of fees for the state.

Common Law

Common law is different from statutory law in that it has evolved from the decisions of previous legal cases that form a **precedent**. These laws represent the accumulated results of the judgments and decrees that have been handed down by courts of the United States and Great Britain through the years. Common law often extends beyond the scope of statutory law. For example, no statutes require a person who is negligent and causes injury to another to compensate that person for the injury. Court decisions that have addressed the same legal issues over and over, such as negligence, however, have repeatedly ruled that the injured person should receive compensation. The way in which each case is resolved creates a precedent, or pattern, for dealing with the same legal issue in the future. The common laws involving negligence or malpractice are most frequently encountered by the nurse.

Common law or case law is law that has developed over a long period. The principle of *stare decisis* requires a judge to make decisions similar to those that have been handed down in previous cases if the facts of the cases are identical. Common law decisions are published in bound legal reports. Generally speaking, common law deals with matters outside the scope of laws enacted by the legislature.

Divisions of Law

In the U.S. legal system, there are many divisions in the law. A major example of such a division is the difference between criminal law and civil law, either of which may be statutory or common in origin.

Criminal Law

Criminal laws are concerned with providing protection for all members of society. When someone is accused of violating a criminal law, the government at the county, city, state, or federal level imposes punishments appropriate to the type of **crime**. Criminal law involves a wide range of **malfeasance**, from minor traffic violations to murder.

Although most criminal law is created and regulated by the government through the enactment of statutes, a small portion falls under the common law. Statutes are developed and enacted by the legislature (state or federal) and approved by the executive branch, such as a governor or the President. Criminal law is further classified into two types of offenses: (1) **misdemeanors**, which are minor criminal offenses, and (2) **felonies**, which are major criminal offenses.

In the criminal law system, an individual accused of a crime is called the defendant. The prosecuting attorney represents the people of the city, county, state, or federal jurisdiction who are accusing the individual of a crime. A **criminal action** is rendered when the person charged with the crime is brought to trial and convicted. Penalties or sanctions are imposed on the violators of criminal law and are based on the scope of the crime. They can involve a range of punishment from community service work and fines to imprisonment and death.

What Do You Think?

Do you know anyone who has filed a malpractice suit or a health-care provider who was the defendant in a malpractice suit? What was the situation that brought the case? How was it resolved? If you have never been involved with a malpractice suit or do not know anyone who has, how would you feel if a lawsuit were to be brought against you?

Nurses can become involved with the criminal system in their nursing practice in several ways. The most common violation by nurses of the criminal law is through failure to renew nursing licenses. In this situation, the nurse is in effect practicing nursing without a license, which is a crime in all states. Nurses also become involved with the illegal diversion of drugs, particularly narcotics, from the hospital. This is a more serious crime, which may lead to imprisonment for the nurse. Recent cases involving intentional or unintentional deaths of clients and assisted suicide cases have also led to criminal action against nurses.

Civil Law

Nurses are much more likely to become involved in civil lawsuits than in criminal violations. **Civil laws** generally deal with the violation of one individual's rights by another individual. The court provides the forum that enables these individuals to have their disputes resolved by an independent third party, such as a judge or a jury of the defendant's peers. The individual who brings the dispute to the court is called the **plaintiff**. The formal written document that describes the dispute and the resolution sought is called the complaint. The individual against whom the complaint is filed is called the **defendant**, who, in conjunction with his attorney, prepares the **answer** to the complaint. In civil cases, the **burden of proof** rests with the plaintiff.

Civil law has many branches, including contract law, treaty law, tax law, and tort law. It is under the tort law that most nurses become involved with the legal system.

Tort Law

A **tort** is generally defined as a wrongful act committed against a person or his or her property independent of a contract. A person who commits a tort is called the **tort-feasor** and is **liable** for **damages** to those who are affected by the person's actions. The word *tort*, derived from the Latin *tortus* (twisted), is a French word for injury or wrong. Torts can involve several different types of actions, including a direct violation of a person's legal rights or a violation of a standard of care that causes injury to a person. Torts are classified as unintentional, intentional, or quasi-intentional.

Unintentional Torts

Negligence is the primary form of **unintentional tort**. **Negligence** is generally defined as the **omission** of an act that a reasonable and prudent person would perform in a similar situation, or the commission of something a reasonable person would not do in that situation. **Nonfeasance** is a type of negligence that occurs when a person fails to perform a legally required duty.[1]

Malpractice is a type of negligence for which professionals can be sued (professional negligence). Because of their professional status, nurses are held to a higher standard of conduct than the ordinary layperson. The standard for nurses is what a reasonable and prudent nurse would do in the same situation: "A registered nurse is charged with utilizing the degree and skill and judgment commensurate with his or her education, experience, and position."[2] For instance, it is reasonable and prudent that the nurse put the side rails up on the bed of a client who had just received an injection of a narcotic pain medication, because the drug causes drowsiness and sometimes confusion. If the nurse gave an injection of a narcotic medication but forgot to put the side rails up, and the client falls out of bed and fractures his hip, the nurse can be sued for the negligent act of forgetting to put the side rail up.

Because of their professional status, nurses are held to a higher standard of conduct than the ordinary layperson.

Four elements are required for a person to make a claim of negligence:

1. A duty was owed to the client (professional relationship)
2. The professional violated the **duty** and failed to conform to the standard of care (breach of duty)
3. The failure to act by the professional was the **proximate cause** of the resulting injuries (causality)
4. Actual injuries resulted from the breach of duty (damages)

If any of these elements is missing from the case, then the client will probably not be able to win the lawsuit (Box 9–2).

Consider the following situation:

Mr. Fagin, a 78-year-old client, was admitted from a nursing home for the treatment of a fractured tibia after he fell out of bed. After the fracture was reduced, a fiberglass cast was applied, and Mr. Fagin was sent to the orthopedic unit for follow-up care. While making her 0400 rounds, the night charge nurse (a registered nurse [RN]) discovered that Mr. Fagin's foot on the casted leg was cold to touch, looked bluish-purple, and was swollen approximately 1½ times normal size. The nurse noted these findings in the client's chart and relayed the information to the day shift nurses during the 0630 shift report. The charge nurse on the day shift promptly called and relayed the findings to Mr. Fagin's physician. The physician, however, did not seem to be concerned and only told the nurse to "Keep a close eye on him, and don't bother me again unless it is an absolute emergency." A short time later, Mr. Fagin became agitated, complained of severe pain in the affected foot, and eventually began

Box 9–2

Malpractice Considerations

Nursing malpractice is based on the legal premise that a nurse can be held legally responsible for the personal injury of another individual if it can be proven that the injury was the result of negligence.[2] Nursing malpractice is based on four elements: (1) duty, (2) breach of duty, (3) causation (the "but for" test), and (4) damage or injury.

Inappropriate work assignment and inadequate supervision are a breach of duty and could be the basis for finding a nurse's actions to be negligent. Failure or breach of duty to delegate is established by proving that a reasonably prudent nurse would not have made a particular assignment or delegated a certain responsibility, or that supervision was inadequate under the circumstances.

The act of improper delegation of tasks or inadequate supervision must be evaluated in light of the "but for" test related to the injury. If the person who performed the injurious act had not been assigned or delegated to perform the task, or had been adequately supervised, the injury could have been avoided. Consequently, the nurse is not being held liable for the negligent act of her subordinate, *but for the lack of competence in performing the independent duties of delegation and supervision.*

Off-site Consideration

Registered nurses who practice in public health, community, or home care settings must rely frequently on written or telephone communication when delegating patient care duties to assistive personnel. The nurse who must supervise from off site has a particular duty to assess the knowledge, skills, and judgment of the assistive personnel before assignments are made. Regular supervisory visits and impeccable documentation will help the registered nurse ensure that care provided by assistive personnel is adequate.[9]

yelling uncontrollably. The charge nurse called the emergency room (ER) physician to come to check on the client. The ER physician immediately removed the cast and noted an extensive circulatory impairment that would not respond to treatment. A few days later, Mr. Fagin's leg was amputated. His family filed a malpractice lawsuit against the hospital, the physician, and both the night and day charge nurses.

Are all the elements present in this case for a bona fide lawsuit? What could have been done to prevent this situation from happening? How should nurses deal with reluctant or hostile physicians?

Malpractice is more serious than mere negligence because it indicates professional misconduct or unreasonable lack of skill in performing professional duties. Malpractice suggests the existence of a professional standard of care and a deviation from that standard of care. A professional **expert witness** is often asked to testify in a malpractice case to help establish the standard of care to which the professional should be held accountable.

A 1988 case in South Dakota presents an example of nursing malpractice. The nurse failed to question the physician's order to discharge a client when she discovered that the client had a fever. In this case, a supervisory nurse provided expert testimony and reported to the judge that the general standard of care for nurses is to report a significant change in a client's condition, such as an elevated temperature. It is the nurse's responsibility to question the physician's order as to appropriateness of discharge. The records on this case indicated that the client's elevated temperature was charted after the physician had completed his rounds. The nurse did not notify the physician of the client's fever; and the client was subsequently discharged. The client was readmitted a short time after discharge and died in the hospital. The nurse was found negligent. The court held that negligence can be determined by failure to act as well as by the commission of an act.

Many other types of actions by nurses can produce malpractice lawsuits. Some of the more common actions include:

- Leaving foreign objects inside a client during surgery
- Failing to assess and observe a client as directed
- Failing to obtain a proper informed consent
- Failing to report a change in a client's condition, such as vital signs, circulatory status, and level of consciousness
- Failing to report another health-care provider's **incompetency** or negligence
- Failing to take actions to provide for a client's safety, such as not cleaning up a liquid spill on the floor that causes a client to fall
- Failing to provide a client with sufficient and appropriate education before discharge

If a nurse is found guilty of malpractice, several types of actions may be taken against the nurse. The nurse may be required to provide monetary compensation to the client for general damages that were a direct result of the injury, including pain, suffering, disability, and disfigurement. In addition, the nurse is often required to pay for special damages that have resulted from the injury, such as all involved medical expenses, **out-of-pocket expenses**, and wages lost by the client while he or she was in the hospital. Optional damages, including those for emotional distress, mental suffering, and counseling expenses that were an outgrowth of the initial injury, may be added to the total settlement. If the client is able to prove that the nurse acted with conscious disregard for the client's safety or acted in a malicious, willful, or wanton manner that produced injury, then an additional assessment of punitive or exemplary damages may be added to the award.

Intentional Torts

An **intentional tort** is generally defined as a willful act that violates another person's rights or property. Intentional torts can be distinguished from malpractice and acts of negligence by the following three requirements: (1) the nurse must intend to bring about the consequences of the act, (2) the nurse's act must be intended to interfere with the client or his property, and (3) the act must be a substantial factor in bringing about the injury or consequences.

The most frequently encountered intentional torts are assault, battery, false imprisonment, abandonment, and intentional infliction of emotional distress. With intentional torts, the injured person does not have to prove that an injury has occurred, nor is the opinion of an expert witness required for adjudication. Punitive damages are more likely to be assessed against the nurse in intentional tort cases, and some intentional torts may fall under the criminal law if there is gross violation of the standards of care.

Assault and Battery. **Assault** is the unjustifiable attempt to touch another person or the threat of so doing. **Battery** is actual harmful or unwarranted contact with another person without his or her consent. Battery is the most common intentional tort seen in the practice of nursing.

For a nurse to commit assault and battery, there must be an absence of consent on the part of the client. Before any procedure can be performed on a competent, alert, and normally oriented client, the client must agree or consent to the procedure being done. Negligence does not have to be proved for a person to be successful in a claim for assault and battery.

A common example of an assault and battery occurs when a nurse physically restrains a client against the client's will and administers an injection against the client's wishes.

False Imprisonment. **False imprisonment** occurs when a competent client is confined or restrained with intent to prevent him or her from leaving the hospital. The use of restraints alone does not constitute false imprisonment when they are used to maintain the safety of a confused, disoriented, or otherwise incompetent client. In general, mentally impaired clients can be detained against their will only if they are a threat to injure themselves or others. The use of threats or medications that interfere with the client's ability to leave the facility can also be considered false imprisonment.

Intentional Infliction of Emotional Distress. Intentional infliction of emotional distress is another common intentional tort encountered by the nurse. To prove this intentional tort, the following three elements are necessary: (1) conduct exceeds what is usually accepted by society, (2) the health-care provider's conduct is intended to cause mental distress, and (3) the conduct actually does produce mental distress (causation). Any nurse who is charged with assault, battery, or false imprisonment is also at risk for being charged with infliction of emotional distress.

A 1975 case is an example of infliction of emotional distress. In *Johnson v. Women's Hospital*, a mother wished to view the body of her baby who had died during birth. After she made the request, she was handed the baby's body floating in a gallon jar of formaldehyde.[1] The Johnson case epitomizes the lack of respect that was shown to the mother. If the mother in this delicate situation had been treated with dignity and respect, the situation would have been avoided.

Because of the nursing shortage, **abandonment** of clients is becoming an important legal and ethical issue for health-care providers. Abandonment occurs when there is a unilateral severance of the professional relationship with the client without adequate notice and while the requirement for care still exists. The nurse-client relationship continues until it is terminated by mutual consent of both parties. From an ethical standpoint, the issue of abandonment falls under the umbrella of beneficence. From the legal view, client abandonment can be considered an intentional tort, breach of contract, or in some cases where injury occurs, malpractice. The key phrase to keep in mind when discussing client abandonment is "without adequate notice." If the client knows that the nurse's shift is scheduled to end at 7:00 P.M., then the client as well as the hospital both have adequate notice. It is not uncommon for nurses in today's health-care system to be approached by nursing supervisors with the statement: "Everyone else called in, so you will have to work a double shift or you could be charged with client abandonment." In this case, the abandonment becomes the hospital's responsibility, not the nurse's. Nurses sometimes feel uncomfortable about going on strike because it seems to imply client abandonment; however, if there is adequate notice about the strike and the facility has had time to make arrangements for care or discharge of clients, then there is no client abandonment. The growing phenomenon of emergency client diversion that occurs when facilities can no longer safely care for emergency clients as the result of lack of space or staffing has the potential to fall under the legal definitions of abandonment.

Quasi-Intentional Torts

A **quasi-intentional tort** is a mixture of unintentional and intentional torts. It is defined as a voluntary act that directly causes injury or distress without intent to injure or to cause distress. A quasi-intentional tort does have the elements of volition and causation without the

Box 9–3

Registered Nurse Licensure

The legislature of each state enacts laws that govern the practice of nursing. The purpose of licensing law is to ensure that the public is protected from unqualified practitioners by developing and enforcing regulations that define who may practice in the profession, the scope of that practice, and the level of education for the profession.

A fundamental premise of nursing practice is that a professional nurse is personally responsible for all acts or omissions undertaken within the scope of practice.

The American Nurses Association defines delegation as "the transfer of responsibility for the performance of an activity from one person to another while retaining accountability for the outcome."[1] Additionally, the nurse is responsible for the adequate supervision of a delegated task to a subordinate. Failure of the nurse to delegate appropriately or supervise adequately and any injuries resulting from the acts of the subordinate may result in licensure ramifications. The state licensing board may take disciplinary actions.

element of intent. Quasi-intentional torts usually involve situations of communication and often violate a person's reputation, personal privacy, or civil rights.

Defamation of Character. Defamation of character, which is the most common of the quasi-intentional torts, is harmful to a person's reputation. Defamation injures a person's reputation by diminishing the esteem, respect, good will, or confidence that others have for the person. It can be especially damaging when false statements are made about a criminal act or an immoral act or when there are false allegations about a client's having a contagious disease. In *Schessler v. Keck* (1954), a nurse was found liable for defamation of character when she told a friend that a caterer for whom she was caring was being treated for syphilis. Even though the statement was false, when the information became public, it destroyed his catering business.[1]

Defamation includes **slander**, which is spoken communication in which one person discusses another in terms that harm that person's reputation. **Libel** is a written communication in which a person makes statements or uses language that harms another person's reputation. To win a defamation lawsuit against the nurse, the client must prove that the nurse acted maliciously, abused the principle of **privileged communication**, and wrote or spoke a lie.

Medical record documentation is a primary source of defamation of character. Through the years, the client's chart has been the basis of many defamation lawsuits. Discussion about a client in the elevators, cafeteria, and other public areas can also lead to lawsuits for defamation if negative comments are overheard.

Invasion of Privacy. Invasion of privacy is a violation of a person's right to protection against unreasonable and unwarranted interference with one's personal life. To prove that invasion of privacy has occurred, the client must show that (1) the nurse intruded on the client's seclusion and privacy, (2) the intrusion is objectionable to a reasonable and prudent person, (3) the act committed intrudes on private or published facts or pictures of a private nature, and (4) public disclosure of private information was made.[3] Examples of invasion of privacy include using the client's name or picture for the sole advantage of the health-care provider, intruding into the client's private affairs without permission, giving out private client information over the telephone, and publishing information that misrepresents the client's condition.

Breach of Confidentiality. **Confidentiality** of information concerning the client must be honored. A breach of confidentiality results when a client's trust and confidence are violated by public revelation of confidential or privileged communications without the client's consent. Most breach of confidentiality cases involve a physician's revelation of privileged communications shared by a client. Nurses who overhear privileged communication or information, however, are held to the same standards as a physician with regard to that information.

Privileged client information can only be disclosed if it is authorized by the client. Most health-care facilities have specific guidelines dealing with client information disclosure. Disclosure of information to family members is also not acceptable unless the client gives permission to do so. For instance, a client may not wish to disclose to a family member a specific diagnosis, such as cancer. If this is the case, the nurse should honor this request; otherwise, it could be considered a violation of that client's privacy.

Use of computerized documentation and telemedicine have led to several lawsuits based on breach of confidentiality and malpractice. (See Chapter 17 for examples.) The legal system has lagged behind in its attempts to keep pace with the use of computers and electronic record keeping. To date, there are no state codes that systematically deal with all the issues raised by computerization. Cases exist in which medical records have been lost because of computer failure. Other issues, such as correction of errors in **charting**, are complicated by use of the computer. In the paper charts, health-care providers had to draw a line through the erroneous entry, initial the entry, and date it. With computerized charting, simply hitting the delete button will completely erase all evidence of a mistaken entry. Understandably, the legal system is very concerned about this practice.

Facing a Lawsuit

Because of the rapid proliferation of lawsuits since the 1990s, there is now a higher probability that a nurse, at some time in his or her career, will be involved either as a witness or as a party to a nursing malpractice action. Knowledge of the litigation process increases the nurse's understanding of the way in which the nurse's conduct is evaluated before the courts.

Statute of Limitations

A malpractice suit against a nurse for negligence must be filed within a specified time. This period, called the **statute of limitations**, generally begins at the time of the injury or when the injury is discovered and lasts until some specified future time. In most states, the limitation period lasts from 1 to 6 years, with the most common duration being 2 years. If the client fails to file the suit within the prescribed time, the lawsuit will be barred.

The Complaint

Filing the suit (also called the complaint) with the court begins the litigation process. The written complaint describes the incident that initiated the claim of negligence against the nurse. Specific allegations, including the amount of money sought for damages, are also stated in the **legal complaint**. The plaintiff, who is usually a client or a family member of a client, is the alleged injured party, and the defendant (i.e., the nurse, physician, or hospital) is the person or entity being sued. The first notice of a lawsuit occurs when the defendant (nurse) is officially notified or served with the complaint. All defendants are accorded the right of **due process** under constitutional law.

The Answer

The defendant must respond to the allegations stated in the complaint within a specific time frame. This written response by the defendant is called the answer. If the nurse had liability insurance in force at the time of the negligent act, the insurer will assign a lawyer to represent the defendant nurse. In the answer, the nurse can outline specific defenses to the claims against him or her.

The Discovery

After the complaint and answer are filed with the court, the discovery phase of the litigation begins. The purpose of discovery is to uncover all information relevant to the malpractice suit and the incident in question. The nurse may be required to answer a series of questions that relate to the nurse's educational background, nurse's emotional state, the incident that led to the lawsuit, and any other information the plaintiff's lawyer deems important. These written questions are called **interrogatories**.

In addition, the plaintiff's lawyer may seek requests for production of documents. These are actual documents related to the lawsuit, including the plaintiff's medical records, **incident reports**, **Kardex**, the institution's policy and procedure manual concerning the specific situation, and the nurse's job description. The plaintiff is also required to disclose information as part of the discovery process that includes the plaintiff's past medical history.

The Deposition

The next step in the process is the taking of a deposition from each party to the lawsuit, as well as any potential witnesses, to assist the lawyers in the trial preparation. A **deposition** is a formal legal process that involves the taking of testimony under oath and is recorded by a court reporter. These are usually wide-ranging in scope and often include information not allowed in a trial, such as **hearsay** testimony. In some cases, videotaped depositions may be used. Nurses can prepare for a deposition by keeping some key points in mind (Box 9–4).

The deposition **testimony** is reduced to a written document for use at trial called an **affidavit**. If a witness during the actual trial changes testimony from that given at the deposition, the deposition can be used to contradict the testimony. This process is called impeaching the witness. Impeaching a witness on a specific issue can create doubt about that witness's credibility and can thus weaken other areas in the witness's testimony. In some situations, witnesses can later be charged with **perjury** if it is proved that they gave false testimony under oath.

The Trial

The actual **trial** often takes place years after the complaint was filed. Once **jurisdiction** is determined, the *voir dire* process, more commonly called jury selection, begins. After jury selection, each attorney presents opening statements. The plaintiff's side is presented first. Witnesses may be served with **subpoenas** that require them to appear and provide testimony. Each witness or party is subject to direct examination, cross-examination, and redirect examination. Direct examination involves open-ended questions by the attorney. Cross-examination is performed by the opposing lawyer, and questions are asked in such a way as to elicit short, specific responses. The redirect examination consists of follow-up questions to address issues that were previously raised during the cross-examination. After both parties have presented their case, the lawyers deliver their closing arguments. The case then goes to a jury or a judge for deliberation. If the facts are not in dispute, the judge may render a **summary judgment**. The decision or ruling made about the case can be appealed if either

Box 9–4

Giving a Deposition

1. Do not volunteer information.
2. Be familiar with the client's medical record and nurse's notes.
3. Remain calm throughout the process and do not be intimidated by the lawyers.
4. Clarify all questions before answering; ask the lawyer to explain the question if not understood.
5. Do not make assumptions about the questions.
6. Do not exaggerate answers.
7. Allow at least 5 seconds after a question is asked before answering it to allow objections from other lawyers.
8. Tell the truth.
9. Do not speculate about answers.
10. Speak slowly and clearly, using professional language as much as possible.
11. Look the questioning lawyer in the eye as much as possible.
12. If unable to remember an answer, simply state "I don't remember" or "I don't know."
13. Think before answering any question.
14. Bring a resume or curriculum vitae to the deposition in case it is requested.
15. Request a break if tired or confused.
16. Avoid becoming angry with the lawyers or using sarcastic language.
17. Avoid using absolutes in the answers.
18. If a question is asked more than once, ask the court recorder to read the answer given previously.
19. Be sure to read over the deposition just before the trial.

Source: Aiken, TJ, and Catalano, JT: Legal, Ethical, and Political Issues in Nursing. FA Davis, Philadelphia 1994.

party is not satisfied. The party appealing the decision is called the **appellant**.

Possible Defenses to a Malpractice Suit

Contributory Negligence versus Comparative Negligence

Damages awarded vary from one state to another and also with the types of injuries sustained. In a state with contributory negligence laws, clients are not allowed to receive money for injuries if they contributed to that injury in any manner. For example, the nurse forgot to raise the bed rail after administering an injection of a narcotic pain medication to a client who had an operation but instructed the client to turn on the call light if he wanted to get out of bed. The client fell while attempting to go to the bathroom; however, because he did not use the call light, he had contributed to his own injuries and thus could not receive compensation.

In a state with comparative negligence laws, the awards are based on the determination of the percentage of fault by both parties. For example, in the aforementioned case, if $100,000 was awarded by the jury, it may be determined that the nurse was 75 percent at fault and the client was 25 percent at fault. In that case, the client would receive $75,000. In general, if the client is 50 percent or more at fault, no award will be made. As can be seen, determination of these types of awards is highly subjective, and an **appeal** is often made to a higher court about the decision. Consider the following case:

Ms. Gouge, a 44-year-old client who weighs

307 lb, was admitted to a large university medical center ER with complaints of chest pain and disorientation and a blood pressure of 208/154. She also displayed aphasia, hemiplegia, and loss of sensation and movement on her right side. After a magnetic resonance imaging (MRI) scan of the head, it was discovered that she had a nonoperative cerebral aneurysm. In addition to appropriate medical treatment for blood pressure and circulation, her family physician told her that she had to lose a significant amount of weight. The nurse in the physician's office instituted a weight loss teaching plan for Ms. Gouge, planned out a calorie-restricted low-fat diet, and gave her a large amount of information about healthy diet and also a videotape of low-impact aerobic exercises. At a follow-up visit 1 month later, Ms. Gouge weighed 315 lb. Six months later, Ms. Gouge's aneurysm ruptured, leaving her in a vegetative state.

Ms. Gouge's family filed a lawsuit against the physician and his office nurse claiming that they had failed to institute proper and appropriate preventive measures and that they had failed to inform the client of the seriousness of her condition.

Did the nurse's decisions or actions contribute to the filing of this suit? Is there any contributory negligence? What is the nurse's role in defending against this suit? What might the nurse have done to prevent the suit in the first place?

Assumption of Risk

When the client signs the informed consent form for a particular treatment, procedure, or surgery, it is implied that he or she is aware of the possible complications of that treatment, procedure, or surgery. Under the assumption-of-risk defense, if one of those listed or named complications occurs, the client has no grounds to sue the health-care provider. For example, a common complication from hip replacement surgery is some loss of mobility and range of motion of the affected leg. Even if a client, after having a hip replaced, is able to walk only using a walker, he or she still does not have any grounds for a lawsuit.

> *When the client signs the informed consent form for a particular treatment, procedure, or surgery, it is implied that he or she is aware of the possible complications of that treatment, procedure, or surgery. Under the assumption-of-risk defense, if one of those listed or named complications occurs, the client has no grounds to sue the health-care provider.*

Good Samaritan Act

Health-care providers are sometimes hesitant to provide care at the scene of accidents, in emergency situations, or disasters because they fear lawsuits. The **Good Samaritan Act** is designed specifically to protect health-care providers in these situations. A health-care professional who provides care in an emergency situation cannot be sued for injuries that may be sustained by the client if that care was given according to established guidelines and was within the scope of the professional's education. For example, a nurse who finds a person in cardiac arrest administers cardiopulmonary resuscitation (CPR) to revive the person. In the process, she fractures several of the client's ribs. The client would not be able to sue the nurse for the fractured ribs if the CPR was administered according to established standards.

Good Samaritan laws do, however, have some limitations. They do not cover nurses for grossly negligent acts in the provision of care or for acts outside the nurse's level of education. For example, in the case of a person choking on a piece of meat, the nurse initially attempts the Heimlich maneuver but without success. As the person loses consciousness, the nurse decides to perform a tracheostomy. The client survives but can sue the nurse for injuries from the tracheostomy, because this is not a normal part of a nurse's education.

Unavoidable Accident

Sometimes accidents happen without any contributing causes from the nurse, hospital, or physician. For example, a client is walking in the hall and trips over her own bathrobe. She breaks an ankle. There were no puddles on the floor or obstacles in the hall, and the client was alert and oriented. Because no one is at fault, there are no grounds for a lawsuit.

Defense of the Fact

This defense is based on the claim that the actions of the nurse followed the standards of care, or that even if the actions were in violation of the standard of care, the action itself was not the direct cause of the injury. For example, a nurse wraps a dressing too tightly on a client's foot after surgery. Later, the client loses his eyesight and blames the loss of vision on the nurse's improper dressing of his foot.[4]

Going through the litigation process can produce high levels of anxiety. Placing every aspect of the nurse's conduct under scrutiny in a trial is very stressful. All aspects of the alleged negligent act will be examined and re-examined. Every word of the nurse's notes and the medical record will be analyzed and questioned. Nurses can survive the litigation process with the help of a good attorney and by being honest and demonstrating that they were acting in the best interest of the client. From this viewpoint, it is easy to see the importance of carrying nursing liability insurance.

Alternative Dispute Forums

Although most lawsuits against nurses are settled through the court system, there are other methods of settling them. Because of the large number of cases and the resultant overload of the judicial system, other methods of resolving disputes have become increasingly popular. These alternative forums of dispute resolution are being used for many types of conflicts and are seen more frequently in the area of torts, contracts, employment, and family law matters. Mediation and arbitration are the most commonly used alternatives to trial.

Mediation

Mediation is a process that allows each party to present his or her case before a mediator, who is an independent third party trained in dispute resolution. The mediator listens to each side individually. This one-sided session is called a caucus. The mediator's role is to find common ground between the parties and encourage resolution of the disputed matters by compromise and negotiation. The mediator aids the parties in arriving at a mutually acceptable outcome. The mediator does not act as a decision-maker, but rather encourages the parties to come to a "meeting of the minds."

Arbitration

Arbitration, in contrast, allows a neutral third party to hear both parties' positions and then make a decision or ruling based on the facts and evidence presented. Arbitration, by agreement or by statutory definition, can be binding or nonbinding. **Arbitrators** or mediators can be, and frequently are, retired judges who work on an hourly-fee basis. They are often attorneys. In the family law areas, they are frequently social workers or specially trained mediators. Negligence and malpractice issues are frequently resolved through arbitration and mediation.

Common Issues in Health-Care Litigation

Informed Consent

Informed consent is both a legal and ethical issue. Informed consent is the voluntary permission by a client, or by the client's designated proxy, to carry out a procedure on the client. Clients' claims that they did not grant informed consent prior to a surgery or invasive procedure can and do form the basis of a small percentage of lawsuits. Although these lawsuits are most often directed against physicians and hospitals, nurses can become involved when they provide the information but are not performing the procedure. The person who is performing the procedure has the responsibility to obtain the informed consent. However, some physicians have gotten into the habit of giving nurses the consent forms and saying, "Get the client to sign this." Informed consent can only be given by a client after the client receives sufficient information on:

- Treatment proposed
- Material risk involved
- Acceptable alternatives
- Outcome hoped for
- Consequences of not having treatment

The physician should provide most of this information. Nurses can reinforce the physician teaching and even supplement the information but should not be the primary or only source of information for the informed consent. It is often difficult to draw a clear distinction between where the physician's responsibility ends and that of the nurse begins.

What Do You Think?

Have you ever had a surgical procedure where you signed an informed consent form? Did it meet all five criteria listed? Which ones were missing?

Exceptions to Informed Consent

There are two exceptions to informed consent:

1. In emergency situations when the client is unconscious, incompetent, or otherwise unable to give consent.
2. In situations where the health provider feels that it may be medically contraindicated to disclose the risk and hazards because it may result in illness, severe emotional distress, serious psychological damage, or failure on the part of the client to receive lifesaving treatment.

Patient Self-Determination Act

The Patient Self-Determination Act of 1990, sponsored by Senator John Danforth, is a federal law that requires that all federally funded institutions inform clients of their right to prepare advance directives. The advance directives seek to encourage people to discuss and document their wishes concerning the type of treatment and care that they want (i.e., life-sustaining treatment) in advance, so that it will ease the burden on their families and providers when it comes time to make such a decision.

There are two types of advance directives: the living will and medical durable power of attorney (Box 9–5). The **living will** is a document stating what health care a client will accept or refuse after the client is no longer competent or able to make that decision. The medical durable power of attorney, or health-care proxy, designates another person to make health-care decisions for a person if the client becomes incompetent or unable to make such decisions.

Each state outlines its own requirements for executing and revoking the medical durable power of attorney and living wills.

Box 9–5

Common Questions about Advance Directives

Q. Which is better—a living will or a medical durable power of attorney for health care or health-care proxy?

A. The documents are different and allow the nurse to do two different things. The living will states what health-care procedures a client will accept or refuse after the client is no longer competent or able to make that decision. The medical durable power of attorney or health-care proxy allows a client to designate another person to make health-care choices for him or her.

Q. If I change my mind and have a living will, can I cancel the living will or durable medical power of attorney?

A. Yes, each state has ways that your advance directives can be cancelled or negated. Most states require an oral or written statement, destruction of the document itself, or notification to certain individuals, such as the physician. Again, each state's statute should be checked for the specific details required.

Q. If I have a living will in one state, is it good in all states?

A. It may or may not be, depending on the requirements for the living will. It is important that you have your living will checked by an attorney in order to determine whether or not it may be effective in the states in which you are traveling or working.

Q. If I have a living will and have medical durable power of attorney who should get copies?

A. Copies should be given to your next of kin, your physician, and your attorney so that more than one person has a copy and knows what your intentions are. Some states will allow you to register your living will with certain state agencies such as the Secretary of State. Also there are national groups that will allow you to register your living will with them so that there is access to it.

Nurses must also teach about advance directives and document all critical decisions, discussions with the client and client's family about such decisions, and the basis for the decision-making process.

Incompetent Client's Right to Self-Determination

The courts are protective of incompetent clients and require high standards of proof before allowing a physician to terminate any life-sustaining treatment for that client.

Nancy Cruzan was 30 years old and in a persistent vegetative state. She had a gastrostomy feeding and hydration tube inserted to assist with the feedings, which was consented to by her husband. Her parents, however, petitioned the court for removal of the tube. In the Cruzan case, the court held that the state had the right to err on the side of life. The U.S. Supreme Court recognized that a living will would have been sufficient evidence of Cruzan's wishes to sustain or to remove her feeding tube.

The issue before the U.S. Supreme Court was whether the state of Missouri could use its own standard of clear and convincing proof for removal of the tube or whether there was a 14th Amendment due process guarantee of a "right to die" that would override the state statute. It was decided that the constitutional right would not be extended and the state procedural requirement would be allowed, at which time the burden of proof was put on Cruzan's family to show that she would not have wanted to continue living in this manner.

The Nurse's Role in Advance Directives

Nurses must know the laws of the state pertaining to advance directives, clients' rights, and the policies and procedures of the institution in which they work. Nurses must inform clients of their right to formulate advance directives and to realize that not all clients can make such decisions. It is important for the nurse to establish trust and rapport with a client and the client's family so that the nurse can assist them in making decisions that are in the client's best interests. Nurses must also teach about advance directives and document all critical decisions, discussions with the client and client's family about such decisions, and the basis for the decision-making process. Discrimination must be also prevented against clients and their families based on their decisions regarding their advance directives. It is important that nurses determine whether or not the client has been coerced into making advance directive decisions against his or her will. Nurses need to become involved in ethics committees at hospitals or nursing specialty groups at local, state, or national levels to better help clients make decisions about advance directives.

> *Although a DNR instruction may be included in an advance directive, DNR orders are legally separate from advance directives.*

Do-Not-Resuscitate (DNR) Orders

Although a DNR instruction may be included in an advance directive, DNR orders are legally separate from advance directives. For the healthcare professional to be legally protected, there should be a written order for a "no code" or DNR order in the client's chart. Each hospital should have a policy and procedure that outlines what is required with regard to a client's condition for a DNR order. The DNR order should be reviewed, evaluated, and reordered. Different facilities have established different time periods for these reviews. Nurses must also know whether there is any law that regulates who should authorize a DNR order for an incompetent client who is no longer able to make this decision. Hospitals often have policies and procedures describing what must be done and which clients fit the requirements for a DNR order. The American Nurses Association (ANA) has published a position statement on nursing care and DNR decisions.

Nurses face many legal dilemmas when dealing with confusing or conflicting DNR orders. For example, it may be difficult to interpret a DNR order when it has been restricted, for instance, "do not resuscitate except for medications and defibrillation" or "no CPR or intubation." Often a lack of proper documentation in the medical records indicating how the DNR decision was reached can be an important and crucial issue if a medical malpractice case is involved and it is disputed whether or not the client or family actually gave consent for a DNR order.

Many facilities have developed DNR decision sheets for recording information about DNR discussions; or the sheets are dated and signed by the client and those family members who took part in the discussion. It then becomes a permanent part of the medical record. It is very important that nurses not stigmatize clients by the use of indicators for DNR orders, such as dots on the wristband or dots over the bed. Health-care providers' attitudes often change because they feel that the client is "going to die anyway." This abandonment can jeopardize the care of a client designated with a DNR order. However, it is also important for the nurses and staff to know whether an order is to be honored and what the policies and procedures are with regard to transfer clients and DNR orders that accompany the incoming client. Information about the DNR status of a client should be obtained during shift report. If there has not been a periodic review, is the order still in effect? If a client is transferred from one facility to another but has a DNR order that is time-limited and has not been reordered, what should a nurse do?

> *Nurses are encountering an increasing number of incidents where conflicts occur between institutional and professional standards, for example in staffing ratios.*

Standards of Care

Standards of care are the yardstick that the legal system uses to measure the actions of a nurse involved in a malpractice suit. The underlying principle used to establish standards of care is based on the actions that would likely be taken by a reasonable person (nurse) who was placed in the same or similar circumstances. The standard usually includes both objective factors (e.g., the actions to be performed) and subjective factors, including the nurse's emotional and mental state. Specifically, a nurse is judged against the standards that are established within the profession and specialty area of practice. The ANA and specialty groups within the nursing profession, such as the American Association of Critical-Care Nurses (AACN), publish standards of care that are updated continually as health-care technology and practices change.

Both external and internal standards govern the conduct of nurses. External standards include nursing standards developed by the ANA, the state nurse practice act of each jurisdiction, criteria from accrediting agencies such as the Joint Commission on Accreditation of Healthcare Organizations, guidelines developed by various nursing specialty practice groups, and federal agency regulations. Nurses are encountering an increasing number of incidents where conflicts occur between institutional and professional standards, for example in staffing ratios. These conflicts are difficult to resolve and may require deliberation and decisions from institutional committees. As a general rule, when a conflict exists, it is safer legally to follow professional standards.

Internal standards include nursing standards defined in specific hospital policy and procedure manuals that relate to the nurse in the particular institution. The nurse's job description and employment contract are examples of internal nursing standards that define the duty of the nurse.

The rationale for advancing standards of care for the nurse is to ensure proper, consistent, and high-quality nursing care to all members of society. When nurses violate their duty of care to the client as established by the profession's standards of care, they leave themselves open to charges of negligence and malpractice. Until recently, nurses were held to the standards of the local community. National criteria have now replaced most **locality rule standards of care**. Individual nurses are held accountable not only to acceptable standards within the local community but also to national standards as well.

Although standards of care may appear to be specific, they are merely guidelines for nursing practice. Because every client's situation is different, the appropriate standard of care may be difficult to identify in a specific case. More than one course of nursing action may be considered appropriate under a proper standard of care. The final decision must be guided by the nurse's judgment and understanding of the client's needs.

The Nurse Practice Act

The nurse practice act defines nursing practice and establishes standards for nurses in each state. It is the most definitive legal statute or legislative act regulating nursing practice. Although nurse practice acts vary in scope from one state to another, they tend to have similar wording based loosely on the ANA model published in 1988. The nurse practice act provides a framework for the court on which to base decisions when determining whether a nurse has breached a standard of care.

Most state nurse practice acts define scope of practice, establish requirements for licensure and entry into practice, and create and empower a board of nursing to oversee the practice of nurses. In addition, nurse practice acts identify grounds for disciplinary actions such as suspension and revocation of a nursing license.[4]

The judicial interpretation of the nurse practice act and its relationship to a specific case provide guidance for decisions about future cases. Many state legislatures have responded to the expanded role of the nurse by broadening the scope of their nurse practice acts. For example, the addition of the term *nursing diagnosis* to many states' nurse practice acts reflects the legislature's recognition of the expansion of the nurse's role. In addition, occupational roles such as nurse practitioner, **nurse clinician**, and clinical nurse specialist are beginning to be included in nurse practice acts. It is important to remember that as the nurse's role expands, so does the legal accountability of the role itself.

Prevention of Lawsuits

What can the nurse do to avoid having to go through the stressful, sometimes financially and professionally devastating, process of litigation? The following guidelines provide some ways to avoid a lawsuit.

Medical Record

The medical record is the single most frequently used piece of objective evidence in a malpractice suit. In preparation for the trial, the lawyers attempt to reconstruct the events surrounding the incident in a minute-by-minute time line. The client's **chart** is the most important source for this time line. Maintaining an accurate and complete medical record is an absolute requirement (Box 9–6). The old adage "if it isn't written, it didn't happen" remains true in most situations; however, recent court trials have recognized some exceptions. Some judges and juries have begun to recognize that charting by exception is a valid form of health-care record keeping. Charting by exception, very closely related to problem-oriented charting, was developed initially to save busy nurses time and to save the facility money by reducing the volume of documents created and stored. In institutions where charting by exception is used, the nurse charts only those elements of client care that are abnormal or unusual or that constitute a health-care problem. If the client is stable and recovering as expected, there may be very little written in the chart about his or her physical or mental assessments.

Trying to recall specific events from 2 to 6 years previously without the benefit of written notes is almost impossible. In general, the client record should *not* contain personal opinion, should be legible, should be in chronological order, and should be written and signed by the nurse. Although opinions have a relatively low value in legal proceedings, the documentation should indicate the nursing judgments made by the nurse. An entry should never be obliterated or destroyed. If a nurse questions a physician's order, record must be made that the physician was contacted and the order clarified.

Box 9–6

Some Documentation Guidelines

Medications

- Always chart the time, route, dose, and response.
- Always chart PRN medications and the client response.
- Always chart when a medication was not given, the reason (client in x-ray, physical therapy, etc.; do not chart that the medication was not on the floor), and the nursing intervention.
- Chart all medication refusals and report them to the appropriate source.

Physician Communication

- Document each time a call is made to a physician even if he or she is not reached. Include the exact time of the call. If the physician is reached, document the details of the message and the physician response.
- Read verbal orders back to the physician and confirm the client's identity as written on the chart. Chart only verbal orders that you have heard from the source not those told to you by an other nurse or unit personnel.

Formal Issues in Charting

- Before writing on the chart, check to be sure you have the correct client record.
- Check to make sure each page has the client's name and the current date stamped in the appropriate area.
- If you forgot to make an entry, chart "late entry" and place the date and time at the entry.
- Correct all charting mistakes according to the policy and procedures of your institution.
- Chart in an organized fashion following the nursing process.
- Write legibly and concisely and avoid subjective statements.
- Write specific and accurate descriptions.
- When charting a symptom or situation chart the interventions taken and the client response.
- Document your own observations and not those that were told to you by another party.
- Chart frequently to demonstrate ongoing care and chart routine activities.
- Chart client and family teaching and the response.

Source: From Tappen, RM, et al: Essentials of Nursing Leadership and Management, ed. 2. FA Davis, Philadelphia, 2001, p. 169, with permission.

Rapport with Clients

Establishing a rapport with the client through honest, open communication goes a long way in avoiding lawsuits. Treating clients and their families with respect and letting them know that the nurse really cares about them may well prevent a lawsuit. Many people are willing to forgive a nurse's error if they have good rapport and a trusting relationship with a nurse who they believe is interested in their well-being.

Current Nursing Skills

Keeping one's nursing knowledge and skills current is vital to prevent errors that may lead to lawsuits. It is better to refuse to perform an unfa-

What Do You Think?

Think about being involved in a legal or courtroom activity, either as a defendant, complainant, witness, or juror. What would your role be in each situation?

miliar procedure than to attempt it without the necessary knowledge and skills. Taking advantage of in-service training, workshops, and continuing nursing education classes is an important part of maintaining the nurse's skill level. Nurses must practice within their level of competence and scope of practice.

Knowledge of the Client

Recognizing the client who is lawsuit-prone can help reduce the risk of litigation. Some common characteristics of this type of client include constant dissatisfaction with the care given, constant complaints about all aspects of care, and negative comments about other nurses. This client often complains about the poor care given by nurses on the previous shift. This client may also have a history of lawsuits against nurses.

Being direct, solving problems with the client, and helping the client become involved in his or her care are helpful to diffuse this negative behavior. Also, even more careful documentation of the care provided and the client's responses to the care can be helpful if a lawsuit is later filed.

Liability Insurance

Maintenance of proper liability insurance is a necessity. Nurses who do not carry liability insurance place themselves at high risk. The nurse's personal assets as well as the nurse's wages may be subject to a judgment awarded in a malpractice action. Even if the client does not win at the trial, the litigation process, including hiring a lawyer and paying the costs of experts, can be financially devastating.

A professional liability insurance policy is a contract with an insurer who promises to assume the costs paid to the injured party in exchange for payment of a premium (Box 9–7). There are two types of malpractice policies: claims-made and occurrence. **Claims-made policies** protect only against claims made during the time the policy is in effect. **Occurrence policies** protect against all claims that occurred during the policy period, regardless of when the claim is made. Generally, the occurrence type of liability insurance offers more protection. Claims-made policy coverage can be broadened by purchasing a tail that is a separate policy that extends the time of coverage.

Some hospitals have liability insurance policies for the nurse as a part of the nurse's employment package with the institution. This hospital policy may be limited to claims arising from the nurse's employment and might not apply in a situation in which a nurse renders care outside the institution, for instance, at an automobile accident site. It is preferable to have liability insurance coverage that includes all situations in which the nurse may be involved. Individual indemnity insurance coverage independent of the facility's policy is recommended for all nurses. With passage of the **Federal Tort Claims Act**, and similar state laws, nurses who were formerly protected from lawsuits by working at federal or state health-care facilities can now be sued for malpractice like nurses at any other facility.

Revocation of License

One of the most drastic punishments that a nurse can experience is revocation of the license to practice nursing. The nursing profession is responsible for monitoring and enforcing its own standards through the state licensing board. These actions may or may not be related to tort law, contract law, or criminal charges. Each state's licensing board is charged with the responsibility to oversee the professional nurse's competence.

The state's nursing board receives its authority to grant and revoke licenses from specific

Box 9–7

What to Look for in an Insurance Policy

The following factors should be reviewed in order to determine what is the best policy for your type of nursing practice:

1. *Type of insurance policy (claims-made or occurrence basis)*
2. *Insuring agreement*

   The insurance company's promise to pay in exchange for premiums is called the insuring agreement. The insurance company agrees to pay a money award to a plaintiff who is injured by an act of omission or commission by a health-care provider who is insured by the company.

3. *Types of injuries covered*

   The language must be scrutinized to determine whether it is broad or limiting. Some companies will agree to pay only if the insured nurse is sued for damages, which means the nurse must be sued for a money amount or award. If the nurse is sued for a specific performance lawsuit or an injunctive relief action, which means that the nurse will either have to perform something or discontinue doing something, that particular insurance policy may not be adequate. Also, most insurance policies do not cover the nurse for disciplinary actions.

4. *Exclusions*

   Items that are not covered by a policy are called exclusions. It is important to review the exclusions. Some of the more common exclusions include sexual abuse of a client, injury caused while under the influence of drugs or alcohol, criminal activity, and punitive damages. Punitive damages are used to punish the defendant for egregious acts or omissions.

Who Is Covered Under the Policy

The purchaser is the named insured and can be an individual, institution, or group. Others who may be covered by the policy are nurses, employees, agents, and volunteers, among others.

Limitations and Deductions

In exchange for payment of the premium, the insurance company agrees to pay up to a certain amount on behalf of the insured. This amount is called the limit of liability. It is usually expressed in two ways: the amount that can be paid per incident (per occurrence), and the amount that will be paid for the entire policy year. For example, if you have a policy that states \$1,000,000/\$3,000,000, it means that the company will pay up to \$1 million per incident and a total of \$3 million per policy year.

The insurance industry relies on the A. M. Best Company to evaluate both the financial size and relative strengths of insurance companies. An A. M. Best rating of A− or better should be a prerequisite for purchase of any policy.

The Right to Select Counsel

Some insurance companies allow nurses to select their own attorneys to represent them in a medical negligence claim. Others retain attorneys or law firms, and the nurse does not have the opportunity to make that selection.

The Right to Consent to Settlement

Some policies allow the nurse to decide whether or not a case should be settled or go to trial, whereas others do not.

statutory laws. The underlying rationale for establishment of a licensing board is to protect the public from uneducated, unsafe, or unethical practitioners. If a nurse fails to adhere to the standards of safe practice and exhibits unprofessional behavior, he or she can be disciplined by the state nursing licensing board. One of the remedies that these boards can use is suspension or revocation of the nurse's license.

A disciplinary hearing is held to review the charges of the nurse's unprofessional conduct. This hearing is less formal than the trial process, and the nurse is allowed to present evidence and be represented by legal counsel at the hearing. Due process requires that the nurse be notified in advance of the specific charges being made. The question of what constitutes unprofessional conduct is an issue frequently dealt with at the disciplinary hearing. Each respective state's nurse practice act provides guidance with regard to the specifics of unprofessional conduct.

Unprofessional conduct can be reported by a nursing peer, supervisor, client, or a client's family. Many cases are dismissed before the hearing takes place if the board finds there is no support for the allegation being made against the nurse. If a hearing is necessary, it is in the best interest of the nurse to seek legal counsel because of the potential risk of license revocation.

The nursing profession is responsible for monitoring and enforcing its own standards through the state licensing board.

License revocation is a serious consequence for the nurse because it removes the nurse's right to practice. Drug abuse, administering medication without a prescription, practicing without a valid license, and any singular act of unprofessional or unethical conduct can constitute grounds for losing a nursing license.

Conclusion

The legal system and its effects on the practice of nursing are ever-present realities in today's health-care system. Nurses need to be aware of the implications of their actions but should not be so overwhelmed by fear that it reduces their ability to care for the client. The more advanced and specialized the nurse's practice becomes, the higher the standards to which the nurse is held. Nurses will be challenged throughout their career to apply legal principles in the daily practice of nursing. An awareness of what constitutes malpractice and negligence will aid in the prevention of litigation.

ISSUES IN PRACTICE

Critical Thinking Exercises

Consider the following case: *Thomas v. Corso* (Md. 1982)
The client was brought to the hospital emergency room (ER) after being involved in an automobile accident. The ER nurse assessed and recorded the client's vital signs and a complaint of numbness in his right anterior thigh. The client was able to move the right leg, and there was no discoloration or deformity. After he was given meperidine (Demerol) for his pain, his blood pressure (B/P) dropped to 90/60 and the nurse notified the ER physician of the change. The physician ordered the nurse to arrange for admission to the hospital, which she did.

The client was transferred to a medical/surgical unit, but he could not be placed in a room because of an influenza epidemic. Rather, the client was placed in the hall next to the nurses' station for close observation. A nurse checked the client's vital signs about 20 minutes after the transfer and noted that the B/P was now 70/50, respiratory rate 40, and pulse 120. His skin was cool and diaphoretic, his breathing was deep and rapid, and he was asking for a drink of water. The client also complained of pain in his leg, but the nurse did not give him more pain medication because of his blood pressure.

The nurse assessed him about 30 minutes later and found his skin warmer, although he still complained of pain and thirst. The nurse also noted a strong odor of alcohol on the client's breath. An assistant supervisor also assessed the client's condition but refused to give him any water because he had obviously been drinking alcohol. She had been told about the low blood pressure by the client's nurse but attributed it to the alcohol and pain medication combination. The nurse checked his vital signs again and found a B/P of 100/89. Thirty minutes later it was 94/70, pulse 100, and respirations 28. When the nurse next assessed the client an hour later, he had a Cheyne-Stokes respiratory pattern, no pulse, and no blood pressure. She started cardiopulmonary resuscitation (CPR) and called a "code blue," but after a lengthy attempt at resuscitation, the client died.

An autopsy was performed and showed that the client had a lacerated liver and a severe fracture of the femur with bleeding into the tissues. The coroner determined that traumatic shock, secondary to the fractured femur and lacerated liver, was the cause of death. His family sued the nurses for poor judgment, and the hospital for malpractice, and won.

- What mistakes were made by the nurses in this case?
- What legal liability did the nurses incur by their actions?
- How can the nurses best prepare for trial in this case?

- What actions could the nurses have taken with this client to prevent a lawsuit?
- What are your feelings toward inebriated clients? Did the nurses' attitudes about inebriation affect their judgments?
- Why are clients who are drunk at higher risk for injury and poor medical outcomes than other clients?

References

1. Guido, G: Legal Issues in Nursing: A Source Book for Practice, ed. 2. Appleton & Lange, E. Norwalk, CT, 1997.
2. Menikoff, J: Law and Bioethics. Georgetown University Press, Baltimore, 2001.
3. Fiesta, J: Legal update, 1995, Part 2. Nursing Management 27(6):24–25, 1996.
4. Aiken, TD: Legal, Ethical, and Political Issues in Nursing. FA Davis, Philadelphia, 1994.

Bibliography

Castledine, G: Professional misconduct case studies. British Journal of Nursing 10(14):902, 2001.

Clark, AP: Legal and ethical dimensions of CNS practice. Clinical Nurse Specialist 15(5):212–214, 2001.

Cox, C: The legal challenges facing nursing. Journal of Orthopaedic Nursing 5(2):78–80, 2001.

Future looks bleak as malpractice premiums continue upward spiral. Healthcare Risk Management 24(1):1–4, 2002.

Geyer, N: Ethics and law. Nursing Update 25(7):20, 2001.

Legal questions: Confidentiality: At a loss for words. Nursing 2001 31(11):32, 2001.

Skyhigh and rising: Limits sought for malpractice in Penn. Healthcare Risk Management 24(3):25–28, 2002.

10

NCLEX: What You Need to Know

Joseph T. Catalano

Learning Objectives

After completing this chapter, the reader will be able to:

- Describe the NCLEX-RN, CAT test plan.
- Discuss the NCLEX-RN, CAT test format.
- Analyze and identify the different types of questions used on the NCLEX-RN, CAT.
- Select the most appropriate means for preparing for the NCLEX-RN, CAT.
- Apply key test-taking strategies to help improve examination grades.

The primary purpose of licensure examinations is to protect the public from unsafe or uneducated practitioners of the profession. When nurses pass the National Council Licensure Examination (NCLEX), it indicates that they have attained the minimal level of competency deemed necessary by the state in order to practice nursing without injury to clients. Licensure is a legal requirement for all professions who deal with public health, welfare, or safety.

All examinations produce anxiety in those who are about to take them. The more important the examination, the higher the anxiety levels. Anxiety is sometimes defined as fear of the unknown. This chapter presents information about the NCLEX test plan, tips for improving the score on multiple-choice examinations, and some suggestions for study. It is hoped that this information will help lower the student's anxiety levels about the NCLEX. There are also several sample practice questions included to give you an idea of how the NCLEX asks about different types of nursing information. Try to answer these questions as you read the chapter. The answers and rationales are found at the end of the chapter.

National Council Licensure Examination Test Plan

The NCLEX is a computerized, **criterion-referenced examination** that is taken after graduation from a school of nursing. Unlike a

ISSUES NOW

Handling Your Anxiety

First, it is perfectly reasonable to be slightly anxious about taking the NCLEX. You have expended plenty of blood, sweat, and tears to come to this point. As one diploma grad told me, "I was in debt up to my ears and running out of money fast when I took the NCLEX. Passing was literally my meal ticket." Even if you're not in such dire financial straits, it's no small thing to be tested on years of accumulated knowledge. You would have to be comatose not to feel butterflies in your stomach at this point. Do not be anxious about being anxious.

Because you cannot go back and change answers, treat each question as an exam in itself; once you hit the enter key the second time, immediately turn your attention to the next question. Tell yourself not to be surprised by anything. You are at a psychological disadvantage if you expect the computer to turn off at a certain number and it doesn't. So if you can, avoid looking at the question number as you answer each question.

If you are distracted by the clicking of other people's computers or other such annoying sounds, you can ask for earplugs. The testing service provides them; they are disposable and not entirely unattractive.

Finally, there are going to be other people close to you or next to you who may sit down at the computer at the same time as you do. They may get up before you, but ignore them. The testing centers administer many different tests, so you can realistically tell yourself that the person next to you who finished in 45 minutes was not even taking the NCLEX. Even if they were taking the NCLEX, you do not need to think about it. A little denial in this situation can go a long way.

Source: Dunham, KS: How to Survive and Maybe Even Love Nursing School. FA Davis, Philadelphia, 2001, pp. 180–181, with permission.

norm-referenced examination, which establishes a passing score based on how others fare in the examination, criterion-referenced examinations compare the test taker's knowledge to a preestablished standard. The examination measures nursing knowledge of a wide range of material. With computerized adaptive tests such as the NCLEX, the computer selects questions in accordance with the examination plan and how well the graduate answered the previous question.

In April 1998, several substantive changes were made in the National Council Licensure Examination–Computerized Adaptive Testing for Registered Nurses (NCLEX-RN, CAT) test plan. The changes included reorganization of the test plan into three primary components: (1) client needs, (2) level of cognitive ability, and (3) integrated concepts and processes. The third component was expanded to include nursing process, caring, communication, cultural awareness, documentation, self-care, and teaching/learning. Additional changes were made in October 2001 and October 2002 to the format and examination test vendor.

Client Health Needs

The NCLEX asks questions about four general groups of material called client health needs:

- Safe and effective care environment
- Physiologic integrity
- Psychosocial integrity
- Health promotion and maintenance needs

Safe and Effective Care Environment

a. Management of care: 7%–13% of NCLEX questions
b. Safety, infection control: 5%–11% of NCLEX questions

Total questions in this category make up between 13 and 24 percent of the total questions on the NCLEX. These questions deal with overt safety issues in client care, such as use of restraints, medication administration, safety measures to prevent injuries (like putting up side rails), prevention of infections, isolation precautions, safety measures with pediatric clients, and special safety needs of clients with psychiatric problems.

This needs category also includes questions about laboratory tests, their results, and any special nursing measures associated with them; legal and ethical issues in nursing; a small amount of nursing management; and quality assurance issues. Questions on these issues are interspersed with other questions throughout the examination.

Physiologic Integrity

a. Basic care and comfort: 7%–13% of NCLEX questions
b. Pharmacologic/parenteral therapies: 5%–11% of NCLEX questions
c. Reduction of risk potential: 12%–18% of NCLEX questions
d. Physiologic adaptation: 12%–18% of NCLEX questions

The physiologic integrity needs are concerned with adult medical and surgical nursing care, pediatrics, and **gerontology**. This category comprises the largest groups of questions, with about 50 to 55 percent of the total number of questions on the NCLEX. The more common health-care problems, both acute and chronic conditions, that nurses deal with on a daily basis include:

- Diabetes
- Cardiovascular disorders
- Neurologic disorders
- Renal diseases

There are also questions about nursing care of the pediatric client, including such topics as:

- Growth and development
- Congenital abnormalities

- Child abuse
- Burn injury
- Fractures

Psychosocial Integrity

a. Coping and adaptation: 5%–11% of NCLEX questions
b. Psychosocial adaptation: 5%–11% of NCLEX questions

Psychosocial integrity needs are those health-care issues that revolve around the client with psychiatric problems. This material also deals with coping mechanism for high-stress situations such as acute illness and life-threatening diseases or trauma. These clients do not necessarily have any psychiatric disorders. This category constitutes approximately 15 percent of the examination and includes questions about the care of clients with anxiety disorders, depression, schizophrenia, and organic mental disease. Also included in the psychosocial needs section are questions about therapeutic communication, crisis intervention, and substance abuse.

Health Promotion and Maintenance

a. Life span growth and development: 7%–13% of NCLEX questions
b. Prevention/early detection of disease: 5%–11% of NCLEX questions

Health promotion and maintenance needs deal with pregnancy, labor and delivery, the care of the newborn infant, growth and development, and contagious diseases, particularly sexually transmitted diseases. This section constitutes approximately 15 percent of the total examination. Teaching and counseling are important parts of the nurse's care during pregnancy, and knowledge of diet, signs and symptoms of complications, fetal development, and testing used during pregnancy is necessary.

Levels of Cognitive Ability

The level of cognitive ability is a component of the NCLEX that measures how information has been learned and how it can be used by the nurse. For the NCLEX, knowledge is tested at three different levels.

Level 1

Level 1 consists of knowledge and comprehension questions. Only approximately 15 percent of the questions are at this level. These questions involve recalling specific facts and the ability to understand those facts in relationship to a pathophysiologic condition; they cover knowledge of specific anatomy and physiology, medication dosage and side effects, signs and symptoms of diseases, laboratory test results, and the elements of certain treatments and interventions. Being able to remember and understand information is the most basic way of learning. Although this type of knowledge is important and underlies the other levels of knowledge, it is not itself sufficient to ensure safe nursing care. An example of a level 1 question is:

Being able to remember and understand information is the most basic way of learning. Although this type of knowledge is important and underlies the other levels of knowledge, it is not itself sufficient to ensure safe nursing care.

1. A client is admitted to the medical unit with respiratory failure. Which of the following is the normal range for the Po_2?
   a. 10–30 mm Hg
   b. 35–55 mm Hg
   c. 10–20 cm H_2O
   d. 70–100 mm Hg

Level 2

Level 2 consists of questions that ask the nurse to analyze and apply the memorized information to specific client care situations. Analysis and application questions are more difficult to answer because they require the nurse to do more than simply repeat the information he or she has learned. Analysis requires the ability to separate information into its basic parts and decide which of those parts are important. Application requires that the nurse be able to use that information in client care decisions. Some examples of this type of question involve interpreting electrocardiographic (ECG) strips, interpreting blood gas values, making a nursing diagnosis based on a set of symptoms, or deciding on a course of treatment. These questions provide a better indication of the nurse's ability to safely care for clients. An example of a level 2 question is:

2. A client is becoming progressively short of breath. The results of his arterial blood gas (ABG) tests are pH, 7.13; PO_2, 48; PCO_2, 53; and HCO_3, 26. These values indicate:
   a. Metabolic acidosis
   b. Respiratory alkalosis
   c. Respiratory acidosis
   d. Metabolic alkalosis

Level 3

Level 3—synthesis, judgment, and evaluation—takes the process a step further. Approximately 85 percent of the questions are at either level 2 or level 3. Questions at the synthesis and judgment level ask the nurse to make decisions about client care. One factor that adds to the difficulty of answering this type of question is that there is often more than one correct answer. The nurse is asked to choose the best, or highest priority, answer from among several correct answers. Questions at this level often ask about the priority of care to be given, the priority of nursing diagnosis formulated, how to best evaluate the effectiveness of care that has been given, and the most appropriate nursing action to be taken. It is believed that the ability of the nurse to make decisions about nursing care at these higher levels is the best indication of the thought processes expected of a nurse demonstrating safe nursing care. An example of a level 3 question is:

3. A client is becoming progressively short of breath. The results of his arterial blood gas (ABG) tests are pH, 7.13; PO_2, 48; PCO_2, 53; and HCO_3, 26. What action should the nurse take first?
   a. Call a code blue and begin cardiopulmonary resuscitation.
   b. Call the physician and report the condition.
   c. Make sure the client's airway is open and begin supplemental oxygen.
   d. Give the ordered dose of 200 mg aminophylline intravenous piggyback (IVPB) now.

Integrated Concepts and Processes

The integrated concepts and processes component includes the following:

- Nursing process
- Concepts of caring
- Therapeutic communication
- Cultural awareness
- Documentation
- Self-care
- Teaching/learning

These concepts are integrated throughout the examination and included as elements in the four needs categories.

Nursing Process

The nursing process has traditionally been a very important part of the NCLEX. The NCLEX-

RN, CAT uses the five-step nursing process: assessment, analysis, planning, intervention and implementation, and evaluation. Each of the questions that the graduate answers falls into one of these five categories. It is important that the graduate keep in mind the steps of the nursing process when answering questions. Often questions that ask "What should the nurse do first?" are looking for an assessment-type answer because that is the first step in the nursing process. Questions on the nursing process are no longer equally divided on the examination. Recent analysis has shown a higher percentage of questions in the implementation phase of the nursing process.

Assessment. The **assessment** phase primarily establishes the database on which the rest of the nursing process is built. Some components of the assessment phase include both subjective and objective data about the client, significant history, history of the present illness, signs and symptoms, environmental elements, laboratory values, and vital signs. Often the examination asks the nurse to distinguish between appropriate and inappropriate assessment factors. An example of an assessment phase question is:

4. A client's respiratory status continues to worsen. Which of the following signs and symptoms would be most indicative of a deterioration of respiratory status?
   a. Increased restlessness and changes in level of consciousness
   b. Bradycardia and increases in blood pressure
   c. Complaints of chest pain and shortness of breath
   d. Rapidly dropping P_{CO_2} and pH

Analysis. The analysis phase of the nursing process involves developing and using nursing diagnosis for the care of the client. The NCLEX uses the North American Nursing Diagnosis Association (NANDA) nursing diagnosis system. Questions concerning nursing diagnosis often ask the graduate to prioritize the diagnoses. An example of an analysis phase question is:

5. A client is admitted to the unit with a diagnosis of bronchitis, congestive heart failure, and fever. The nurse assesses him as having a temperature of 101.8°F, peripheral edema, dyspnea, and rhonchi. The following nursing diagnoses are all appropriate, but which one has the highest priority?
   a. Anxiety related to fear of hospitalization
   b. Ineffective airway clearance related to retained secretions
   c. Fluid volume excess related to third spacing of fluid (edema)
   d. Ineffective thermoregulation related to fever

Planning. The planning phase of the nursing process primarily involves setting goals for the client. Included in the planning phase are such factors as determining expected outcomes, setting priorities for goals, and anticipating client needs based on the assessment. An example of a planning phase question is:

6. A client is found to be in respiratory failure and is placed on oxygen. Which of the following goals has the highest priority for this client?
   a. Walk the length of the hall twice during a nurse's shift.
   b. Complete his bath and morning care before breakfast.
   c. Maintain an oxygen saturation of 90% throughout the shift.
   d. Keep the head of the bed elevated to promote proper ventilation.

Intervention and Implementation. The **intervention** and **implementation** phase of the nursing process involves identifying those nursing actions that are required to meet the goals stated in the planning phase. Some of the material in the intervention and implementation phase includes:

- Provision of nursing care based on the client's goals
- Prevention of injury or spread of disease
- Therapy with medications and their administration
- Giving treatments
- Carrying out procedures
- Charting and record keeping
- Teaching about health care
- Monitoring changes in condition

An example of an intervention/implementation phase question is:

7. When the nurse ambulates a client who has been on bed rest for 3 days, he suddenly becomes very restless, displays extreme dyspnea, and complains of chest pain. Which of the following would be the most appropriate nursing action?
   a. Call a code blue.
   b. Continue to help the client walk, but at a slower pace.
   c. Give the client an injection of his ordered pain medication.
   d. Return the client to bed and evaluate his vital signs and lung sounds.

Evaluation. The **evaluation** phase of the nursing process determines whether or not the goals stated in the planning phase have been met through the interventions. The evaluation phase also ties the nursing process together and makes it cyclic. If the goals were achieved, it is an indication that the plan and implementation were effective, and new goals need to be established. If the goals were not met, then the nurse has to go back and find the difficulty. Were the assessment data inadequate? Were the goals defective? Was there a deficiency in the implementation? Evaluation is a continual process. Material in the evaluation phase includes comparison of actual outcomes to expected outcomes, verification of assessment data, evaluation of nursing actions and client responses, and evaluation of the client's level of knowledge and understanding. An example of an evaluation question is:

8. A client is being prepared for discharge. He is to take theophylline by mouth at home for his lung disease. The nurse will know that her teaching concerning theophylline medications has been effective if the client states:
   a. "I can stop taking this medication when I feel better."
   b. "If I have difficulty swallowing the time-released capsules, I can crush them or chew them."
   c. "If I have a lot of nausea and vomiting or become restless and can't sleep, I need to call my physician."
   d. "I need to drink more coffee and cola while I am on these medications."

> *Contrary to rumor, no graduates are randomly selected to take all 265 questions.*

NCLEX Examination Format

The NCLEX is a multiple-choice test taken on a personal computer. The questions are all constructed similarly and usually include a client situation, a stem or stem question, and four answers or distractors. All the questions on the NCLEX stand alone, although a similar situation may be repeated. Occasionally a single question may be included without a case situation.

The graduate is asked to select the best answer from among the four possible choices. No partial credit is given for a "close" answer; there is only one correct answer for any particular question. The questions are totally integrated from the content areas previously discussed in the approximate percentages identified. Each question carries an equal weight or value toward the final score.

The graduate may take between 75 and 265 questions. Contrary to rumor, no graduates are randomly selected to take all 265 questions. Graduates can pass or fail the test with either 75 or 265 questions or any number in between. The average number of questions taken over the past 5 years is 119, and the average time is just over 2 hours. There is a maximum time limit of 5 hours for the entire examination, although there is no minimum time limit. The test is graded on a statistical model that compares the graduate's responses with a pre-established standard. The graduate who demonstrates a knowledge level consistently above that standard passes the examination.

Because the NCLEX-RN examination is given by computerized adaptive testing (CAT), increases in the passing standard does not necessarily require a higher number of items to be answered correctly by the graduate. However, it does require that the graduate answer questions correctly at a slightly higher difficulty level than last year's graduates. Questions are assigned a difficulty value on a 7-logit (unit) scale called the NCLEX-RN logistic scale, ranging from the easiest (–3), which all graduates should answer correctly, to the most difficult (+3), which almost all graduates would be expected to miss (Box 10–1).

Box 10–1

NCLEX-RN Logistic Scale

Logits

+3	Most difficult
+2	
+1	
0	Approximate pass level
−1	
−2	
−3	Least difficult

The difficulty level of the questions is determined by the question writers and question reviewers and is based on factors such as when the material is usually presented in nursing programs (material presented earlier is considered less difficult) and the complexity of the material.

Example – Low-Difficulty-Level Question:

9. What blood test does the nurse evaluate as the best measure of a client's long-term control of diabetes mellitus?
   a. Fasting blood sugar
   b. Arterial blood gases
   c. Glucose tolerance test (GTT)
   d. Glycosylated hemoglobin (Hgb A_{1C})

Example – High-Difficulty-Level Question:

10. While monitoring a client with a pulmonary artery catheter, the nurse notes catheter fling artifact on the pressure tracing. Identify the nursing measure that best compensates for this problem.
    a. Record only mean pressures.
    b. Ask the physician to reposition the catheter.
    c. Irrigate the catheter forcefully with heparinized saline solution.
    d. Level and zero the transducer before taking readings.

Remember that it is probably a good sign that you are getting difficult questions. It means that your level is above the standard level. Also keep in mind that the NCLEX is designed so that no one can answer all the questions correctly. Even your most knowledgeable nursing instructor would not be able to answer some of the questions on the exam.

The National Council last revised the passing standard of the NCLEX-RN, CAT in 1998. The passing standard is –0.35 on the NCLEX-RN logistic scale, 0.07 logit (unit) above the previous standard of –0.42. This increase is similar to past increases in the difficulty level that occurred in

1995 (0.06-logit increase) and in 1992 (0.04-logit increase).

The new passing standard was established by a nine-nurse member panel that included diverse representation (regional, nursing specialty, minority, educator, new RNs) in conjunction with the results of a survey of nursing professionals such as nursing administrators of all types of facilities and directors of nursing. After consideration of all the data, including current trends in health care, the National Council Board of Directors determined that safe entry-level practice for RNs required a higher level of knowledge, skills, and abilities than was required in 1995. The passing standard and test content was again evaluated in 2001 to maintain the current 3-year cycle of revision, although no changes were made.

As of October 2002, the new test vendor for the NCLEX is VUE, a subsidiary of NCS Pearson Professional Centers. The tests will be given at the new state-of-the-art Pearson Professional Centers. The test items and the format of the examination will not change because the exam is owned by the National Council of State Boards of Nursing, which contracts with vendors to administer the examination.

After graduates have completed their nursing program, they apply to the state board of nursing. Appointments at the examination sites are made on a first-come, first-served basis. The centers are required to schedule the examination within 30 days from the time the graduate applies. Each state establishes its own time interval for application after graduation, generally within 1 year. There are both morning and afternoon sessions of 5-hour duration. Depending on the size of the center, between 8 and 15 graduates may be accommodated at one time.

The computer skills required are minimal. As of May 2002, only the mouse is used for all parts of the examination. A digital picture is taken at the time the graduate enters the examination room, and that picture, along with the graduate's information, appears on one of the computer screens in the room. The graduate then sits at the computer with his or her picture on it, completes a three-question tutorial on the use of the mouse, and then uses the mouse to select the answers to the questions on the rest of the exam. After the examination is completed, there is a short personal data questionnaire and an evaluation of the examination site facility.

The computer screen is split with the situation and stem question on the left side and the answers on the right (see example in Box 10–2). After an answer is selected, the question is replaced with another question and answers. No question is ever repeated, nor is the graduate able to change the answer once it has been selected.

As of October 2001, a drop-down calculator was added to the program for use in answering dosage calculations questions. Up to that time, no calculators were allowed, and all calculations had to be performed on scrap paper. It is probably safe to assume that the difficulty level of future calculation questions will increase markedly.

The NCLEX is graded on a pass-fail basis. If the student has failed the examination, the entire examination must be taken again. The National Council of State Boards of Nursing (NCSBN) requires a 90-day waiting period before repeating the examination, and first-time takers are given preference over those who are repeating the

Box 10–2

While assessing a man in the ER, the nurse notes that he has Kayser-Fleischer rings on the corneas of both eyes. Which lab value alterations can the nurse anticipate?	a. Sodium 135; potassium 4.2 b. BUN 2.2; creatinine 0.22 c. Total protein 7.2 d. SGOT 84; total bilirubin 5.4

examination. A number of states have restricted the number of times the graduate can re-take the test, usually to three. Check with your state board of nursing for the particular regulations.

The exam results are sent to the graduate 7 to 10 days after the examination has been completed, although this time frame varies from state to state. Many states are offering on-line results within a few days after the exam. Check with your state board of nursing to make sure they are offering this service and how to access the site. A new service is being offered by the NCSBN where the graduate can obtain unofficial results by telephone 3 days after taking the examination. The telephone number is 900-225-6000; the cost for the call is $7.95. You can also access the NCSBN on the Web at www.nclex.com/store.asp. Not all states participate in the service, and your employment agency may or may not accept the results.

Study Strategies

There are several ways to prepare for examinations, including the NCLEX. To attempt to take the examination with an attitude of "If I don't know it by now, I never will" is to court failure. Carefully directed study and preparation will considerably increase the chances of passing the examination.

Review Books

The material covered by review books is the key material found on the NCLEX. These books usually follow the NCLEX Test Plan very closely. A review book is, however, just that; it reviews the material that graduates should already know. Reviewing is important to reinforce learning and recall unused information.

Review books are not really designed to present any new information about key material. If a graduate is totally unfamiliar with the material in a particular section of the review book, then reading a more complete textbook on that particular subject area will be necessary.

Another important function that a review book serves is to point out areas of weakness. If the graduate finds sections that seem to contain "new" material, it is important to investigate that particular section in more detail. If graduates find most of the material familiar and easy to grasp, then they are probably prepared for the NCLEX.

What Do You Think?

When was the last time you sat in on a group study session? List three of the problems you encountered at the session? How can they be solved?

Group Study

Group study can be an effective method of preparation for an examination such as the NCLEX. To optimize the results of group study sessions, there are several rules that should be followed.

Rule 1. *Be very selective when choosing the members of the study group.* They should have a similar frame of mind and orientation toward studying. They should be nurses who are also going to be taking the NCLEX. The ideal size for a study group is between four and six people. Groups larger than six become difficult to organize and handle. After the group has been formed and has begun its study sessions, it may be necessary to ask an individual to leave the group for not participating or for being disruptive to the study process or displaying negative attitudes about the examination.

Rule 2. *Have each individual prepare a particular section for each group study session.* Study groups generally meet once or twice a week. For example, if next week the group is going to study the endocrine system, assign group member #1 the anatomy and physiology of the system, #2 the pathologic conditions, #3 the medications used for treatment, and #4 the key elements of nursing care. When the group comes together, have each individual present his or her prepared section. This type of preparation prevents the "What are we going to study tonight?" syndrome that often plagues group study sessions.

By following this process, the study group is organized and allows for more in-depth coverage of the topic. It also permits the members of the group to ask questions of the other members, thereby reinforcing the information being discussed.

> *No matter what other study and preparation methods are used, individual preparation for the NCLEX is a necessity.*

Rule 3. *Limit the length of the study session.* No single study session should be longer than between 90 and 120 minutes. Sessions that go for longer tend to get off the topic and foster a negative attitude about the examination. Try to avoid making group study sessions into party time. A few snacks and refreshments may be helpful to maintain the energy level of the group, but a real party atmosphere will detract significantly from the effectiveness of the study session.

Rule 4. *Use role play to reinforce information.* The more senses you can involve in the learning process, the better the learning.

Rule 5. *Remain positive.* Although group study times should not be party times, relax and have some fun with the study.

Individual Study Tips

No matter what other study and preparation methods are used, individual preparation for the NCLEX is a necessity. This preparation can take several forms.

Tip 1. As previously discussed, use of a review book is valuable to indicate areas of deficient knowledge. Reading and studying the appropriate textbooks and study guides can be helpful if it is approached correctly. It is important that the graduate mentally organize the information being read into a format similar to that found in the NCLEX. After reading each page of a textbook or study guide, the graduate should be able to ask three or four multiple-choice questions about that information. These questions can be asked silently or actually written out and should answer the question "How might the NCLEX test my knowledge of this material?"

Tip 2. Practice answering questions similar to those found on the exam you are going to take or the NCLEX itself. When practice questions are answered, several important mental processes occur. First, the graduate is becoming more familiar with and therefore more comfortable with the format of the examination. In research, this process is termed the practice effect; it must be accounted for when analyzing the results from pretest/post-test-type research projects. Individuals will have better results after a test even without any type of intervention because of having practiced answering questions on the pretest. Similarly, the score on the NCLEX may increase by as much as 10 percent through answering practice questions.

A second result of answering practice questions is that it reinforces the information already studied. Although it is unlikely that a question on the NCLEX examination will be identical to a practice question, there are many similarities in the questions. Realistically, only a limited number of questions can be asked about any given subject. After a while, the questions will begin to sound very similar.

A third advantage of answering practice questions is that it reveals subject areas that will require more study. It is relatively easy to say, "I understand the renal system pretty well." It is quite another to answer correctly 10 or 15 questions about that system. If the questions are answered correctly, then the graduate can move on to the next topic. If the majority of the questions are missed, however, then further review is required.

In order to obtain the optimal benefit from working practice questions, it is probably best to spend 30 to 45 minutes each day working 10 to 20 questions rather than trying to do 100 questions on 1 day during the week.

After the questions are answered, the student reviews them and compares them with the answers the study book provides. The student should also look at the rationales and the categories into which the questions fall. Try to understand why you missed the questions you did. Was it lack of knowledge? Didn't read the question carefully? Didn't use critical thinking?

Tip 3. Study using images. Studies have shown that among all the types of learning, visual learning is the most effective. Some ways to enhance visual learning is to outline the pictures in the book with a highlighter, color in the pictures, and draw your own pictures. Act out situations when group studying or even with individual study.

Tip 4. Don't cram! Of course, it is very difficult to cram for the NCLEX. You would have to cram all the information from the previous 2 to 4 years of nursing school. But even in everyday tests, cramming is counterproductive. The experts recommend that, before each class, you review the notes from the previous class at a rate of 15 minutes per hour of class. It has been shown that this type of study improves memory of content by 30 to 50 percent. Also, asking questions during class reinforces memory. Students who do well often play "stump the instructor," where they try to think of questions that the teacher probably will not know the answer to.

Tip 5. Make notes about key concepts. Create your own flash cards that include information you find difficult to remember. For example, make medication cards with the name of the medication on one side and the dosage and side effects on the other. Make sure to summarize what you have read or heard in class on the cards and think about the material; don't just memorize it.

Tip 6. Never leave a class if you do not clearly understand the content. The instructor is getting paid to explain the material so that you can understand it. Don't be afraid to keep asking questions until the content is explained in a way that is clear and makes sense to you. If the teacher seems to be unable to do this in class, make an appointment with him or her outside of class. If you don't understand the content, you never will be able to remember it.

Tip 7. Get rid of negative thoughts when you study. If you think any of the following to yourself when you are studying, you are guilty of negative thoughts:

- "I'm always anxious during a test."
- "I'm a loser because I can't remember all the details."
- "If there is a question about _______, I'm dead."
- "My family will think I'm stupid if I don't get an *A*."
- "My classmates will think I'm stupid if I don't get an *A*."
- "I'll think I'm stupid if I don't get an *A*."
- "No one ever understands what this teacher is talking about."
- "I just know I'll forget everything when I get to the exam."
- "Everyone knows I won't pass this exam, so why even try."
- "I'm not smart enough to be a nurse."
- "This teacher asks such tricky questions that it doesn't matter if I study. I miss them anyway."
- "I'll be happy if I can make a C-minus."

Formal NCLEX Reviews

The NCSBN does not endorse or sponsor any review courses for the NCLEX directly, but many companies offer reviews shortly after graduation. There is an on-line comprehensive review course for the NCLEX-RN examination found on the NCSBN Web site that is offered by an independent company (http://www.nclex.com). These review courses range from 2 to 5 days and basically cover the information found in review books. They are rather expensive, and the quality of NCLEX reviews varies. In general they are only as good as the people who are presenting the material. Also, look at the reported pass rate of the graduates after they take the review. Those with higher pass rates are probably better.

Test-Taking Strategies

The multiple-choice question test format is one of the most commonly used. Of course the best way to get a good grade on any exam is to know the material. There is no substitute for knowledge. However, some individuals seem always to do well on multiple-choice question tests, whereas others seem to have problems with that test format. The individuals who always do well are not necessarily more intelligent; rather, they may have intuitively mastered some of the strategies or "tricks" necessary to do well on multiple-choice tests. Fortunately, once graduates become aware of these strategies and master them, they also will be able to score well on this type of examination format.

The best way to get a good grade on any exam is to know the material. There is no substitute for knowledge.

Knowing how to take a multiple-choice examination and optimizing the selection of the correct answers is a skill that can be mastered.

Knowing how to take a multiple-choice examination and optimizing the selection of the correct answers is a skill that can be mastered. When mastery of this skill is combined with knowledge of the key material, the probability of passing the NCLEX increases greatly. The following section lists and describes these important test-taking strategies. Strategies 1 to 6 work best when the test taker knows the material well and is fairly confident about the correct answer. Strategies 7 to 27 can be used when the test taker is unsure of the answer or does not know the answer at all.

Strategy 1. Think positive and avoid test anxiety. The night before the exam and the morning before the exam, sit back, relax, and say the following to yourself: "I am intelligent and I will pass." "I'll show the instructor that I can do it." "I can do well on this exam." Avoid negative people; don't even talk to them!

Strategy 2. Cover up the answers and read the question carefully trying to formulate your own answers. Looking at the answers right away pulls your attention away from the question. As you read the question and answers, try to understand what knowledge the question is asking for. Look for and make note of any key words, qualifiers, or statements that may help select the correct answer or eliminate the incorrect ones. Ask yourself: "What is this question really asking?" "What information do I need to have to answer this question?" "Is the information I need in the client situation or the stem?" Restate the question in your own words to see if you really understand it.

Treat each question individually. Use only the information that is provided for that particular question in answering. Don't make the client any sicker than he or she already is. Even though there may be client situations somewhere else in the examination that are similar to the one currently on the screen, avoid returning mentally to these previous items for help. You should also be careful about reading into a question information that is not actually provided. There is a tendency to recall exceptions or unusual clients that the nurse may have encountered. By and large, questions on the NCLEX ask for "textbook" levels of knowledge of the material.

Strategy 3. Uncover the answers one by one and ask yourself "Does it answer the question?"

Eliminate the incorrect answers and then leave them alone. Read ALL the answers carefully. Priority-type questions may have more than one correct answer. Many mistakes are made on this type of examination because the person taking the test did not read all parts of the question carefully. Look for the most specific answer to the question.

Strategy 4. Take the time to do the test well the first time. After you select an answer, go back and read the question to make sure they match. On your class tests, do NOT go back at the end and re-read all the questions and answers. Mark the ones you are unsure of and go back and look only at those.

Sample question for strategy 4:

11. Select the nursing action that is most helpful in relieving the pain from an episiotomy in a 1 day postpartum client.
    a. Increase fluid intake to 2000 to 3000 mL per day.
    b. Encourage the client to breast-feed the infant every 3 hours or on demand.
    c. Apply cold compresses to the perineum every 2 hours.
    d. Administer methylergonovine (Methergine) as prescribed PRN.

Strategy 5. Don't change your answers! Trust intuition. When a question and answers are read for the first time, an intuitive connection is made between the right and left lobes of the brain. The end result is that the first answer selected is usually the best choice. When a question is read too many times, you may start to read into it elements that are really not there. On the NCLEX, once an answer is selected, it cannot be changed; but on class tests, change answers only when you are 100 percent sure that the answer you are changing it to is correct. If there is any doubt at all, don't change your answer.

Strategy 6. Don't spend a lot of time on questions you don't know. Monitor and manage your time, but don't rush. Although the examination, strictly speaking, is not timed, the graduate is never sure how many questions will need to be answered. If the graduate plans on taking all 265 questions in 5 hours, he or she will need approximately 70 seconds per question. Actually, most individuals who take this type of test average approximately 45 seconds per question; thus, it is likely that the student will be finished well before the time limit is reached. Take a watch along to the examination. If any question takes more than 2 minutes, put an answer down and move on. Theoretically, the graduate could sit in front of the computer screen for 5 hours with the same question. There is a mandatory 10-minute break at 2½ hours, and another optional break at 4 hours. Of course, breaks can be taken any time during the exam, but that time is lost from the total allowed time.

Strategy 7. An educated guess is better than no answer at all. There is no penalty for guessing on the NCLEX, and you do have to put an answer down in order to move on to the next question. If you are unable to make any decision at all about the correct answer, you should just select one and move on. There is at least a one-in-four chance of choosing the correct answer. Studies have shown that answer *c* has the highest probability (30%), answer *b* the next highest, answer *d* the third highest, and answer *a* the lowest probability of being the correct answer. Wild guessing for large numbers of questions, of course, will have a negative effect on the total score.

Strategy 8. If you know the other three answers are wrong, then the one that is left is correct. Use the process of elimination to select the correct answer. Usually there are one or more of the answers that can easily be identified as being incorrect. By eliminating these from the possible choices, you will be better able to focus attention on the answers that have been identified as having some chance of being correct. Go back and read the stem question over again to try to determine exactly what type of information is being asked. If you are still unable to decide which of the remaining two answers is correct, select one and move on. Using this method increases the probability of choosing the correct answer to 1 in 2.

Sample question for strategy 8:

12. What action should the nurse take for a client who is developing Stevens-Johnson syndrome?
    a. Place tight tourniquets in the antecubital spaces of both arms.
    b. Give all medications through the client's arterial line.
    c. Hold the client's next dose of Bactrim and notify the physician.
    d. Inform the family that the client will die within 24 hours.

Strategy 9. Pay attention to where the client is in the disease/recovery process. One day postoperative clients have different needs and complications than a 5-day postoperative client. The assessment is different for a client who has been taking antibiotics for 7 days and one who has just started taking an antibiotic. The teaching required for a client who has been a diabetic for 10 years is different than for a client who was just diagnosed.

Sample question for strategy 9:

13. Identify the assessment of a client who had a Wilms' tumor removed 3 hours ago that would require immediate intervention by the nurse.
    a. Diminished appetite
    b. Pinkish urine
    c. Temperature of 99.4°F
    d. Dressing soaked with bright red blood

Strategy 10. If part of the answer is incorrect, the whole answer is incorrect. One incorrect part of a multi-part answer makes the whole answer incorrect.

Sample question for strategy 10:

14. Identify the side effects a nurse should evaluate for a client who is receiving oral prednisone (Deltasone).
    a. Edema, hypotension, mood swings
    b. Dehydration, hyperglycemia, hirsutism
    c. Unstable moods, moon face, hypoglycemia
    d. Euphoria, hyperglycemia, hypertension

Strategy 11. Look for qualifying words in the question stem. There are some important words that can help determine what type of information is being elicited in the answer. Some of these words are:

First
Best
Most
Initial
Better
Highest priority

When words like these appear in the question stem, it is an indication that more than one of the choices are correct. The task then becomes to select the one answer that should be first or the answer that ought to receive the highest priority. Remember Maslow, the ABCs of cardiopulmonary resuscitation (CPR), and nursing diagnosis.

Sample questions for strategy 11:

15. A client is admitted with the symptoms of anthrax infection, including fever of 102°F, severe dyspnea, tachypnea, and chest pain. Which nursing diagnosis has highest priority?
    a. Anxiety related to fear of death
    b. Pain related to pressure on the sternum
    c. Hyperthermia related to bacterial infection
    d. Ineffective airway clearance related to retained respiratory secretions

16. A 62-year-old client who has a history of coronary heart disease is brought into the emergency room (ER) complaining of chest pain. What action should the nurse take first?
    a. Give the client nitroglycerin gr 1/150 sublingual now.
    b. Call the client's cardiologist about his admission.
    c. Check his blood pressure and note the location and degree of chest pain.
    d. Place the client in an elevated Fowler's position after loosening his shirt collar.

Strategy 12. Look for the answer that has the broader focus. Another method that may be used when the choices have been narrowed down to two is to examine the answers and try to determine whether one answer may include the other. The answer that is broader, that includes the other answer, is the correct one.

Sample question for Strategy 12:

17. Select the finding by the nurse that best identifies when a 10-year-old child with acting-out behavior requires help.
    a. Frequent fights with peers
    b. Multiple aspects of the child's life are affected
    c. Grades start to decline
    d. Stressful relationships with siblings and parents

Strategy 13. Watch for similarities in the content of the options. When answers are grouped by similar concepts, activities, or situations, select the one that is different. If three of the four choices have some common element that makes them similar, and the fourth answer lacks this element, the different answer is probably correct.

Sample question for strategy 13:

18. How can the nurse best help a 7-year-old boy diagnosed with acute lymphoblastic leukemia cope with the fear of dying?
    a. Instruct the parents to avoid bring up the subject of death.
    b. Re-direct the child's questions to safe topics when he mentions death.
    c. Answer the child's questions at the level of his understanding.
    d. Emphasize that nurses are not allowed to make prognosis about death.

19. A woman has been treated for severe chronic emphysema for several years using bronchodilators and relatively high doses of prednisone (Deltasone). Which of the following activities would pose the least risk for this client in relation to the side effects of prednisone therapy?
    a. Shopping at the mall on Saturday afternoon.
    b. Spring-cleaning her two-story house.
    c. Attending Sunday morning church services.
    d. Serving refreshments at her 6-year-old son's school play party.

Strategy 14. Look for negatives in the question stem. Although there are very few negative questions on the NCLEX, negative words or prefixes in the question stem change how the correct answer is selected. Some common negatives include:

Least
Unlikely
Inappropriate
Unrealistic
Lowest priority
Contraindicated
False
Except
Inconsistent
Untoward

All but
Atypical
Incorrect
Not

In general, when a negative question is asked, it indicates that three of the choices are correct and one is incorrect. The incorrect choice is the answer. When a negative question appears, the test taker needs to ask: "What is it they don't want me to do in this situation?" Sometimes negative questions are disguised.

Sample question for strategy 14:

20. Identify the client statement about taking aspirin at home for arthritis that requires further discharge instructions.
    a. "I need to take it with food or milk."
    b. "A small amount of blood in my urine is normal."
    c. "I should call the clinic if I develop large black-and-blue areas on my body."
    d. "Ringing in my ears may mean that I am taking too much medication."

Strategy 15. Do not panic if a totally unfamiliar question is encountered. Examinations such as the NCLEX are designed so that it is very difficult, if not impossible, for anyone to answer all of the questions correctly. As a result, there are questions that are very complex, which deal with disease processes, medications, and laboratory tests that may be unfamiliar to the graduate. Questions like this may be encountered no matter how much review or study has been done.

Nobody knows everything! When encountering these types of questions, it is important to avoid panic. It is just one question out of many. Use some of the strategies already discussed in this chapter to select the best answer. Remember that nursing care given is very similar in many situations even though the disease processes themselves may be quite different. Select the answer that seems logical and involves general nursing care. Common sense can go a long way on this type of examination.

Sample question for strategy 15:

21. What is the best action for the nurse to take when she or he discovers that a 9-year-old girl has a positive Rovsing's sign?
    a. Have the child rest quietly and assess the vital signs.
    b. Call a code blue and begin CPR.
    c. Inform the child's parents that she only has 3 months to live.
    d. Confront the child about which adult member of the family had been sexually molesting her recently.

Strategy 16. Other factors being equal, watch the length of the answers. The average length answer is most often correct. The NCLEX is difficult because the material itself is difficult, but the examination is not designed to be "tricky" or difficult for the sake of confusing the test taker. On the other hand, the test question writers are not going to make the correct answer completely obvious. Therefore, if one answer is much longer or shorter than the other three, it is probably not the correct choice. Be wary of answers that sound like they are trying to rationalize the correct choice by using a lot of explanation, particularly when the other answers do not. Such answers are probably incorrect. You should also avoid answers that are different from the other three because of measurements or the way in which they are presented.

Sample question for strategy 16:

22. How can the nurse best administer tetracycline oral liquid suspension to an 8-year-old child?
    a. Quickly
    b. Through a drinking straw
    c. With milk or antacid to prevent stomach irritation and vomiting
    d. Hidden in the child's food so that the bitter taste will be disguised and the child will complete the full course of treatment

Strategy 17. If there is a lengthy client situation or case study, read the stem question before reading the case study. Reading the question first will help you focus on the information you will need to obtain from the case study. It is a way to save a little time. On the NCLEX, the amount of space for the client situation is limited to half the computer screen.

Strategy 18. Avoid automatically passing the decision or intervention to the physician. The NCLEX is for nurses and deals with conditions and problems that nurses should be able to resolve independently. Often a nursing action can and should be taken prior to notifying the physician; however, it is an important element of nursing knowledge and judgment to know when notifying the physician is appropriate.

Sample question for strategy 18:

23. A post lobectomy client pulls out his chest tube while going to the rest room. What is the appropriate initial nursing action?
    a. Call the physician immediately.
    b. Position the client on the operative side.
    c. Insert a new sterile chest tube and reconnect it to underwater seal drainage.
    d. Cover the insertion site with an occlusive dressing.

Strategy 19. Avoid selecting answers that have absolutes in them. Answers that have absolutes in them are almost always incorrect choices. Some absolute words to be aware of include:

Always
Every
Only
All
Never
None

Humans are very complex biochemical entities. Every person is different and almost every rule will have an exception.

Sample question for strategy 19:

24. Which factor should the nurse include in the teaching plan of a client with a home prescription for reserpine (Serpalan)?
    a. Walk 2 miles every day.
    b. Never eat any candy or ice cream.
    c. The physician is the only one who can cut your toenails to prevent bleeding.
    d. Try to take the medication at the same time each day.

Strategy 20. Avoid answers that make the client seem inferior, immoral, unworthy, or ignorant. Nurses are obligated by the code of ethics to treat all clients equally, regardless of race, sex, lifestyle preferences, disease process, or economic status. Be careful of cultural differences and biases that can color the way the nurse interacts with a client. Also be particularly cautious in situations that are emotionally charged, such as child abuse, drug or alcohol addiction, spousal abuse, teen pregnancy, HIV, sexually transmitted disease (STD), or homosexuality.

Sample question for strategy 20:

25. Identify the most therapeutic statement by the nurse to a 14-year-old girl who admits she is sexually active and has just been informed that she has gonorrhea and is 3 months pregnant.
    a. "You obviously lack the intelligence to understand how to use the birth control pills and condoms you were given at the clinic at your last visit."
    b. "Tell me how you think your pregnancy will affect your life."
    c. "I hope you now understand the consequences of your lack of moral standards."
    d. "Tell me how you feel when your classmates call you a slut behind your back."

Strategy 21. Look for answers that have words identical or similar to those in the question stem. If there is no other way to determine the correct answer, similarities to the stem may act as a clue to the correct answer. With therapeutic communication questions, look for the answer that reflects or restates the emotions the client is expressing.

Sample questions for strategy 21:

26. Which assessments indicate to the nurse that a client was developing steal syndrome after the insertion of an AV graft in the left forearm?
    a. Hypotension and irregular pulse
    b. Weak radial pulses and mottled fingers of the left hand
    c. Elevated temperature and purulent urinary drainage
    d. Bruit and thrill over the surgical site

27. Select the most therapeutic response when a client says to the nurse: "That stupid doctor of mine makes me so mad I could spit nails! I want to leave this dump now!"
    a. "You seem very angry. Tell me why you want to leave."
    b. "If you sign the AMA sheet, you can go home now."
    c. "It is your right to change to a new physician if you are not satisfied with your care."
    d. "If there is no one to care for you at home, legally the hospital cannot release you."

Strategy 22. Watch for grammatical clues that may be a tip-off to the correct answer. All the options should be grammatically consistent with the question stem; however, question writers tend to pay more attention to this detail with the correct answer. Answers that grammatically do not match the stem or disagree in number (singular/plural) are usually incorrect. When the stem is an incomplete statement, the options should complete the sentence in a grammatically correct manner.

Sample questions for strategy 22:

28. Identify the assessments that would lead the nurse to suspect that a newly admitted client was developing Kugelberg-Welander disease.
    a. Compression fracture of L4
    b. Blood-tinged urine
    c. Muscle atrophy and twitching of the extremities
    d. Grade 3 pansystolic murmur over the PMI

29. An important therapeutic measure for the nurse to take when treating a client with a *Dracunculus medinensis* is to:
    a. Maintain a steady traction by winding around a small object like a pencil
    b. Keeping the client on strict bed rest throughout the treatment period
    c. Soaking the affected area in warm bath water several times a day
    d. Active and passive range of motion every 4 hours

Strategy 23. Look for qualifiers in the answers. The answer that includes a qualifying word when the others do not is often the correct answer. Qualifying words include:

Generally
Tends to
Usually
Often
May
Might
About
Approximately
Most
Many

Sample question for strategy 23:

30. What is the most accurate information for the nurse to provide to the parents of an infant with gray syndrome?
    a. Gray syndrome is always caused by a genetic defect.
    b. You can take the baby home after 2 weeks' treatment with antibiotics.
    c. The baby will require open heart surgery to live past age 3.
    d. Approximately 40% of newborns with gray syndrome die by the fifth day of life.

Strategy 24. When two of the answers are opposites, one of them is usually correct. Look for answers that, when considered, cover all the possibilities of action. One of the answers must be correct and you have improved your odds to 50-50.

Sample question for strategy 24:

31. What should the nurse conclude when she or he finds a positive scarf sign while assessing a newborn infant?
    a. The infant was born after 30 weeks' gestation.
    b. The mother of the infant used cocaine during her pregnancy.
    c. There is a genetic predisposition for sickle cell disease.
    d. The infant was born before 30 weeks' gestation.

Strategy 25. When asked about numerical values or dates, the one in the middle range is more often correct. Numerical ranges can be from large to small or small to large. Dates can range from present to past or past to present. Extremes in numerical values or dates are usually incorrect.

Sample question for strategy 25:

32. Identify the serum medication level that indicates to the nurse that a client with seizure disorder was taking his/her clonazepam (Klonopin) as prescribed.
    a. 142 ng/mL
    b. 112 ng/mL
    c. 72 ng/mL
    d. 12 ng/mL

Strategy 26. Avoid looking for a pattern in the selection of answers. The questions and answers on the NCLEX are arranged in a random fashion without any particular pattern. If something appears to be in a pattern, ignore it. Any pattern is just coincidental. For example, if question 6 had answer *a*, question 7 had answer *b*, question 8 had answer *c*, question 9 had answer *d*, question 10 had answer *a*, and question 11 had answer *b*, you might expect that question 12 would require answer *c*. This is probably not the case. Here is another example of a pattern-type situation that sometimes occurs with answers on this type of test. Questions 22 to 29 all have *c* as their correct answers. The answer to question 30 also seems to be *c*, but the tendency may be not to select it because of all the other choice *c* answers on the previous questions. The correct answer may very well be *c*, and if that is the best choice, go ahead and select it. It is important that each question be treated individually.

Strategy 27. Be positive about the examination! Motivational research has shown that people who have a positive attitude about an examination score higher on the examination than people who are negative about it. Believe in yourself. Think positive thoughts all the time. Not only will you do better on tests, but you will be a happier and friendlier person too!

> *Think positive thoughts all the time. Not only will you do better on tests, but you will be a happier and friendlier person too!*

Conclusion

Taking and passing the NCLEX-RN, CAT is a necessary step in the process of becoming a professional registered nurse. Like all licensure examinations, its purpose is to protect the public from undereducated or unsafe practitioners. The examination is comprehensive and includes material from all areas of the graduate's nursing education. Although most graduates have some anxiety about taking this examination, knowledge about its format and content and strategies for taking the examination can lower anxiety to an acceptable level.

In addition, many of these test-taking strategies can be applied to the student's course examinations during the nursing program. Although nothing is as effective for passing an examination as paying attention in class, good note taking, and thorough study, awareness of these important test-taking strategies may improve the student's overall score.

Answers to Questions in Chapter 10

1. The correct answer is *d*. You either have or do not have the knowledge for this particular laboratory test.
2. The correct answer is *c*. Not only does the nurse have to know the normal values for each of the blood gas components given, he or she must also be able to use that information in determining the underlying condition.
3. The best answer to this question is *c*. Choices *b* and *d* are also actions that should be carried out; but at this particular time, opening the airway and oxygenating the client must receive highest priority. Not only does this question require that the nurse know the normal values and interpretation, but it also requires that a decision be made about the seriousness of the condition (analysis) and a selection of the type of care to be given from several correct options (judgment).
4. The correct answer is *a*. The brain is one of the first organs to be affected by a decrease in oxygenation. Restlessness and changes in level of consciousness indicate this decrease. All the other choices are assessments for other conditions.
5. The correct answer is *b*. Nursing diagnoses that deal with airway always have highest priority.
6. The correct answer is *c*. Choice *a* is unrealistic for this client; choice *b* is not client-centered; and choice *d* is a nursing intervention, not a goal. Maintaining an oxygen saturation of 90% is realistic and within normal limits.
7. The correct answer is *d*. These are symptoms of a pulmonary embolism, which is a common complication of prolonged bed rest.
8. The correct answer is *c*. Answer *c* lists some side effects of theophylline medications that may indicate the onset of toxicity. The physician needs to know about these so that the theophylline level can be determined and the dosage adjusted accordingly. Other instructions that the client could be given when taking theophylline medications include to avoid excessive amounts of caffeine, never to suddenly stop taking the medication, to take it with a full glass of water and a small amount of food, and to watch for interactions with over-the-counter (OTC) medications.
9. The correct answer is *d*. Laboratory tests and their significance are considered basic knowledge and are taught in the early part of most nursing programs.
10. The correct answer is *a*. The question asks about how to compensate for the problem, not correct it. Invasive hemodynamic moni-

Critical Thinking Exercises

- Obtain an NCLEX-RN, CAT review book. Analyze the questions in the practice examination for type, cognitive level, and level of difficulty.
- Identify three to five other students in your class with whom you would feel comfortable working in a study group. Organize a study group session before the next major course examination.
- When you get the results of your next course examination, identify why you missed the questions you did and what strategies might have been used to answer those questions correctly.

toring is considered advanced medical/surgical nursing and is usually presented during the last year of nursing school.

11. The correct answer is *c*. Although the other answers may be appropriate nursing measures, they do not address the problem of pain relief.
12. The correct answer is *c*. Stevens-Johnson syndrome is a type of erythemic edema that is commonly seen in clients who are taking Bactrim for urinary tract infections. The other three answers are things that the nurse should never do.
13. The correct answer is *d*. One of the key assessments during the immediate recovery period after surgery is to make sure the dressing is dry and intact. The other findings would be considered normal for a 3-hour postoperative client.
14. The correct answer is *d*. Prednisone causes fluid retention, resulting in hypertension and edema; raises the blood sugar, resulting in hyperglycemia; affects the mood, causing instability; and causes abnormal fat distribution, resulting in moon face and buffalo hump.
15. The correct answer is *d*. Airway-related nursing diagnoses have highest priority (ABCs of CPR).
16. Correct answer is *c*. The first step in the nursing process is assessment. Always look for an assessment type answer when asked what to do first.
17. Correct answer is *b*. It includes all of the other answers.
18. Correct answer is *c*. All the other answers try to avoid talking about death with the child.
19. Correct answer is *b*. All the other answers place the client at risk for infection by exposure to large groups of people in open public areas.
20. Correct answer is *b*. The other three answers would be considered correct for a client taking aspirin. There should never be any blood in the urine.
21. Correct answer is *a*. Rovsing's sign is an indication of appendicitis. The child should rest quietly until she can go to surgery.
22. Correct answer is *b*. Tetracycline liquid stains the teeth and is best given to children through a straw. Note that answer *a* is very short, and answers *c* and *d* have long rationales.
23. Correct answer is *d*. Covering the site quickly is an acceptable nursing action and will prevent the pneumothorax from becoming larger. The physician can be called later.
24. Correct answer is *d*. The other three choices all have absolute words in them.
25. Correct answer is *b*. Good therapeutic communication answers reflect or explore the client's feelings. The other three answers all make judgments about the girl's moral character or intelligence.
26. Correct answer is *b*. Steal syndrome occurs when too much of the arterial blood is shunted away from the hand. Note that answer *b* is the only one with the word *left* in it, matching the stem question that has the word *left*.
27. Correct answer is *a*. Good therapeutic responses reflect the emotions and content of the client's statements.
28. Correct answer is *c*. Kugelburg-Welander disease is a neuromuscular disorder that affects primarily teenagers, leading to loss of coordination and paralysis. Note that answer *c* is the only plural answer matching grammatically the question that asks for "assessments."
29. Correct answer is *a*. A *Dracunculus medinesis* is a type of parasitic worm that infects the upper part of the leg. It can be removed by maintaining a slow steady traction force on it

over a period of time. Note that answer *a* is the only one of the answers that grammatically completes the open-ended statement of the stem question.

30. Correct answer is *d*. Gray syndrome occurs in infants who were treated with chloramphenicol during the newborn period and is highly lethal. Note that answer *d* is the only one with a qualifying word, *approximately*.

31. Correct answer is *d*. Scarf sign is elicited when the elbow of the infant can be drawn across the chest without resistance. It is a sign of prematurity. Note that answers *a* and *d* cover all the possible options for age.

32. Correct answer is *c*. Therapeutic range for clonazepam is 20 to 80 ng/mL. Answer *c* is in the middle of the extremes of the answers.

Answer to Computer Screen Box 10–2: *d* – Kayser-Fleischer rings are caused by the deposition of a golden brown pigment from an increased copper level secondary to hepatolenticular disease, a familial disorder of abnormal copper metabolism. The liver is damaged, and the tests related to the liver are abnormally high. Other symptoms include dysphasia, dysarthria, rigidity, and coarse resting tremors (wing-beating tremors).

Bibliography

Beeman, PB, and Waterhouse, JK: NCLEX-RN performance: Predicting success on the computerized examination. J Prof Nurs 17(4):158–165, 2001.

Dimitrov, DM, and Shelestak, D: Learning outcomes related to success on NCLEX-RN. Nurse Educator 26(3):108, 2001.

Kleinpell, RM, and Marks, C: Evolving nursing practice prompts changes to licensure exam. Nursing Spectrum 14(4):5, 2001.

Mills, LW, et al: A holistic approach to promoting success on NCLEX-RN. Journal of Holistic Nursing 19(4):360–374, 2001.

National Council of State Boards of Nursing: NCLEX-RN Test Plan, April 2001.

Oklahoma selected for NCS Pearson Beta Test. Oklahoma Board of Nursing Newsletter 12(1):1, 2002.

Siktberg, L, and Dillard, NL: Assisting at-risk students in preparation for the NCLEX-RN examination. Nurse Educator 26(3):150–152, 2001

Washington, LJ, and Perkel, L: NCLEX-RN strategies for success. ABFN Journal 12(1):12–16, 2001.

Wendt, A: End-of-life competencies and the NCLEX-RN examination. Nurs Outlook 49(3):138–142, 2001.

11

Reality Shock in the Workplace

Joseph T. Catalano

Learning Objectives

After completing this chapter, the reader will be able to:

- Describe the concept of reality shock.
- Define burnout and list its major symptoms.
- Discuss the key factors that produce burnout.
- List the important elements in personal time management.
- Analyze how the nurse's humanity affects nursing practice.
- List at least four health-care practices nurses can use to prevent burnout and to improve their professional performance.

Most nursing students, if asked what they wanted most in the world, would likely answer, "to graduate and practice real nursing in the real world." To some extent, they are correct in assuming that the world of nursing school and education is not the real world. Although nursing school is demanding physically, mentally, and emotionally and raises the anxiety levels of nursing students a great deal, it is also a place where the student is sheltered from the realities of the workplace and provided with relatively clear goals for advancement. Students are given a constant stream of reinforcement and always have someone to turn to if they have a question. Things are different in the "real world." The transition from nursing student to registered nurse is referred to as transition shock or reality shock.

Nursing Shortage

A lack of qualified nurses has been present in the health-care system for so long that the term *nursing shortage* has become a truism. However, as recent history has demonstrated, the demand for nurses increases and decreases with changes in the health-care system. In addition, the demand for nurses is to some extent regional. Some areas of the country have a high demand for registered nurses, and others may have fewer available jobs. However, studies about employment opportunities project that there will be a shortage of nurses well into the twenty-first century.[1]

The demand for nurses is finally being recognized by high-school counselors and employment agencies. Encouraging young people to enter nursing schools increases enrollment. After several years of decline in nursing school enrollments that reduced the number of graduates by almost 30 percent nationally, nursing schools are starting to see increases in enrollment. Drops in enrollment tend to occur when the economy is strong. Simply stated, when the economy is strong, there are more opportunities outside of the traditional female employment areas for young women to pursue. Also, overall enrollment in higher education also decreases during periods of strong economic growth and increases when the economy takes a downturn.

> *Studies about employment opportunities project that there will be a shortage of nurses well into the twenty-first century.*

There are many reasons for the decrease in professional nursing positions that occurred in the past. The primary reason is increased concern for cost reduction in the health-care system. Although no comprehensive **national health insurance** or health-care reform bills have ever been passed, the writing is on the wall. Health care is going to have to become more efficient and reduce the cost of operations.

One of the most obvious areas facilities have tried to cut costs is in personnel. Although a reduction in nursing positions may greatly reduce the costs in the short term, health-care facilities are finding that the long-term effects to the quality of health care are devastating. It is obvious that exchanging qualified nurses for lower-paid unlicensed technicians will eventually have an effect on the quality of client care.[2] Hospitals and other health-care facilities are experiencing the results of personnel cutting practices by experiencing reduction in the number of clients seeking care at these facilities as well as closing units and losing revenue.

Certain groups of nurses are in higher demand than ever, such as nurses who can practice independently in several different settings, **multiskilled practitioners,** home care nurses, community nurses, and hospice nurses.[3] A major trend in health care today is to move the care out of the hospital and into the community and home settings. Provision of nursing services in these settings often requires that a nurse have at least a bachelor's degree or even higher education. Fewer than 50 percent of all new graduate nurses today are graduating from bachelor's degree programs.[4]

Another area of health care in which there is not an oversupply of nurses is in the realm of the nurse practitioner. Advanced practice nurses are able to provide various services that were traditionally kept within the physician's scope of practice.

Although most nurse practitioners are currently based in community clinics, there is an ever-expanding opportunity for them to become involved in the care of hospitalized clients. A key element in many of the proposed health-care reform plans is that clients would be required to be evaluated by a primary health-care provider before they could be referred to secondary health-care providers or specialists. The advanced-practice education of nurse practitioners would make them eminently qualified to fill this role of primary health-care provider.

Certain specialty areas (e.g., intensive care units, neonatal units, and burn units) are always seeking nurses. As with community nurses, nurses who provide care in specialty units must be able to work independently and to draw from a large base of theoretical knowledge.

The nursing profession and nursing educators need to increase their vigilance in times when there are nursing shortages to maintain the high quality of the profession.

Making the Transition from Student to Nurse

At any point in their lives, most people fulfill several different roles simultaneously. For a nursing student, the biggest role conflict might occur during the transition from student to registered nurse. The roots of the conflict may lie in integrating three distinct aspects of any given role: the **ideal role image**, the **perceived role image**, and the **performed role image**.

In the academic setting, the student is generally presented with the ideal of what a nurse should be. The ideal role projects society's expectations. It clearly delineates obligations and responsibilities as well as the rights and privileges that those in the role can claim. Although the ideal role presents a clear image of what is expected, it is often static and somewhat unrealistic to believe that everyone in this role will follow the expected patterns of behaviors.

The ideal role of nurse might require someone with superhuman physical strength and ability and unlimited stamina and also one who possesses superior intelligence and decision-making ability, yet remains kind, gentle, caring, and able to communicate with any client at any time. Ideal nurses function independently, know more than the physician, and are able to prevent the physician from making grievous errors in client care while continuing to be responsive to client requests and to carry out any physician's order with unerring accuracy and absolute obedience. Some perceptive students, early in their clinical experiences, may begin to suspect that this ideal role of nurse is not the way that it actually is in the real world.

The perceived role is an individual's own definition of the role, which is often more realistic than the ideal role. When individuals define their own roles, they may reject or modify some of the norms and expectations of society in establishing the ideal role. Intellectually, though, the ideal role is often used as the yardstick against which the perceived role is measured.

After a minimal amount of clinical experience, the nursing student may realize that nurses do not possess extraordinary physical strength or intellectual ability but may continue to cling to the idea. Many students accept unconditionally, as part of their perceived role, that nurses must be kind, gentle, and understanding at all times with all clients. The perceived role is the role with which the nursing student usually graduates.

What Do You Think?

Think of some nurses who you know or have met in the past. Do any of them fit the title of the "ideal nurse"? What characteristics do they have?

Reality shock occurs when the ideal or perceived role comes into conflict with the performed role. The performed role is defined as what the practitioner of the role actually does. Many new graduate nurses soon realize that the accomplishment of role expectations depends on many factors other than their perceptions and beliefs about how nursing should be performed. The environment has a great deal to do with how the obligations of the role are met.

In nursing school, where students are assigned to care for one or two clients at a time, there is plenty of time to practice therapeutic communication techniques; to provide completely for the physical, educational, and emotional needs of the client; and also to develop an insightful care plan. The realities of the workplace may dictate that a nurse be assigned to care for six to eight clients at a time. In this situation, the perceived role of the nurse as an expert communicator may have to be set aside for the more realistic performed role of the nurse as expert task organizer. Meeting all the client's physical and emotional needs becomes impossible, and the care plan may be forgotten.

Such situations can produce what is called cognitive dissonance in many new graduate nurses; that is, they know what they should do and they know how they should do it, yet the circumstances do not allow them to carry it out. The end result is increased anxiety. High levels of anxiety, left unrecognized or unresolved, can lead to various physical and emotional symptoms. When these symptoms become severe enough, a condition called burnout may result.

The reality shock that new graduates often experience can be reduced to some extent. Some schools of nursing have instituted a **preceptor** clinical experience during the last semester of the senior year. The main goal of this type of clinical experience, which occurs just before graduation, is to help the student feel more comfortable in the role of registered nurse. Preceptor experiences allow the student to experience the employment situation before actually graduating.

A student who works with a preceptor is assigned to one registered nurse for supervision for most of the semester. The student experiences the role of the registered nurse by working the same hours and on the same unit as the nurse to whom he or she is assigned. As the role expectations of the workplace are absorbed by the student during the preceptor experience, the student's perceived role expectations also change, allowing movement from the student role to that of practicing professional with less anxiety and stress.

> *Employers are still looking for the best of the best for the positions they have available.*

Another experience that lessens role transition shock is called an internship. Internships are available to students between the junior and senior years at some hospitals. Internships allow the students to work in a hospital setting as nurses' aides, while permitting them to practice, with a few restrictions, at their level of nursing education. These experiences are invaluable for gaining practice in skills and for becoming socialized into the professional role.

Employment in Today's Job Market

Currently, the health-care industry is in dire need of registered nurses and it is projected that the need will only increase well into the twenty-first century.[5] However, employers are still looking for the best of the best for the positions they have available.

In addition, **employers** are looking for graduates who can function independently, require little retraining or orientation, and can supervise a variety of less educated and unlicensed employees.

Although these requirements may seem daunting, some strategies can be used to increase the chance of being hired. Students should take advantage of preceptor and "extern" experiences in their senior year and attempt to meet their clinical obligations in the institution where they desire employment. In this way, the student can evaluate the hospital closely and observe its working conditions and the type of care provided to clients. The hospital, on its part, has the opportunity to examine closely the student's knowledge, skills, personality, and ability to relate with clients and staff. The hospital benefits by getting **employees** who are familiar with the hospital before employment starts, thus decreasing the overall time of paid adjustment (referred to as "orientation").

What Do You Think?

Have you ever been on a job interview? What were some of the mistakes you made? How can you correct these mistakes in the future?

Resumes

In today's job market, the **resume** is often the institution's first contact with the nurse seeking employment, and it has a substantial effect on the whole hiring process. First impressions are important. Preparing a neat, thorough, and professional-looking resume is worth the time and effort. If you have access to a computer, a good-looking resume can be prepared at almost no cost. If a computer is not available, it is a good idea to spend a few dollars to have the resume professionally prepared and reproduced.

The goal of a resume is to provide the hospital with a complete picture of the prospective employee in as little space as possible. It should be easy to read and visually appealing and have flawless grammar and spelling. Although various formats may be used, all resumes should contain the same information. There are many books available in local bookstores that can serve as a guide in organizing the information for a resume. Many new computers now come from the factory loaded with software for the preparation of resumes in different formats. Keep an electronic copy of the resume for future use or reference. The required information includes the following:

- Full name, current address (or address where the person can always be reached), and a telephone number (including area code).
- Educational background (all degrees), starting with the most recent first, naming institution, location, dates of attendance, and degrees awarded.
- Former employers, again starting with the most recent. Give dates of employment, title of position, name of immediate supervisor, supervisor's telephone number, and a short description of the job responsibilities.
- Describe any scholarships, achievements, awards, honors, or activities that have been received, starting with the most recent.
- List professional memberships, offices held, dates of the memberships.
- List any publications. If both books and journal articles were published, list the books separately, starting with the most recent.
- Include an "Other" category to describe any unpublished materials produced (e.g., an internal hospital booklet for use by clients), research projects, **fellowships**, grants, and so forth.
- Provide professional license number and annual number for all states where licensed, along with the date of license and expiration date.

Each area of information should have a separate heading (Box 11–1). References should be included on a separate sheet of paper. Most institutions require three references. After obtaining permission from the individuals listed as references, the nurse preparing the resume should make sure to have accurate titles, addresses, and telephone numbers. When selecting individuals for references, it is important that the individual know the applicant well, either in a professional or personal capacity, have something positive to say about the applicant, and be in some type of position of authority. The director of the nursing program, esteemed nursing faculty, supervisory level personnel at a health-care facility, and even a physician make good references. It is best not to list relatives, unless the hospital is asking for a specific personal reference.

A cover letter should be sent with every resume (Box 11–2). Like the resume itself, it should be neatly typed without errors and should be short and to the point. Although a friendly, rambling letter might provide insight into a prospective employee's underlying personality, most personnel directors or directors of nursing are too busy to read through the whole document. The letter should be written in a business letter format and should include the name and title of the person who will receive the letter. Letters beginning "To Whom It May Concern" do not make a favorable impression. The statement of interest and the name of the position should constitute the opening paragraph of the letter. The prospective employee should mention where he or she heard about the position. This should be included in the first paragraph as well as a date when the applicant would be able to begin working.

The second paragraph should give a brief summary of any work experience or education that qualifies the applicant for this position. Newly graduated nurses will have some difficulty with this part, but they should include their graduation date, the name of the school that they graduated from, the prospective date for taking the NCLEX, and the name of the director of the program. This paragraph should also state which shifts the applicant is willing to work.

The third paragraph should be very short. It should express thanks for consideration of the nurse's resume and a telephone number. Both the

Box 11–1

Sample Resume

Mary P. Oak
100 Wood Lane, Nicetown, PA 22222 Telephone (333) 555-1234 (H)

Objectives
Obtain an entry-level position as a Registered Nurse; deliver high-quality nursing care; continue my professional development.

Skills

- Good organizational and time management skills
- Communication and supervisory ability
- Sensitivity to cultural diversity

Education

Mountain University, Nicetown, PA
Bachelor of Science in Nursing, May, 2003

Experience

Supercare Hospital, Hilltown, PA
Nursing Assistant, 1999 to present
Responsibilities: Direct client care, including bathing, ambulation, daily activities, feeding paralyzed clients, assisting nurses with procedures, charting vital signs, and entering orders on the computer.

Big Bob's Burgers, Hilltown, PA
Assistant Manager, 1996–1999
Responsibilities: Supervised work of six employees; counted cash-register receipts at end of shift; inventoried and ordered supplies.

Awards

Nursing Student of the Year, 2000
Mountain University, Nicetown, PA

Pine Tree Festival Queen, 1996
Hilltown High School, Hilltown, PA

Professional Membership

National Student Nurses Association, 1999 to present
Mountain University, Nicetown, PA

Box 11–2

Sample Cover Letter

Mary P. Oak
100 Wood Lane
Nicetown, PA 22222

May 25, 2003

Mr. Robert L. Pinc
Director of Personnel
Doctors Hospital
Gully City, PA 44444

Dear Mr. Pine:

I am interested in applying for the Registered Nurse position in the General Medical/Surgical Unit. I have five years of experience in providing care for a variety of clients with medical/surgical health-care problems as a nursing assistant. I completed my baccalaureate degree in nursing on May 9, and am scheduled to take the NCLEX examination on June 3. Enclosed find my resume.

I believe that my organizational and time management skills will be a great asset to your fine health-care facility. I work well with all types of staff personnel, and having been a nursing assistant for the past five years, I can appreciate the problems involved in their supervision.

Thank you very much for consideration of my resume and application. I will call you within the next few days to arrange a date and time for an interview. Feel free to call me at home anytime (333) 555-1234.

Sincerely,

Mary P. Oak

letter and the resume should be sent by first-class mail in a 9-by-12-inch envelope so that the resume will remain unfolded, thus making it easier to handle and read.

Waiting for a reply can be the most difficult part of the whole process. Resist the urge to call the hospital too soon. Because most health-care institutions recognize the high anxiety levels of new graduates, they return calls within 1 to 2 weeks after receipt of the application. If no response is given after 3 weeks, the nurse should call the hospital to see whether or not the application was received. Mail does get lost. If the application has been received, the applicant should make no further telephone calls. Harassing the personnel director or director of nursing about a job is not usually an effective employment strategy.

Interviews

The next important step in the process is the interview. The interview allows the institution to obtain a firsthand look at the applicant, as well as an opportunity for the applicant to obtain important information about the institution and position requirements. The interview often produces high levels of anxiety in new graduates, who are interviewing for what might be their first real job.

Again, first impressions are important. The interview starts from the moment that the applicant enters the office. Conservative business clothes that are clean, neat, and well pressed are recommended. Similarly, a conservative hairstyle and a limited amount of accessories, jewelry, and makeup produce the best impression. Smoking, chewing gum, biting fingernails, or pacing nervously do not make good first impressions. The interviewer recognizes that interviews are stress producing and will make allowances for certain stress-related behaviors. Arriving a few minutes early allows time for last-minute touch-ups of hair and clothes and gives the applicant a chance to calm down. Carrying a small briefcase with a copy of the resume, cover letter, references, and information about the hospital also makes a favorable impression (Box 11–3).

> *First impressions are important. The interview starts from the moment that the applicant enters the office.*

Mental preparation is as important to a successful interview as physical preparation. Most interviewers start by asking about the resume, thus a quick review just before the interview is helpful. Expect questions about positions held for only a short time (less than 1 year), gaps in the employment record (longer than 6 months), employment outside the field of nursing (e.g., waitress, clerk), educational experiences outside the nursing program, or unusual activities outside the employment setting. Answer the questions honestly but briefly. Most personnel directors or directors of nursing are busy and do not appreciate long, detailed, chatty answers. Applicants can anticipate being asked:

- Why do you want this position?
- Why have you selected this particular facility?
- Why do you think that you are qualified for the position?
- What unique qualifications do you bring to the job to make you more desirable than other applicants?
- Where do you see yourself 5 years from now? Ten years from now?

Because of the emphasis placed on discrimination issues in recent lawsuits, there are a number of areas that prospective employers are not supposed to discuss, but sometimes do anyway. These include questions about sexual preferences or habits, age, race, plans for a family, personal living arrangements, **significant others**, and religious or political beliefs. If these questions are asked, the applicant needs to consider the implications of not answering them. Although there is no legal obligation for the applicant to answer, refusal to do so or pointing out that the question should not have been asked in the first place may be unwise. If these personal questions that violate an individual's right to privacy or seem discriminatory are answered by the graduate and then the graduate is not hired for the position, there may be grounds for some type of legal action based on discrimination.

At some point in the interview, usually toward the end, applicants are asked whether they have any questions. Although most do have questions, many applicants are afraid to ask. In fact, asking questions can be seen as a demonstration of independence, initiative, and intellectual curiosity—all traits that are highly valued by health-care providers. It is important that the first questions are not about salary, vacations, and other benefits. Questions that indicate interest in the institution are included in the Box 11–4.

After these questions have been answered, the applicant may want to ask, in passing, about

Box 11–3

Fashion Do's and Don'ts of Interviews

Do's

Men

1. Do shave or trim facial hair closely.
2. Do use after-shave and/or cologne sparingly (a little goes a long way).
3. Do carry a money clip or leather wallet, and a small, plain functional briefcase.
4. Do wear leather shoes that are polished and in good repair. Lace-up or slip-on shoes are best.
5. Do wear calf-length dark socks.
6. Do wear a tailored suit (blue, gray, beige are best) with a dress shirt (lighter in color than the suit). Do wear a conservative tie.

Women

1. Do apply perfume or cologne sparingly (a little goes a long way).
2. Do invest in a good haircut/perm. Clean, neat, and conservative is best.
3. Do wear shoes that are polished and in good repair. Plain pumps with medium heels are best.
4. Do carry a briefcase or simple (small) handbag that matches your shoes.
5. Do wear hose that coordinate in color, style, and texture with your shoes and outfit. Do take an extra pair for emergencies.
6. Do apply makeup lightly and carefully.
7. Do apply conservatively colored nail polish carefully.
8. Do dress conservatively.
9. Do wear colors that make a strong statement, such as shades of gray in medium to charcoal, or blue in a medium to navy.
10. Do wear small, conservative earrings.

Don'ts

Men

1. **Don't** overstuff wallet, money clip, or briefcase.
2. **Don't** carry a can of smokeless tobacco in your back pocket or pack of cigarettes in a shirt pocket.
3. **Don't** wear sandals, running shoes, or cowboy boots.
4. **Don't** wear socks that are lighter color than your trousers.
5. **Don't** wear green or flashy colors.

Women

1. **Don't** wear sneakers, sandals, cowboy boots, or heels more than 1½ inches high.
2. **Don't** overstuff your handbag or briefcase.
3. **Don't** apply makeup so that it looks artificial and heavy.
4. **Don't** use black or bright or dramatic colored nail polish.
5. **Don't** wear skimpy or low-cut outfits, leather, or fringe apparel.
6. **Don't** wear large, dangling earrings or have other body piercing such as nose rings, lip rings, tongue rings, multiple earrings.

Sources: Dunham, KS: How to Survive and Maybe Even Love Nursing School. FA Davis, Philadelphia, 2001, pp.222–225.

Leyen-Witzig, M: Starter kit—Interviewing 101. Magazine for Healthcare Travel Professionals 9(2):30–31, 2001.

Box 11–4

Questions Interviewee's Should Ask

- What are the responsibilities involved in the position?
- Who are the other staff or personnel working on this unit?
- What is the typical client-to-staff ratio for the unit?
- Are their any mandatary rotating shifts, weekend obligations, overtime, or floating?
- Does the hospital offer opportunities for continuing education, **clinical ladder,** advancement, or movement to other departments?
- Please describe the facility's policies for employee health and safety.

salary, raises, vacations, and other benefits, although it may be best not to ask about these at all. The applicant should also ask for written material on the nurse's contract with the agency, including benefits and job descriptions. Often the interviewer will provide this information without being asked in the course of answering some of the other questions.

It is appropriate to close the interview by asking for a tour of the facility. This allows first-hand evaluation of the workplace and a chance to observe the staff and clients in a real work setting. The interviewer may not be able to provide a tour at that time and so may ask another individual (e.g., a secretary) to take the applicant on the tour. It would also be wise to inform the interviewer of the dates scheduled for the National Council Licensure Examination (NCLEX) so that arrangements can be made for time off.

As with the resume, making frequent calls about the results of the interview is unwise. It is,

Box 11–5

20 Worst Job Interview Mistakes

1. Arriving late
2. Arriving too early (10–15 minutes is ok)
3. Dressing wrong (see fashion do's and don'ts)
4. Smoking
5. Drinking alcohol prior to the interview
6. Chewing gum and/or blowing bubbles
7. Bringing along a friend, relative, or children
8. Not being prepared for the interview
9. Not having an interview "dress rehearsal"
10. Not knowing your strengths and weaknesses
11. Asking too many questions of the interviewer (a few are ok)
12. Not asking any questions at all
13. Asking about pay and vacation as the first questions
14. Accusing the interviewer of discrimination
15. Bad-mouthing your present/former boss/employer
16. Name-dropping to impress the interviewer
17. Appearing lethargic and unenthusiastic
18. Weak, "dead fish," or bone-crusher handshake
19. Looking at your watch during the interview
20. Losing your cool or arguing with the interviewer

Sources: Dunham, KS: How to Survive and Maybe Even Love Nursing School. FA Davis, Philadelphia, 2001, pp. 225–228.

Zamboni, AM: Emergency assistance for the interviewee. Emergency Medical Services 30(3):59–60, 2001.

Beach, RS: Interviewing 101. Family Practice Management 8(1):38–40, 63–64, 2001.

Box 11–6

Sample Follow-up Letter

Mary P. Oak
100 Wood Lane
Nicetown, PA 22222

June 20, 2003

Mr. Robert L. Pine
Director of Personnel
Doctors Hospital
Gully City, PA 44444

Dear Mr. Pine:

Thank you very much for considering my resume and for the interview on June 3, 2003. I learned a great deal from the interview, and from my tour of the hospital after the interview.

I am writing to let you know that I am still interested in the position and was wondering about the status of my application. If at all possible, I would appreciate it if you could either call me or write a note relating to my potential employment at your facility.
Feel free to call me at home anytime (333) 555-1234.

Sincerely,

Mary P. Oak

however, appropriate for the applicant to send a letter within 1 week after the interview to thank the interviewer for his or her time and express appreciation for being considered for the position (Box 11–6). The applicant should also acknowledge how much it would mean to him or her to become a member of the staff at such a fine agency or hospital. If the position is offered, a formal letter of acceptance or refusal should be sent to the institution. Hospitals will not hold positions indefinitely, and failure to accept the position formally may cause the hospital to offer it to someone else. In today's health-care system, many applicants are often in search of a few positions.

Issues After Employment

Burnout

The **burnout syndrome** has existed for many years and has been recognized as a problem that can be reduced or even prevented. A widely accepted definition of burnout is a state of emotional exhaustion that results from the accumulative **stress** of an individual's life, including work, personal, and family responsibilities. Although the term is not often applied to students, many of the symptoms of burnout can be observed in these aspiring nurses.[6]

The people who are most likely to experience burnout tend to be more intelligent than average, hard-working, idealistic, and perfectionist. There are certain categories of jobs and careers that tend to produce a higher incidence of burnout: situations and positions in which there is a demand for consistently high-quality performance, expectations are unclear or unrealistic, there is little control over the work situation, and the financial rewards are inadequate. These jobs or careers tend to be very demanding and stressful, with little recognition or appreciation of what is being done. Also, jobs in which there is constant contact with people (customers, clients, students, or criminals) rank high on the burnout list.

Even with the most superficial knowledge of nursing, it is easy to see that many of these elements are present in the nurse's work situation. It is possible to recognize nurses who are in the early stages of burnout by identifying some classic behaviors (Box 11–7).

One of the earliest indications is the attitude that work is something to be tolerated, rather than eagerly anticipated. Nurses in the early stages of burnout often are irritable, impatient, cynical, pessimistic, whiny, or callous toward coworkers and clients. These pre-burnout nurses take frequent sick days, are chronically late for their shifts, drink too much, eat too much, and often are not able to sleep. Eventually, as their idealism erodes, their work suffers. They become careless in the performance of their duties, uncooperative with their colleagues, and unable to concentrate on what they are doing, and they display a general attitude of boredom and **apathy**. If allowed to continue, burnout may lead to feelings of helplessness, powerlessness, purposelessness, and guilt.[7]

Despite this bleak picture, nurses do not have to fall victim to the burnout syndrome. There are many nurses who practice their profession for many years, manage to deal with the stress, and find great personal satisfaction in what they do. These satisfied and motivated nurses have developed ways to deal with the stress of their careers while maintaining their goals and purpose as nurses.

The first step in dealing with burnout is to be able to recognize its signs. Many nurses who are burning out use denial and rationalization to block recognition of burnout, because it is just too painful for them to think that they put so much time, money, and effort into preparing for a career that they no longer want or enjoy. It is important to realize that it is not the career that is producing the burnout, but rather the difficulty in coping with the stresses the career is producing. Although it may not be possible to change the requirements of the profession significantly, it is possible to learn how to cope more effectively with stress.

Box 11–7

Symptoms of Burnout

- Extreme fatigue
- Exhaustion
- Frequent illness
- Overeating
- Headaches
- Sleeping problems
- Physical complaints
- Alcohol abuse
- Mood swings
- Emotional displays
- Anxiety
- Poor-quality work
- Anger
- Guilt
- Depression

Managing Stress and Time

Although there are many schools of thought about stress and time-management techniques, several common threads run through many of these theories. These views include setting personal goals, identifying problems, and using strategies for problem solving.

ISSUES IN PRACTICE

Critical Incident Stress Debriefing Teams: Responding to Major Stressful Events

Nurses are familiar with the stresses routinely found in their daily work and usually develop skills that are successful to some degree in dealing with it. Most nurses believe that traumatic events in their work setting are a part of the job and that they should be able to handle them without difficulty. However, as recent history has shown, major and overwhelming stressful events, such as the devastation of the World Trade Center, can strike without warning. As individuals and a nation, we experience a sense of horror, helplessness, and powerlessness in addition to the normal stress responses of shock, disbelief, anger, and grief. The end result may well be a complex of symptoms similar to burnout syndrome, including physical symptoms, depression, and chronic anxiety.

In response to major tragedies that have occurred over the past decade, the critical incident stress debriefing (CISD) process was developed to help people deal with major acts of violence and traumatic disasters. The American Red Cross has been instrumental in training and providing resources for local CISD teams that are made up of mental health professionals specially trained in crisis intervention, stress management, and post-traumatic stress disorders (PTSDs). After a major incident, employers often call for the formation of the teams to support their workers though the immediate post-trauma period.

To be most effective, the CISD teams need to be on site within 2 to 3 days after serious events ranging from the death of coworkers, natural disasters such as tornados, or acts of terrorism. The goal of the team is to encourage the participants to verbalize their feelings and thoughts, identify and develop their coping skills, and generally lower overall grief and anxiety levels. One of the keys when working with nurses is to have them recognize that they are not expected to be able to handle all situations and that it is appropriate to ask for help. Although nurses study the stress response and grieving process in nursing school, it is sometimes hard for them to apply the information about normal stress reactions to themselves. When nurses do not recognize that they are having difficulty in responding to traumatic stress, they increase their risk for developing long-term stress reactions. When they do not seek help, they can develop the symptoms of PTSD anywhere from a few days to as long as 6 months after the event.

Warning signs of PTSD include:

1. Recurring nightmares and inability to sleep
2. Intrusive and vivid flashbacks
3. Prolonged depression
4. High levels of anxiety
5. Maladaptive coping behaviors such as drug and alcohol abuse

The CISD session generally requires up to 3 hours. Sessions can be longer or shorter depending on the nature of the event and the number of people affected. In addition to the opportunity to express emotions and feeling, the participants are educated in some ways to reduce anxiety and promote mental and physical health that include:

1. Not watching televised replay of the event over and over
2. Staying with friends as much as possible
3. Avoiding unhealthy, high-fat diets
4. Engaging in regular aerobic exercise as much as possible
5. Avoiding excessive dependence on alcohol and drugs for sleep
6. Getting back to a comfortable routine as soon as possible
7. Feeling comfortable seeking professional help when needed

During the CISD sessions, nurses are asked for their input about the process. If the team feels it necessary, additional referrals for long-term treatment may be recommended.

Although they do have a number of skills that help them deal with traumatic events in their workplace, nurses are not super-people and should not expect that they can handle all stressful events without help. The CISD process was developed to allow individuals, including nurses, to obtain help soon after the event to promote coping and resolution of major traumatic events.

Sources: Antai-Otong, D: Overwhelming stressful events: Proactive response key to coping. American Nurse 34(1):9, 2002.
McGown, B: Self-reported stress and its effects on nurses. Nursing Standard 15(42):33–38, 2001

Setting Personal Goals

Goals and goal setting are an important part of client care. Nursing students—and by extension, practicing nurses—are highly proficient in the planning stage of the nursing process, in which goal setting is the primary task. They know that a good set of goals should be client centered, time oriented, and measurable and that they should write these goals with every care plan they prepare.

It is important to realize that it is not the career that is producing the burnout, but rather the difficulty in coping with the stresses the career is producing.

In their personal lives, however, these nurses may rush full-tilt into one erratic day after another, subordinating their own needs to the needs of others, working long, hard hours, but without accomplishing very much and feeling frustrated about it. What is the problem here? Very simply, nurses can prepare realistic, beneficial goals for their clients, but they seem to be unable to do the same for themselves.

Personal goals should include both long-term and short-term goals. Typically, personal long-term goals look into the future at least 10 years and include a statement about what the nurse wants to achieve during his or her lifetime. Some examples are going back to school to obtain an advanced degree, becoming a director of nursing, or even writing a book about nursing. Practicing nurses who are caught up in the whirlwind of everyday life find it difficult to formulate statements about the future. One other important characteristic of long-term goals is that they need to be flexible. As life circumstances change, modifications are required.

Short-term goals are those that the nurse expects to accomplish in 6 months to 2 years. These goals should be aimed primarily at making the nurse's professional or personal life more satisfying and fulfilling. Like long-term goals, they do not need to be related to work. Perhaps visiting a foreign country, a skiing trip in the mountains, even learning how to paint a picture or play the piano may be achievable in a relatively short time. In the professional realm, joining a professional organization, becoming a head nurse, or changing an outdated hospital policy all are goals that can be achieved in a short time. The fact that everyone ages over time cannot be altered, but that time can also be used to achieve personal satisfaction in life and increase knowledge and accomplishments.

Although goal setting is an important first step in dealing with the stress that leads to burnout, any good nurse recognizes that a plan without implementation is useless. As difficult as goal setting may be for nurses, carrying it out may be even more difficult. Although goal achievement requires a degree of hard work and personal sacrifice, when people are working toward something they really want, the effort that it takes to achieve the end actually becomes enjoyable. At first glance, this process may seem like a lot of work (and it is), but it actually becomes an exciting adventure in its own right.

Identifying Problems

Another important step in dealing with burnout is to identify the actual problems that are producing the stress. Again, nurses are taught as students that they need to identify client problems so that they can work toward solving them. Formulation of a nursing diagnosis is nothing more than precisely stating a client's problem. One thing that nurses realize early in the learning process is that what may appear to be an obvious problem may in reality not be a problem at all. And, conversely, something that may only be mentioned in passing by a client may turn out to be the real source of the client's nursing needs. Perhaps nurses should look at their own lives and attempt to formulate nursing diagnoses that deal with their stress-related problems (setting the North American Nursing Diagnosis Association list aside).

For example, a new graduate has just completed a shift where he has been assigned to eight complete-care clients. He has had to supervise two badly prepared nurses' aides and has put in 55 minutes of overtime (for which he will not be paid) to complete the charting. This nurse is feeling tired, frustrated, and even a little bit guilty because of an inability to provide the type of care that he was taught in nursing school. What is the problem? A possible nursing diagnosis might be: Alterations in personal satisfaction related to excessive workload, evidenced by sore feet, headache, shaky hands, feelings of guilt, frustration, and small paycheck.

Now that the problem has been identified, goals and interventions can be introduced to solve the problem. The goals may range from better organizing time to refusing to take care of so many complete-care clients. Interventions, depending on the goals, can include activities such as attending a time management seminar, talking to the head nurse, or changing a policy in the policy and procedure book. Nurses already know the nursing process as a client problem-solving technique. Why not apply the same knowledge and skills to personal problems? The stress level only increases if problems are left unsolved.

Strategies for Problem Solving

Although specific problems may require specific solutions, several widely accepted methods exist

What Do You Think?

List three tasks that you have put off today. Why did you avoid doing these? How can you get them done sooner?

to deal with the general stresses produced by everyday work and personal life. Included in these methods are activities such as recognizing that nurses are only human, improving time-management skills, practicing what is preached, and decompression.

Improving Time-Management Skills. In modern life there is often not enough time to do everything that needs to be done. The key to time management is setting priorities. In the world of nursing and client care, nurses are often required to do many tasks. Multitasking, the process of doing several tasks at the same time, tends to fragment the nurse's attention and concentration. Nurses need to recognize that only some nursing activities are essential to the safety and well-being of clients. These include ensuring that the clients get their medications on time, that their comfort needs are met, and that accidental injuries are prevented. Beyond these actions, nurses really have a great deal of discretion in what they can do when providing care to clients.

Burnout results mainly from personal and professional dissatisfaction. If nurses feel fulfilled in what they are doing, burnout is much less likely to occur. Activities that may increase nurses' satisfaction include spending time talking with clients, learning new skills, and decreasing the anxiety of families through teaching and listening. After such activities have been identified, time should be set aside for them during the shift. The real secret in using time management to prevent burnout is for the nurse to use the time left for those nursing activities that bring the most professional and personal satisfaction.

Several skills need to be developed to be able to allow time during a shift for these preferred activities. First, the nurse must learn to delegate by letting the licensed practical nurses (LPNs) or aides do those tasks that they are supposed to be able to do. Many nurses graduate from nursing school with the attitude that if you want it done right, you need to do it yourself. After becoming familiar with the LPN and nurse's aide job descriptions, nurses need to give others a chance to prove themselves.[8]

Another necessary skill is overcoming procrastination. Most people have a natural tendency toward procrastination, particularly when unpleasant or difficult tasks are involved. The primary reasons that people postpone or delay doing something is because they either do not want to begin or do not know where to begin the task. More time and energy are expended in inventing excuses for putting off tasks than would actually be taken in doing the task.

The best way to overcome procrastination is by starting the task, even if it is only a small step. An effective method is to select the most distasteful task to be done that day and to commit just 5 minutes to it. After 5 minutes are over, the task can be either set aside or continued. It is very likely that once the task is started and momentum builds, the task will be carried to completion.

Tasks can be prioritized by listing them in three categories. Category A tasks (e.g., passing out medications, treatments, and dressing changes) are those that need to be completed on time. Category B tasks (bath, linen change, lunch break, charting) can be postponed until later in the shift. Category C tasks (cleaning up the room, attending to personal grooming tasks other than those that are absolutely required) are tasks that can wait until the next day.

For daily tasks, both pleasant and unpleasant, the best time to do them is immediately. If achievement of the plan requires delegation, then it needs to be done at the beginning of the shift, not at the middle or end of the shift. Often nurses have a built-in fear of taking chances. As a result, they avoid doing things if there is a chance for failure, in the hope that somehow the problem will resolve itself. Any time that an important decision is made, there is a chance that someone will disagree or that the decision will be incorrect. These types of situations need to be viewed as a challenge or an opportunity, rather than a life-altering risk to be avoided. Although mistakes in health care do have the potential to be fatal, learning from mistakes is one of the most fundamental ways of increasing knowledge.

Time management, like other skills, requires some practice. Once a nurse masters this skill, his or her life becomes more satisfying.

Practice What You Preach. Because nursing is oriented toward keeping people healthy as well as curing illness, nurses spend a large amount of their time teaching clients about eating well; getting enough sleep; going for regular dental, eye, and physical examinations; avoiding too much drinking and smoking; and exercising regularly. It might make an interesting project for a student taking a nursing research course to have nurses rank themselves on how well they have incorporated these health maintenance activities in their own lives. The results would probably indicate a low overall score on the "practice what you preach" scale.

Nurses know all about the food pyramid, but they do not translate that knowledge into feeding themselves properly. In reality, there are going to be some busy days when it is impossible to eat right. But it should be possible, at least occasionally, to follow a diet that will promote health and reduce the buildup of fat plaques in the arteries.

It is important to get enough sleep to avoid chronic fatigue. People can adjust to a state of fatigue, but it tends to decrease the enjoyment that they find in life, as well as make them irritable, careless, and inefficient. Most people need between 5 and 8 hours of good sleep each night. It also probably would not hurt for nurses to take a short nap during the afternoon on their day off.

Many nurses feel that they get enough exercise during their busy shifts. And, in truth, the average staff nurse will walk between 2 and 5 miles during each 8-hour shift. Unfortunately, this type of walking does not qualify as the type of aerobic exercise recommended for an improved cardiovascular condition. Exercise, in order to be beneficial, must be done consistently and must raise the heart rate above the normal range for an extended period. The short sprint-type walking involved in client care does not accomplish this goal.

Walking 1 to 2 miles a day outside the hospital is a beneficial, simple exercise that will improve health. Nurses can also use a wide variety of exercise equipment for those days when walking outside is undesirable. The important requirement is that the exercise be done consistently and frequently. Regular exercise not only improves the cardiovascular system but also helps improve stamina, raise self-image, and promote a general sense of well-being.

Time to Decompress. The profession of nursing is stressful, even under ideal circumstances. Nurses are required to deal with other people constantly and to carry out numerous tasks that are potentially dangerous. At the end of any shift, even the most skilled and best-organized nurse has a sense of internal tension. This tension must be released or it will eventually cause a major explosion or (if turned inward) produce anxiety.

Tension must be released or it will eventually cause a major explosion or (if turned inward) produce anxiety.

Establish a Daily Decompression Routine. It may take a little time to discover, through trial and error, what works to reduce the tension built up during the shift. Some effective techniques include setting aside approximately 30 minutes of private, quiet time to dream and reflect about the day's activities. Perhaps relaxing in a tub of hot soapy water or sitting in a favorite reclining chair might meet the need for decompression. Relaxation activities, such as swimming, shopping, or even going for a drive, can help reduce tension and act as a time for decompression. Of course, stress-management techniques learned at seminars (e.g., self-hypnosis or meditation) can be used by those who have developed these skills. Finally, meeting with a nurse support group can help the nurse vent feelings and make constructive plans for solving problems.

Critical Thinking Exercises

- Make a list of the characteristics that would be found in the "perfect nurse." Make a second list of characteristics found in nurses observed in actual practice. Discuss how and why these lists differ from each other.

- Outline a plan for implementing a preceptor clinical experience for the senior class of a nursing program. Make sure to include how many hours of practice are required, criteria for the selection of preceptors, student objectives from the experience, and methods of evaluation.

- Write at least three long-term and five short-term personal or professional goals. Develop a realistic plan and time frame for achieving these goals. Make sure to include what is required to achieve these goals.

- Complete this statement, using as many examples as possible: "I feel most satisfied when I am done with my shift in knowing that. . . ." Analyze these answers and discuss how they can be implemented in everyday practice.

- Think of at least three situations in which you were asked to do something that you really did not want to do. How did you handle these situations? How could they be handled in a more assertive manner?

Conclusion

Although transition shock and burnout are realities of the nursing profession, they can be reduced or even avoided altogether. Nurses should be able to recognize the causes and early symptoms of transition shock and burnout in order to prevent them from developing into a problem. Therefore, nurses should use techniques to prevent these disorders from becoming insurmountable obstacles. In doing so, nurses will be able to practice their profession proficiently and gain the satisfaction that only nursing can provide.

References

1. Brewer, C, and Kovner, CT: Is there another nursing shortage? What the data tell us. Nurs Outlook 49(1):20–26, 2001.
2. Nursing shortage puts patients at risk and creates liability problems. Health Care Risk Management 23(6):61–65, 2002.
3. Sellack, JP, and O'Neil, EH: Recreating nursing practice for a new century. Nursing and Health Care Perspectives 21(1):14–21, 2001.
4. Manthey, M: Continuing the case for the baccalaureate. J Prof Nurs 18(1):7, 2002.
5. Pontious, JM: Where have all the nurses gone? The Oklahoma Nurse 17(1):1, 18, 2002.
6. Peir, JM, et al: Does role stress predict burnout over time among health care professionals? Psychology and Healthcare 16(5):511–525, 2001.
7. Garrett, DK, and McDaniel, AM: A new look at nurse burnout: The effects of environmental uncertainty and social climate. J Nurs Adm 31(2):91–96, 2001.
8. Wheeler, J: How to delegate your way to a better working life. Nursing Times 97(36):34–35, 2001.

Bibliography

Balevre, P: Professional nursing burnout and irrational thinking. Journal for Nurses in Staff Development 36(2):206–214, 2001.

Coffey-Love, M: Said another way: The nursing shortage: What is your role? Nursing Forum 36(2):29–35, 2001.

Evers, W, et al: Effects of aggressive behavior and perceived self-efficacy on burnout. Issues in Mental Health Nursing 22(4):439–454, 2001.

Five tips to avoid burnout and stay motivated. J Psychosoc Nurs Ment Health Serv 39(10):10, 2001.

Greenwalt, BJ: Can branding curb burnout? Nursing Management 32(9):26–31, 2001.

Harrington, D, et al: Job satisfaction and burnout. Administration in Social Work 25(3):1–16, 2001.

Rode, D, et al: The therapeutic use of technology. Am J Nurs 98(12):32–35, 1998.

3

Leading and Managing

12

Principles of Leadership and Management

Joseph T. Catalano

Learning Objectives

After completing this chapter, the reader will be able to:

- Identify and discuss the three major theories used to explain leadership.
- Define and distinguish between the three styles of leadership.
- Discuss the relationship of transformational and situational theories to leadership style.
- Identify the key behaviors and qualities of effective leaders.
- Distinguish the differences between management and leadership.
- Identify and discuss the two major theories of management.

In today's health-care system, even new graduates who have an "RN" after their name will be placed quickly in positions of leadership and management.

Leadership

The old saying that "Leaders are born, not made" implies that at birth a person either is a leader or is forever relegated to the rank of follower. Not many agree with this statement. Although some people may have an easier time filling the leadership role than others, most experts believe that almost everyone can develop leadership skills.

Many definitions of leadership refer to the ability of an individual to influence the behavior of others. When nurses exert leadership, they inspire other health-care workers to work toward one or more of several goals that include providing high-quality client care, maintaining safe working environment, developing new policies and procedures, or increasing the power of the profession.

Some leadership theories try to explain why some people are leaders and others are not, but as yet none covers all the possibilities. That may be because leadership requirements differ depending on the situation. In the intensive care unit (ICU), for example, where quick decisions are a matter of life and death, the leader is the nurse with highly developed critical thinking and analytical skills and the confidence to make decisions under pressure. In quality management, where the problems are often long term and complicated, the leader tends to be a nurse who is well organized and can methodically sift through a mountain of information and statistics to develop a policy that covers the widest range of possibilities. Several of the better known leadership theories are discussed here.

Trait Theory

The trait theory identifies qualities that are common to effective leaders (Box 12–1). Trait theory by itself is limited, because it focuses only on the traits of the individual and does not take into account how the person acts in specific situations. The question left unanswered is why everyone who has these traits does not become a leader.[1]

The old saying that "Leaders are born, not made" implies that at birth a person either is a leader or is forever relegated to the rank of follower.

Leadership Style Theory

One of the best-known theories of leadership looks at three styles of leadership:

1. Laissez-faire
2. Democratic
3. Authoritarian

Although they are discussed separately, they are a continuum of leadership style ranging from a mostly passive approach to a highly controlling one (Table 12–1).

The **laissez-faire** (French for "leave it alone") leadership style is also described as permissive, nondirective, or passive. The laissez-faire style leader allows the group he or she is leading to determine their own goals and the methods to achieve them. There is little planning, minimal decision making, and a lack of involvement by the leader. This style works well in only a few settings, for example, in a research laboratory that is staffed by self-motivated scientists who know what they want to achieve and are familiar with the means of achieving it. The laissez-faire style works best when the members of the group have the same level of education as the leader and the leader performs the same tasks as the group members. In most situations, however, the laissez-faire leadership style can leave people feeling lost and frustrated because of the lack of direction by the leader. When they do try to achieve some goal, often the only input from the leader is that they are doing it incorrectly. When faced with a difficult decision, laissez-faire leaders usually avoid making a decision in the hopes that the problem will resolve itself.

In a **democratic** (also called supportive or participative) leadership style, all aspects of the process of achieving a goal from planning and goal setting to implementing and taking credit for the success of the project are shared by the group. The democratic leadership style is based on four beliefs:

1. Every member of the group needs to participate in all decision making.
2. Within the limits established by the group, freedom of expression is allowed to maximize creativity.
3. Individuals in the group accept responsibility for themselves and for the welfare of the whole group.
4. Each member must respect all the other members of the group as unique and valuable contributors.[2]

The leader using the democratic style provides guidance to the group, and all members share control. This style works best with groups whose members have a relatively equal status and who know each other well because they have worked together for an extended period. Democratic leadership can be time consuming and inefficient in some situations, particularly when group members disagree strongly, but in the end, when a goal is achieved or a decision

Box 12–1

Key Leadership Traits

- High level of intelligence and skill
- Self-motivation and initiative
- Ability to communicate well
- Self-confidence and assertiveness
- Creativity
- Persistence
- Stress tolerance
- Risk taking
- Ability to accept criticism

made, there is a strong sense of ownership and achievement by the whole group. Many leaders are uncomfortable with this style of leadership because of the minimal control they have over the group.

The leader with an **authoritarian** (also called controlling, directive, or autocratic) style maintains strong control over all aspects of the group and its activities. Authoritarian leaders provide direction by giving orders that the group is expected to carry out without question. The final decision-making authority rests with the leader alone, although input from the group may be considered.

A leader using a dictatorial authoritarian style has no regard for the feelings and needs of the group members. Achieving the goal is the only thing that matters, and the leader will use any means, including harsh criticism, to do so. A

What Do You Think?

Have you ever had to be a leader in a group? What type of leadership style did you use? How successful was the outcome of the group work?

military mission to destroy a terrorist group by a SEAL (*s*ea *a*ir *l*and) assault team is an example of this type of leadership.

The benevolent authoritarian leader uses a more paternalistic approach to achieving the goal. That leader attempts to include the group's feelings and concerns in the final decision, but ultimately he or she makes the decision. Some group members may feel that the benevolent leader is condescending and patronizing.

The authoritarian leadership style works best in emergency situations, where clear directions are required to save a life or prevent injury, or in situations where it is necessary to organize a large group of individuals. Although highly efficient in achieving goals and completing tasks, the authoritarian leadership suppresses the creativity of the group members and may reduce the long-term effectiveness of the group. Authoritarian leadership also reduces the motivation levels of the group and may lead to passive-aggressive type behavior by the members that will further reduce the effectiveness of the group. Although some people can accept the need for the total control exerted by an authoritarian leader, most in a long-term work relationship with this type of leadership style will become frustrated and even rebellious at some point.

Table 12–1

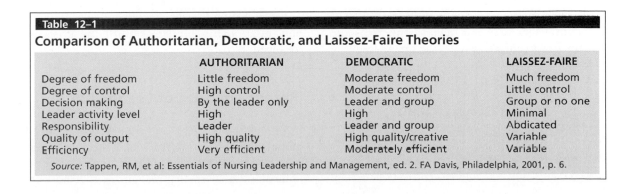

Comparison of Authoritarian, Democratic, and Laissez-Faire Theories

	AUTHORITARIAN	DEMOCRATIC	LAISSEZ-FAIRE
Degree of freedom	Little freedom	Moderate freedom	Much freedom
Degree of control	High control	Moderate control	Little control
Decision making	By the leader only	Leader and group	Group or no one
Leader activity level	High	High	Minimal
Responsibility	Leader	Leader and group	Abdicated
Quality of output	High quality	High quality/creative	Variable
Efficiency	Very efficient	Moderately efficient	Variable

Source: Tappen, RM, et al: Essentials of Nursing Leadership and Management, ed. 2. FA Davis, Philadelphia, 2001, p. 6.

In reality there are few leaders who use only one style. Most leaders use multiple leadership styles depending on the situation. Many factors may influence what type of leadership style is used at any given time, including external regulations and requirements, the ability of the group members, the work setting, and the problem being solved. For example, a nurse manager on a hospital unit may use a highly democratic style in most of the routine activities of the unit, but when a client goes into cardiac arrest, she may revert to a highly authoritarian style while directing the staff through a code.

Relationship-Task Orientation

Another commonly used theory of leadership rates leaders on whether they are more oriented toward establishing relationships or achieving assigned tasks and resolving problems. A leader with a high relationship–low task orientation is usually well liked by the group because of her or his acceptance of the group members as individuals, consideration of their feelings, encouragement, and promotion of good feelings among all the group members. However, the leader often sacrifices the achievement of the task or resolution of a problem when it conflicts with the feelings or goodwill of the group. This leader often allows the group to make its own decisions without regard to the task at hand and ultimately may not achieve the goals the group was organized to do in the first place.

> *The authoritarian leadership style works best in emergency situations, where clear directions are required to save a life or prevent injury, or in situations where it is necessary to organize a large group of individuals.*

The opposite extreme is the leader with a low relationship–high task orientation. This form of leadership is similar to the authoritarian style where the leader does all the planning with little regard to the input or feelings of the group, gives orders, and expects them to be carried out without question. Various forms of punishment are often used by this leader, ranging from verbal putdowns to poor performance evaluations that are used to determine pay raises.

The worst leader is the person with a low relationship–low task orientation that simulates the laissez-faire leadership style where the leader is uninvolved, does no planning, has little concern for the group members' feelings, and accomplishes little. On the other hand, the best leader is the one with a high relationship–high task orientation. This leader combines the best of both worlds in that he or she is open to input and actively communicates with the group members, provides constructive direction, quickly resolves conflicts, and ultimately achieves creative and effective solutions to problems. Certainly, perfect leaders are difficult to find. Most use a combination of styles and adjust them to the circumstances surrounding the problem. Again, think of the nurse manager who uses a high relationship–high task orientation for managing the unit in most of the day-to-day operations. In the cardiac arrest situation, this nurse manager may quickly change her or his orientation to one of low relationship–high task until the crisis is resolved.

What Do You Think?

Think of the best leader you have ever worked with. What traits did that person have? Now think of the worst leader you ever worked with. What traits did that person have?

Recent Theories of Leadership

Although the behavior and trait theories remain popular, researchers have come to the conclusion that leadership is really a more complex process. The situational theory recognizes that no one approach works in all situations. The leader needs to acknowledge this fact and adjust the leadership style and behavior to the situation, considering the many variables that may be involved. Good leaders seem to do this instinctively. One of the key factors is the type of organization in which the group is located. The environment is always important when exercising leadership.

The transformational theory takes the situational theory one step further. This theory recognizes that there are multiple intangibles that exist whenever people interact. Factors such as sense of meaning, creativity, inspiration, and vision all are involved in creating a sense of mission that exceeds good interpersonal relationships and rewards. Although this is true in most work settings, health care and nursing, where care of human beings is the primary goal, require that nurses do something positive. In many health-care facilities, nursing leaders are expected to inspire excitement and commitment in nurses who often must provide care to very ill clients in less than ideal circumstances.

Key Leadership Behaviors

Traits are characteristics that an individual possesses. Traits may or may not lead to the actions or behaviors that are required for successful leadership. It is also possible to lack leadership traits, yet be able to carry out successful leadership behaviors.

Critical Thinking. The ability to think critically is a multistep process similar to the nursing process. Critical thinkers must be able to analyze data, organize and plan, and use creativity in the resolution of problems (see Chapter 6). Leaders must often make important decisions based on incomplete data.

Problem Solving. Being able to use the problem-solving process effectively is essential to effective leadership. Leaders in the health-care setting face problems that arise from many sources, including staffing and personnel, scheduling, administrative, budget, and client demands.

Acknowledgment and Respect for Individual Differences. Personality is the sum total of people's experiences. Because no two people have identical experiences, each one has different needs, feelings, and orientations. The effective leader recognizes these differences and is able to direct the people to their highest level of achievement given their varying orientations.

Active Listening. To be effective, leaders must be able to hear not only the words that the person is saying but also the body language and underlying emotions and meaning. The experts tell us that only 7 percent of communication is verbal; 93 percent is all the other nonverbal content. Leaders often fail in their leadership roles when they do not listen to the full message of the individuals they are attempting to lead.

Skillful Communication. Communication is a complex process that involves an exchange of information and feedback (see Chapter 13). Mistakes happen on both sides when the information being shared is incomplete or confusing. Providing frequent and positive feedback is one of the best methods for leaders to determine how well they are communicating and how open the communication channels remain. It also can boost morale and improve the working environment. Effective leaders should also be able to give and use negative feedback to improve performance. If negative feedback is given in a nonthreatening and encouraging manner, the person receiving it will often appreciate the chance to improve his or her skills.

> *Leaders often fail in their leadership roles when they do not listen to the full message of the individuals they are attempting to lead.*

Establishment of Clear Goals and Outcomes. The old question that asks, "How do you know when you've arrived if you don't

ISSUES NOW

Nurses and hospital administrators are not the only ones who have noticed the nursing shortage. Increasingly, physicians are feeling the crunch of not having enough qualified nurses to provide care for their hospitalized clients, who are sicker and have more complicated health-care problems than even a few years ago. The traditional answer is to merely educate more nurses. But the other side of the coin is to reduce the drain of experienced nurses from the hospital to the private sector, home health, freestanding one-day surgery hospitals, or any one of a number of the newest entrepreneurial health-care schemes.

Physicians are beginning to wonder if there is any cure for the nursing shortage. In Oklahoma, a number of physicians have started to recognize that they might actually be part of the problem. Some of the physician members of the State Medical Association have proposed a nonmandatory set of guidelines for working with nurses:

- Treat nurses as professionals, and respect and honor the care they provide for your clients.
- Teach your clients to do the same thing.
- Advocate for educational opportunities for nurses.
- Treat nursing students with respect, and teach them every time you have an opportunity to do so.
- Include nurses in your plan of care for clients.
- Advocate for reasonable documentation practices (i.e., cut down on nurse's paperwork).
- When frustrated with nursing care, look for ways to improve the system rather than berate nurses.
- Tell your nursing colleagues when they have done a good job.
- Advocate for funding for nursing education.
- Advocate innovative workplace modifications with more open scheduling ideas

As nurses, we would likely respond as a group: "It's about time!" Physicians also need educating. Have you done anything recently to educate a physician about the nursing shortage?

Source: Pontious, JM: Where Have All the Nurses Gone. The Oklahoma Nurse 47(1):1–2, 2002.

Box 12–2

Keys to Leadership

Key Qualities	Key Behaviors
• Integrity	• Critical thinking
• Courage	• Problem solving
• Initiative	• Acknowledgment and respect for individual differences
• Energy	• Active listening
• Optimism	• Skillful communication
• Perseverance	• Establishment of clear goals and outcomes
• Well rounded	• Continued personal and professional development
• Coping skills	
• Self-knowledge	

Source: Adapted from Tappen, RM, et al: Essentials of Nursing Leadership and Management, ed. 2. FA Davis, Philadelphia, 2001, p. 8.

know where you are going?" is a truism that all leaders must address at some point by establishing clear goals and outcomes for the group. Groups who lack clear goals often feel frustrated and lost. Initially, leaders must clearly identify their goals. Then they must identify the goals shared by the group and use them to motivate the group. Successful outcome is often a thoughtful melding of the vision of the leader and the group.

Continued Personal and Professional Development. One of the most valuable lessons that nursing students can learn while in nursing school is that education does not end when they graduate, it just begins. One of the primary goals of the nursing education process should be to teach the student how to learn. Lifelong learning is a goal that effective leaders seek not only for themselves but also for those whom they are leading. Leaders can function as teachers in certain settings, but a more effective means of encouraging others to continue to learn is to set a good example. It is important to recognize that learning takes place not only in a formal school-like setting, but in all those encounters and situations that affect attitudes, beliefs, and behavior.

KEY LEADERSHIP QUALITIES

No matter what style a leader favors, successful leaders have common qualities (Box 12–2).

Integrity. For many years, nursing has been ranked among the top five professions that are most respected by the public in the annual Gallup Poll (in 2002, nurses ranked second behind firefighters). One of the keys to this respect is the integrity of the profession as it is perceived by clients and their families. The public expects nurses, as a group, to be honest, trustworthy, ethical, moral, and professional. The American Nurses Association (ANA) Code of Ethics for Nurses (see Chapter 7) is directed toward promoting and maintaining the integrity of the profession. If a group observes less than complete integrity in their leader, that person's ability to lead is markedly diminished.

Courage. Although having the courage to maintain one's convictions in the face of adversity is a quality all leaders must have, certain leadership positions may require a higher degree of courage. Nurses who are in what are called middle management positions, such as unit managers, house supervisors, or quality control coordinators, often find themselves caught in a no-man's-land between two opposing worlds.[3] For example, higher management may be attempting to implement a plan or procedure that the staff nurses strongly object to, or the staff nurses may be complaining about some issue, such as staffing, that the middle manager has little control over. The leader in this situation may need to take the risk of offending one or the other of the groups to resolve a difficult problem.

Initiative. Effective leadership demands that the leader be a "self-starter" and have the ability to start projects without pressure from above. Often the group relies on the leader to begin the process of completing a task or resolving a problem.

Energy. Energy refers not only to the ability to do work but also to the display of that energy in the form of enthusiasm for the work. Energetic people are contagious. Charismatic leaders are the ones who are the most energetic and enthusiastic. The group needs to see that the leader is willing to work as hard as they are being asked to work. However, energy has to be rationed carefully to maintain the optimum levels.

Optimism. A positive attitude is also contagious. Conversely, so are negative attitudes, which often lead to discouragement and failure (Table 12–2). A leader who has an overall positive attitude and views new problems as opportunities for success will be much more successful than the leader who constantly complains about each new crisis.

Perseverance. Leaders need to be able to continue to work through difficult problems in difficult circumstances, even when others feel like quitting. Again, if the leader sets the example for the group with a "there's more than one way to skin a cat" attitude, the group will be encouraged to find new and creative solutions.

Well Rounded. Leaders, as well as those they are leading, live multifaceted lives. It is important to develop and foster nonwork relationships with friends and family. The time at work should be balanced with recreational, spiritual, social, and cultural activities that complete the person and round out the personality. Time must also be invested in maintaining good health through proper nutrition and regular exercise that will also help prevent burnout (see Chapter 11).

Coping Skills. All jobs have some degree of stress, although people in leadership positions often experience higher levels. Stress can be handled in two ways: unconsciously, through defense mechanisms; or consciously, by bringing learned coping skills into play. A more productive way to deal with stress is to use coping skills developed in dealing with past stressors to promote a positive and healthy resolution to the stress. Some people learn how to use the stress they experience to motivate them and to tap into the energy it generates to achieve at a higher level of functioning.

Self-Knowledge. Leaders who do not know and understand themselves are less able to understand those who are working for them. Self-awareness is the beginning of self-acceptance as a thinking, feeling person who interacts with other thinking, feeling persons. Unless leaders understand and accept their motivations, biases, and perceptions, they will not be able to understand why they feel and react to certain individuals and situations.

Table 12–2

Winner or Whiner—Which One Are You?

A WINNER SAYS...	A WHINER SAYS...
We have a real challenge here.	This is a big problem.
I'll do my best.	Do I have to do this?
That's great!	That's nice, I guess.
We can do it.	It can't be done, it's impossible.
Yes.	Maybe, when I have some time.

Source: Tappen, RM, et al: Essentials of Nursing Leadership and Management, ed. 2. FA Davis, Philadelphia, 2001, p. 8.

Management

Unlike the development of leadership theory, which primarily focused on the leader, the early study of management was aimed toward influencing employees to be as productive as humanly possible. Two schools of thought address and define management.

Time-Motion Theory

Time-motion theory developed out of the early industrial age in which theorists concentrated on ways to complete a task most easily and efficiently. Often their efforts resulted in increased productivity but a decrease in employee satisfaction. From this viewpoint, management can be defined as planning, organizing, commanding, coordinating, and controlling the work of any particular group of employees. The time-motion approach holds the belief that providing the right incentives to the employee, primarily money, can increase employee productivity. Although the weaknesses of this approach make it less desirable in today's society, variations of it served as the harbingers of many of the business techniques currently in use.

Human Interaction Theory

Early on in the study of management, the limits of the time-motion approach became evident. Researchers observed that some lower-paid employee groups had higher levels of productivity than others with higher pay who were doing the same jobs. It appeared that factors such as employee attitudes, fears, hopes, personal problems, social status in the group, and visions strongly influenced how they worked. From this perspective, management can be defined as the ability to elicit from employees their commitment, loyalty, creativity, productivity, and continuous improvement.

Managers who favored the human interaction theory were required to develop a different set of management skills, including understanding human behavior, effective counseling, increasing motivation, using effective leadership skills, and maintaining productive communication. Just being a "nice guy" was not enough to guarantee employee cooperation and commitment. To be effective, management needed to be able to recognize and respond to employee concerns and needs, gain their acceptance, and protect workers from pressures from higher administration.

It is also important to keep in mind that different management forms are necessary for different work settings. A predominantly time-motion approach may still work best in an area such as manufacturing of automobiles or washing machines. Using the same approach would be inappropriate and probably ineffective when attempting to manage a group of registered nurses (RNs) working in an intensive care unit of a busy city hospital.

As is commonly the case, good managers use a combination of the two theories along with additional factors, including motivational and needs theory.

Motivational theory can be defined as the ability to influence the choices people make among a number of possible choices open to them. For example, what factors would motivate a new graduate nurse to work at one hospital when there are four facilities that are offering him or her a job? Are the pay and benefits better? Maybe it is closer to home. Perhaps the shifts are better and the facility does not require mandatory overtime.

Several theorists have attempted to explain this phenomenon. Probably the best known is Abraham Maslow, who developed the Hierarchy of Needs Theory. Although nursing students are taught and use this theory to deal with client needs, the theory also has application in the realm of leadership and management. Maslow believes that human needs are arranged in a hierarchy from the most basic and essential to those that are more complex. Most basic are the physiologic and safety needs, and until these are met in at least a satisfactory fashion, the person is less likely to deal with the higher needs such as social relationships, self-esteem, or self-actualization. For example, if a nurse was not being paid a salary that would meet the needs for food, housing, and clothing, that would become the nurse's primary concern rather than delivering quality client care. Realistically, needs are never fully met, but they have to be accommodated to a degree where the person feels comfortable enough to move up in the hierarchy.

Some of the more important satisfiers that have been identified include elements that tend to expand the work challenges and scope, such as career advancement, increased responsibility, recognition for achievements, and opportunities for professional growth.

Another theory that has become popular is Herzberg's Motivation-Hygiene Theory. Although there are some similarities between Maslow's and Herzberg's theories, particularly in their applications, Herzberg believes that people have two different categories of needs that are fundamentally different from each other.

The first category is referred to as needs dissatisfiers or hygiene factors. According to Herzberg, if these needs are not met, the person feels dissatisfied with his or her job and focuses more on the environment than the work that is supposed to be performed. Hygiene factors are related to the work environment and include factors such as salaries and benefits, job security, status in the organization, work conditions, policies, and relationships with coworkers. Hygiene factors are related to the conditions under which the work is performed and not to the work itself. Hygiene factors only serve as negative motivators, in that when they are not met, work productivity is reduced. However, if they are satisfied, there is no guarantee that increased productivity and higher quality performance will result.

The second category of needs according to Herzberg, are called satisfiers or needs motivators. Unlike the hygiene factors, satisfiers focus primarily on the work itself. Some of the more important satisfiers that have been identified include elements that tend to expand the work challenges and scope, such as career advancement, increased responsibility, recognition for achievements, and opportunities for professional growth. The satisfiers can have both a positive and negative motivation effect. If they are satisfied, they can motivate workers to increased productivity and higher quality work. If they are not satisfied, they often have the opposite effect.

Herzberg concludes that employers must satisfy the hygiene factors as a minimum requirement before there is any increase in productivity. Then programs to promote job enrichment will be effective in upgrading the achievement, roles, and satisfaction of employees. In the hospital setting, career or clinical ladder programs provide nurses with the recognition for achievement and opportunity for advancement, along with financial rewards (hygiene factor), and allows them to remain in direct client care.

It is important for RNs to understand and be able to use motivation techniques, even if they are not in a designated management role. The ability to motivate is one of the keys to success in delegation at any level, and in reality, the success of RNs is often assessed by how well people on the health-care team they are supervising perform their jobs. Successful motivation is the door to successful leadership because these are the people who can make things happen in an organization.

Making Changes Successfully

Motivating people to change is one of the most challenging and most important functions of leadership. Simply stated, change is the process of transforming, altering, or becoming different from what was before.[4] Although change is a constant in health care and nursing, it is surprising how resistant nurses can be to even minor changes in their work environment.

There are two primary forces that bring about change: external forces that originate from outside the person or organization, and internal forces that start from within the individual or organization. A primary example of external change is what happens when governmental agencies pass down new rules and regulations that affect health care. An example of internal change would be a hospital increasing salaries or eliminating mandatory overtime from the work action of a group of nurses.

Change can also be planned or unplanned. Planned change is more productive and occurs when there is a directed and designed implementation of some element within the organization. Change can affect all aspects of an organization, including policies, goals, organizational philosophy, work environment, or even structure. Planned change can be used for all sorts of projects, ranging from minor to the most complex.

Unplanned change, sometimes called reactive change, occurs when some problem forces a person or organization into a situation in which it must respond. These are often minor in nature, but sometimes can involve projects that are large in scope and complexity. Examples in nursing include changes in staffing due to nurses who call in sick, clients who experience cardiac arrest, or even equipment failures, such as when the electricity fails or a water main breaks.

Nurses often take on the role of the change agent, that is, the one who is bringing about the change (Box 12–3). All change requires the ability to overcome resistance to change (called restraining forces) by a driving force that pushes toward change. When the driving and restraining forces are equal, then no change occurs and the status quo is maintained. Change can occur only when the driving force is greater than the restraining force. Those who want to change have a tendency to push, but those who are being asked to change tend to push back to maintain things as they were. It is important when attempting to implement change to identify the restraining forces and ways to overcome them. Habit, comfort, and inertia are the three most common restraining forces.

Planned change works best when it is well organized, proceeds at a steady pace, and has a definite date for achievement. There is a level of excitement that raises energy levels when a change is near completion, but postponing the date for the change can drain that energy and leads to disappointment.

Group Dynamics

All successful leaders and managers understand and are able to use the principles of group dynamics. A group exists when three or more people interact and are held together by a common bond or interests. Groups are open systems that interact with the environment to achieve a goal (see Chapter 4). The individuals who make up the group are its subsystems and interact with each other as well as the environment. Group dynamics provides the principles that underlie team building, which is so essential to the success of nursing units. Establishing and sharing common goals is the starting point for successful team building.

Box 12–3

Characteristics of an Effective Change Agent

- Well organized
- Identifies restraining forces
- Ability to motivate
- Demonstrates and maintains commitment to change
- Develops trusting relationships
- Responsive to feedback and negotiation
- Goal directed
- Good communicator
- Optimistic

Table 12–3

Do's and Don'ts of Effective Change Agents

DO'S	DON'TS
Do develop a sense of trust.	Don't have a hidden agenda.
Do establish common goals.	Don't be unpredictable.
Do facilitate effective communication.	Don't miss or reschedule meetings frequently.
Do establish a strong team identity.	Don't use threats or bluffs to manipulate members.
Do contribute as much as possible.	Don't volunteer to be the record keeper.
Do find reasons to celebrate and recognize accomplishments.	Don't follow the rest of the crowd.

When the common goal is to help one another, effective team building results. Members of the team respond most positively when they feel they are included in the decision making and when they realize that their input is valued by the other team members. It is important that the leader always ask team members for their ideas about the goal that the team is working toward achieving. A strong team spirit is crucial to the success of the team.

Similarly, the team will only function smoothly when the members understand their role and the role of the other members. It identifies their place on the team and establishes the expectations from each member. In order to be successful, the leader must establish the belief that all the roles are of equal importance and value for the achievement of the goals or purposes of the group. Team members also need to realize that they are not merely responsible for their own personal roles, but need to be supportive of the roles of the other members. Although the leader establishes the goals to be achieved, it is important that the team members be allowed to achieve their tasks in ways that are most appropriate for them, particularly when working with self-motivated professionals such as nurses.

Ongoing or complicated projects require a long-term commitment that is sometimes difficult to maintain. Effective team leaders are good at finding accomplishments along the way that the team can celebrate and enjoy. It allows the team to feel good about what they have achieved to this point and motivates them to accomplish more in the future. A good leader also recognizes the accomplishments of others and rewards them appropriately. Often even simple statements of praise can be effective.

Finally, establishing a sense of team identity and trust completes the group dynamic and team building process. Some degree of creativity may be required for establishing team identity, ranging from similar uniforms to buttons or pins. Trust allows the team members to be more open to communications from other members and more willing to take risks. Trust empowers the members, allowing them to make independent decisions and promoting the smooth functioning of the team (Table 12–3).

Care Delivery Models

No place are the elements of groups dynamics reflected better than in the nursing units of the hospital or health-care facility. The organizational structure found in the nursing units of a facility reflects how the nursing department interacts with coworkers and participates in the delivery of client care. Various models may be used in the delivery of nursing care. Many health-care facilities have made a transition from one model to another and may even be incorporating several different models at the same time. The nurse must recognize which model is being used as well as its strengths and weaknesses. These models include functional nursing, team nursing, primary care nursing, and modular nursing (Table 12–4).

Table 12–4

Comparison of Common Models for Delivering Client Care

MODEL	NURSES ARE CALLED	DESCRIPTION	WHERE MODEL IS USED
Functional	Charge nurse Medical nurse Treatment nurse	Nurses are assigned to specific tasks rather than specific clients	Hospitals Nursing homes Nurse consultants Operating rooms
Team	Team leader Team member	Nursing staff members are divided into small groups responsible for the total care of a given number of clients.	Hospitals Nursing homes Home care Hospice
Primary Care	Primary nurse Associate nurse	Nurses are designated either as the primary nurse responsible for clients' care or as the associate nurse who assists in carrying out the care.	Hospitals Specialty units Hospice Dialysis Home care
Modular	Care pair	Nurses are paired with other less trained caregivers. Generally involves cross-training of personnel.	Hospitals Home health care Transport teams

Functional Nursing

Functional nursing has as its foundation a task-oriented philosophy—each person performs a specific job that is narrowly defined according to the needs on the unit. The medication nurse, for example, focuses on the duties concerned with administering and documenting medications for the assigned group of clients. In this organizational unit, the nurse manager is called the charge nurse, whose main responsibility is to oversee the various workers. Charge nurses are also appointed for each shift to manage the care during that time. This model relies on ancillary health workers such as nurses' aides and orderlies. Some believe this model fragments care too much. Because many people have specific tasks, coordination can be difficult, and the holistic perspective may be lost.

Team Nursing

Team nursing has a more unified approach to client care, with team members functioning together to achieve client goals. The team leader functions as the person ultimately responsible for the clients' well-being. More cohesiveness is present among the members of the team than is found in the functional model. Rather than having a narrow task to accomplish, team members focus on team goals under the coordination of the team leader. The team conference provides for effective communication and follow-up between and among team members and is the key to successful team nursing.

Primary Care Nursing

The primary care nursing model provides nurses the opportunity to focus on the whole person. The **primary care nurse** provides and is responsible for all of the client's nursing needs. The nurse manager in this model becomes a facilitator for the primary care nurses. Primary care nurses are self-directed and concerned with the consistency of care. The primary care model is similar to the case management model, which has one nurse caring for one client. Many home-health-care agencies use this method of assigning a registered nurse to work with an individual or family for the duration of the services rendered.

Modular Nursing

Modular nursing, also called client-focused care, is one model that was developed in response to professional nursing personnel shortages and to the downsizing of professional nursing staffs. This model is based on a decentralized organizational system that emphasizes close interdisciplinary collaboration. Redesigning the method of nursing care delivery takes much planning and input from the various departments involved, such as nursing, respiratory therapy, physical therapy, radiology, laboratory, and dietary.

Important aspects of modular nursing include relying on unlicensed assistive personnel (UAP), also called unit service assistants, for the provision of direct care; grouping clients with similar needs; developing **relative intensity measures (RIMs)**; and emphasizing team concepts in small groups that remain constant. Cross-training of personnel is another important aspect of modular nursing; for example, using this system, respiratory therapists do not just provide respiratory treatments but also help clients to the bathroom and turn bedridden clients. Nurse managers in this system are responsible for providing explicit job descriptions, maintaining the work group's cohesiveness, carefully monitoring each staff person's abilities, delegating tasks as appropriate, and evaluating the effectiveness of care.

The role of UAPs is one area of the client-focused care model that needs more definition, particularly in relation to the registered nurse's accountability and responsibilities in supervising these workers. State boards of nursing across the country are in the process of considering possible changes in nurse practice acts necessitated by the use of UAPs.

Benefits of this care delivery model include decreased staffing cost and greater autonomy of cross-trained personnel. The nurse manager must be a strong leader for this model of care delivery to succeed. Consistent collaboration between the nurse manager and physician is of utmost importance in planning client care.

Leadership versus Management

There are several questions that arise when people speak about leadership and management.

Are Leadership and Management the Same Thing?

Leadership can be exerted either formally or informally. Often the most effective leaders in a group are not the ones who are officially designated as the leader. On the other hand, managers are given the title by some higher authority and have formally designated authority to supervise a group of employees in the achievement of a task. Similarly, managers can be held formally responsible for the quality, quantity, and cost of the work that the supervised employees produce.

Must Managers Possess Good Leadership Skills to Perform Their Job?

The most effective managers will have highly developed leadership skills; however, by virtue of their title and position, even managers with poor leadership skills are still the official authority, although their effectiveness is reduced. Often, in groups where the manager is not a good leader, unofficial leaders emerge and exert either a strong positive or negative influence on the achievement of the group's task. If the unofficial leader is generally supportive of the manager's and administration's goals, then the work group can be highly productive and the organization's goals will be achieved. Conversely, if the unofficial leader's goals are opposed to those of the manager and administration, productivity may decrease to a point where the manager is asked to leave the position by higher level management.

Are People with Leadership Ability Always Good Managers?

A person who has leadership ability may not have good management skills. This phenomenon is often seen in nursing when a highly effective and skilled staff nurse who functions as the unofficial unit leader is taken out of that role and promoted to an official management position. Some do well, others may require additional training in management principles and skills. Management and leadership skills complement each other. As with all skills, they can be learned and require practice and experience to be developed fully. Even new graduate nurses can be effective leaders within their new nursing roles. As they gain experience and develop new skills, their ability and opportunities to provide leadership will also increase. Learning and improving skills in one area will increase the ability in the other.

A person who has leadership ability may not have good management skills. This phenomenon is often seen in nursing where a highly effective and skilled staff nurse who functions as the unofficial unit leader is taken out of that role and promoted to an official management position.

Functions of the Nurse Manager

Nurse managers often find themselves located on the organizational chart between employees and upper-level management. The functions and duties of nurse manager roles depend to a great degree on how the institution defines the role. One of the first activities of a new nurse manager is to make sure he or she understands the job description, responsibilities, and levels of authority the position has in the institution where he or she is employed. Some of the tasks that have been identified as being a regular part of a nurse manager's position are listed in Box 12–4.

Box 12–4

Common Tasks for Nurse Managers

- Conduct orientation of new staff
- Evaluate staff
- Terminate employees with unsatisfactory work performance
- Develop time schedules that cover the unit safely
- Make team and staff assignments
- Develop a realistic budget for the unit
- Justify the number of nursing hours used by the unit
- Call in nurses on their days off when staffing falls short
- Attend nursing management meetings
- Hold regular meetings with unit staff to resolve problems, implement new policies and procedures
- Set unit goals for staff
- Contribute to facility goals
- Communicate regularly with physicians about unit problems
- Conduct quality assurance studies
- Provide rewards for high-quality care

In today's health-care system, nurse managers continue to follow the trend of moving away from the close supervision of the staff nurse's work to a role of helping them complete their work safely and effectively. As this role evolves in the future, the emphasis will shift from traditional management functions to highly supportive functions as are seen in the leadership role.

Conclusion

Over the years, there has been one constant in the changing health-care system, and that is that the RN is still expected to provide leadership and management skills to direct and ensure the high quality of the health care given to clients. Both leadership and management require sets of skills that can be learned. Nurses who learn these skills will become successful managers and the leaders of the health-care system in the future.

Successful leaders and managers know and often combine the best aspects of the many theories that deal with leadership and management. Knowledge of one's strengths and weakness provides the basis for successful management. Developing effective leadership and management skills is a lifelong, ongoing process. Learning from books and articles, as well as from other successful nurse managers, presents an opportunity for professional and personal growth.

ISSUES IN PRACTICE

Jill, an RN, was recently appointed as the evening charge nurse on a busy post-surgical unit. She has been an active participant in the hospital's quality assurance committee for the past 2 years since her graduation. One of the issues the committee identified as a problem was the higher than average surgical wound infection rate on Jill's unit. After some research, Jill identified that a major component of the high infection rate was the procedures that were used when changing postoperative dressings. After obtaining permission from the unit manager and hospital education director, Jill developed a new procedure for dressing changes incorporating the most current research. She presented the changes in a short in-service program to the unit personnel, several times to each of the three shifts to make sure that all the nurses and staff on the unit were familiar with the new changes. The expectation was that there would be a 25% reduction in wound infections after using the new procedures for 1 month.

At the end of the first month of using the new dressing change procedures, the postoperative wound infection rate showed no improvement over the previous month's rate. At the monthly staff meeting, Jill discovered that the licensed practical nurses (LPNs) on the unit were refusing to use the new procedures because they "took too much time" and had reverted back to the procedures they had always used before.

Critical Thinking Questions

1. What was the style of leadership and management that Jill used when attempting to initiate the dressing procedure change?
2. Other than the stated reason, why do you think the LPNs did not want to use the new procedures?
3. How can Jill increase the level of compliance by the LPNs on the unit?
4. What is the role of the unit manager in initiating the the new dressing change procedures?

References

1. Tappen, RM: Nursing Leadership and Management, ed. 4. FA Davis, Philadelphia, 2001.
2. Kerfoot, K: On leadership. From motivation to inspiration leadership. Pediatric Nursing 27(5):530–531, 2001.
3. Bissett, L: Perspectives in leadership. The manager's list. Nursing Spectrum 5(2):9, 2001.
4. Duffin, C: Training to plug gaps in management skills. Nursing Standard 16(4):8, 2001.

Bibliography

Bobulski, ED: Perspectives in leadership. A message for managers: Care, teach, connect. Nursing Spectrum 13A(3):NJ4, 2001.

Gray, W: Clinical governance: Combining clinical and management supervision. Nursing Management 8(6):14–17, 2001.

Manion, J: Managers forum. Cutting-edge discussions of management policy and program issues in emergency care. Journal of Emergency Nursing 27(5):498–499, 2001.

Nohre, A: Spotlight on. Soul + spirit + resources + leadership = results. J Nurs Adm 31(16):287–289, 2001.

Robotham, M: How to handle complaints. Nursing Times 97(30):25–28, 2001.

Tappen, RM, et al: Essentials of Nursing Leadership and Management, ed. 2. FA Davis, Philadelphia, 2001.

13

Communicating Successfully

Joseph T. Catalano

Learning Objectives

After completing this chapter, the reader will be able to:

- Explain the importance of understanding human behaviors.
- Describe conflict resolution and relationship tools.
- Identify communications styles.
- Analyze and apply problem-solving and conflict-resolution tools.
- Discuss the use of the nursing process in conflict resolution.
- Formulate coping strategies to handle difficult people.

Good communication skills are often advertised as the answer to many of the problems encountered in everyday life. Television personalities, instructors, and psychologists promote improved communication skills as the answer to parental, marital, financial, and work-related problems. The nursing profession recognizes communication as one of the cornerstones of its practice. Nurses must be able to communicate with clients, family members, physicians, peers, and associates in an effective and constructive manner to achieve their goals of high-quality care. Good communication is essential for good leadership and management.

In today's rapidly evolving health-care system, registered nurses (RNs) are called on to supervise a growing number of assistive and unlicensed personnel. One of the keys to good supervision is the ability to communicate to the individual what he or she must do to provide the required care and, often, how the care should be given. It is not always easy. Many of the people whom nurses supervise are poorly trained, lack the theoretical and technical knowledge base of the nurse, and may display attitudes that make them resistant to direction. However, nurse supervisors can be and often are held legally responsible for the actions of those individuals who work under their direction.

Factors that Affect Communication

Change

How people deal with change can affect how they respond to the environment and communicate with others. Change is one of the few absolute certainties in today's health-care system. Change can produce many emotions, ranging from excitement and anticipation to stress, fear, and anxiety. At minimum, change makes most people feel uncomfortable. Any change can be simultaneously positive and negative. During the process of learning new skills, treatments, or techniques, most people feel a sense of accomplishment at the same time as they feel afraid of making mistakes, being judged by others, or being labeled as "slow learners." An example is when a new graduate nurse starts his or her first day at work and is very excited about the new experience and the potential for career development. However, at the same time the nurse is worried about being accepted into the group, being able to practice what was learned in nursing school, and being able to learn the new skills required by the unit. Almost everyone has a sense of dread when moving away from activities with which they have become comfortable. Setting realistic personal goals and time lines for learning new information helps reduce the fear and stress when making major changes.

Change affects communication in various ways. People may be afraid to ask questions about new procedures or policies because they fear that they might appear "stupid" in front of their colleagues. Fear of being criticized closes individuals off to positive suggestions and new ideas. Others may hesitate in sharing ideas because they are afraid of being labeled as being confrontational. For example, a nurse is reassigned from the medical/surgical unit to the intensive care unit (ICU). This nurse will initially be somewhat fearful in the new environment with the highly trained and assertive expert unit nurses who always seem to be in control. A more positive approach would be for the new nurse to utilize the unit nurses' expertise and learn from their example. The new nurse needs to remember that everyone on that unit was a novice at one time. In the current health-care system, almost everyone is fearful much of the time of making mistakes and of falling short of the high standards of the profession.

People may be afraid to ask questions about new procedures or policies because they fear that they might appear "stupid" in front of their colleagues.

Change can have both positive and negative effects. Often a staff that is initially resistant to a change and fights to prevent it, once they have gone through the process, would never go back to the old way of doing things. All change involves some risk taking, and some people are better at risk taking than are others. Consider the following case study:

> After analysis of the needs of the clients and the nursing workload of a busy medical unit, the unit manager decided to change the work shift times. In addition to the standard 7 A.M. to 3 P.M., 3 P.M. to 11 P.M., and 11 P.M. to 7 A.M. shifts, she decided to add a 5 A.M. to 1 P.M. shift to increase coverage during the busiest period of the shift. The RN assigned to the new shift recognized the benefits to the unit and clients, thus she accepted and supported the change with few objections. Also, the change in shift times allowed her to alter her personal schedule so that she could take extra courses toward her master's degree at a local college. For the RN, the change in shifts was a positive experience.
>
> However, the licensed practical nurse (LPN) assigned to this new shift was upset with the change. She was a "late sleeper" and did not want to come in so early. She liked the

shifts the way that they were and did not see any advantages to changing things needlessly.

After the new shift was initiated, the LPN was usually 15 to 30 minutes late, called in sick frequently, and was "grumpy" and hard to talk to when she did come in to work. For this LPN, the change was negative and unacceptable.

Nurses need to keep in mind that the communication abilities of clients who are experiencing change will be affected in very much the same way as nurses who are experiencing change. As a result of disease, trauma, or surgery, many clients face sudden and major alterations in their bodies, as well as changes in their ability to function and carry out daily self-care activities. For example, a client with a new colostomy must adapt to major physiologic, psychological, and emotional changes. Most clients who have surgical procedures that result in major body function alterations go through the stages of the grief process: denial, anger, guilt, depression, and resolution. Communication with a client in the anger stage of the grief process, who is hostile, critical of his care, and verbally abusive, will be much different than communication with a client in the depression stage, who is withdrawn, reticent, and sleeps most of the time. Recognition of the communication behaviors of each of the grief stages is essential in understanding why clients are acting in a particular way. A decision must then be made regarding the most effective communication technique to use when providing care.

Stress

Stress is produced by many factors and always affects an individual's ability to communicate. Some common causes of stress for health-care workers include institutional restructuring, group interaction and dynamics, unilateral management decisions, or personal issues and experiences. Regardless of the source, stress usually decreases people's ability to interact and communicate and increases the demands on their coping mechanisms. When people are unable to cope with a stressful situation successfully, they may experience an increased state of tension or anxiety; they may develop physiologic symptoms such as nausea, stomach cramps, diarrhea, or palpitations; and, in extreme cases, they may even become paranoid or psychotic. Uncontrolled, high levels of stress on a nursing unit may lead to competition among the nurses that affects their teamwork, productivity, and the quality of the care given.

Physicians who are stressed by worry about a severely ill client or threats to their autonomy, practice, and income by changes in reimbursement policies may become tense and highly critical of or even verbally abusive toward nurses. The hospital management may also experience increased stress owing to the escalating responsibility of maintaining high-quality services with ever-shrinking revenues. Management often deals with its stress by becoming more autocratic, making increased demands on the nursing staff while reducing the control that nurses have over their practice, and becoming closed off to input from nurses and physicians. At some point, one group's stress always affects another group's stress level, whose stress in turn increases another group's stress. The process becomes a destructive circle of cause-and-effect responses that increases the stress levels for everyone in the facility.

Stress in the health-care environment is not just experienced by health-care providers. Stress for clients starts when they first come into contact with the health-care system, peaks when they have to undergo physical examinations, surgery, or invasive treatments, and continues throughout the recovery period. The fear that a nurse may not respond to clients' needs increases clients' stress levels, and they sometimes become more demanding of care, which, in turn, increases the nurse's stress levels. If the nursing

What Do You Think?

List four factors or situations that made you angry when in the hospital or health-care setting. Why did these make you angry? How did you deal with the anger?

staff is experiencing high stress levels, clients often sense this subconsciously, and as a result, clients' stress levels will increase also.

Several techniques can be used to reduce clients' stress levels so that they can better communicate and become more receptive to teaching. Stress reduction techniques range from very simple measures that everyone can use, such as distraction with music or simple activities, exercise, or reduction in stimuli, to more advanced techniques such as meditation, **biofeedback**, and even antianxiety medications.

Nurses need to be able to identify situations that produce stress, recognize the symptoms shown by someone in a stressful situation, know how to reduce stress, and be able to use appropriate communication techniques with someone under stress. Of course, if possible, the best way to reduce stress is to eliminate the stressful situation. For example, the hospital management has just sent a memo to all the hospital units that a new client assessment form they have developed is to be implemented next week. This new form is in addition to the ones that the nurses already fill out each day. The new form is to be completed by RNs only and must be done each shift on every client and then sent to the house supervisor so that management can track acuity. Because of recent facility restructuring and changes in staffing patterns, often there is only one RN on the 3 P.M. to 11 P.M. and 11 P.M. to 7 A.M. shifts to cover a 42-bed unit. This extra, time-consuming, and seemingly redundant paperwork increases the stress of the staff RNs to an unacceptable level. They meet as a group with management and propose that the assessment forms that they already are using be modified so that they include the data that management wants on the new forms. Photocopies of the revised "old" form could then be made by the unit clerk for each shift and given to the supervisors, thus eliminating the new form. Management notes the high stress levels of the RNs, recognizes that increased stress lowers the quality of care, and decides to follow the RNs' proposal, thus eliminating the primary source of the RNs' stress. Although all sources of stress cannot be eliminated completely, in most situations it can be reduced to a manageable level. However, high stress levels should never be used as an excuse for destructive anger and behaviors, failure of communication, or abuse of individuals.

Anger

In addition to being one of the stages of the grief process, anger can be a symptom of personal frustration, lack of control, fear of change, or feelings of hopelessness. Anger is one of the strong primitive natural emotions that helps individuals protect themselves against a variety of external threats. Although everyone experiences anger, how it is expressed often depends on a person's family and ethnic background, life experiences, and personal values. In some cultures, loud and physically expressive outbursts are the norm for the expression of anger, whereas in other cultures, anger is internalized and expressed only as a "controlled rage."

As with most of the other factors that affect communication, anger can be either positive or negative. When anger is used in a positive, productive manner, it can promote change and release tension. Anger can be used positively to increase others' attention, initiate communication, problem solve, and energize the change process. Sensitivity to internal anger can warn individuals that something is wrong either within themselves or with someone or something in the external environment.

Many individuals have difficulty expressing and using their anger in a positive manner. Anger that is used negatively is very destructive. It hinders communication, makes coworkers fearful, and erodes relationships with others. Anger expressed by abusive behaviors such as pounding on nursing station counters, throwing charts or surgical instruments, verbal outbursts, or even in violent physical contact is never acceptable and may lead to civil or criminal actions against the perpetrator. The negative expression of anger may cause the person who is the object of the anger to retaliate or seek revenge. But probably the most destructive form that negative anger can take is when it is internalized and suppressed. Long-term, suppressed anger has been associated with a number of physiologic and psychological problems ranging from gastric ulcers and hypertension to myocardial infarctions, strokes, and even psychotic rage episodes.

Nurses who understand what makes both themselves and others angry are better able to either avoid anger-producing situations or cope effectively with their own anger or with that of others. For example, even new graduate nurses soon learn that there are some situations that will almost always evoke an angry response from hospitalized clients. These include serving meals that are cold or poorly cooked, not answering call lights in a timely manner, waking up soundly sleeping clients at midnight to give them a sleeping pill, or taking 10 attempts to start an intravenous (IV) line. Similarly, unit managers and hospital administrators quickly learn that some of the things that they do will almost always produce angry responses from the staff. These actions include unilateral changes in the work schedule, additional paperwork, reduction in staffing levels, or refusal for requests for vacation or time off.

Even new graduate nurses soon learn that there are some situations that will almost always evoke an angry response from hospitalized clients.

It is important that nurses understand that anger is a normal human emotion. Once it is recognized, it should be dealt with and then let go. There are times when situations are not going to change, no matter how angry the person becomes, and other times when no amount of anger will prevent changes from occurring.

Group Dynamics

The power of the group over an individual's behavior should never be underestimated. Groups establish and exert their power through a set of unique behaviors or norms that their members are expected to follow. These norms may be formal or informal, written or unwritten, promulgated or merely understood. Unfortunately, in most nursing units the norms are often not clearly expressed, yet they may be used as judgment tools or standards for evaluating work behaviors. When new nurses begin work on a particular unit, in order to function effectively they must quickly learn the unwritten unit norms and identify the informal leaders.

As with most elements in communication, group dynamics may be positive or negative. Nurses who do not learn and fail to display the expected group behaviors may be ostracized from the group, thus making the work environment psychologically uncomfortable and perhaps even physically difficult. For example, nonconforming nurses may find that there is no one around when they need help ambulating an unsteady client. Or a particular nursing unit staff may have a strong team approach. If the new nurse is highly independent and prefers to work alone, he or she may not "fit in" and experience hostility or sarcasm from the other nurses on the unit.

Consider the following scenario demonstrating group dynamics:

> The ICU has the responsibility for on-call coverage for the recovery room for unscheduled postoperative clients on the evening shifts, night shifts, and all of the weekend shifts. There is no formal written policy, but coverage has traditionally been handled on a voluntary, rotating basis. Because it is "voluntary," one of the ICU nurses has decided that he does not want to take call any more. He is the only member of the ICU staff who does not take call. Soon after he announces his decision, he begins to sense anger and experi-

ence alienation from his peers. Although he is very knowledgeable, has highly developed nursing skills, and provides consistently high-quality care to assigned clients on his regular shifts, on his semiannual peer evaluation, he receives low ratings from his coworkers based on the informal call coverage standard and expectations. The unit nurses feel that he is no longer a team player.

The nurse becomes angry because he feels that the use of unclear, unwritten standards is an unfair way to evaluate his ability as a nurse. He soon finds that the other ICU nurses accidentally "forget" to invite him to group functions. He also seems to be assigned the most difficult and largest number of clients during any given shift, seemingly to compensate for not taking call.

Group dynamics involves many factors, including methods of communications, professional behaviors, professional growth, flexibility, problem solving, participation, and competition. The ability to understand and use the elements of group dynamics has a direct relationship on the behaviors, cooperation, and effectiveness of the team. Often, when a team labels an individual member as "difficult," it most likely means that the individual is not following one or more of the informal, unwritten group norms.

Competition

Competition can be a very powerful element in group dynamics and communication. Depending on how it is channeled, expressed, and used, competition can be a positive or negative force within the group. The various forms of competition can be individual, team, or unit focused. A common expression of competition in the group setting is peer evaluations. For peer evaluations to be a positive form of competition, the unit must decide ahead of time on the norms and expectations that they value and then design an objective measurement tool to evaluate whether the individual is meeting the norms. Also, each individual being evaluated must be aware of the criteria before the evaluation is conducted. The evaluation team must be educated on evaluation techniques and must be as objective and professional as possible.

The power of the group over an individual's behavior should never be underestimated.

In the health-care setting, it is important for all professionals, unit groups, and management to promote competition in a positive, progressive, and supportive environment. When competition is channeled positively, it leads to new and creative ideas, better programs, increased growth, more productive interactions, and higher quality client care. When the competition is negative, it often produces failures, depression, sabotage, unit turf conflicts, decreased productivity, and lower quality care. For example, the competition on a nursing unit turned negative when the nurses on the 7 A.M. to 3 P.M. shift began competing with the nurses on the 3 P.M. to 11 P.M. shift in order to appear more knowledgeable about client care to the nurse manager. In order to "look better," the nurses on the 7 A.M. to 3 P.M. shift intentionally withheld selected client laboratory test results during shift report. As a result of this action, several tests scheduled for the 3 P.M. to 11 P.M. shift were not done, angering the physicians, potentially threatening the safety of the clients, and making the nurses on the 3 P.M. to 11 P.M. shift appear incompetent. In addition, the nurses on that shift had to complete several incident reports on the errors that occurred on their shift. One informal component of the staff nurses' performance evaluations used by the unit manager is the number of incident reports that a nurse must file. The more incident reports, the poorer will be the nurse's performance evaluation. To the unit manager, the nurses on the 7 A.M. to 3 P.M. shift appear to be more competent because of the seemingly poor care, indicated by a large number of incident reports, that is being given on the

3 P.M. to 11 P.M. shift. However, when the nurses on the 3 P.M. to 11 P.M. shift discovered what really happened, they devised several ways to "get even" with the nurses on the 7 A.M. to 3 P.M. shift.

What Do You Think?

Have you ever been in a situation where others have intentionally sabotaged your work? What was the situation? How did you feel? How did you deal with it? Did you try to retaliate?

Working Environment

The delivery of health care is currently in a rapid transition from a fee-for-service to a managed care environment. Health care is shifting from acute, inpatient care to long-term outpatient care and from being illness based to a prevention and wellness focus. The changes produced by this transition are creating a high degree of stress at all levels of the health-care system. As discussed earlier, both change and stress are major barriers to effective communication.

One measure that can be taken to both alleviate some of the stress caused by the current changes in health care and improve unit communication is to encourage all members of the health-care team to participate in the renovation of their work environment. Through active participation, workers have an opportunity to have an impact on and direct the changes that are being made. Some people mistakenly believe that if they do not become involved, the changes will not happen. Unfortunately, when people are not actively involved in the restructuring process, others who are probably less qualified will make the changes anyway.

Increased fear, high stress levels, angry outbursts, and feelings of insecurity all are potential results of a work environment where the workers do not participate in the change process. Difficult behaviors resulting in unclear communication become more evident during times of change and stress. Ugly rumors, feelings of resentment, and increased insecurity often result when intergroup communications are not clear. An open, interactive work environment increases the probability of successful communication and adaptation to change.

Understanding what motivates a person's behavior permits the individual to design a plan or develop coping mechanisms for communicating based on sound interpersonal techniques. When individuals are able to separate themselves from the difficult situation, they are less likely to take things personally and more likely to begin to focus on the underlying issues causing the problems rather than the other person's difficult behavior. The interaction becomes less judgmental and threatening to the other person. However, understanding the other person's motives never excuses unacceptable behaviors such as sarcasm, angry outbursts, and abusive language. Rather, it allows for direct confrontation of the behavior in a more controlled and less emotional way.

All professional nurses need to develop coping mechanisms in order to deal with the behaviors demonstrated by difficult people. The very nature of the profession exposes nurses to a large number of people who are experiencing change, are under stress, and have a wide range of backgrounds and values as well as varying expectations. By understanding communication, using **behavior modification**, developing **assertiveness**, avoiding submissive and aggressive behaviors, and appreciating diversity, the nurse can develop the coping skills required for problem solving, handling conflict in the work setting, and confronting the unacceptable behaviors of difficult people.

Understanding Communication

Communication is an interactive sharing of information. It requires a sender, a message, and a receiver. After the sender sends the message, the receiver has a responsibility to listen to, process, and understand (encode) the information and then to respond to the sender by giving feedback (decoding). The encoding process occurs when the receiver thinks about the information, understands it, and forms an idea based on the message.

Several factors can interfere with the encoding process. On the sender's side, these can be factors such as unclear speech, monotone voice, poor sentence structure, inappropriate use of terminology or jargon, or lack of knowledge about the topic. On the receiver's side, factors that may interfere with encoding include lack of attention, prejudice and bias, preoccupation with another problem, or even physical factors such as pain, drowsiness, or impairment of the senses. For example, a staff nurse is in a mandatory meeting where the unit manager is discussing a new policy that will be starting the next month. However, the nurse is thinking about an important heart medication that her client is to receive in 5 minutes. The nurse's primary concern is to get out of the meeting in time to give the medication. After the meeting, the nurse has only a minimal recollection of what was said because she did not encode the information well. The following month when the new policy is started, the staff nurse is confused about what she should do and makes several errors in relationship to the new policy.

There are two primary methods of communication—verbal and nonverbal. **Verbal** communication is either the written or spoken word and constitutes only about 7 percent of the communicated message. **Nonverbal** communication, which makes up the other 93 percent of communication, is everything else, including body language, facial expressions, gestures, physical appearance, touch, vocal cues (tone, pauses), and spatial territory (personal space). When the verbal and nonverbal messages are congruent, then the message is more easily encoded and clearly understood. If the verbal and nonverbal messages are conflicting, the nonverbal message is probably the most reliable. It is relatively easy for people to lie with words, but nonverbal communication tends to be unconscious and more difficult to control. For example, the nurse suspects that the mother of a newborn infant may be experiencing postpartum depression. The nurse asks the mother how she feels about her new baby. The mother responds in a low volume, very slow-paced monotone voice: "I'm so happy I have this baby," while looking down at her feet in a slouched-over posture. The message from the mother is conflicting. The words are saying she is happy, but all the nonverbal signs indicate that she is depressed. The nurse concludes that more assessment for depression is required.

Effective communication requires understanding that the perceptions, emotions, and participation of both parties are interactive and have an effect on the transmission of the message. Nurses often encounter situations that require clarification of the information for accuracy and encoding. The following is an example of client teaching requiring a return demonstration:

> A nurse gives a teaching session to a client who is being sent home with a T-tube after surgical removal of gallstones from the common bile duct. After the nurse finished, she asked the client whether he understood how to empty the drainage bottle and measure the drainage. The client looked very confused, but mumbled "yes," while shaking his head back and forth. The nurse recognized that although the verbal response was positive, the nonverbal responses indicated that he really did not understand. The nurse surmised that further explanation or demonstration was required for proper encoding of the message by this client.

Nurses should recognize the many barriers to clear communication as well as the benefits of clear communication. Once the barriers to communication are identified, they can be overcome and the benefits of clear communication will result. These barriers and benefits that result when they are overcome are outlined in Box 13–1.

Communication Styles

There are two predominant styles of communication—assertive and nonassertive. Nonassertive communication can be either submissive or

Box 13–1

Barriers to Clear Communication	Benefits of Clear Communication
Unclear/unexpressed	Clear expectations
Confusion	Understanding
Retaliation	Forgiveness
Desire for power	Recognized leadership
Control of others	Companionship
Negative reputation	Respect
Manipulation	Independence
Low self-esteem	Realistic self-image
Biased perceptions	Acceptance
Inattention	Clear direction
Mistrust	Trusting relations
Anger	Self-control
Fear/anxiety	Comfort
Stress	Motivation/energy
Insecurity	Security
Prejudice	Increased tolerance
Interruptions	Increased knowledge
Preoccupation	Concentration

aggressive. Individuals develop their communication styles over the course of their lives in response to many personal factors. Although most people have one predominant style of communication, they can and often do switch or combine styles depending on the situation in which they find themselves. For example, a unit manager who uses an assertive communication style when supervising the staff on her unit may revert to a submissive style when called into the director of nursing's office for her annual evaluation. Recognizing which communication style a person is using at any given time, as well as a person's own style, is important in making communication clear and effective.

Assertive Communication Style

Assertive communication involves interpersonal behaviors that permit people to defend and maintain their legitimate rights in a respectful manner that does not violate the rights of others. Assertive communication is honest and direct and accurately expresses the person's feelings, beliefs, ideas, and opinions. Respect for self and others constitutes both the basis for and the result of assertive communication. It encourages trust and teamwork by communicating to others that they have the right to and are encouraged to express their opinions in an open and respectful atmosphere. Disagreement and discussion are considered to be a healthy part of the communication process, and negotiation is the positive mechanism for problem solving, learning, and personal growth.

Assertive communication always implies that the individual has the choice to voice an opinion, sometimes forcefully, as well as not to say

What Do You Think?

Consider the health-care providers whom you have worked with in the recent past. What were their communication styles? How did it affect the way you communicated with them?

anything at all. One of the keys to assertive communication is that the individual is in control of the communication and is not merely reacting to another's emotions.

Assessing Self-Assertiveness

Answer the following questions to assess your self-assertiveness:

- Who am I and what do I want?
- Do I believe I have the right to want it?
- How do I get it?
- Do I believe I can get it?
- Have I tried to be assertive with a person I am having difficulty communicating with?
- Am I letting my fears and perceptions cloud my interactions?
- What is the worst that can happen if we communicate?
- Can I live with the "worst"?
- Will communications have a long-term effect?
- How does it feel to be in constant fear of alienation or rejection?

Rules for Assertiveness

Anyone can learn to use an assertive communication style and develop assertiveness. When first developing this skill, people often feel frightened and overwhelmed. However, once individuals become comfortable with assertiveness, it helps reinforce their self-concepts and becomes an effective tool for communication. There are a few rules to keep in mind while developing an assertive communication style and assertiveness:

- It is a learned skill.
- It takes practice.
- It requires a desire and motivation to change.
- It requires a willingness to take risks.
- It requires a willingness to make mistakes and try again.
- It requires an understanding that not every outcome sought will be obtained.
- It requires strong self-esteem.
- Self-reward for change and positive outcomes is essential.
- Listening to self is necessary for identifying needs.
- Constant re-examination of outcomes helps assess progress.
- Role-playing with a friend prior to the interaction builds skill and confidence.
- Goals for assertiveness growth need to be established beforehand.
- It requires recognition that change is a gradual process.
- Others should be allowed to make mistakes.

Personal Risks of Assertive Communication

There are always personal risks involved in learning any new skills or in attempting to change behavior. Learning assertive communication is no exception. People often fear that they may not choose the "perfect" assertive response. However, even seasoned assertive communicators may err from time to time, because every encounter is unique, involving different people and situations. The person who is new to assertive communication needs to recognize that it is a skill that takes practice.

Assertiveness does not mean that a person will always get his or her way in every situation, and it is likely the individual will handle some situations better than others. Remember that the goal of assertive communication is not to have an "I win, you lose" situation, but rather an "I win, you win" outcome. A "win-win" goal is achieved when both parties have the ability and willingness to negotiate even though they do not get all that they want. However, there may be situations when personal goals are not achieved. Some questions to consider when this occurs are:

- How do I feel about losing?
- Did I express my opinion clearly? Why not? How could I make it more clear?

- Did I do the best I could do? How could I have done better?
- Was I in control when responding to the situation? When did I lose control? What should I have done to regain control?
- Did I stay focused on the issues? What side issues distracted me? How could I have avoided distractions?
- Did I allow the situation to get personal? Did the other person initiate the personal attack? How could I have redirected it away from the personal?
- Was what I asked for under my control? If not, why did I ask for it? What would have been more realistic?

Reviewing these questions and analyzing the answers will help when attempting to be assertive in future communications. For example, if the answer to the last question was yes, then during the next communication, a special effort can be focused on avoiding personal attacks during the encounter. Learning to communicate assertively is a process of continual improvement.

Another risk factor that quickly becomes evident when changing to an assertive communication style is the impact that it has on those who know the person best. Sometimes family, friends, peers, and coworkers become barriers to change. As mentioned earlier, change always produces some degree of stress. Those individuals who are closest to the person trying to initiate changes may feel uncomfortable because they have become accustomed to the old communication styles and behaviors over a long time. They can no longer anticipate and depend on the person responding and reacting in the usual way. In addition, they will have to develop new communication patterns of their own to match the changes caused by assertive communication. Sometimes family, friends, peers, and coworkers become so uncomfortable that they may try to sabotage the person's attempts at assertive communication. It is important to recognize why and when these sabotage efforts occur and also to remember that assertiveness is an internal, personal process. Everyone has a right to change, and it must be respectfully communicated to others that their support for these changes is important.

It is also important to know and periodically review the rights and responsibilities of assertiveness to help reinforce the assertive communication process. The rights and responsibilities of assertiveness are listed in Box 13–2.

Practice and reinforcement of assertiveness skills may be required, especially when preparing

Box 13–2

Rights and Responsibilities of Assertiveness

- To act in a way that promotes your dignity and self-respect
- To be treated with respect
- To experience and express your thoughts and feelings
- To slow down and make conscious decisions before you act
- To ask for what you want
- To say "No"
- To change your mind
- To make mistakes
- Not to be perfect
- To feel important and good about yourself
- To be treated as an individual with special values, skills, and needs
- The right to be unique
- To have your own feelings and opinions
- To say "I don't know"
- To feel angry, hurt, frustrated
- To make decisions regarding your life
- To recognize that your needs are as important as others

for an anticipated conflict negotiation or a confrontational meeting with another. Although a confrontational situation always produces anxiety, rather than being feared, it should be recognized as having the potential to be highly productive. Box 13–3 lists several behaviors that, if practiced and used, will help increase confidence and assertiveness skills during anticipated confrontational meetings.

Nonassertive Behavior/Communication

There are two types of interpersonal behaviors that are considered to be nonassertive. These are submissive and aggressive behaviors.

Submissive Behavior/ Communication

When people display submissive behavior, they allow their rights to be violated by others. When people use submissive behavior and submissive communication, they surrender to the requests and demands of others without regard to their own feelings and needs. Many experts believe that submissive behavior and communication patterns are a protective mechanism that helps insecure persons maintain their self-esteem by avoiding negative criticism and disagreement of others. In other situations, it may be a means of manipulation and the basis for passive-aggressive behavior.

Because of their great fear of displeasing

Box 13–3

Conflict Resolution Tips

In nursing practice, good communication and conflict management skills are essential. The following tips may help resolve communication problems:

Improve Your Conflict Management Skills

- Seminars
- Books
- Mentors

Change Your Paradigm

- Focus on the positive not the negative.
- Realize that appropriately confronting is a risk-taking activity for:

  Better communication
  Improved relationships
  Improved teamwork
  Mentoring

Understand Your Values

- Focus on a win-win.
- Be willing to negotiate/compromise.
- Be direct and honest.
- Focus on the issues.
- Do not attack the person.
- Do not make judgments.
- Do not become the third person; encourage peers to go direct.
- Do not spread rumors.

Set Personal Guidelines

- Confront in private, never in front of anyone else.
- Confront the individual, do not report him or her to the supervisor first.
- Do not confront when you are angry.
- Start with an "I" message.
- Express how you feel and your opinions.
- Allow the other person to talk without interruptions.
- Listen attentively.
- Set goals and future plans of action.
- Let it go!
- Keep it private and confidential.

others, personal rejection, or future retaliation, submissive communicators dismiss their own feelings as being unimportant. However, at a deeper level, submissive behavior and communication merely reinforce negative feelings of powerlessness, helplessness, and decreased self-worth. Rather than being in control of the communication or relationship, the person is trading his or her ability to choose what is best for the avoidance of conflict. Every communication by a submissive person becomes an "I lose, you win" situation.

Aggressive Behavior/ Communication

Sometimes there is only a very fine line separating assertiveness from aggressive behavior and communication. Whereas assertive communication permits individuals to honestly express their ideas and opinions while respecting the rights, ideas, and opinions of others, aggressive communication strongly asserts the person's legitimate rights and opinions with little regard or respect for the rights and opinions of others. Aggressive communication can be used to humiliate, dominate, control, or embarrass the other person or lower the other person's self-esteem and creates an "I win, you lose" situation. The other person may perceive aggressive behavior or communication as a personal attack. Aggressive behavior and communication is viewed by some psychologists as a protective mechanism that compensates for a person's own insecurities. By demeaning another person, aggressive behavior allows the person to feel superior and helps inflate his or her own self-esteem.

Aggressive communications can take several different forms, including screaming, sarcasm, rudeness, belittling jokes, and even direct personal insults. It is an expression of the negative feelings of power, domination, and low self-esteem. Although outwardly aggressive persons may seem to be in control, in reality they are merely reacting to the situation to protect their self-esteem.

Diversity

Diversity is a multifaceted issue that involves many areas of people's lives, including culture, values, life experiences, instinctual responses, learned behaviors, personal strengths and weaknesses, and native abilities or skills. Each time two people interact, they bring the sum total of all these elements into their communication. In order to communicate effectively, both parties need to first recognize that the other person is different, then understand how these differences affect the communication, and finally accept and build on these differences. Rather than being divisive, diversity, when recognized and used correctly, can promote teamwork, improve communication, and increase productivity. Recognizing diversity helps people better understand each other as well as themselves. The ultimate goal of diversity recognition is to use each individual's strengths, rather than emphasizing the weaknesses, to build a stronger, more self-confident, and productive environment. For example, consider the following scenario:

> Anne B., RN, is a nurse in your unit who has a reputation as being a "nitpicker." She is constantly judging her peers and criticizing their actions based on her own personal standards. Her judgments of others are not well accepted by her coworkers, who try to avoid her as much as possible.
>
> Betty A., RN, another nurse on the unit, always seems to be coming up with ideas to change things in the unit, but then avoids joining the committees that are formed to put the ideas into practice. When she does join a committee, she quickly gets bored and does not follow through on her responsibilities. The other committee members become angry and frustrated by Betty's behavior. They feel that because it was her idea in the first place, she should work as hard as everyone else to make the change.
>
> You have been selected as the chairperson for a committee that has been formed to design a new client care documentation tool.

Box 13–4

Assertiveness Self-Assessment Evaluation

Statement	Communication Behavior
1. I didn't say what I really wanted to say at the last staff meeting.	______________
2. I always express my opinion because it is better than everyone else's.	______________
3. I have the courage to speak up almost all the time.	______________
4. I wish someone else would speak up at the meetings besides me.	______________
5. I am not intimidated by the high-pressure tactics of supervisors, physicians, and/or teachers.	______________
6. I have trouble stating my true feelings to those in authority.	______________
7. I really put that know-it-all aide in her place last shift.	______________
8. After the last meeting with my unit director I felt hopeless, resentful, and angry.	______________
9. I speak up in meetings without feeling defensive.	______________
10. When I need to confront someone, I avoid the problem because it will usually resolve itself.	______________
11. When I need to confront someone, I address them directly.	______________
12. When I confront someone, I let them know in no uncertain terms that they are wrong and need to change their behavior.	______________
13. When I'm reprimanded, I keep silent even though I'm seething inside.	______________
14. The last time I was asked to stay over for another shift, I said "no" and didn't feel guilty.	______________

Both Anne and Betty are on the committee. The other committee members are upset because Anne and Betty are on the committee. Everyone knows about Anne's and Betty's personality quirks. As chairperson of the team, you need to utilize everyone's strengths while recognizing his or her diversities in order to develop a new, comprehensive yet easy-to-use form. If you perform well in your chairmanship role, each team member's self-esteem should be enhanced, and the morale of the group should improve.

At first glance, these may not seem like diversity issues. However, Anne is a detail-oriented person, whereas Betty is a visionary. Although their interests and abilities are very diverse, neither one is right or wrong. Persons who are preoccupied with details are left-brain dominant; creative, visionary individuals are usually right-brain dominant.

Two primary tasks are required to complete the project:

Task 1. Brainstorming sessions must be conducted with staff members, physicians, and ancillary personnel to develop a general concept of what the documentation should include and how the form should look.

Task 2. Work with the printshop to design the specific layout and content of the final form.

Plan. *Task 1:* It would be most appropriate to include Betty in the group that directs the brainstorming groups and collects different ideas. She probably has no preconceived form in mind before starting the process and will feel comfortable investigating and researching a variety of different possibilities. Anne would have difficulty with this task. The lack of structure of the brainstorming process would make her feel out of control and would probably frustrate her urge to consider all the details of the project. Anne would most likely already have a good idea of the form she wanted. *Task 2:* Anne would be much better at this task because of her orientation to structure and detail. Working with the printshop, she could focus her attention on each item on the form, decide where it should be placed, how much room it should be given, and how it flows in the document. She would make sure that the form met all the standards and regulatory requirements of the Joint Commission as well as ensuring that it was error free. Betty, on the other hand, would very quickly become bored with this aspect of the project. To her, all the attention given to the details would seem like a waste of time, and she would probably start recommending changes in other unit forms.

Results of Committee Work. Placing the right person in the right working environment that corresponds with his or her strengths ensures success for the project. The project will be a successful experience for the nurses and will promote positive changes in peer relationships.

For many people, working with diversity can be difficult, especially when individuals feel insecure about their skills or abilities. When people feel insecure, they may revert to submissive or aggressive behavior or communication styles to hide their weaknesses or differences. Because assertive persons recognize that everyone, including themselves, have both strengths and weaknesses, they feel comfortable with diversity and are more likely to accept and support others by recognizing and using their strengths. Focusing on the strengths of people provides them with positive feedback and helps them grow personally and professionally. Focusing on weaknesses and differences tears down an individual's self-esteem, creates an uncomfortable work atmosphere, and makes people defensive and sometimes hostile.

Problem Solving

Problem solving is a process that everyone uses all the time. For example, on the way to work, a tire goes flat on a person's car. That is a problem. How the person solves the problem depends partially on critical thinking skills, partially on past experiences, and partially on physical abilities. If the person with the flat tire is a 250-lb 33-year-old male construction worker in good health, he most likely has changed tires before and will probably be physically able to remove the flat tire and put on the spare without difficulty. However, if the person with the flat tire is a 90-lb, 67-year-old female church organist who is unable to distinguish a lug nut from a tire valve, her solution to the problem will likely be different. She will probably call the automobile association and have someone come and change the flat for her.

One of the primary activities for nurses in the work setting is problem solving using the nursing process. It really does not matter whether the problem is client centered, management oriented, or an interpersonal issue, the nursing process is an excellent framework for problem resolution. It focuses on the goals of mutual interaction and communication to establish trust and respect. Using the process of assessment, analysis, planning, implementation, and evaluation helps the nurse organize and structure interpersonal interactions in a way that will produce an "I win, you win" situation.

The basic problem-solving steps of the nursing process form the framework for successful conflict management. Many people experience less anxiety when practicing personal problem solving than when they are involved in conflict management. Problem solving is often perceived as less emotional and more structured, whereas conflict management is considered to be more emotionally charged with the potential to produce hostility. However, the steps of conflict management are almost identical to those of the nursing process. The one additional element that must be included in conflict resolution is the ability to use assertive behaviors and communication when discussing the issues. Nurses who are good problem solvers using the nursing process also tend to be good at conflict resolution, and nurses who are good at conflict resolution tend to be excellent problem solvers. Rather than avoiding conflict in the work setting, it should be considered as an opportunity to practice and grow in the use of problem-solving skills.

Conflict Management

Everyone experiences conflict at one time or another as a part of daily life. Often people feel more comfortable addressing the conflict that arises in their personal lives rather than the professional conflicts that arise from the job setting. A common situation that causes conflict is when nurses feel overworked or overwhelmed by their assignments. The overloaded nurse might say something like "I have such a heavy load today, why isn't anyone helping me?" rather than asking a particular individual for help. When the person who is expected to help fails to comply with the implied request for help, the overworked nurse becomes angry and resentful. The other person may not understand where this anger is coming from and often avoids addressing the angry person for fear of making him or her angrier. This type of poor communication and lack of direct, respectful conflict management produces tension among workers, deterioration of working relationships, decreased efficiency, and, ultimately, poor client care.

There are many reasons why individuals are uncomfortable handling or addressing conflict, including:

- Fear of retaliation
- Fear of ridicule
- Fear of alienation of others
- Mistaken belief that they are unable to handle the conflict situation
- Feeling like they do not have the right to speak up
- Past negative experiences with conflict situations
- Family background and experiences
- Lack of education and skills on conflict resolution

There are several different strategies that can be used to resolve workplace conflicts. Depending on a person's communication style and personality traits, different outcomes may occur:

Strategy 1: Ignore the Conflict

- Submissive personality: Person avoids bringing the issue to the other because he or she is afraid of retaliation or ridicule from others if he or she confronts and expresses honest feelings or opinions.
- Aggressive personality: Person has decided not to pursue the conflict because the other person is "too stupid to understand" or it would just be a "waste of their time."

Strategy 2: Confront the Conflict

- Submissive personality: Person does not handle the situation directly but refers the problem to a supervisor or to another person for resolution.
- Assertive personality: Person sets up a time and place for a one-on-one meeting. At the meeting, the two parties focus on the issues that caused the conflict and negotiate to define goals and problem solve.
- Aggressive personality: Person confronts the other loudly, in front of an audience, and attacks the other's personality rather than the issue. Person either walks away before the other can speak or keeps talking without stopping and does not allow the other person to respond. The communication is strictly one-sided and very negative.

Strategy 3: Postpone the Conflict

- Submissive person: Person keeps "count" of the issues until they reach a critical point, then dumps all the issues at one time on the offender in a highly aggressive manner. The other person generally has no idea why he or she is being attacked and may respond with anger or submission.
- Aggressive personality: Person waits until he or she can either use the incident as a threat or blackmail or until the conflict can be expressed in front of an audience.

Professional nurses need to be assertive and feel comfortable when handling conflict situations and confronting others. The conflict situations that nurses may encounter range from uncooperative clients and lazy coworkers to hostile, insecure, but influential physicians. Practicing assertiveness skills during confrontational situations helps increase the nurse's confidence in handling daily work-related conflicts and allows the honest but respectful expression of opinion and ideas. Keep in mind that unresolved conflicts never really go away. Ignoring a conflict situation may postpone it, sometimes for a long time, but it will not resolve the issue. Unresolved conflicts often fester until they either reach the boiling point or are manifested in negative behaviors or feelings. Some of the feelings and behaviors that are symptoms of unresolved conflicts include:

- Tension and anxiety manifested as sudden angry outbursts
- Generalized distrust among the staff members
- Gossiping and rumor spreading
- Intentional work sabotage
- Backstabbing and lack of cooperation
- Isolation of certain staff members
- Division and polarization of the staff
- Low-rated peer evaluation reports

Often, when conflict is handled appropriately, it produces much less anxiety than was initially anticipated. An individual who prepares for a confrontational meeting by expecting the worst-case scenario may be pleasantly surprised when the actual meeting and discussion take place. Many conflicts turn out to be merely errors in perception, simple misunderstandings, or misquotes of something that was said. If a situation is cleared up at an early stage, this prevents the development of the symptoms of unresolved conflict (listed earlier) and improves staff relationships. Individuals feel more confident and have better self-esteem when they resolve the conflicts in an adult and productive manner.

Another advantage of good conflict management is the improvement in communication skills. As with any skills, the more these skills are practiced, the easier they will become to use. Some tips for conflict resolution are listed in the Issues in Practice box at the end of the chapter.

Difficult People

All nurses recognize that obtaining a thorough history and understanding the underlying disease processes better prepare them for the care of their clients. Similarly, when working with difficult people, a knowledge of their backgrounds and understanding of the underlying personality traits better prepare the individual to deal with the important issues. It would seem that nurses should be better at handling conflict and difficult people, because an understanding of cause and effect and the intricacies of human nature are skills that are used daily in the care of clients. Shifting the communication paradigm from one of instinctual response to one that uses the nurse's relationship skills should make dealing with difficult people a much less difficult task. Remember that the behavior displayed by a difficult person is really a symptom of a deeper problem, just as an assessment of shortness of breath is a symptom of a respiratory disease. Identification of the cause of the problem permits the nurse to treat the disease rather than just the symptoms. The problem will not be cured by merely ignoring it or dealing only with the symptoms. In the long term, it usually only makes things worse.

Box 13–5

Assertive Communications Suggestions

- Maintain eye contact.
- Convey empathy; stating your feelings does not mean sympathy or agreement.
- Keep your body position erect, shoulders and back straight.
- Speak clearly and audibly; be direct and descriptive.
- Be comfortable with silence.
- Use gestures and facial expressions for emphasis.
- Use appropriate location.
- Use appropriate timing.
- Focus on behaviors/issues; do not attack the person.

Identifying Difficult People

Most of the time, it is rather easy to identify when a person is being "difficult." However, there are some behaviors of difficult people that may not be evident at first glance. Each type of difficult person requires a different strategy for dealing with his or her behaviors.

There are four basic behavioral pattern types of communication: (1) in control and responsive pattern, (2) in control but unresponsive pattern, (3) uncontrolled and responsive pattern, (4) and the uncontrolled and unresponsive pattern of communication.

Anyone who has been employed in or even associated with the health-care setting for any length of time soon becomes aware of a variety of different personality types among the staff members. These personality types can be identified by their predominant behaviors and also require different strategies for communication. Keep in mind that these are stereotypes that tend to batch individuals into groups based on predetermined characteristics. In reality, people may have an overlapping or combination of characteristics that may require combining the listed strategies for communication (Box 13–5).

The various types of characterizations, behavioral patterns, and stereotypes all are interrelated and based on individual communication styles. An increased awareness of the various identifying characteristics and strategies for communication will help develop the coping skills and communication techniques necessary for communicating with difficult people.

Development of Coping Skills

Just as developing communication skills requires a willingness to change and a lot of practice, so does the development of coping skills. Coping skills can be used to resolve crisis situations, deal with anxiety, and resolve difficult issues of communication. Everyone has at least a fundamental set of coping skills that they have developed during their lives, and these can be used as the foundation for adding to or building new coping skills for future problems. Presented here are some strategies that will help in the development of coping skills to use in communicating with difficult people.

First, separate the person from the problem by focusing on the issues without personally attacking the person. Having the facts about the situation makes people much more receptive to resolution of the problem than attacking their personality. When situations are made into personal attacks, it makes people feel defensive, responsible, or persecuted and either blocks or closes off the communication.

One way to avoid making a conversation into a personal attack is to use "I" rather than "you" messages. Avoid starting a conversation by saying, "You made a mistake," or "You said this about me," or especially "You always do this." People are less likely to perceive a communication as a personal attack when the conversation begins by explaining a personal view of the situation or even how feelings were affected. Statements such as "I thought it was done this way," or "I heard something the other day," or even "I feel hurt when people judge me" are a more productive way to begin an exchange of ideas and information. For example:

> During shift report on a particular client, the 11 P.M. to 7 A.M. nurse forgot to tell the 7 A.M. to 3 P.M. charge nurse, Gail L., RN, that the client had fallen out of bed during the night shift. Later in the day, both the client's physician and family confronted Gail to find out what happened and why the client was not placed on "fall protocols." Later, when Gail confronts the night nurse about the omission, she has two options for initiating the discussion of the incident with the responsible night nurse. Which approach would the night nurse probably take as a personal attack?

Option 1: Gail: "I was taken off guard and unprepared when the family and physician asked me about this client's fall, and I felt unprepared to explain the problem or a solution to them. My lack of knowledge about the fall really made me feel incompetent."

Option 2: Gail: "You failed to tell me about his fall last night. Because of you, I was not aware of the incident and was not prepared to answer questions. You always make me look like a fool!"

Another way to avoid making issues into personal attacks is to avoid focusing on what a person "should" have done based on a personal standard. This type of statement becomes an arbitrary judgment call. Instead, ask the person for his or her ideas on how the situation could have been handled differently or what other options were available. One should especially avoid becoming personally or verbally abusive.

A second important strategy for developing communication-related coping skills is to be willing to actively listen to and respect the other person's perspectives, ideas, or opinions. Active listening can help minimize the misunderstandings or erroneous perceptions that cause much of the tension seen on nursing units. As mentioned earlier, active listening involves "listening" not only to the words but also to the body language in order to hear the real meaning of the communication and understand the underlying message. When a person is focused in on the communication, he or she is not preoccupied with other issues or preparing mentally a response or a defense. Allowing the other person to say all he or she has to say without interruption before responding provides for an atmosphere where honest and open communication can occur. In some situations, merely allowing a person to ventilate emotions by using active listening reduces the levels of anger and animosity and sometimes even solves the conflict situation. Also, when intelligent people are allowed to speak openly and freely, they may be able to develop a new solution to the problem that they had not considered previously.

Before responding to a person, it is important to ask clarifying questions that validate the person's concerns, feelings, and perceptions. Validating will help ensure that the responses address the real issues. Also, avoid reflex type reactions to hostile or aggressive statements. It is a human instinct to become defensive when one is attacked and to attack the person back. However, this behavior only escalates the anger and tension and blocks effective communication.

A third strategy that is useful in developing communication coping skills is to always make a conscious decision about the importance of the issue that needs to be discussed. When individuals can identify the issues that really matter and focus their efforts on them, they gain credibility among their peers and develop a reputation for caring and realism. Again, it is a very human tendency to become preoccupied with trivial and unimportant issues. If a person is spending a large portion of his or her energy in dealing with trivia, he or she will have little energy left to deal with the major issues when they come along. By establishing and analyzing the outcomes to be attained and by being open to negotiations and compromise, both parties will leave the confrontation with a sense of accomplishment and fair resolution even if they did not get everything they wanted.

Setting the Stage

After a decision is made to deal with a difficult issue or person, it is important to set the stage for a positive experience. The location for the exchange should be private. The format of the meeting needs to be established ahead of time, including an explanation to the other person that each party will take turns expressing his or her opinions and feelings without interruption.

Establishing Trust

An important issue in conflict negotiations is the establishment of trust. In addition to showing respect for the other person's opinions and ideas, trust can be established by talking first and directly to the person about the problem issue rather than everyone else on the unit. Being talked about behind one's back tends to make people resentful and defensive. Trust is reinforced when a person makes it known that all he or she wants is to resolve the issue and then move on. When the threat of retaliation is removed, people are more likely to express themselves honestly, as well as becoming more open to the other side's ideas. Once two people begin to trust each other, even if they disagree about some of the issues, they are much more likely to come to a satisfactory resolution of the problem.

Box 13–6

Seven Principles of Communication

1. Information giving is not communication.
2. The sender is responsible for clarity.
3. Use simple and exact language.
4. Feedback should be encouraged.
5. The sender must have credibility.
6. Acknowledgment of others is essential.
7. Direct channels of communication are best.

Source: Adapted from Tappen, RM: Nursing Leadership and Management Concept and Practice, ed. 3. FA Davis, Philadelphia, 1995, with permission.

The Actual Exchange

When the actual exchange takes place, it is important to avoid the "I" language and be direct by focusing on the facts and issues. Remember that active listening is a two-way street. A person's own body language, tone of voice, and eye contact can say much more than the actual words (Box 13–6). Showing the other person that his or her opinion is respected, even if not agreed with, helps develop that important sense of trust between the two parties.

After each person has had a chance to express himself or herself and validate the communication, they begin to address the issues and develop a solution for the problem. Sometimes there is a need to set goals for, or at least agree on, how the issues are to be approached and settled. It is fairly common that some issues will remain unresolved after the first meeting. A decision about when and where the second meeting will take place needs to be made before leaving the first meeting. Also, before leaving the first meeting, each party should summarize what they agreed to and how they felt about the exchange. This summarization will help clarify any miscommunications and give each party one last chance to introduce any issues that remain unresolved.

Dealing with difficult people and conflict resolution are never pleasant undertakings. However, like most skills, the more it is practiced, the more comfortable the individual will become using the communication techniques discussed. The importance of handling problematic situations in a timely, honest, and caring manner is self-evident. The anxiety and fear provoked by confrontation are part of the price that nurses must pay in order to do their jobs well and provide high-quality client care.

Conclusion

A person's professional and personal life is influenced by communication styles and behavioral patterns. The ability to analyze personal strengths, weaknesses, and communication behaviors is particularly important when dealing with difficult people.

Certain specific communication qualities and skills are essential when interacting with difficult people. First of all, it is important to develop the skill of assertive communication, which allows people to express themselves openly and honestly while respecting the other person's opinions and ideas. Being able to identify submissive and aggressive behavior is also essential when trying to resolve problems, as well as recognizing issues of diversity, which underlie many problems in communication. Difficult situations are ultimately resolved through the practice of conflict management. Because it is an outgrowth and extension of the problem-solving method, nurses should be able to quickly grasp its structure and master its use.

ISSUES IN PRACTICE

Julie H., RN, has been working the 7 P.M. to 7 A.M. shift in a busy, 32-bed surgical unit of a large university hospital since her graduation from a small bachelor of science in nursing (BSN) program 6 months ago. Although Julie was told by the unit director when she was hired that she would have at least a full year of training before she had to work as charge nurse, tonight the other two RNs who usually work the shift called in sick, and Julie was left in charge. The 7 P.M. to 7 A.M. shift is always busy because the unit has to both discharge clients who are ready to go home after surgery as well as admit clients who are going for surgery the next day. The hospital policy requires that the RN make and sign both the discharge and admission assessments.

Although Julie is nervous about this new role as charge nurse, she feels that she can handle the responsibility if she has some additional help. Normal staffing for the unit on this shift is three registered nurses (RNs), three licensed practical nurses (LPNs), and three unlicensed assistive personnel (UAP). Julie calls the house supervisor to see if she can get some help. The only place in the hospital that is not busy that night is the obstetrics (OB) unit, so the supervisor sends two of the OB unit's UAPs to the surgical unit to help Julie.

It was not the help Julie really wanted, but she feels that she can handle the responsibility. However, when Julie begins to make assignments, the older of the OB unit UAPs, Hanna J., informs Julie that she, for the past 15 years, had worked only in the newborn nursery and does not know anything about the care of adult clients who had surgery. In addition, Hanna states that she has a bad back and cannot lift or turn adult clients and is afraid that she might catch some disease from the adults that she would take back to the babies. Julie asks Hanna, "What do you feel you are qualified to do on the surgical unit?" In response, Hanna crosses her legs, folds her arms across her chest, puts her head down and mumbles under her breath, "A lot more than a new know-it-all RN like you."

Critical Thinking Exercises

- What messages, both verbal and nonverbal, are being communicated? How should Julie respond to this comment? What should she do to rectify the situation?
- Using the various tables in the chapter, identify the personality type of each of the persons involved in the situation.
- How can the RN best communicate with this UAP? What were some of the communication mistakes that the RN made?
- What background, cultural, and diversity factors played a part in this situation?
- Develop a strategy for resolution of this conflict.

- Make a list of your values and where they came from. Describe how each value affects your work ethic and life.
- List your communication strengths and weaknesses. Rank them on a scale of 1 to 10—10 being the highest. Determine which weaknesses you want to change, and create an improvement plan.
- Identify your primary communication style and character type.
- Complete this statement, using as many situations or statements as possible: "In a conflict situation, I have difficulty saying __________." Analyze reasons that prevent you from saying it. What would have been the worst thing that could have happened to you if you had said it? Create a phrase that you feel comfortable with that you could use the next time you want to say something difficult to the members of your team.
- Identify the communication and behavior characteristics of your work group or team. List areas of diversity for each member, including yourself. Identify their strengths and weaknesses. Identify methods for using the team members' diversity to enhance the team.

Bibliography

Brown, G: Cultural diversity in nursing: An impact on communication and learning. Journal of Cultural Diversity 8(1):16–20, 2001.

Cornell, D: Say the words: Communication techniques. Nursing Management 24(3):24, 1993.

Dreger, V: Communication: An important assessment and teaching tool. Journal of the American Society of Ophthalmic Registered Nurses 26(2):57–62, 2001.

Hargrave, J: Nonverbal communication, 2001. Available at: www.janhargrave.com/index.html.

Hunt, P, and Pearson, D: Motivating change. Nursing Standard 16(2):45–52, 2001.

Munro, NL: Apply the rules of "people ethics." AACN News 15(11):2–15, 1998.

Sutherland, K: Speak carefully. Journal of Christian Nursing 18(3):36, 2001.

Tappen, RM: Nursing Leadership and Management, ed. 4. FA Davis, Philadelphia, 2001.

Tappen RM, et al: Essentials of Nursing Leadership and Management, ed. 2. FA Davis, Philadelphia, 2001.

Williams, CA, and Gossett, MT: Nursing communication: Advocacy for the patient or physician? Clinical Nursing Research 10(3):332–340, 2001.

14

Delegation and Supervision in Nursing

Joseph T. Catalano

Learning Objectives

After completing this chapter, the reader will be able to:

- Apply the principles of delegation to nursing practice.
- Analyze and identify situations where delegation is used improperly.
- Discuss the legal implications of delegation in the current health-care setting.
- Distinguish between delegation and supervision.

In today's health-care system, delegation has become an essential component of client care and management of nursing units. It allows health-care managers to maximize the use of caregivers who are educated at multiple levels in a variety of programs. Delegation, if performed properly, permits nurses to meet the requirements of quality care for all clients and has become a basic skill that registered nurses (RNs) must learn. Delegation is used to meet the cost restraints of limited health-care budgets by using less expensive personnel, to maximize the use of time by RNs, and to promote team building.

Delegation versus Supervision

Although delegation and supervision are closely related concepts, they are different. **Delegation** is recognized as assigning or designating a competent individual the responsibility of carrying out a specific group of nursing tasks in the provision of care for certain clients. Delegation includes the understanding that the authorized person is acting in the place of the RN and may be carrying out tasks that generally fall under the RN's scope of practice. Supervision, on the other hand, is the initial direction and periodic evaluation of a person performing an assigned task to ensure that he or she is meeting the standards of care. Although delegation almost always requires supervision, it is possible to have supervision without delegation. When nurses delegate nursing tasks to non-nurses, the RNs are always legally responsible for supervising that person to ensure that the care given meets the standards of care. However, if the facility, or the state board of nursing, or some other official body has a predesignated list of tasks that non-nursing personnel may undertake in the care of clients, then the RN is responsible only for supervising them to make sure the tasks are carried out safely.

Legally, the power to delegate is restricted to professionals who are licensed and governed by a statutory practice act. RNs are considered professionals and can delegate independent nursing functions to other personnel.

Nursing Responsibilities When Delegating

Although it is now a buzzword, the concept of delegation has been a part of health care since the time of Florence Nightingale, when she instructed her nurse "... to look to all these things yourself does not mean to do them yourself."[1] In more recent times, as the delegation phenomenon has grown, the American Nurses Association (ANA) addressed and defined delegation in 1991 when it was beginning to become a more widespread phenomenon in health care and further refined the definition in 1997. The ANA defines delegation as "the transfer of responsibility for the performance of an activity from one individual to another while retaining accountability for the outcome."[2] The ANA stresses the belief that even though the leader or manager delegates a task to another employee, he or she remains responsible and accountable for the care that is provided.

> *In today's health-care system, delegation has become an essential component of client care and management of nursing units.*

What Do You Think?

Is delegation used in the facility where you have clinicals? Who does the delegation on the unit? Does it work well?

Prior to delegating any task, RNs should give careful consideration to the condition of the client and his or her health-care needs. Assessing clients is a designated **responsibility** of registered nurses. Without a thorough assessment, it is likely that critical needs may remain unidentified by less trained personnel, leading to potential errors in care. Clients who are relatively stable and not likely to experience drastic changes in health-care status are the most suitable for delegation. Also, the tasks being delegated must be routine in nature, performed without varying from policy or procedure, and should not require the use of nursing judgment while being performed.

The nurse delegating needs to know the availability of staff and the education and competency levels of the personnel to be assigned. These factors must be matched with the level of care required by the client. Key information to obtain in relation to delegation is how often the delegatee has performed the required tasks or cared for this type of client, what units they have been working on and feel comfortable in, and the organizational abilities of the person.

The RN needs to know both the institution's official position description for the unlicensed assistive personnel (UAP) as well as the UAP's actual abilities. For example, the position description may state that the UAP can care for postoperative clients who have multiple wound drains. However, when the RN assigns a specific UAP to such a postoperative client, he or she discovers that the UAP has worked only in the newborn nursery for the past 5 years and has no knowledge of how to care for complicated postoperative clients. If the RN assigns this UAP anyway, and some major complication develops with the client as a result of the UAP's lack of competence (even though the position description states that this is an appropriate function for

Box 14–1

Barriers to Effective Delegation

A. Internal barriers (person delegating):
   1. Lack of experience delegating
   2. Lack of confidence in others
   3. Personal insecurity
   4. Demanding perfectionism
   5. Poor organizational skills
   6. Indecision
   7. Poor communication skills
   8. Lack of confidence in self
   9. Fear of not being liked by everyone
   10. Micromanaging management style

B. External barriers (circumstances or person being delegated to):
   1. Unclear policies about delegation
   2. Policies that do not tolerate mistakes
   3. Management-by-crisis model for facility
   4. Unclear delineation of authority and responsibilites
   5. Poor staffing
   6. Lack of competence
   7. Overdependence on the person delegating
   8. Unwillingness to accept responsibility for one's own practice
   9. Immersion in trivia and gossip
   10. Work overload

Source: Tappen, RM, et al: Essentials of Nursing Leadership and Management. FA Davis, Philadelphia, 2001.

the UAP), the RN is held legally responsible for the poor outcome. When the RN determines that the client's needs match the skills and abilities of the UAP or licensed practical nurse (LPN), only then should that person be assigned.

RNs who delegate are also responsible for educating the UAP about the task that is to be done. If the person is unfamiliar with what needs to be done, the RN is required to demonstrate how the tasks or procedures are performed and then document the training. Education also includes telling the UAP what is expected in the completion of the task and which possible complications to watch for and report to the RN. The ANA suggests that the RN watch the UAP perform the designated task at least initially, then make periodic observations throughout the shift to ensure safe and competent care for the client.[3] Furthermore, the RN must always be available to answer questions and help the UAP whenever assistance is required. Consider the following situation:

Elsie Humber, RN, is the evening charge nurse on a busy oncology unit of the county hospital. On one particularly busy evening, she discovers during shift report that one of the scheduled LPNs has called in sick, and there are no other LPNs available to take her place. Ms. Humber assigns the LPN's duties and clients, including a heat lamp treatment for a decubitus ulcer, to a UAP who has worked on the unit for several months. The UAP protests the assignment, but Ms. Humber rebukes her saying, "I have no one else. If you don't care for these clients, they won't get any care this shift." In setting up the heat lamp treatment, the UAP knocks the lamp over and burns the client. Because of his suppressed immune system from chemotherapy and generally debilitated condition, the burn does not heal and develops into an infection. The client later sues the hospital for malpractice. The hospital in turn attempts to shift the legal responsibility for the burn to Ms. Humber. Who is legally responsible for the incident? Does the client have grounds for a successful case?

When delegating tasks, the outcomes of performing the tasks should be expected and predictable. For example, when a UAP is assigned the task of feeding a client who has suffered a stroke and has hemiplegia, the predicted outcome will be that the client will eat and not choke on the food. The task should also not require excessive supervision, complex decision making, or detailed assessment during its performance. If any of these elements are required, then it needs to be reassigned to an RN.

> *It is important to remember that when nurses delegate nursing tasks they are not delegating nursing.*

It is important to remember that when nurses delegate nursing tasks they are *not* delegating nursing. Professional nursing practice is both a science, based on a unique body of knowledge, and an art, guided by the nursing process. It is not merely a collection of tasks. Of all health-care workers, professional nurses are the most qualified to provide holistic care of the client by promoting health and treating disease. Nurses' education and experience provide them with the skills and knowledge to coordinate and supervise nursing care and to delegate specific tasks to others.

Although mastering delegation skills can seem like a daunting task, there are a number of common sense steps a nurse can use to attain this skill. As a nursing student or nursing assistant, you have had tasks delegated to you from RNs. You probably noted that some of the RNs were good at delegation and others were not as good.

Developing Delegation Skills

In developing your own delegation skills, try to emulate the good delegators. Develop good communication and interpersonal relationship skills. Make eye contact with the other person, be pleasant, and ask for suggestions. However, avoid allowing the person to whom you are delegating tasks to control the exchange by intimidation or resistance. After delegating a task, if one does not already exist, make a written list of the responsibilities that you expect from the person. The list will help clarify what is expected and head off possible misunderstandings. It is also important to be flexible. Clients' conditions change, new clients may be admitted, or other clients may be discharged. The original assignments may have to be modified in response to changes in the environment. Monitor those to whom you have delegated tasks. Are they doing what they should be doing? Do they understand the responsibilities involved in the client's care? Help them if you determine they need help. Teach them if you determine they have a lack of knowledge. And most important, at the end of the shift, say "Thank you. I appreciate the hard work (good job) you've done today."

There are certain delegation situations that may place the RN at an increased risk for liability. Try to avoid the following when delegating:

- Assigning tasks that are highly invasive or have the potential to cause significant physical harm to clients
- Assigning tasks that are designated under the scope of practice or standards of care as belonging exclusively to the RN
- Assigning tasks that the person is not trained for or lacks the knowledge to safely complete
- Assigning tasks when there is inadequate time to safely monitor or evaluate the practice of the person performing the tasks[4]

The long-term effect of the growing trend to delegation on the quality of client care remains to be seen. However, the knowledge and judgment of the professional nurse will remain essential elements in any health-care system reforms,

What Do You Think?

What qualities have you observed in good delegators? What qualities made the poor delegators ineffective?

Box 14–2

Delegation Decision Tree

1. Are there laws and rules in place supporting the rules of delegation?
2. Is the task within the scope of practice of the UAP, LPN/LVN, RN, or new graduate?
3. Has there been an assessment of the client's needs?
4. Is the UAP, LPN/LVN, RN, or new graduate competent to accept the delegation?
5. Does the ability of the caregiver match the care needs of the client?
6. Can the task be completed without requiring nursing judgments?
7. Is the result of the task somewhat predictable?
8. Can the task be safely performed according to directions?
9. Can the task be performed without repeated assessment?
10. Is appropriate supervision available?

Source: Tappen, RM: Nursing Leadership and Management, ed. 4. FA Davis, Philadelphia, 2001.

including clinical integration, case management, outsourcing practices, **total quality management (TQM)**, and **continuous quality improvement (CQI)**.

Legal Issues in Delegation

The health-care system's headlong rush to managed care has increased nurses' liability for lawsuits in the area of supervision and delegation. In the search for cost-effective client care, current managed care strategies attempt to make optimal use of relatively expensive RNs by replacing them with less costly and less educated personnel. As more and more health-care facilities move toward restructuring, the use of less-educated UAPs who have minimal education and experience will continue to increase. Although RNs have always been responsible for the delegation of some tasks and the supervision of less-qualified health-care providers, it is now one of the primary functions of RNs in today's health-care system.

Delegation does have some advantages. It is an RN extender in that a quantitatively larger amount of care can be given to more clients than can be given by one RN. Delegation can free the RN from those lower-level time-consuming tasks so that more time can be spent planning for care and performing those skills that less prepared individuals would be unable to perform. For those to whom tasks are delegated, it can serve as an incentive to learn additional skills, increase knowledge, and develop a sense of initiative and perhaps to seek further formal education. Delegation, if performed properly, maintains accountability and decision making where it belongs—with the RN.

Who Can Delegate — Legally?

Most state practice acts do *not* give delegatory authority to **dependent practitioners** like licensed practical nurses/licensed vocational nurses (LPNs/LVNs) or UAPs. In addition, professionals who delegate specific tasks retain accountability for the proper and safe completion of those tasks as well as responsibility for determining whether the assigned personnel are competent to carry out the task. One exception is when the person who is assigned a task also has a license and the tasks fall under that person's scope of practice.[5] Then, again, the RN is responsible only for supervision of the other licensed person;

this is often seen in situations where there are LPNs/LVNs assigned to client care.

The delegation and supervision responsibilities of RNs have been and continue to be a major concern for the nursing profession, both ethically and legally. The ANA Code of Ethics for Nurses states, "The nurse is responsible and accountable for individual nursing practice and determines the appropriate delegation of tasks consistent with the nurse's obligation to provide optimum patient care" (statement 4).[6] From the ethical view, RNs have an obligation to refuse assignments that they are not competent to carry out and also to refuse to delegate tasks to individuals whom they believe are incapable of or unprepared to perform particular nursing tasks.

Most state practice acts do not give delegatory authority to dependent practitioners like licensed practical nurses/licensed vocational nurses (LPNs/LVNs) or UAPs.

The legal side of the delegation issue has also been addressed by the ANA in a publication *ANA Basic Guide to Safe Delegation.* This document makes a distinction between direct delegation, which is a specific decision made by the RN about who can perform what tasks, and indirect delegation, which is a list of tasks that certain health-care personnel can perform that is produced by the health-care facility.[3] The **consensus** among many experts is that indirect delegation is really a form of covert institutional licensure. Lists of activities from the facility allowing non-nursing personnel who do not have the education of the RN to carry out professional nursing functions is a de facto permission to practice nursing without a license. Indirect delegation places RNs in a precarious legal position.

Basically, indirect delegation takes away much of the authority of the RN to assign personnel tasks, yet the RN remains accountable for the safe completion of the tasks under the doctrines of **respondent superior** and **vicarious liability**. Although some states are beginning to address the UAP and delegation issues in their nurse practice acts, many states either have no official standards for UAP delegation or include UAP standards under the medical practice act.

Box 14–3

Five Rights of Delegation

- Right task
  Do the tasks delegated follow written policy guidelines?
- Right person
  Does the person have the proper qualifications for the tasks?
- Right direction or communication
  Are the instructions and outcomes clearly stated? When should the person report changes?
- Right supervision or feedback
  How can the delegation process be improved? Are the client goals for care being achieved?
- Right circumstances
  Are the tasks that are being delegated free from requiring independent nursing judgments?

Sources: Fisher, M: Do you have delegation savvy? Nursing 2000 (9):58–59, 2000.

Tappen, RM: Nursing Leadership and Management, ed. 4. FA Davis, Philadelphia, 2001.

Wheeler, J: How to delegate your way to a better working life. Nursing Times 97(36):34–35, 2001.

Critical Thinking Exercises

- Obtain a copy of your state's nurse practice act. Review the section that deals with delegation. Apply those criteria to the case study at the beginning of this chapter.
- As a student, you have had tasks delegated to you. Identify how delegation has changed in regard to your leaning and level of skills as you have progressed through your program.
- Obtain a copy of the policy on delegation from at least two of the clinical sites where you practiced. How do these policies differ? How are they similar? What are the reasons for the similarities and differences?

Conclusion

With the increased use of less educated and unlicensed personnel present in today's health-care system, it is essential that the nurse develop effective delegation and supervision skills. The nurse needs to be mindful that the tasks that can be delegated can change based on work setting, client needs, position descriptions, institutional training of personnel, and the ever-changing requirements of nurse practice acts and professional standards. Nurses also need to know when delegation is inappropriate.

References

1. Nightingale, F: Notes on Nursing. What It Is and What It Is Not. Harrison and Sons, London, 1859, p. 17.
2. American Nurses Association: Position Statement: Registered Nurse Utilization of Unlicensed Assistive Personnel. ANA, Washington DC, 1997.
3. American Nurses Association: Registered Professional Nurses and Unlicensed Assistive Personnel, ed. 2. ANA, Washington, DC, 1996.
4. Wheeler, J: How to delegate your way to a better working life. Nursing Times 97(36):34–35, 2001.
5. Wissmann, J, et al: Assessing nurse graduate leadership outcomes. Nurse Educator 27(1):32–36, Jan/Feb 2002.
6. ANA Code of Ethics for Nurses, 2001. Available at: www.ana.org.

Bibliography

American Nurses Association: Policy Series: Regulation of Unlicensed Assistive Personnel. ANA, Washington, DC, 1996.

Creighton, H: Law Every Nurse Should Know, ed. 5. WB Saunders, Philadelphia, 1986.

Fisher, M: Do nurses delegate effectively? Nurse Manager 99(5):23–25, 1999.

Fisher, M: Do you have delegation savvy? Nursing 2000 (9):58–59, 2000.

Sullivan, TJ: Collaboration: A Health Care Imperative. McGraw-Hill, New York, 1998.

Tappen, RM: Nursing Leadership and Management, ed. 4. FA Davis, Philadelphia, 2001.

Tappen, RM, et al: Essentials of Nursing Leadership and Management, ed. 2. FA Davis, Philadelphia, 2001.

Wheeler, J: How to delegate your way to a better working life. Nursing Times 97(36):34–35, 2001.

Wissmann, J, et al: Assessing nurse graduate leadership outcomes. Nurse Educator 27(1):32–36, Jan/Feb 2002.

15

Collective Bargaining and Governance

Joseph T. Catalano

Learning Objectives

After completing this chapter, the reader will be able to:

- Define collective bargaining.
- Analyze the key issues that concern nurses in collective bargaining.
- Identify the steps in the contract negotiation process.
- Distinguish between a mediator and an arbitrator.
- Delineate the important elements in a contract.
- Name alternative forms of governance.
- Analyze the effect governance has on collective bargaining.

As nursing moves toward achieving its full status as a profession, the issue of collective bargaining becomes more important. Since the early 1960s, the number of nurses who have joined unions has increased steadily, yet the question remains: Is professionalism compatible with membership in a union? Union members still have the image of male workers in blue-collar, heavy industry jobs. However, not only are registered nurses (RNs) joining unions at a faster pace than most other categories of workers, they are also more militant and aggressive in their demands.[1]

Nursing practices have often been defined and controlled by other groups, such as physicians and hospital administrators. These groups saw the potential power of an organized large group of well-educated and dedicated nurses and feared the time when they would become independent. Even today, most hospital management reacts to any unionization attempts on the part of nurses with hostility and resistance. As nurses begin to accept the independence, authority, and responsibility of the profession, they need to consider whether or not joining a union will help them reach their goal of full professionalism. Without a doubt, this is one of the most highly charged issues that a nurse might face in professional practice.

The image of nursing has always been one of dedication, service to clients, and selflessness. In the past, nurses' pay and working conditions were often secondary considerations, and many nurses felt that too much emphasis on money demeaned the profession. In today's society, nurses are beginning to realize that professionals with a career should have a say in matters that affect their practice, including working conditions, staffing patterns, benefits, and income. They need to be able to express these concerns without loss of status or reputation with the general public and other health-care professionals.

Perspective on Collective Bargaining

Collective bargaining is the uniting of employees for the purpose of increasing their ability to influence their employer and to improve working conditions.[2] Collective bargaining is based on the principle that there is greater strength in large numbers. Its primary goal is to equalize the power between labor and management. The primary collective bargaining unit is the union.

Initially unions were formed to protect workers from exploitation by greedy and insensitive employers. Although confronted with much opposition, they did accomplish their goals and became very powerful entities themselves. Recently, unions have received a more negative image because of the use of destructive and sometimes illegal practices in the quest for additional power. The end result is that the union movement itself is now in a fight for survival because of decreasing membership.[3] For some, unions and collective bargaining arouse images of picket lines, rowdy strikes, and violence. Many professionals, including nurses, do not regard this as activity that professionals should be involved in and tend to reject the idea of union membership outright.

Legislative Development of Collective Bargaining

Although the informal roots of collective bargaining can be traced back to the middle 1800s, formal collective bargaining in this country was first legally recognized in 1935 with passage of the National Labor Relations Act (NLRA). This act granted employees the right to self-organization and to form, and help in the organization of, labor unions that could then bargain collectively through representatives. The representatives would be appointed by the union and bargain with management for the purpose of collective bargaining, mutual aid, and protection.[4] Under the NLRA, the National Labor Relations Board (NLRB) was established to supervise the implementation of the act.[1]

Originally, the NLRA included nonprofit hospitals and other health-care providers under its authority. In its attempt to protect unions, the NLRA prevented some employers from reducing wages, in hopes that higher paid workers would spend more and decrease the severity of the depression. One negative result of NLRA was that many employers who did not have enough income to pay the higher wages went bankrupt. The NLRA was amended in 1947 by the Taft-Hartley Act, also called the Labor Management Relations Act (LMRA), with the goal of restoring equality between the unions and management. Taft-Hartley excluded nurses in nonprofit hospitals from coverage under the NLRA, legally preventing nurses from organizing collective bargaining units and going on strike. It was not until 1974 that the Taft-Hartley Act was amended to cover nurses in nonprofit hospitals, thus allowing nurses to form collective bargaining units.[1]

In April of 1991, the U.S. Supreme Court ruled that the NLRB had the authority to define bargaining units for health-care providers in all settings, including acute care hospitals. Under this ruling, the NLRB defined eight separate bargaining units that were appropriate for use in hospitals (Box 15–1).[5]

Ultimately, this ruling by the Supreme Court permitted "all registered nurses (RNs) bargaining units" to be formed so that work issues important to professional nurses could be addressed. The current major representative for nurses is the Service Employees International

What Do You Think?

How do you perceive unions? Do unions have any place in health care?

Box 15–1

Eight Bargaining Units for Use in Hospitals

1. Nurses
2. Physicians
3. All professionals except nurses and physicians
4. All technical employees
5. All skilled maintenance employees
6. All business office clerical employees
7. All guards
8. All other nonprofessional employees

Union, which represents almost 500,000 nurses and health-care providers nationwide. The American Nurses Association (ANA) has been active in the support of collective bargaining throughout its history.

Although the ANA does not serve as a bargaining agent, it does support the state nurses associations (SNAs) to function as bargaining agents. As early as 1944, the ANA ruled that the SNAs could engage in collective bargaining. In response to the attempt to regulate nursing from the outside, the ANA presented a position paper in 1946 that stated the importance for nursing to assume responsibility for advancing the social and economic security of its practitioners rather than leaving it to organizations outside the profession.[6] Today the SNAs represent approximately 140,000 RNs in some 840 individual bargaining units across the United States. Since the ruling by the Supreme Court in 1991, there has been an increased interest in organizing additional bargaining units.[7] The Workplace Advocacy Initiative was also initiated in 1991 to help RNs improve the work environment and gain more control over professional practice.

Goals of Collective Bargaining

Although the basic goal of collective bargaining is to equalize power between management and employees, the inequality of power between the two groups is not so great as it initially appears. In many organizations management relies on employees who are near the bottom of the power structure hierarchy to carry out the work of the organization. Employees are vital to the growth, development, and even the survival of the organization. Employees also far outnumber individuals in management. Collective bargaining takes advantage of these two factors when attempting to produce change in the organization. An individual employee is highly vulnerable when attempting to force the employer to change.

The main area of concern of collective bargaining is basic economic issues such as salaries and benefits. In some hospital settings, nurses are paid less than other individuals in the hospital who have less education and fewer responsibilities. Collective bargaining attempts to balance these inequities.

Other concerns of collective bargaining include shift differentials, overtime pay, holidays, personal days off, the number of hours required in a work week, sick leave, maternity and paternity leave, uniform reimbursements, lunch and coffee breaks, health insurance, pension plans, and severance pay.[2] These elements all are found in the employment contract and may vary greatly depending on the hospital and the power of the bargaining unit.

One of the most important goals of a bargaining unit is to protect the employee against arbitrary treatment and unfair labor practices. These can be anything from working five weekends in a row to being fired because a physician felt the nurse was acting in an insubordinate manner. Other issues that might be considered unfair labor practices include being passed over for promotion without an explanation, unreasonable staffing and scheduling policies, excessive demands for overtime, rotating shifts, unfair on-call time, transfers, layoffs, seniority rights, and failure to post job openings. The collective bargaining unit establishes a grievance procedure by means of which the employee can bring a complaint against management without fear of reprisals. These grievance procedures also allow a mechanism for the employee to follow up on the complaint to a satisfactory conclusion.

An important goal of collective bargaining is to maintain and promote professional practice. Often overlooked by management, this goal is one way nurses can keep and increase control over their own professional practice. For example, some nurses' bargaining units have been able to include the entire ANA Code of Ethics into the contract with the hospital. Other units have been able to address issues such as staffing, standards of care, and quality of care in the contract negotiations.

> *Although the basic goal of collective bargaining is to equalize power between management and employees, the inequality of power between the two groups is not so great as it initially appears.*

Interest-Based Bargaining

Traditionally, collective bargaining has been viewed as a struggle between two groups, one (usually employees) attempting to gain more power and another (usually management) attempting to retain power. This type of struggle often resulted in hurt feelings or impasses in negotiations.

Interest-based bargaining, also called mutual gains, win-win, and best-practice bargaining, is based on the idea that the way to achieve a mutually beneficial contract is to create an environment in which all parties can openly discuss all issues to the fullest extent. In interest-based bargaining, a highly structured six-step process is followed:

1. Selection of issues
2. Discussion of interests
3. Generation of options
4. Establishment of standards to measure the options
5. Measurement of the options
6. Development of solutions

This step-by-step process prevents the parties involved in the bargaining from reverting to the traditional power struggle. All steps are done jointly, and even the 2-day training session that precedes negotiations requires participation by both management and labor.

An issue that is central to the contract negotiations is ensuring that the role of the registered nurse as the primary assessor and planner of care be maintained. The contract spells out what the RNs role will be, including activities such as assessing, planning, and evaluating the client's nursing care needs. To ensure that nursing issues are addressed adequately in contracts, RNs need to participate in facility committees that establish priorities for labor-management relations, nurse staffing, client-care standards, and health and safety policies. This partnership between nurses and hospital administrators allows for joint decision making when issues of nursing practice and delivery of care are involved.

Interest-based bargaining seems to be gaining momentum and may be the trend for the future, particularly in the health-care industry. Traditional collective bargaining methods are primarily adversarial and often leave the parties involved with deep-seated feelings of hostility toward each other. The old methods sometimes result in strikes or other types of work actions that harm the reputations of both nurses and the hospitals. Interest-based bargaining allows participants an opportunity to negotiate without hostility and to develop a more positive relationship after the contract has been agreed on.

What Do You Think?

Who are the people who hold governing power in your clinical institution? What process can employees in health-care facilities use to affect the quality of care that they provide?

Nurses' Questions About Collective Bargaining

Although large numbers of RNs have successfully unionized, there remain some fundamental questions about collective bargaining. These questions are at the heart of what makes collective bargaining an ethical issue for many nurses.

Is It Unprofessional?

Nurses have a great deal of difficulty in adjusting their image to that of a union member or a striker. It just does not seem to be professional. For many nurses it seems that there must be other ways to achieve the same goals without collective bargaining.

Organizers of collective bargaining units stress that many other professionals, such as pilots, teachers, and even physicians, are members of unions. The NLRB defines nurses as professionals because their work requires advanced and specialized education and skills. They also make critical judgments that affect the health and well-being of others. Union organizers contend that it is even less professional to accept low pay and poor working conditions than it is to join a union to improve these elements. They also feel that collective bargaining will give nurses control over their practice, which is one of the keys to professionalism.

> *The collective bargaining unit establishes a grievance procedure by means of which the employee can bring a complaint against management without fear of reprisals. These grievance procedures also allow a mechanism for the employee to follow up on the complaint to a satisfactory conclusion.*

Is It Unethical?

One of the major beliefs of nurses is the priority of the clients' health and well-being over the personal needs and gains of the health-care provider. This concern conflicts with the methods commonly used by collective bargaining units, such as strikes or work slowdowns. There is a feeling among many health-care providers that these types of actions constitute abandonment of their clients and therefore violate the code of ethics. Those who support collective bargaining stress that poor or intolerable work conditions are as much a threat to that client's health and well-being as the work actions taken to correct these conditions. The ability of nurses simply to threaten to strike, even though it may never materialize, is often powerful enough to bring about change.[8] Law requires that there must be a 10-day notice given before a strike takes place. This gives the hospital a chance to prepare for the strike and to make changes to ensure client safety, such as transferring critical care clients to another hospital, eliminating elective surgeries, and refusing to admit new clients.

In the few times when nurses have gone on strike, client safety and well-being have not been affected. The institutions involved were always given enough lead time to discharge or transfer the majority of the clients. The few remaining clients were cared for by management personnel who are not covered by unions.

Is It Divisive?

Does the process of collective bargaining set nurse against nurse? The process of collective bargaining is adversarial by nature. It sets two groups, management and employees, against each other. Although this relationship can result in conflict, it allows the staff nurses to be heard and to initiate changes that affect the practice of nursing. Nurses have been attempting for years to improve working conditions in the health-care setting, and to achieve **comparable worth**. Administrators pay little attention to an individual nurse or to a small group of concerned nurses. When a collective bargaining unit speaks for all of the nurses, however, administration will listen.[1]

> The chief executive officer (CEO) of a large home health agency in a southwestern resort area called a general staff meeting. She reported that the agency had grown rapidly and was now the largest in the area. "Much of our success is due to the professionalism and commitment of our staff members," she said. "With growth comes some problems, however. The most serious problem is the fluctuation in patient census. Our census peaks in the winter months when seasonal visitors are here and troughs in the summer. In the past, when we were a small agency, we all took our vacations during the slow season. This made it possible to continue to pay everyone his or her full salary all year. However, with the pressures to reduce costs and the large number of staff members we now have, we cannot continue to do this. We are very concerned about maintaining the high quality of patient care currently provided, but we have calculated that we need to reduce staff by 30 percent over the summer in order to survive financially."
>
> The CEO then invited comments from the staff members. The majority of the nurses said they wanted and needed to work full-time all year. Most supported families and had to have a steady income all year round. "My rent does not go down in the summer," said one. "Neither does my mortgage or the grocery bill," said another. A small number said that they would be happy to work part-time in the summer if they could be guaranteed full-time employment from October through May. "We have friends who would love this work schedule," they added.
>
> "That's not fair," protested the nurses who needed to work full-time all year. "You can't replace us with part-time staff." The discussion grew louder and the participants more agitated. The meeting ended without a solution to the problem. Although the CEO promised to consider all points of view before making a decision, the nurses left the meeting feeling very confused and concerned about the security of their future income. Some grumbled that they probably would begin looking for new positions "before the ax falls."
>
> The next day, the CEO received a telephone call from the nurses' union representative. "If what I heard about the meeting yesterday is correct," said the representative, "your plan is in violation of our collective bargaining contract." The CEO reviewed the contract and found that the representative was correct. A new solution to the financial problems caused by the seasonal fluctuation in patient census would have to be found.
>
> (Tappen, RM, et al: Essentials of Nursing Leadership and Management, ed. 2. FA Davis, Philadelphia, 2001, pp. 106–107, with permission.)

Administrators pay little attention to an individual nurse or to a small group of concerned nurses. When a collective bargaining unit speaks for all of the nurses, however, administration will listen.

Different collective bargaining units have different requirements for membership, which are often included in the negotiations. Many unions negotiate a *closed shop* or *agency shop* clause in the contract. A closed shop institution requires that all the employees pay membership dues whether they belong to the union or not. The rationale behind the closed shop approach is that because all the employees benefit from the union's negotiations, they should all pay for it. It also encourages employees to join the union because they are already paying the dues. However, many states have *right to work* laws that make closed shop contracts illegal. In these states, the *open shop* collective bargaining model is used, and only those employees who desire to be members join the union and pay dues. There is more chance for nurse-to-nurse conflicts in open shop institutions because of the divisions between those who belong to the union and those who do not. Collective bargaining does not have to be adversarial, and in facilities where administration is open to change and the collective bargaining unit is realistic in its requests, the process can be very smooth and amicable.

Is There a Threat to Job Security?

Although the main goals of collective bargaining are improvement of working conditions and protection from unfair labor practices, it can itself pose a threat to job security. In some cases, employees who are active in the collective bargaining process become well known to management and may become the targets for reprisals, particularly if the collective bargaining fails. Facilities sometimes suggest that granting RNs higher wages and benefits will cause bankruptcy and closure of the facility or that the higher RN wages will at least drain the organization's resources so much that it has to cut back the number of other employees. In reality, recent changes in contract law have resulted in job losses. Nurses can be replaced during strikes, and even if a settlement is reached, they are hired back only after new employees leave or openings occur. If no settlement is reached, striking nurses may never be hired back.

Taking an action always carries risk. Nurses involved in collective bargaining have to weigh the risk-to-benefit ratio before they take action. Are the working conditions so poor and the pay so inadequate that they overshadow the risk of possible job loss? The first attempts at organizing a collective bargaining unit are usually the most dangerous in terms of job security. Initial attempts at organizing nurses are usually made outside the hospital between representatives of the SNA and the union. This type of activity prevents any individuals from becoming targets of management's anger and makes management's reprisals more difficult. In addition, there are also some legal protections for nurses who organize collective bargaining. There are grievance procedures that can be followed under the unfair labor practices rules that vary somewhat from state to state.

The Contract

After a collective bargaining unit has been selected, the next important step is to develop or negotiate a contract between the nurses and the hospital. The contract is a legal document that is binding for both management and the union.[2] Contracts can be very specific and include just a few items, or very broad and include many. Contracts often contain requirements for union membership by the employees and set the cost of dues for that membership.

Negotiating teams are selected by both management and employee groups. One member of each of these teams is designated as the spokesperson who will be the main representative for the group. Before negotiations start, each team meets separately to decide on its position on various issues and on what they are willing to compromise. A list of demands is exchanged by the two sides; it should include everything each might possibly want.

Generally, management is reluctant to give up power or relinquish money. The employees' group tries to gain some of management's power and gain benefits for its members. Often many meetings between the two groups are required before they discover the key issues and determine where compromise is possible. Posturing and showmanship play a big part in the initial negotiations. Later, when serious issues are discussed and dealt with, final agreements may be reached behind closed doors.

The law requires that each side bargain in good faith. Good faith bargaining requires that both parties must agree to meet at reasonable times, to send individuals to the negotiations who can make binding decisions, and to be willing to bargain with the other side.[2] A lack of willingness to negotiate is not bargaining in good faith.

When the sides are unable to reach a settlement, a stalemate occurs. Stalemates are sometimes resolved through mediation, in which a neutral third party provided by the Federal Mediation and Conciliation Service meets with each side. After determining the nature of the conflict, the mediator brings the two sides together to attempt to work out a settlement. Both sides must work with the mediator, but they are not required to accept the mediator's recommendations.

If mediation fails, the Federal Mediation and Conciliation Service may appoint a fact-finding panel to investigate the conflict and to make recommendations. The panel's report is made public and can exert pressure on both sides to accept the recommendations of the mediator.

In some situations, an arbitrator with binding power may be appointed. This person is a neutral third party who, like the mediator, investigates the conflict, meets with both sides, and makes a recommendation for settlement. Unlike that of the mediator, however, the arbitrator's recommendation must be accepted by both sides. Both labor and management try to avoid binding arbitration because it limits their negotiating powers and they may lose something gained during previous negotiations.

When all else fails, the final step in the contract negotiation process is work slowdowns or stoppages (strikes). Although strikes are usually the tool used by employees to gain power, management can use a form of enforced strike called a lockout, whereby employees are not permitted to enter the work facility.

The prospect of a strike is usually accompanied by more intense negotiations that may lead to a last-minute settlement. Strikes are detrimental to both sides. Employees lose pay and benefits during a strike, and management loses income. In addition, the overall public image of strikes is negative, and they have little support. Some collective bargaining units have developed alternative ways of achieving their goals without a strike. Methods such as disruption of services on a random basis or boycott of an organization can achieve the same effects as a full-blown strike without damaging the image of the union.

After a settlement has been reached, the contract must be ratified. The collective bargaining unit takes the contract back to the employees, who must approve it (Box 15–2). Once it is approved by a majority of the employees, the contract becomes legally binding for both management and the employees.

What Do You Think?

Did you ever sign a contract for employment? Did you read the contract? Were all the elements of a good contract present?

Concerns

Representation

One of the most difficult decisions that nurses have to make is who shall represent them as a collective bargaining unit. It is reasonable to conclude that only a professional organization, such as the state nurses association (SNA), that understands the complex and varied needs of the profession will be able to represent that profession in a collective bargaining situation.

Over the years, SNAs have developed into skilled representatives able to negotiate contracts with considerable success. However, nonprofessional unions have years of experience with negotiations and large sums of money to spend on developing skilled individuals whose only job is negotiating contracts. The union must be able to convince the group of nurses that it is able to represent the interests of the nurses more effectively than the SNA.

Union groups who attempt to represent nurses soon find that nurses have difficulties in forming a consensus concerning problems and issues. Individuals outside the nursing profession have difficulty understanding issues such as quality and standards of care, ethical dilemmas, or even the different levels of nursing education.

Box 15–2

Elements of a Good Contract

- A statement outlining the objectives of both management and the employees
- A description of the official collective bargaining group
- A description of the benefits included in the contract, such as wages and salary, overtime pay, holiday pay, shift differentials, differentials for advanced education or certifications
- A description of other benefits, such as health insurance, life insurance, retirement, legal benefits, among others
- A description of acceptable in-house labor practices, such as transfers, promotions, seniority, layoffs, **grievance** procedures, and work schedules
- A description of the procedure to be used when employees have disciplinary problems or when there is a **breach of contract**
- A description of the grievance procedures and the due process to be followed
- A description of what is expected of the professional, including standards of care and codes of ethics

Nurses should also be concerned about the public image of the collective bargaining unit they select to represent them. Some nurses' groups have been represented by a machinists' union, a teamsters' union, or even a meat cutters' union. Although these unions are highly proficient at negotiating contracts to gain benefits for their members, some feel the image of nursing is tarnished in the process.

Nursing Supervisors—Employees or Management?

Everyone is familiar with the idea of the traditional nursing supervisor. This is the older, more experienced nurse who guides the less experienced nurses. Nursing supervisors make sure staffing is adequate for their assigned shifts, resolve problems that are beyond the skills of the staff nurse, act as mediators between physicians and nurses, and use their higher skill levels to assist the staff nurses with code blues or complicated procedures. The term *nursing supervisor* also includes nurse educators, directors of nursing, head nurses, unit supervisors, assistant head nurses, and sometimes even charge nurses on the 3 P.M. to 11 P.M. or 11 P.M. to 7 A.M. work shifts.

Under the amendments to the Taft-Hartley Act of 1974, a supervisor was defined as any individual with authority to hire, transfer, suspend, lay off, promote, assign, reward, or discipline another employee.[2] From this legal viewpoint, nursing supervisors were no longer employees but really members of the management. Management cannot be involved in collective bargaining activities and is therefore prevented from joining units. A careful reading of the definition of a supervisor as presented in the Taft-Hartley Act makes the category of supervisor open to interpretation. Anybody who assigns a task to another nurse could be considered a supervisor.

Management has sometimes used this provision in the Taft-Hartley Act in the attempt to control the organization and function of collective bargaining units. Management, if so inclined, can use this distinction to induce tension between nursing staff and supervisors, thus reducing the cohesion of the group. Supervisors often serve on important hospital committees to develop standards of care, foster professional recognition, and support nurse advancement. When contracts are negotiated, the supervisors are on the opposite side of the table from the staff nurses. Often in the heat of negotiation, things are said that foster negative feelings. After the negotiations have ended, it is difficult to re-establish that sense of unity that contributes to high-quality client care.

Attempts have been made by some health-care institutions to categorize all of their RNs and licensed practical nurses (LPNs) as supervisors, thus preventing any of them from organizing into a collective bargaining unit.

1994 Supreme Court Decision

In a 5-to-4 vote, the Supreme Court of the United States supported the decision that LPNs at the Heartland Nursing Home in Urbana, Ohio, should be considered supervisors because they directed the work of nurses' aides "in the interest of the employer." Under this ruling, these LPNs were not protected under the NLRA. This ruling has been of great concern to all nurses, but particularly to the ANA's Department of Labor Relations and Workplace Advocacy committee.

The implications of this decision are far-reaching and pose a direct threat to the ability of RNs to pursue collective bargaining. Employers have already begun to use this ruling to fight nurses in collective bargaining units from Alaska to Washington, DC. The ANA has been working toward developing language that would follow the description of a supervisor as found in the NLRA and the Taft-Hartley Act (see earlier discussion). Since the passage of the NLRA, nurses who provide client care have been considered to be acting within the professional nature of nursing and not in the interests of the employer (as a supervisor would primarily be).

Under the ANA's proposed revisions, the scope of the definition of supervisor would be narrowed to include only employees of health-care institutions. This change would allow the NLRB to continue to determine, on a case-by-case basis, whether nurses were supervisors or professional or technical employees. This legislation, introduced to Congress in 1996, was initially tabled. Although never officially acted upon, recent court rulings have supported the position that all RNs are not supervisors with resulting successful work actions and strikes nationwide.[4]

Governance

The term *governance* has a variety of meanings in different contexts. In general, the term describes the arrangement of the hierarchy of power within an organization and how that power flows through the organization. In relationship to nursing, governance has been defined as "the establishment and maintenance of social, political, and economic arrangements by which nurses maintain control over their practice, their self-discipline, their working conditions, and their professional affairs."[9] The traditional structure of authority in the health-care industry has been based on the triad of the board of directors, the administrator, and the medical staff.

Authority is a type of power that has its origins in the position that an individual holds within an organization.[2] This individual has this power only because others are willing to accept the decisions made by the person in that position. This allows relatively few people in the organization's hierarchy to control large numbers of employees as well as the directions and functions of the rest of the organization.

At the top of the governance hierarchy is the board of directors, also called the trustees or governors. The board of directors is usually composed of influential business people who are considered community leaders. Although they retain the ultimate legal and ethical responsibility for the operation of the organization, generally the day-to-day operation is delegated to the administrator. The board's main function is to set general policies and to plan for the long-range development of the organization. Most boards become directly involved in the facility's operations only when there is a crisis, such as a financial shortfall or a major lawsuit.

The administrator is usually the highest ranking member of the hierarchy who actually becomes involved in the daily operation of the facility. The administrator has the education and knowledge required to direct the highly complex and technologically advanced elements that are an essential part of today's health-care system.

In most health care facilities, the medical staff also exerts a great deal of control over the governance structure. The medical staff also has its own internal governance structure with higher- and lower-level members. Traditionally, the physicians in a facility had a great deal of influence in the facility because they were neither employed nor controlled by the facility. However, the advent and spread of managed care has markedly altered the traditional physician-institution relationship in many facilities. In a managed care setting, physicians are hired and salaried employees just like nurses, housekeepers, administrators, or security personnel. Their practice and productivity are monitored and evaluated, and they can be terminated from the facility for poor performance.

Nurses' Role in Governance

In the recent past, nurses had little say in the governance of their facility or agency. Because of their traditional ideology of professionalism, nurses were more oriented toward loyalty and respect than autonomy of practice and independent decision making about the quality of care.[1] Nurses often accepted the work hours assigned to them without question, withstood disrespect and abuse from physicians and administrators as part of the work environment, and were satisfied with the meager salaries paid to them because theirs was a profession of caring and dedication. This situation has, however, changed drastically since the 1970s.

Self-governance is a concept that is important to all professions. The most powerful professional groups are those that maintain a strong sense of self-governance for their members. The American Medical Association (AMA) is a classic example of the power that an organized group can exert. Much of the physicians' power to affect institutional governance, and even broader issues such as managed care, comes from the AMA. Membership in a powerful organization can be an alternative to unions. Up to this time, the ANA has split its activities and focus between self-governance and collective bargaining. It has been successful in most of its efforts at collective bargaining but somewhat limited in its success for self-governance.

As nursing responsibilities increased with advancing technology and changes in the health-care system, nurses began to recognize that their responsibilities far exceeded their authority to influence their practice. They started to view professional autonomy, authority, and accountability as essential elements in high-quality client care. One approach to gaining these elements was to change the organizational structure of the health-care facilities where they were employed.

Nurses have challenged the traditional governance structure at a number of levels with varying amounts of success. Nursing service administrators are the leaders of the largest single group of health-care professionals in most health-care organizations—generally about 50 percent of all the employees.[2] Because of their education and experience, many nursing administrators have moved into positions of power in the health-care system and are no longer willing to accept the traditional role to which nurses were relegated. As middle managers, nursing administrators are often caught in the middle of conflicting expectations. For example, the chief administrator may want to cut the budget by reducing staffing, whereas the nurses on the units recognize that they can no longer provide high-quality nursing care because the staffing levels are already too low.

Staff RNs often view themselves as located at the bottom of the hierarchy with very little power. This is rarely the case. Depending on the organization of the facility, RNs have positional authority over LPNs, nursing assistants, and individuals from the laboratory and radiology department.

Nurses have gained greater control over their practice by fostering change in the organizational structures of health-care facilities and agencies. The changes include decentralization of authority, identification of professional nurses as peers, agreement on the philosophy and goals of nursing care, and increased responsibility for directing and planning the care given to clients while they are in the facility.[10]

Alternative Models for Governance

In an attempt to redistribute power and authority within health-care organizations, several alternative forms of governance have been developed. Some of these work better than others, depending on the facility and the willingness of the individuals involved to cooperate.

Board of Nursing Model

In this model of governance, the nursing staff structure is similar to the medical staff structure. There is a general board of trustees at the top and, immediately below, at the same level, a medical board of directors, a nursing board of directors, a board of directors representing other professionals, and the hospital administration itself.[2] The nursing board of directors deals with such matters as credentials and standards of care and also promotes cooperation between nurses and the other professionals of the facility. Although this type of structure places nurses on an equal administrative footing with the physicians, administration, and other professionals in the facility, it does have the tendency to create a large number of administrative personnel. A tendency for conflicts to arise between the different board members does exist.

> *Nurses have gained greater control over their practice by fostering change in the organizational structures of health-care facilities and agencies. The changes include decentralization of authority, identification of professional nurses as peers, agreement on the philosophy and goals of nursing care, and increased responsibility for directing and planning the care given to clients while they are in the facility.*

Contracting for Nursing Services Model

The **fee-for-service** model proposes that clients be billed for nursing care as a separate item, much the same way that they are billed for medical care by the physicians. Currently, when a client receives a hospital bill, the care provided by nurses is included in the overall room charge. In order to make this model work, nurses select individual clients for whom they wish to care and then accept responsibility for providing that care. Some type of scale would need to be developed so that the nurse could charge a higher rate for taking care of more seriously ill clients with more complex health-care needs. Nurses would take responsibility for scheduling and for self-management. And as with physicians, there would have to be a **peer review** mechanism to monitor the quality of health care provided.

Although this model supports primary care and the expansion of the nurse's role and responsibility, it would be very difficult to implement. Some of the problems include establishing acceptable pay scales, ensuring adequate staffing, and paying ancillary help such as orderlies and nursing assistants. Probably the most significant single factor that affects the implementation of this model is the hospital administration's loss of control over the nursing staff. If the nurses' pay were to come directly from the client, rather than the hospital, nurses would tend to place the client's needs before the needs of the facility. This model is still unacceptable to most facilities.

Shared Governance Model

In the shared governance model, power and authority are transferred to the nursing staff rather than being seated primarily in nursing administration. The key to shared governance is decentralization of the nursing administration structure. Its goal is to involve professional nurses in the decision-making process at all levels to ensure that their knowledge and expertise are used to deliver the highest quality care possible.[1]

Shared governance allows the nurse autonomy in decisions about nursing practice, working conditions, staffing levels, standards of care, and other areas. It gives professional nurses the chance to be held accountable and responsible for their clinical judgment and the care they give to clients. It allows their peers a chance to recognize their knowledge and competence as true health-care professionals.

In general, shared governance locates the source of power in the clinical areas rather than in the **administrative** areas. Several different types of shared governance exist.

In the congressional shared governance model, a group of professional nurses is organized into a congress. This congress develops bylaws, elects representatives, and forms committees to govern the activities of the nursing staff.[9] Composed entirely of professional nurses, the committees oversee professional practice, evaluate quality of care, provide continuing education, plan for staffing, conduct research, and discipline errant nurses. Although this is a highly effective method to provide nursing care and to increase the autonomy of nurses, it does require a tremendous initial expenditure of time, effort, and money. Many institutions are not willing to make that commitment.

In the unit-based model, the shared governance is on a smaller scale. Groups of nurses on each unit form councils for professional practice that perform many of the functions that the professional congresses perform. In order to make this model succeed, there must be a real transfer of decision-making power from the head nurse or unit supervisor to the staff nurses.

Shared governance is a model that the staff is willing to undertake, rather than being forced into it by the administration. Unfortunately, many facilities that profess a shared governance structure really are using a traditional hierarchy structure with somewhat more open lines of communication.

Shared governance is a model that the staff is willing to undertake, rather than being forced into it by the administration. Unfortunately, many facilities that profess a shared governance structure really are using a traditional hierarchy structure with somewhat more open lines of communication. The test of a true shared governance model quickly becomes evident when difficult decisions have to be made. For example, if the staff nurses decide that more staffing is needed for their unit, but the administration refuses to make money available for new nurses, then it is not a true shared governance model.

Governance and Collective Bargaining

Forms of governance directly affect which issues are likely to be involved in nurses' collective bargaining. Although salary and benefits are important considerations in professional nursing, issues of autonomy, accountability, and control of practice are gaining importance for many nurses. In a health-care facility with a form of governance that allows nurses to have a relatively large degree of control over their practice, the issues discussed at the bargaining table are more likely to revolve around a professional agenda. In facilities with a rigidly structured hierarchy of authority that gives nurses little autonomy, accountability, or control over their practice, collective bargaining is more likely to center on control and power issues.

Nurses are highly educated professionals. They recognize that they can practice autonomously and can make sound decisions about client care. They also recognize that an increased understanding of the governance process requires many of the same skills used in collective bargaining. Key elements in both processes are an understanding of negotiation, compromise, and consensus building to attain one's goals. Changes in methods of governance also will require major changes in the health-care system. Professional nurses have the power to produce those changes and the ability to deal with the future of health care successfully.

ISSUES IN PRACTICE

Deciding to Go on Strike

Sharon S., RN, was completing her charting on another busy 3 P.M. to 11 P.M. shift. While she was walking down the hall toward the time clock, she wondered who would be taking her place for the rest of the week. Like most of the other nurses at the Medical Center, she had decided to go on strike starting with the 7 A.M. to 3 P.M. shift the next day. The decision to strike had not been an easy one and had been reached only after much discussion (arguments?), many hours of meetings and conferences with the hospital negotiators, and animated discussion among the nurses' negotiating team.

Sharon could see both positive and negative sides to a strike. On the positive side, increased salaries, better fringe benefits, and improvements in working conditions and staffing would be a plus for all the nurses and clients at the Medical Center. Sharon herself had felt increasingly stressed during the past year because of the hospital's measures to reorganize. From what Sharon was able to see, reorganization meant saving money by cutting professional staff and partially replacing them with less-trained, unlicensed individuals. This pattern of restaffing had led to longer hours, increased responsibilities for the RNs, and fewer support services. She also felt that the overall quality of care had decreased noticeably.

On the negative side, Sharon was experiencing a real ethical and emotional dilemma about going on strike. The quality of care was sure to deteriorate even further because of the reduced services caused by the strike. Was it really fair to decrease the services and care for clients who had nothing to do with the issues that brought on the strike? Of course, during the past 3 days, the clients who had been well enough were sent home early in anticipation of the strike. Some whose conditions were too complicated for them to be cared for at home were sent to other facilities. The hospital had severely restricted admissions, reducing the census to an all-time low.

Yet there were several clients who were too ill to transfer or send home. Mrs. Anderson, a 78-year-old client with renal failure, congestive heart failure, and a recent colostomy for a bowel obstruction, came to mind. Mrs. Anderson and a number of other clients like her, who had no family nearby and few resources, were highly dependent on the nursing staff to meet their needs of care. Mrs. Anderson was just beginning to be taught how to care for her colostomy. Even if she was discharged to a nursing home, there was no way to ensure that she could receive the teaching needed for her eventual self-care. Although there was to be a skeleton crew of nurses left in the facility, they would be stretched very thin in trying to care for the remaining clients.

Sharon also thought about the ANA Code of Ethics for Nurses she had been taught in nursing school, particularly the passage that stated "the nurse participates in the profession's effort to establish and maintain conditions of employment conducive to high-quality nursing care." The reason for the strike was to bring about improved working conditions that would benefit future clients in the hospital. But should these measures be carried out when nursing services were already operating at a reduced level of care and at a minimal level of safety? Didn't that somehow contradict the first statement in the Code, that "the nurse provides services with respect for human dignity"? When Mrs. Anderson was admitted to the hospital 4 days before, she came with the expectation of the best possible care under any circumstances. The Code seemed to have a split personality on strikes. While calling for service to the profession to maintain high standards and quality of care, the Code also insisted that the health, welfare, and safety of the clients should be the nurse's first consideration.

What should Sharon do? Does the overall welfare of the profession ever supersede the obligation to provide client care?

Conclusion

Although few issues elicit such strong emotions among nurses as collective bargaining, it is a reality in today's health-care system. Nurses are beginning to realize that they are not in a strictly altruistic profession, but rather one in which they use their knowledge and skills to provide high-quality services to clients. The knowledge and skills used in client care are gained at the cost of years of expensive education in schools of nursing and of dedication to an often underappreciated profession. Nurses no longer need to apologize or feel guilty about seeking payment for their work on a level commensurate with their knowledge and skills.

Negotiation is the process of give and take between groups with the goal of reaching an agreement acceptable to both sides. Negotiations may be formal or informal, hostile or friendly. A cooperative atmosphere fostered by both sides that recognizes the similarity of each side's demands will be the most productive in reaching a satisfactory contract.

Although not a new concept for nursing, collective bargaining is an issue that is still hotly debated among professional nurses. Collective bargaining is viewed by some as unprofessional, unethical, divisive, and a fundamental threat to job security. However, the goals of collective bargaining, including improvement of economic benefits, better staffing and scheduling, fair treatment for all nurses, and improved quality of care for clients, are common to all health-care providers. Nurses must decide at some point in their careers whether joining a collective bargaining unit will best help them to achieve these goals. This is not an easy decision to make, and each nurse should gather as much information as possible about the situation before making a decision.

Nurses need to recognize that the time has arrived to elevate the profession to a new level. Change in forms of governance is one method that nurses can use to change the health-care system. Nursing as a profession now has the opportunity to gain tremendous power and take its rightful place as an indispensable force in the health-care system. All that is required is for nurses to become educated in the issues involved and to take an aggressive stance in the shaping of the future.

Critical Thinking Exercises

- Develop a position paper either supporting or opposing collective bargaining.
- A nurse on your unit states one day: "Membership in the state nurses association is a waste of time and money. They can't help you make a better living!" How would you respond to this nurse?
- Develop an ideal contract for nurses. Which elements would receive the highest priority?
- Develop a plan for shared governance in a facility you are familiar with. How would the organizational process take place? What are some of the major difficulties in developing this plan?

References

1. O'Grady, P: Collective bargaining: The union as partner. Nursing Management 32(6):30–32, 2001.
2. Tappen, RM: Nursing Leadership and Management, ed. 4. FA Davis, Philadelphia, 2001.
3. Abelson, R: With nurses in short supply, patient load becomes a big issue. New York Times, May 7, 2002. Available at: www.newyorktimes.com.
4. DeMass-Martin, S: Striking nurses win from coast to coast. American Nurse 34(2):8–10, 2002.
5. Gray, W: Clinical governance: Combining clinical and management supervision. Nursing Management 32(6):14–17, 2001.
6. Tappen, RM, et al: Essentials of Nursing Leadership and Management, ed. 2. FA Davis, Philadelphia, 2001.
7. Bissett, L: Perspectives in leadership: The manager's list. Nursing Spectrum 5(2):9, 2001.
8. Costa, L: As union activity surges, it pays to be alert to workplace disruptions. Patient Care Management 16(4):10–11, 2001.
9. McKeown, C, and Thompson, J: Clinical governance: Implementing clinical supervision. Nursing Management 8(6):10–13, 2001.
10. Stephenson, C: Management function analysis: Learning from the expert. Nursing Forum 36(3):9–11, 2001.

Bibliography

Costa, L: As union activity surges, it pays to be alert to reduce workplace disruptions. Patient Care Management 16(4):10–11, 2001.

Cross, LL: Protected whistle-blowing or a legal firing? The Oklahoma Nurse 47(1):14–16, 2002.

DeMass-Martin, S: Striking nurses win from coast to coast. American Nurse 34(2):8–10, 2002.

Kennedy, MS, et al: To supervise of unionize? That is the question: A Supreme Court ruling may limit nurses' ability to form unions. Am J Nurs 101(8):21, 2001.

Oregon nurses strike for pay, health care. American Nurse 34(1):7, 2002.

Tammelleo, AD: Do union contracts preempt emotional distress claims? Nursing Law's Reagan Report 42(2):1, 2001.

Trossman, S: Illinois nurse loses job for helping Sept. 11 victims. American Nurse 34(1):1–2, 2002.

UAN advocates of patients and nursing practice. Oregon Nurse 66(3):9, 2001.

16

The Health-Care Delivery System

Deborah L. Finfgeld

Learning Objectives

After completing this chapter, the reader will be able to:

- Analyze the evolution of the health-care delivery system in the United States.
- Evaluate the factors that are influencing the evolution of the health-care delivery system.
- Synthesize the concerns surrounding the uninsured in this country.
- Analyze industry efforts to manage health-care costs.
- Evaluate the efforts being made to ensure quality cost-effective health care.

Historically, hospitals were thought of as places where people went to die. As technology evolved and the growing pharmaceutical industry began to offer lifesaving medications, hospitals evolved into acute care facilities where people went to be treated, cared for, and recover from illness. Gradually, acute care of the sick, which is known as **secondary intervention**, was moved from the home to the hospital setting.

Another layer of care developed when technology provided the resources necessary to perform advanced procedures, such as open-heart surgery and organ transplants. To meet the demand for these types of interventions, centralized hospitals offering advanced services were developed to draw clients from large geographical areas. These facilities provide what are known as **tertiary interventions**. Unfortunately, as tertiary and acute care facilities became more popular, less attention was devoted to **primary intervention**, which focuses on health promotion, illness prevention, early diagnosis, and treatment of common health problems.

To a great extent, delivery of health care became centralized within hospitals, where professionals were thought to hold the key to well-being through technology. Individual responsibility was minimized, and concerns about cost were diminished because **third-party reimbursers** were responsible for paying a large proportion of the bills. Health care was essentially removed from the hands of consumers, and clients' needs became secondary in an expansive, expensive, and highly technical system.

Consumers, health-care providers, and third-party reimbursers remained relatively satisfied with this system until it became obvious that health-care costs were out of control and millions of Americans had little or no access to care. It also became evident that failure to focus on promoting health and preventing illness was resulting in countless cases of unnecessary suffering and death. To solve these problems, the health-care industry is gradually moving toward a decentralized system in which more and more care is being provided on an outpatient basis; emphasis is being placed on health promotion, illness prevention, and responsible self-care practices; and health-care providers are implementing cost-containment measures (Table 16–1). Within today's highly competitive marketplace, health care is being provided in a more coordinated and comprehensive manner along the wellness to illness and acute to chronic continua.

During the current period of rapid change, provider roles and reimbursement practices are being drastically overhauled. It is important for nursing students to understand these changes in the health-care delivery system to ensure that their services will be fully used and that their ability to function independently and autonomously is protected. In addition, third-party reimbursers must be cognizant of the important role that nurses fulfill and the importance of fair reimbursement practices.

Demographics Affecting the Health-Care Delivery System

Age

Between now and the year 2050, the number of persons 65 years of age or older is expected to double, so that by 2050, one in five Americans will be elderly, and their numbers will reach an estimated 80 million.[1] Of this number, many will eventually become more dependent on the health-care delivery system as a result of chronic health problems.

Although aging Americans constitute a sizable number of persons who will potentially require expensive long-term health care, their community activism and powerful influence at the ballot box may provide them with better access to health care than other less vocal and politically savvy groups. Additional at-risk groups consist of persons residing in urban areas with limited incomes as well as individuals living in remote rural areas where access to care is limited.

Chronicity

Another factor that is influencing the climate of health-care delivery in the United States is the long-term and expensive nature of many health problems. Although significant strides have been

Table 16–1

Health-Care Delivery System Changes

FROM	TO
Hospital-based care	Community-based care
Acute care	Illness prevention, health promotion, long-term and rehabilitative care
Incidental fragmented care	Comprehensive, continuous, coordinated care
Patients as passive participants	Patients assuming responsibility for self-care with support of family members
Expensive high-tech care	Cost-effective care provided at an appropriate level
Health-care delivery system	Competitive health-care marketplace monopoly
Service use increases profits	Service use decreases profits

made in the treatment of some acute infectious diseases, many challenges still exist in the management of health concerns such as cancer, heart disease, Alzheimer's disease, diabetes, chronic obstructive lung disease, and human immunodeficiency virus (HIV). Additional concerns include environmental and occupational safety, drug abuse, and mother and child health care.

Health Promotion

In light of the health problems that were faced in the late twentieth century, the United States Department of Health and Human Services (DHHS) outlined proactive strategies for the year 2000 and beyond in the areas of health promotion, protection, and prevention. **Health promotion** priorities include physical fitness, adequate nutrition, reduced use of tobacco and other harmful substances, family planning, preservation of mental health, avoidance of violence and abusive behavior, and community support services. Health protection priorities include reduced numbers of accidents, occupational safety and health, improved oral health, improved environmental quality, and food and drug quality.[2]

Between now and the year 2050, the number of persons 65 years of age or older is expected to double so that by 2050, one in five Americans will be elderly, and their numbers will reach an estimated 80 million.

In addition, mother and child health, heart disease, stroke, cancer, sexually transmitted diseases, HIV, and other infectious diseases were targeted for new preventive strategies. Finally, emphasis was placed on access to health-care services and the importance of individual, family, employer, community, and government responsibility in improving the profile of the nation's health.

In the mid-1990s, the DHHS reported that 8 percent of these stated objectives had been reached, and progress was being made toward another 40 percent. The greatest progress had been made in heart disease, stroke, cancer, and unintentional injuries. However, in 18 percent of the targeted areas, there had actually been a decline in rate of goal achievement.[3] Areas in which there was movement away from the target objectives included diabetes and other chronic conditions, occupational safety and health, physical activity, mental health and mental disorders, and violence and abusive behavior. Finally, the gap between infant mortality among minority and nonminority groups widened, with minorities experiencing an increasing number of infant deaths.

Managed Care

Managed care is a term used to describe health-care services that are administered to enhance their efficient and effective use. The primary purpose of these business ventures is to deliver, finance, buy, and sell quality health-care services as economically as possible. In theory, costs are limited by reducing the number of hospitalizations, decreasing the length of inpatient stays, providing more home care, and offering health promotion and illness prevention services.

One way that managed care is being enacted is through the use of precertification. **Precertification** requires that health-care **providers** receive preapproval from third-party reimbursers for a plan of care before it is initiated. This practice enables managed care organizations to cut costs by eliminating unnecessary procedures and encouraging practitioners to adhere to efficacious practice guidelines. Precertification approval also assures the client and provider that expenses will be covered. Nurses are frequently responsible for communicating with reimbursers

Table 16–2

Comparison of Indemnity Insurance and Some Managed Care Options

	INDEMNITY INSURANCE	HMO	IPA (HMO)	PPO
Copayment	Yes	Nominal	Nominal	Varies
Fee for service	Yes	No	Yes	Yes
Limited number of providers	No	Yes	Yes	Yes
Out-of-plan provider option	N/A	Emergencies only	Emergencies only	Penalty applies
Utilization guidelines	No	Yes	Yes	Yes

to solicit precertification approval for a treatment plan. Although precertification is in widespread use, disconcerting questions loom regarding potential conflicts of interest. These conflicts include the impact that financial analysts have on making health-care decisions based on cost.

The actual advantages of managed care systems have yet to be fully determined owing to a lack of data that fully reflect actual health-care outcomes and the comprehensive cost of health promotion, illness activities, and home care services. The total cost of administering a comprehensive managed care system, which services the chronically ill with complex health problems as well as healthy individuals who merely access the system for acute care, is yet to be determined.

Managed care systems consist of administrators, providers, and the physical facilities in which health care is delivered. Many times hospitals are the focal point of managed care organizations, with ancillary services providing an array of complementary care. These delivery systems are of interest to nurses, particularly advanced practice nurses, because of the autonomous practice opportunities they offer.

Several different administrative structures are characteristic of managed care arrangements.

What Do You Think?

Are you currently covered by a health-care plan? How would you rate it? How do you pay for your health care?

Some of the more common structures include **health maintenance organizations (HMOs)**, **independent practice associations (IPAs)**, **independent practice organizations (IPOs)**, **preferred provider organizations (PPOs)**, and **point-of-service (POS) plans** (Table 16–2). It should be noted that these systems are in a state of flux, and efforts are continually being made to refine them. To reduce costs, private insurance companies have had a major role in encouraging their development.

Health Maintenance Organizations

HMOs can be organized according to one of two ways: the staff model and the group model. In the staff model, the employees of the HMO both provide health-care services and function as administrative personnel to supervise and manage the organization. With the group model, there is a medical group that accepts a contract from an HMO to provide health-care services for its participants. The administrative functions are carried out by individuals from the HMO's own administrative staff. Regardless of their structures, the primary purpose of HMOs is to ensure profits by decreasing referrals to specialists, restricting diagnostic studies, decreasing client hospitalizations, reducing lengths of hospital stays, and using a capitated payment system.

In a **capitated payment system**, participants pay a flat rate, usually through their employer, to belong to an HMO for a prescribed period of time.

Expenses incurred by the HMO in excess of the capitated rate during the contract period are considered financial losses. Amounts that remain after services have been rendered and costs have been covered are profit. In short, health-care practitioners who function within an HMO have strong incentives to keep costs down and ensure profits. The uniqueness of this system is that health-care providers share in the financial risk. The ideal HMO is one in which there is a large pool of healthy members who require few services and relatively few unhealthy clients who require more and expensive care.

HMOs appear attractive to clients for two reasons. First, after premiums are paid, care is free or requires only a small copayment if a designated HMO provider is used. Second, cost-containment incentives are in place to keep expenses down. Less attractive aspects of HMOs include a limited number of providers under contract at any one time. Clients must select a practitioner from a list of providers (**provider panel**) that may exclude the client's preferred clinician. If individuals choose to use providers who are not included in their HMO's panel, they must pay for those services themselves. The only exception is in emergency situations, such as when an individual is injured in a car accident away from home.

Independent Practice Associations

A variation of the traditional HMO is the IPA, which is usually organized by physicians. Within this structure, HMOs contract with physicians and hospitals to provide care for their members. Physicians are paid on a fee-for-service basis at rates that are usually predetermined and attractive to payers. **Fee for service** means that IPA members are charged for each service at the time care is provided, unlike most HMO plans, in which members pay premiums and are not charged for each service individually. As with traditional HMOs, IPAs do not reimburse for payments to nonmember providers. Finally, hospitals and physicians must adhere to **utilization guidelines** to contain costs, which limit the number of services they can provide. Independent practice organizations (IPOs) are a variation of IPAs in which a group of providers deals with more than one payer at a time.

Preferred Provider Organizations

PPOs are another type of managed care organization that can be sponsored by providers, insurance companies, or employers. Contracts are established with a limited number of health-care facilities and professionals, and lower-than-customary rates are usually negotiated. In an attempt to contain costs, providers are required to adhere to PPO utilization guidelines. In return for these concessions, provider services are used by greater numbers of clients.

Within PPO systems, physicians are reimbursed on a fee-for-service basis and members are charged each time care is provided. In addition to the fee-for-service arrangement, some PPO plans require participant copayments in which individuals pay a percentage of the cost of services. The copayment requirement is thought to decrease client use and thus reduce costs.

A critical difference between HMO and PPO plans is that use of the PPO providers is encouraged through preferential rates; however, benefits extend beyond the use of these services. Penalties apply if providers are used outside of the PPO, but their use is not prohibited.

Point-of-service (POS) plans are similar to the PPOs, in that they allow clients to access designated practitioners outside the prescribed panel of providers for an additional fee. This option is provided to ensure comprehensive care. Americans have traditionally valued the freedom to choose their health-care providers, making

PPOs and POS options more popular than traditional HMO plans.

Current and Future Managed Care

One of the primary goals of managed care is to reduce costs. Studies suggest that this goal is being achieved in some instances as a result of fewer hospital admissions, shortened lengths of stay, and expanded home care services. In spite of these optimistic projections, health-care expenditures continue to rise at a rate higher than inflation.

Additional expenses that may not have been accounted for in this total include the comprehensive costs of running managed care operations and the actual price of providing care in the home. The problem of determining home care costs stems from the fact that a standardized and accurate system for pricing, billing, and reimbursement is still in the state of development. As solutions to these problems emerge, the overall effectiveness of managed care will be more clearly determined and the health-care delivery system will continue to evolve.

For most consumers, as well as many health-care providers, the current health-care delivery system has become a confusing alphabet soup of options, some of which include HMOs, IPAs, IPOs, PPOs, and POS plans. Health-care providers need to remain informed about health-care delivery options to ensure the best possible practice environments and to promote the most efficacious and cost-effective delivery system for clients. It is also important to be knowledgeable about these issues in order to talk informatively to legislators and make wise decisions at the ballot box.

Issues that still require resolution include the following: Should privatization of the health-care delivery system be continued, with an emphasis on fewer and less confusing options? Will increased government-controlled interventions make the health-care system more cohesive and comprehensive? Should the current dual-track system, consisting of government and private sector options, be maintained but with the goal of streamlining the system? Health-care providers need to become involved in these issues and can play an important part in the transformation process occurring in the health-care system.

In the current health-care system, managed care has become a primary model for care delivery in an attempt to hold down health-care costs. Many health-care insurers have woven managed care into their payment programs, ranging from restricting the medications that can be prescribed to designating where the client can receive care and what procedures are deemed unnecessary. Although managed care programs began with the idea that keeping clients healthy would reduce health-care costs, they are finding it increasing difficulty to achieve that goal as the population ages and more and more clients are being treated for long-term serious illnesses.

Costs

Rising costs are also affecting health-care delivery in this country. In 2001, health-care spending exceeded $1.3 trillion, which represents an average of $4608 per person in the United States. Although overwhelming, these figures actually reflect a slowdown in the overall annual increase in spending to less than 5 percent.[4]

Many factors account for this spending pattern. Among them is the way third-party payers customarily reimbursed health-care services with little attention paid to cost-control measures. Other factors include the high cost of innovative technology, the increased need for long-term care, providers who have not always delivered care in the most cost-conscious manner, care provided to uninsured individuals, and the limited ability and motivation of consumers to compare health-care prices.

Who Pays for Health Care?

There is no simple answer to the question of who pays for health care. The health-care system currently in use is one of the most fiscally complex health-care systems in the world. Paying for health care involves all levels of government, private enterprise, and innovative commercial financing structures.

As of 2002, approximately 68.4 percent of Americans have some kind of private health insurance.

It is important to be familiar with health-care reimbursement practices for several reasons. Judgments about whether or not to perform diagnostic tests or to use certain treatment strategies are sometimes based on third-party payer guidelines. Decisions relating to how long a client is allowed to stay in a care facility are frequently determined by reimbursement policies. Plans of care based purely on financial incentives may raise legal and ethical questions.

The type of care individuals seek depends to some degree on the health-care benefits they have. For example, it is common for people who lack adequate coverage to seek care in an emergency department rather than using more economical primary care agencies such as community health centers or physicians' offices.

As client advocates, nurses must understand reimbursement practices in order to offer clients appropriate advice and to make necessary referrals. Finally, advanced practice nurses need to understand reimbursement practices so that they can confidently negotiate fair salaries for themselves and lobby for appropriate reimbursement legislation.

Private Health-Care Insurance

As of 2002, approximately 68.4 percent of Americans have some kind of private health insurance.[5] These plans are most commonly offered by employers and are **retrospective payment systems** based on actual care rendered. This type of insurance is often used by the working population and covers more than 34 percent of hospital costs, 47 percent of physician services, and 47 percent of dental services. These policies cover a much smaller proportion of home care (13 percent) and nursing home expenses (3 percent).[5] An attractive aspect of most private health insurance is that the consumer can choose any health-care facility or physician and still receive the same insurance benefit. Private health insurance is offered through two primary mechanisms: commercial insurance companies and Blue Cross and Blue Shield.

Blue Cross and Blue Shield

Blue Cross and Blue Shield plans evolved during the Great Depression. Financial hardships among the rich resulted in fewer philanthropic donations, and nonprofit hospitals were forced to seek out new sources of revenue. The Blue Cross plan was sponsored by hospitals, and subscribers received hospital services in exchange for their **premiums**, hence the term **point-of-service plans**. Physicians became involved when they saw an opportunity to guarantee payment for their services and to deter the government-sponsored national health insurance movement. As a result, Blue Shield coverage became readily available.

From the beginning of the Blue Cross and Blue Shield programs, the physician's role in managing these plans raised questions. Traditionally, Blue Cross was controlled by hospital boards, which consisted mainly of physicians. Likewise, physicians made up a large percentage of the Blue Shield governing bodies. Moreover, physicians on Blue Cross and Blue Shield boards also frequently administered federal Medicare and state Medicaid programs.

In short, those receiving payments had the most control over establishing prices. In recent years, sensitivity to this conflict of interest has led to an increased number of community representatives on Blue Cross and Blue Shield boards and in more private insurance companies administering these programs.

Another criticism of Blue Cross and Blue Shield plans is that they have traditionally been oriented toward treating illness, with little emphasis placed on health promotion or illness prevention. Because of their size, Blue Cross and Blue Shield have had a significant impact on health-care legislation, but unfortunately, they have not led the way toward a primary health-care focus.

Commercial Insurance Companies

Commercial insurance companies, such as Metropolitan Life, Travelers, and Aetna, gained popularity after World War II, when unions began to promote benefit packages in lieu of wage increases. A common feature of these **indemnity insurance** plans is that the client is responsible for a copayment. **Copayments** are charges the client is expected to pay when services are rendered. The insurer then directly reimburses either the consumer or provider for the balance of charges. Traditionally, these companies have avoided introducing cost controls except in cases where there appeared to be excessive use or abuse of services.

Unlike most traditional Blue Cross and Blue Shield companies, commercial insurance companies are **for-profit**, versus **not-for-profit**, and surplus income is paid to shareholders rather than automatically put back into the operating budget of the company. For-profit status raises concerns for some in that loyalties to stockholders may be perceived as more important than providing the highest quality care possible to clients. In spite of this concern, more and more Blue Cross and Blue Shield companies have been moving toward for-profit status in recent years.

Self-Insurance Arrangements

In an attempt to reduce costs, approximately 75 percent of the larger employers in this country are choosing to become self-insured. This means that businesses are taking on the financial risk of offering their own self-funded health-care plans.

Employers perceive that there are several advantages to self-funded plans. First, under the **Employee Retirement Income Security Act (ERISA)** of 1974, outside regulators who supervise private insurance plans are eliminated. Second, employer self-funded plans are shielded from state regulations and can act as a tax shelter for the company. As a result of these exclusions, the cost of insuring employees is reduced.

Despite the advantages of self-insured plans, authorities have expressed concern about the lack of regulation and consumer protection. Although employers may fabricate other reasons for not hiring someone, there is the possibility that they may reject potential employees based on existing health problems, although this practice has become much more difficult under the Americans with Disabilities Act. However, the question remains whether these types of criteria should determine the nation's workforce.

Government-Funded Health Care

The creation of Blue Cross and Blue Shield in the 1930s only temporarily slowed the movement toward government involvement in health-care financing. By the mid-1960s, it became clear that changes needed to be made to ensure adequate health care for the elderly and the indigent. In 1965, legislation was passed that resulted in the establishment of the Medicare and Medicaid programs. Currently these two programs finance more than one-third of the nation's total health-care bill.

Medicare

Medicare is a federally run program that is financed primarily through employee payroll taxes. This program covers any individual who is 65 years of age or older as well as permanently disabled workers of any age and their qualifying dependents. In addition, persons with end-stage renal disease are covered under this plan.

Medicare consists of two parts. Part A of Medicare is free in most instances and covers acute hospital, nursing home, hospice, and home care services. Part B may be purchased for a monthly premium, and 97 percent of the individuals participating in Part A are enrolled in the program. Participants are covered for physician services, outpatient hospital care, laboratory tests, durable medical equipment, and certain other selected services. Although Medicare was designed for older Americans, long-term care is not covered, and health promotion and illness prevention benefits are limited. In addition, the cost of outpatient medications is not covered, which can account for a considerable portion of an elderly or disabled person's total monthly income. For this reason, it is estimated that a large majority of middle-income and upper-income individuals purchase private insurance, also known as **Medigap policies**, to cover these expenditures.

Medicare was originally designed so that many services were fully covered. This arrangement did not provide cost-containment incentives, nor was the cost-benefit ratio of services taken into consideration. For example, heroic and costly measures were used to extend life with little consideration given to the quality of that existence, precipitating a financial crisis that peaked in the middle 1980s. Since then, cost-control measures have been implemented.

In 1983, a **prospective payment system (PPS)** was implemented in which hospitals are reimbursed based on a fixed rate, with incentives to reduce the length of hospital stays. At the core of this program is a classification system made up of hundreds of **diagnosis-related groups (DRGs)**. Based on the particular DRG in which a client is placed, hospitals are reimbursed for a predetermined amount. In the event that a client is discharged early or costs are kept under the allotted amount, the hospital keeps the difference. In contrast, if a client's bill exceeds the maximum reimbursable amount, the hospital absorbs the cost.

What Do You Think?

Have you ever received services from advanced practice nurses? How would you rate their abilities and the care that they provide?

From the outset, developers of the DRG classification system feared that quality of care might be compromised in favor of cost containment. To prevent misuse of the DRG prospective payment system, the **Medicare Utilization and Quality Peer Review Organization (PRO)** was instituted. The purpose of this group is to ensure quality care and prevent misuse of the system.

Cost shifting has become a common practice since the implementation of the DRG prospective payment system. For example, to make up for lost revenues for clients on the DRG system; clients with other forms of insurance have been charged inflated amounts for health-care services. Reports of paying $7 or more for an aspirin tablet are not uncommon.[6]

Under the DRG prospective payment system, physician reimbursement remained untouched. Physicians continued to be reimbursed based on **customary, prevailing, and reasonable charges**. In other words, what physicians in a given geographical area normally charged is what they received for their services. If a physician charged more than the customary, prevailing, and reasonable rate for a service, he or she could bill the client for the remaining amount that Medicare did not pay. Attempts to control physician costs were resisted strongly by the American Medical Association (AMA), and as a result, between 1961 and 1991 the price of physician services increased more than sixfold.

In an attempt to contain physician costs, Congress passed legislation in 1989 to establish (1) a standardized physician reimbursement schedule, (2) limits on **out-of-pocket expenses** for clients, (3) ceilings on the volume of services provided by physicians annually, and (4) federal practice guidelines to identify the most effective and efficient means of managing client care.[6]

In part, because uniform practice guidelines were established, clinical nurse specialists (CNSs) and nurse practitioners (NPs) argued that, in addition to physicians, they too should receive direct Medicare reimbursement. Their rationale was that both advanced practice nurses (APNs) and physicians perform the same procedures using the same practice guidelines; thus, there should be no barriers to equitable and direct reimbursement for nurses. Thanks to the ardent efforts of many nurse lobbyists, Medicare legislation was passed in 1997 such that nurses now receive unrestricted Medicare reimbursement. In the past, only CNSs and NPs in rural areas could receive direct payments.

> *Medicare is currently in a state of change because of the enormous number of "baby boomers" who will soon become eligible for Medicare benefits and the diminishing numbers of individuals who will be supporting the program through payroll taxes.*

Medicare is currently in a state of change because of the enormous number of "baby boomers" who will soon become eligible for Medicare benefits and the diminishing numbers of individuals who will be supporting the program through payroll taxes. It is thought that to sustain the Medicare program in a similar form, national health-care insurance is inevitable. Many proponents of national health-care insurance point to the success that the Canadian health-care system has had. Even though Americans are divided on the issue of a national health-care system, Congress appears to be incrementally moving the country in this direction. For example, in an attempt to avoid Medicare fraud and cut costs, Congress passed legislation that severely penalizes physicians for accepting out-of-pocket payments for Medicare-reimbursable services. Physicians who accept such payments are subsequently ineligible to receive Medicare reimbursement for 2 years, a penalty that would seriously affect most practices.

This legislation has caused considerable confusion among the public, who perceives the Medicare program to be financially vulnerable but feels compelled to seek services within the parameters of the system. Individuals who have tried to provide insight into this situation suggest that this legislation is essentially a covert movement toward national health insurance. Other interesting developments that support this notion are overall growth rates in Medicare spending versus diminishing growth rates of employer-sponsored health insurance premiums and initiatives to lower the Medicare eligibility age from 65 to 55. Although purported to be self-supporting through participant premiums, this latter initiative has the potential to greatly increase costs and force total reform of the Medicare financing mechanism.

Although Medicare has traditionally been a fee-for-service benefit, and individuals have typically been able to freely choose their health-care providers, managed care initiatives have begun to change these practices. This is an example of a private sector initiative affecting a government program. The full impact of this trend is still unknown; however, it may foretell the emergence of a unique, albeit complex, reimbursement system that blends private and government reimbursement strategies. This trend also compels NPs and CNSs to join a **panel of approved providers** to ensure their reimbursement eligibility under Medicare.

Medicaid

Medicaid is a state-administered entitlement program that is designed to serve the poor. Funds are generated at the federal, state, and local levels; and each state has the freedom to customize its program based on the needs of its residents. Because the financial status of each state is different, Medicaid eligibility and services vary from place to place. States with more money tend to offer better benefit packages or cover more people than states that have limited resources. In fiscal year 1996, Medicaid paid out $147.7 billion for health services and supplies.

Services that are typically covered include hospitalization, diagnostic tests, physician visits, and rehabilitative and outpatient care. Medicaid often covers long-term nursing home costs after personal funds have been exhausted. States can opt to offer services such as home care, for which they receive federal matching funds. Because Medicaid covers the poor and may reimburse at relatively low levels, some practitioners are reluctant to treat patients covered under this program.

The uninsured tend to be from minority groups, less well educated, unemployed or working part-time, foreign born, poor, and between 18 and 24 years of age.

Although Medicaid was originally developed to serve the poor, some states are changing their eligibility requirements. In some areas of the country, individuals who are classified as medically indigent qualify for Medicaid benefits. **Medically indigent** refers to individuals who, if faced with medical expenses, would experience financial hardships. For all practical purposes, however, they are not considered poor. Some analysts have suggested that this is one more way in which health-care financing is moving toward a government-controlled system.

Managed care initiatives are beginning to have an impact on Medicaid programs, and participants in some states are being asked to select from a panel of approved providers rather than having unlimited freedom to choose a practitioner. Capitated versus fee-for-service payment systems are also being instituted. Unfortunately, direct reimbursement under Medicaid is not guaranteed to qualified nurses; thus, continued lobbying efforts are necessary on a state-by-state basis.

What Do You Think?

Is health care a right or a privilege? How would each one affect the cost of health care?

Uninsured

Despite what may appear to be a plethora of reimbursement options, it is estimated that there are well over 40 million U.S. citizens who currently have no health insurance.[7] It is a common misconception that these individuals receive adequate care through charitable donations. In reality, the insured receive 54 percent more ambulatory care services and 90 percent more hospital care than the uninsured.

The uninsured tend to be from minority groups, less well educated, unemployed or working part-time, foreign born, poor, and between 18 and 24 years of age. Employees of small businesses (fewer than 25 individuals) also tend to be less well insured. On the whole, white-collar workers have better health-care benefits than blue-collar workers and workers in service industries. Those in manufacturing still have relatively good benefits. Preexisting or long-term health problems can preclude some individuals from receiving coverage at reasonable rates. One of the reasons that the movement toward substantial health-care reform gained so much momentum during the 1990s was because of the large number of uninsured.

Group Practice Arrangements

A precursor to many of the ongoing changes in the health-care delivery system was the development of group practices. A **group practice** usually consists of three or more physicians, or nurse practitioners, who are formally organized to provide medical care. They distribute income according to a prearranged plan and jointly use equipment, records, and personnel.

Group practice arrangements are thought to be advantageous for a number of reasons. First, they preserve the ideal of private entrepreneurship while cutting overhead. Second, they are attractive to providers who prefer to hire professional managers. This arrangement enables practitioners to spend more time caring for clients and less time worrying about the mechanics of running a business. Group practice arrangements are also appealing because they offer providers more time off, better client coverage, and professional camaraderie. Finally, group practices frequently employ an array of specialists, and consumers are offered convenient, centralized, and comprehensive services. Because of these advantages, the number of group practices is continuing to increase.

Most group practices were originally set up such that individuals paid for services at the time care was rendered. As early as the 1890s, however, prepaid service contracts were offered by physicians working within group practices. Under these arrangements, potential clients prepaid a flat yearly fee in return for health-care services. At the time care was actually rendered, there were no additional costs to the client. As such, physicians were ensuring a certain level of income for the practice, but they were also accepting a calculated risk that they would procure enough prospective payments to generate a profit. In retrospect, these creative financing ventures foreshadowed current industry efforts to ensure a profitable health-care industry.

The Effect of the Nursing Shortage on Health-Care Costs

The origins of the current nursing shortage can be traced directly back to the implementation of managed care in the 1990s as a method of controlling health-care costs. Managed care companies required many procedures to be performed outside the hospital, leading to clients being sicker when they do enter the hospitals. In addition, health-care facilities trying to cut costs hired fewer expensive registered nurses (RNs) in favor of less-expensive personnel. Nursing service at most facilities is the largest single budget item, averaging between 50 and 60 percent of the overall operating budget. At first glance, this seemed like a promising way to control health-care cost, but in the long run it turned out to be a very expensive mistake. RNs who were employed in acute care settings moved in droves to the home-health-care and primary care settings. At the same time, the U.S. population was aging, resulting in a need for more nurses who can deliver high-quality specialized care in the acute care facilities. As a result, the health-care industry has seen a trend to closing hospital units because of a lack of RNs. It is estimated that a closed 20-bed general medical/surgical unit will cost a hospital approximately $3 million in lost revenue per year.

The nurses who remain are finding working conditions to be less than ideal. Mandatory overtime, short staffing, and increased client acuity all are adding to the stress that these nurses experience. As a result, they call in sick more often or leave for other facilities that have fewer demands. Sick time, recruitment, and orientation costs for many facilities have skyrocketed as a result.

The other area where health-care institutions feel the cost of the RN shortage is in lawsuits and rising insurance costs. During periods when there is a shortage of RNs, the quality of health care decreases, clients become dissatisfied with the care they are receiving, and serious mistakes are made in care, resulting in injury or death of clients. It only takes a relatively few of these cases with awards in the range of tens of millions of dollars to re-emphasize the correlation between RN care and quality care.

One proposed solution to the nursing shortage problem is the passage of mandatory staffing ratio laws (Box 16–1). Of course, hospital associations see these as increasing operating costs. However, the presumption is that more RNs will equate to higher quality of care and ultimately reduced long-range health-care costs. Currently

ISSUES NOW

More RNs Equals Better Care

To most people, it would seem logical to conclude that a hospital with more RNs would be able to provide higher quality care than a hospital with fewer RNs. However, some managers in the health-care industry have been refuting the logic behind this deduction.

A new study, funded primarily by the U.S. government, set out to determine whether there was a correlation between the RN-to-client staffing and the quality of the care provided. The massive study reviewed the outcomes of more than 6 million clients at some 799 hospitals in 11 states, 5 million of whom had medical problems and 1 million who had surgery.

The results show that in regard to certain elements of care, the presence of more RNs increased the quality of care. A comparison between those hospitals with the highest RN-to-client ratios as compared with those with the lowest RN-to-client ratios revealed the following results:

Client Care Area	Results of Increased RN Staffing
Length of stay (surgical)	Reduced by 3% to 5%
Postoperative complications	Reduced by 2% to 9%
Length of stay (medical)	Reduced by 3.5%
Urinary tract infections	Reduced by 9%
Gastrointestinal bleeding	Reduced by 5.1%
Pneumonia	Reduced by 6.4%
Cardiac arrest	Reduced by 9.4%
Survival after serious complications	Increased by 2.5%

This study is the latest and most comprehensive in a series of studies that looked at RN staffing ratios and client outcomes. It validates what the American Nurses Association has been saying since the early 1990s—that there is a direct correlation between the care provided by RNs and positive client outcomes. The American Hospital Association has formally acknowledged that RNs are key and critical to ensuring good client care. However, they still resist the move toward mandatory staffing ratios, characterizing them as an "oversimplistic" solution to a complex problem. It is evident, however, from this study that in hospitals with low numbers of RNs, clients are more likely to stay longer, suffer more complications, and die from complications that, if they were identified and treated sooner, would be survivable.

California and Florida have passed such laws. Nursing groups envision the mandatory staffing ratio laws as a way to solve staffing shortages by enticing inactive nurses or nurses who have sought employment in other health-care areas to return to the bedside in acute care facilities.

Not everyone, including some in the nursing profession, is convinced that enforced staff-to-client ratios will cure an ailing health-care system. One of the key issues is a lack of documented research that demonstrates that more RNs per clients equals higher quality care. Intuitively, it would seem that putting more RNs back into the hospital would improve client care, yet more than 3 years ago the Institute of Medicine identified a dearth of information about the quality of care being delivered in the nation's acute care facilities. The documentation and research have been painfully slow to develop. Leaders of the nursing profession hope that the new staffing ratio laws will help demonstrate the important and critical part nurses play in providing high-quality care.

Nursing groups envision the mandatory staffing ratio laws as a way to solve staffing shortages by enticing inactive nurses or nurses who have sought employment in other health-care areas to return to the bedside in acute care facilities.

Some in nursing are concerned that the managed care facilities will use the mandated staffing ratio as a ceiling number rather than the minimum number of nurses required to provide safe care. There is also a fear that the facilities will look only at the numbers and not at the educational, skill, and experience levels of the nurses they use to meet their quotas. Without consideration of the acuity of the clients on a unit and the care needs related to their illnesses, staffing ratios may actually lower the quality of care and threaten the safety of the clients. In addition, some fear that facilities that find the staffing ratio laws unworkable will merely close units where more acute clients are being treated, thus reducing access to care.

Some farsighted nursing leaders see the passage of staffing ratio laws as an important, but short-term solution to a much broader problem. Decreasing nurse-to-patient ratios are really just a symptom of a much more acute systemic problem in the health-care industry. The underlying problem revolves around an overly aggressive policy of cost cutting by managed care often at the expense of the very clients who are supporting the system with their insurance premiums. Passing staffing ratio laws may be a quick fix to an emotional and dramatic concern, but it does not address a much wider range of problems hospitalized clients face every day. What is needed to ultimately cure the industry is a long-range plan for systemic reform based on client needs, not the needs of a profit-motivated insurance industry.

Clients educated to understand what quality care is, and how it can best be achieved, will ultimately be the most powerful force for attaining the care they require. When managed care facilities begin to really listen to the clients they are supposed to be serving, nurse staffing ratio laws will no longer be necessary. The facilities will meet the quality expectations by making sure that however many nurses are needed are there to provide the care the client expects.

It is likely that other states will follow California's lead in mandating nurse-to-client ratios. At the beginning of 2000 there were 21 staffing-related bills that had been introduced in 15 states. Although these laws may not be the ultimate solution to a much deeper problem, at least clients in the states with staffing ratio laws will be reassured to know that they will have a well-educated, skilled professional nurse nearby who can act as an advocate for their needs and monitor the care they are receiving when they are most vulnerable.

Continuous Quality Improvement

Quality assurance initiatives are essential when efforts are being made to cut costs and, at the same time, maintain high standards of care. In order to ensure high-quality care, the health-care industry borrowed the philosophy of **continuous quality improvement (CQI)** from the busi-

Box 16–1

Hospital Administrators Square Off with Nurses Over Staffing

Recent data show that as many as 13% of hospital nursing jobs remain unfilled, particularly in acute care areas such as intensive care units, obstetric units, emergency departments, and general medical/surgical floors. As a result, many nurses report that they are caring for too many clients at a time and, subsequently, placing those clients at risk. Nurses feel that these working conditions are unacceptable and actually contribute to the nursing shortage by forcing nurses away from acute care to areas such as community health and home health care. Current statistics show that 41% of nurses work outside of the hospital setting, primarily because of the working conditions they experience in the hospitals.

Nursing organizations nationwide are pushing for contracts with hospitals that spell out specific nurse-to-client ratios. In states with more active and powerful nursing organizations, these efforts have been targeted at state legislatures with varying degrees of success.

In some extreme cases, nurses have gone on strike to make their point. Tenet Healthcare, the nation's second largest for-profit hospital chain, was sued in May 2002 for unsafe working environment. The nurses accused the chain of making them work through meal breaks without pay because they did not have enough staff to allow them leave the floor. Others, such as those nurses at St. Vincent's Hospital in Manhattan, held a protest march outside the hospital to accentuate their concerns.

Some hospital administrators are putting up resistance to the nursing efforts to increase staffing. They argue that fixed staffing ratios are really useless because of the great differences between hospitals and the clients they serve. They feel that they have the best vantage point to determine what the staffing ratios need to be and how to best use the employees. They also feel that there is nothing they can do to fill the nursing positions they have vacant because the nurses just are not there. They calculate the cost of meeting staffing ratios such as are found in the California legislation at $400 million per year, forcing them to cut services and close units.

Hospitals are reluctant to reveal how many nurses they have working on units or what the nurse-to-client ratio is for the whole facility. Many argue that ratios have very little relevance to the quality of care; however, the death of a client at Mount Sinai Medical Center in the liver transplant unit is an example of what can happen when nurses are assigned too many critically ill clients at a time. The results of a subsequent review by the State Health Department indicated that the there were not enough qualified nurses to care for the 34 transplant recipients who were on the unit at that time.

In facilities where hospital administration is willing to listen, amicable agreements have been reached. Nurses and management at Crouse Medical Center in Syracuse, New York, have been able to reach an agreement regarding staffing levels facility wide. Crouse has also agreed to pay nurses overtime when they are consistently asked to work in short-staffing situations. Northridge Hospital in Los Angeles negotiated an agreement with the nurses belonging to the Service Employees International Union to form committees to address staffing ratio issues. The agreement is similar to one that was implemented at 17 other California hospitals. The nation's largest nonprofit managed care provider, Kaiser Permanente, is using its staffing ratio plan as a recruitment tool for attracting nurses. They guarantee that no nurse will be assigned more than four clients on any of its general medical/surgical units. Although Kaiser estimates that the additional cost will be more than $200 million for staff per year, they expect to regain the costs in lower nurse turnover, less sick time, better client outcomes, and higher occupancy rates of their units.

There are no simple solutions to this problem. The rapidly changing face of health care is affected both by an aging population and the nursing shortage. It is a challenge to all nurses. However, working together with hospital administrators by pooling resources and sharing information can create a positive work environment and a place where nurses can achieve satisfying and long careers.

Source: Abelson, R: With nurses in short supply, patient load becomes a big issue. New York Times, May 6, 2002, Available at: www.newyorktimes.com.

ness world. The **Joint Commission on Accreditation of Healthcare Organizations (JCAHO)** was so impressed with its potential to improve health-care delivery that in 1994 it began requiring hospitals to implement CQI strategies.

CQI, also known as **total quality management (TQM)**, is based on the belief that the organization with the higher-quality service will capture a greater share of the market than competitors with lower-quality services. Emphasis is placed on not only meeting the expectations of the customer (in this case, the health-care consumer) but exceeding those expectations. Within the CQI philosophy, there are internal customers and external customers. The external customers are clients and their families; internal customers are individuals working within the health-care setting. Delivering high-quality services is valued above all else, and the ideal goal is that every constituent be completely satisfied with the services provided.

CQI requires that the process used to deliver services receive close and constant scrutiny, and everyone is encouraged to generate ideas for improving quality. Although change based on systematically documented evidence is encouraged, standardization of the process is also valued so that efficiency is maximized. CQI is proactively oriented so that the emphasis is placed on anticipating and preventing problems rather than reacting to them after the fact.

Nurses are in an excellent position to implement CQI strategies. On a daily basis, they assess how the health-care delivery system is functioning and the effectiveness of specific treatment approaches. For example, based on evidence that inexpensive saline is as effective as heparin in keeping intermittent intravenous catheters patent, nurses at one hospital implemented a new protocol and saved $70,000 within 1 year.[8]

Case Management Protocols

Another mechanism that has been instituted for monitoring cost-effective quality care has been outcomes-based case management protocols, also known as **clinical pathways**. The development of clinical pathways grew out of a need to assess, implement, and monitor cost-effective quality client care in a systematic manner. Clinical pathways were an outgrowth of nursing care plans but had the advantages of streamlining the charting process, encouraging documentation across multidisciplinary team members, and systematically monitoring variances from prescribed plans of care. The ability to identify how client care and progress varied from a predetermined plan enabled more accurate assessment of client care costs and maintenance of quality control measures. Integration of clinical pathways into practical usage has been enhanced by computerization of client records and on-line, bedside documentation.

Care Delivery

Outpatient Care

In recent years, several factors have led to greater demand for outpatient services, also known as alternative ambulatory services. First, implementation of the Medicare prospective payment system resulted in shorter hospital stays. Second, private insurers and managed care companies encouraged use of ambulatory versus inpatient services to reduce costs. Third, new technology made procedures that were formerly complicated or dangerous available on an outpatient basis. Finally, consumers demanded less expensive and more user-friendly health-care services.

Some hospitals are embedding themselves within a cluster of outpatient services. Others are establishing satellite clinics in surrounding suburbs and rural communities. Outpatient facilities are also cropping up in retail malls, where families can shop or eat lunch while significant others are receiving health-care services. Services commonly provided in ambulatory care settings include general medical examinations; treatment of injuries; diagnoses

ISSUES IN PRACTICE

Future Health-Care Costs Projected to Skyrocket

A report by the Health and Human Services' Centers for Medicare and Medicaid Services projected that in the year 2011 Americans will be spending approximately $9216 per person for health care—almost double the cost in 2000. The growth rate is estimated to be more than 7% per year between now and the year 2011.

The total cost of health care could reach $2.8 trillion, which represents about 17% of the gross national product, second only to defense spending. The report noted that the year 2000 marked the end of what was previously considered an era of reasonable health-care costs. The dramatic increases in cost are related to increased spending on prescription medications, hospital care, and long-term care. Additionally, hospitals and health-care providers have been able to attain an increased bargaining power for higher insurance payments coupled with loosening of governmental regulations. The aging of the population, particularly of the "baby boomer" generation, has seen an increased demand for use of high-tech tests, equipment, and procedures, as well as high-priced medications. However, it is projected that spending on prescription medications will gradually slow over the same time period, dropping by some 7%.

The initial cost-cutting effects of managed care are beginning to wane as health-care providers learn how to manipulate the plethora of rules and regulations. An indication of this trend is the decrease in private spending for health care that has already started. In the year 2000, private spending was at an all-time high of 9.4%. By 2011, it is projected to be at 5.9%. These numbers may be affected by economic factors such as slowing of the economy.

Source: www.dhhs.gov.

of illnesses such as upper respiratory infections, hypertension, and otitis media; and medication therapy.

Nursing Homes and Other Long-term Care Facilities

Today, more senior citizens need long-term care. In addition, individuals of all ages are managing their lives with conditions such as HIV, traumatic head injuries, and other debilitating problems. Such individuals require extended care and rehabilitative services. Hospitals and nursing homes are attempting to meet these demands by developing units to accommodate the long-term needs of these clients.

The trend of hospitals providing care in home-like atmospheres continues. Large client rooms, comfortable dining areas, and space for activities are important to meet the psychosocial needs of clients who stay for extended periods of time. Emphasis is also being placed on interacting with family members and involving them in the client's care. Because the restorative process may be slow, priority is placed on long-term goals and adjusting to ongoing health concerns.[9]

> *Assisted living centers are becoming increasingly appealing to both the public and those in the health-care industry as the need for a comprehensive continuum of cost-effective health-care services grows.*

Nursing homes are another place where long-term health care is being provided. Although clients in these settings experience complex health problems, acute care is usually not necessary. Nursing homes generally provide care for two types of clients. Some individuals are admitted to recuperate after being hospitalized and generally stay fewer than 90 days. They may be recovering from surgery and require assistance until they are able to manage independently. Other clients need care for lengthier periods of time because they are more disabled or do not have significant others who can assist them at home. They may require services ranging from help with activities of daily living to skilled nursing care.

The nursing home industry has experienced considerable growth in recent years, and there are now more beds in these facilities than in acute care hospitals. Traditionally, nursing homes were nonprofit agencies sponsored by organizations such as churches. Today, the overwhelming majority of nursing homes are for-profit institutions, and they rely heavily on Medicaid and Medicare reimbursements.[5] Medicare benefits may be limited, and private insurance frequently pays the balance charged.

Assisted Living Centers

Assisted living centers are becoming increasingly appealing to both the public and those in the health-care industry as the need for a comprehensive continuum of cost-effective health-care services grows. Assisted living centers have the advantage of allowing clients to maintain the greatest amount of independence possible, while providing a protective living environment where assistive services are available as needed. Individuals in these centers frequently maintain their own private living quarters; prepare some or all of their own meals; and may transport themselves via their own vehicles to shopping malls, church, and social events.

These centers are increasingly being developed or bought by integrated long-term care companies so that as client acuity levels rise, individuals who require care can be easily integrated into company-owned nursing homes. Likewise, when less acute care is required, clients can be easily transferred back to their assisted living quarters.[9]

Adult Day Care Centers

In an attempt to meet the health-care and psychosocial needs of a growing number of individuals in the community, adult day care centers are becoming more common. These centers provide services primarily for elderly clients who need supportive care for physical problems, organic brain dysfunction, or mobility problems that make them vulnerable to social isolation. Care is available during the day, and clients return to supervised home settings at night. Adult day care services may provide an alternative to more expensive nursing home residency or home care services.

Comprehensive adult day care centers provide holistic services, including nursing care, rehabilitation therapy, assistance with activities of daily living, transportation, social services, and recreational activities. As such, they employ a wide array of professional staff such as dietitians, art therapists, social workers, physical and occupational therapists, as well as nurses. Some adult day care centers have a more narrow focus, such as those that provide care for individuals with mental health problems. More and more, adult day care centers are becoming vertically integrated into a coordinated network of health-care services that helps to ensure a client referral base for all agencies involved. The vertical integration allows clients with changing health-care needs to move easily from one level of care to another. For example, a client diagnosed with the early stages of Alzheimer's dementia may initially require minimal supervision in an adult day care center. As the disease process progresses and the client requires more care, the client can move with relative ease to the next level, assisted living, and then later, to the skilled nursing care level, all under the same health-care provider's umbrella.

In the past, it has been common for adult day care centers to be funded by government agencies, philanthropic organizations, and private payments. Today, these facilities are relying less on government and philanthropic subsidies and are looking more toward traditional third-party payment sources. Currently Medicaid is assuming a large portion of the cost of these services, whereas Medicare has not traditionally reimbursed for such care. Commercial long-term care insurers have been slow to reimburse for adult day care; however, there is increased interest in this option versus more expensive alternatives such as nursing home placement. The general public is also expected to put more pressure on commercial insurers to reimburse for these services because of their growing popularity.

Home Care Agencies

More and more, nurses employed by home care agencies are assuming responsibilities in private residences that public health nurses previously assumed. These nurses may work for hospital-based or local independent agencies, regional-national chains, or private duty registries. In recent years, many independent home care agencies have been vertically integrated into health-care system networks. Home care agencies have benefited from this restructuring because it provides them with a continual source of client referrals. Likewise, parent agencies have benefited by being able to enhance continuity of client care. In the past, home care agencies focused on the provision of long-term care. However, this focus has shifted more toward short-term care that can be funded through Medicare or other payment sources. To supplement home-health-care services, home health aide and homemaker assistance may also be available. Homemakers typically do not help with bathing and grooming but provide services such as housekeeping, meal preparation, and transportation.

Hospice

The philosophy behind hospice care originated in Great Britain and has grown in popularity in this country over the last few decades. Today, hospices are designed to offer compassionate care to terminally ill clients and their family members. Services are provided in homes or institutional settings, usually by nurses and homemakers. Psychological support, respite care for family members, and comfort and pain control measures are common interventions. Preservation of client and family dignity, integrity, and overall well-being is of utmost importance. Medicare provides reimbursement for hospice services if clients meet the guidelines for care.

Community Health Centers

Community health centers provide services primarily for medically underserved and disadvantaged individuals. Based on their philosophical origins, community health centers make a special effort to tailor services to meet local needs, and community members are intimately involved with their operation, development, and governance. These centers are supported by federal funds, and their focus is on health promotion and disease prevention. Some centers offer emergency assistance, home care, mental health counseling, and rehabilitative support. Diagnostic, laboratory, and pharmaceutical services may also be available.

> *Hospices are designed to offer compassionate care to terminally ill clients and their family members. Services are provided in homes or institutional settings, usually by nurses and homemakers.*

Community health centers use a team approach, and nurses along with physicians and physicians' assistants are the main care providers. The variety of ambulatory services offered tends to vary as government funding fluctuates. As Medicare and Medicaid funding declines, **sliding-scale fees** are relied on more heavily. Using sliding-scale fee schedules, clients pay differing amounts depending on their income. Along with public hospitals, community health centers are being influenced by the capitated payment movement, and some fear that their long-term survival is in jeopardy unless they incorporate with integrated health-care delivery agencies and managed care operations.

School-Based Health Care

Nurses provide a variety of services within local school systems. These services include screenings, health promotion and illness prevention programs, and treatment of minor health-care problems. Emphasis is placed on physical, social, and psychological well being. Concerns relating to self-esteem, stress, drug abuse, and adolescent pregnancy are frequently addressed by the school nurse. In addition, children and adolescents with long-term health problems often attend school, and it is not uncommon for the nurse to be consulted about such issues as seizure management, colostomy care, or gastric tube feedings.

Students who have health concerns are frequently referred to providers within the community; and an important role of the school nurse is that of community liaison. For this reason, the nurse must be knowledgeable about community resources and adept at getting clients into the system in a timely and efficient manner.

Workplace Health Centers

As a result of rising health-care costs and lost productivity related to health problems, employers are increasingly supporting workplace health promotion, illness prevention, and safety programs. It is estimated that 80 percent of businesses employing 50 workers or more have some sort of health program.[5] Some programs are mainly educational; others provide health screenings and referrals; and still others offer classes on topics such as stress management, nutrition, exercise, and substance abuse. In industrial settings, health-care services are typically more comprehensive, and preliminary emergency services may be provided in the event of an accident. Nurses usually staff industrial health-care centers; however, company health promotion programs are commonly run by health educators.

Nurse-Run Health Centers

Similar to community health centers, nurse-run health centers tend to focus on health promotion and disease prevention. Historically, they have been service rather than profit oriented and remain so today. Nurses who are interested in autonomous practice often work in these settings.

Several types of nurse-run health centers have been identified. Among these are community health and institutional outreach centers. These facilities may be freestanding or sponsored by a larger institution, such as a university or public health agency. Primary care services are generally offered to the medically underserved, and these centers are typically funded by public and private sources. Wellness and health promotion clinics are another type of nurse-run clinic that offer services at work sites, schools, churches, or homeless shelters. Many of these centers are affiliated with schools of nursing, providing health-care services while offering educational experiences for nursing students. A final type of nursing center includes faculty practice, independent practice, and nurse entrepreneurship models. These facilities are owned and operated by nurses and may be solo or multidisciplinary practices. Services are typically reimbursed through fee-for-service, grant monies, and insurance. The ability of nurses in these centers to secure payments through the newly emergent and complex health-care reimbursement network will in large part determine the future financial viability of these types of clinics.[10]

Public Health Departments

Epidemics in the eighteenth and nineteenth centuries forced community leaders to take measures to prevent and control communicable diseases in their communities. Along with this mission came an emphasis on public education and home care. Today, public health departments are administered by state, county, or city governments. The emphasis of public health departments is now on prevention and the management of acute and chronic conditions among the population rather than home care. Foci include prenatal care, children's health, detection and treatment of tuberculosis, control of sexually transmitted diseases, and mental health problems. Although a large percentage of clients seen in these settings are indigent, receive Medicaid, or are Medicare recipients, the services are available to all members of the community. A new emphasis for public health departments is preparation for acts of bioterrorism. In many areas of the country, health department personnel are designated as the front line contact in potential bioterrorism threats and have regular bioterrorism practice drills to prepare for such events.

Parish Nurses

It is estimated that approximately 2000 parish nurses throughout the country are attempting to meet the needs of individuals who are without adequate primary care or who are experiencing escalating health-care costs. Many of these nurses work part-time or are volunteers, and some work in conjunction with community-based programs. Churches are engaging parish nurses to:

- Serve as health educators and counselors
- Do health assessments and referrals

- Organize support groups
- Make visits to parishioners who are sick or elderly
- Serve as client advocates or case managers[11]

Parish nurses are in a unique position to exercise their skills as case managers. As nurses, they possess clinical knowledge and skills, understand the health-care delivery system within their communities, and know many of the key health-care providers. As members of their parish, they are intimately familiar with their communities, understand the cultural climate of their clientele, and are familiar with the services that are available. Moreover, as members of the church community that they serve, they are likely to be familiar with the spiritual, psychosocial, and financial needs of their clients. However, direct reimbursement is not yet available for parish nurses.[11]

Voluntary Health Agencies

Since their inception in 1892, voluntary health agencies have experienced steady growth to the point where they currently number more than 100,000. The first voluntary health agency was the Anti-tuberculosis Society of Philadelphia. Some of the more well known agencies that exist today include the American Cancer Society, The American Heart Association, The National Foundation for the March of Dimes, The National Easter Seal Society for Crippled Adults and Children, and the Alliance for the Mentally Ill. These agencies provide many valuable services, some of which include fundraising in support of cutting-edge research and public education. Others, such as the American Cancer Society, which has a strong emphasis on education and research, also help individuals secure special equipment such as hospital beds for the home and wigs for chemotherapy patients. The Alliance for the Mentally Ill is very politically active and organizes support groups for the mentally ill and their families. These groups are not-for-profit organizations, so that all revenue in excess of cost goes toward improving services.

Rural Health Care

Delivery of health care in rural areas presents unique challenges. These challenges result from low numbers of physicians, nurses, and allied-health-care professionals who are willing to live and practice in remote areas; decreased access to advanced medical technology; and the fact that rural hospitals often have more expenses than revenues. In recent years, many rural hospitals have been forced to close or severely curtail their services.

Rural health-care delivery problems are being overcome through integrated delivery networks that provide primary, secondary, and sometimes tertiary care to residents in designated regions. Rural health-care providers are often employees of large multilayered networks and function under the aegis of a single administrative staff. These systems are composed of physicians, nurse practitioners, nurses, physicians' assistants, and other ancillary health-care personnel who provide local primary health care. To receive secondary and tertiary care within the network, rural residents must frequently travel considerable distances. Although complex and sometimes inconvenient, this layering of services under the same administrative umbrella makes rural health care financially feasible.

Paying for health-care services is another concern for rural residents. Many of these individuals are farmers or employees of small businesses that do not offer health benefits. To overcome this problem, the use of **health insurance purchasing cooperatives (HIPCs)** has been proposed. These are large groups of people or employers who band together to buy insurance at reduced costs. HIPCs may be organized by private groups or the government. A typical concern in establishing such groups is estimating the minimum number of individuals necessary to make the organization financially viable. For example, taking into consideration the health status of the population in question, it is important to correctly estimate the minimum number of individuals who will need to pay into the system to cover the resultant costs of those who need services.

Conclusion

The health-care delivery system in this country offers a variety of care facilities, payment plans, and providers. Nurses have traditionally played key roles as direct care providers. As the call for change in the health-care delivery system grows louder, the roles that nurses play will be expanded and transformed. Nurses will be an important part in the coordination of health care as case managers. Care provided in the home and through various community-based delivery systems will place a high demand on nurses who can function independently and make critical decisions. Nurses remain one of the bastions of client advocacy by speaking out for clients in the face of a powerful health-care system.

Nobody really knows what the health-care delivery system of the future will look like. The reforms proposed in the 1990s were never implemented. Several recent bills considered by the United States Congress were not passed. Several state legislatures started working on bills to provide more coordinated health care, but with the downturn in the economy, most of these plans were shelved due because of lack of resources. The prevailing philosophy seems to be that the free marketplace will eventually sort things out. Unfortunately, the free marketplace often tends to overlook those who are most needy and least able to fend for themselves. Nurses and nursing have always been committed to these groups, and the future of health care will demand an even more concentrated effort to support initiatives that focus on caring.

Critical Thinking Exercises

- Select three clients you are familiar with who have different health-care needs. Describe these clients' medical histories, current problems, and future health-care needs, then determine which health-care setting and which health-care practitioners would be most appropriate for them. Identify any difficulties that might be encountered during their entry into the health-care system. How can the nurse facilitate the process?

- Skilled nursing facilities, subacute care facilities, and assisted living facilities all are forms of long-term or extended health care. Identify five specific problems that nurses working in such facilities encounter. What is the best way to resolve these problems?

- Identify cost-cutting measures used at a health-care facility with which you are familiar. Have these measures affected the quality of client care? What other measures to cut costs can be implemented? How have changes within the health-care delivery system altered nursing practice?

- Identify four health-care priorities that may be initiated by the year 2010. How are these likely to affect the profession of nursing?

- Describe the advantages and disadvantages of various health-care reimbursement plans. Which ones will produce the highest quality care? Which ones are best for the profession of nursing? Are there any payment plans that do both?

- Identify those elements in health-care reform that are most necessary. Should nurses support these changes and why?

References

1. Bellack, JP, and O'Neil, EH: Recreating nursing practice for a new century: Recommendations and implications of the Pew Health Professions Commission's Final Report. Nursing and Health Care Perspectives 21(1):14–21, 2002.
2. Davidson, SB, et al: Legislative and regulatory update: Statutory and regulatory recognition for clinical nurse specialists. Clinical Nurse Specialist 15(6):276–283, 2001.
3. United States Census Bureau: Statistical brief, 2002. Available at: http://www.census.gov/socdemo/www/agebrief.html.
4. Health Care Financing Administration: Highlights: National health expenditures, 2002. Available at: http://www.hcfa.gov/stats/NHE-OAct/hilites.htm.
5. Higgs, ZR, et al: Health care access: A consumer perspective. Public Health Nurs 18(1):3–12, 2001.
6. Lindeman, CA: The future of nursing. J Nurs Educ 39(1):5–12, 2000.
7. Burke, RJ: The ripple effect: Staffing post restructuring. Nursing Management 33(2):41–43, 2002.
8. Congressional Budget Office: Trends in Health Spending: An Update. U.S. Government Printing Office, Washington, DC, 2001.
9. Milio, N: Health care reform: What went wrong? Am J Nurs 101(12):69–71, 2001.
10. National Center for Health Statistics: Monitoring health care in America—Spotlight on ambulatory care in the U.S. Available at: http://www.cdc.gov/nchswww/releases/97facts/97sheets/mhc0697.htm.
11. Hughes, CB, et al: Primary care parish nursing: Outcomes and implications. Nursing Administration Quarterly 26(1):45–59, 2001.

Bibliography

Bellack, JP, and O'Neil, EH: Recreating nursing practice for a new century: Recommendations and implications of the Pew Health Professions Commission's Final Report. Nursing and Health Care Perspectives 21(1):14–21, 2002.

Brewer, C, and Kovner, CT: Is there another nursing shortage? What the data tell us. Nurs Outlook 49(1):20–26, 2001.

Burke, RJ: The ripple effect: Staffing post restructuring. Nursing Management 33(2):41–43, 2002.

Carlson, ED: Welfare reform: Policy implications for health. Texas Journal of Rural Health 19(2):42–48, 2001.

Davidson, SB, et al: Legislative and regulatory update: Statutory and regulatory recognition for clinical nurse specialists. Clinical Nurse Specialist 15(6):276–283, 2001.

Emerson, B: Hospital in the home. More than just a cost cutting mechanism. ACCNS Journal for Community Nurses 6(2):13–15, 2001.

Higgs, ZR, et al: Health care access: A consumer perspective. Public Health Nurs 18(1):3–12, 2001.

Tappen, RM: Nursing Leadership and Management, ed. 4. FA Davis, Philadelphia, 2001.

17

Nursing Informatics

Kathleen Mary Young

Learning Objectives

After completing this chapter, the reader will be able to:

- Discuss the impact of the information revolution on society in general and on health care specifically.
- Define nursing informatics.
- Explain the importance of nursing informatics to nursing practice.
- Analyze the availability of resources and references in the practice site.
- Evaluate the importance of human factors engineering on equipment design.
- Compare the electronic health record to the paper record system.

A worldwide information revolution is exploding the systems of modern culture. Although no one can predict the full effect of the current information revolution, it is easy to see the changes that it creates in our daily lives. The information revolution changes both the way that teachers teach and the way that learners learn. Teaching in the public school, and even in colleges, now demands fast-moving, entertaining lessons that capture the student's attention, because the classroom teachers must compete with television and the computer games with which this generation has been raised. School children and college students no longer read whole books. Technology has accustomed them to 30-second "sound bites" of information. Libraries are evolving from repositories of hardbound volumes and journals to providers of Internet access to on-line journals and books.

Technology and Communication

The information revolution has changed both the form and the format of communication. Before the advent of the telephone, people communicated through the written word. Letter writing was an art. Before television and the computer were invented, people gathered together in neighborhoods and developed a sense of community. Today the whole world is the community, and every corner can be reached from a home computer. Senior citizens in Blacksburg, Virginia, use their computers not only to chat but also to organize get-togethers. "It's like wandering into the town center to meet friends and to check the bulletin board," says Dennis Gentry, a retired Army officer. "Only you can do it in pajamas anytime you want."[1]

The award of the Nobel Prize in economics in 1996 and 2001 illustrates the increasing role of information in today's society. Microeconomic theorists won the prizes for explaining how the lack of information helps shape modern business decisions. The theorists study an area of economics called asymmetric information. According to the Royal Swedish Academy of Sciences, "Many markets are characterized by asymmetric information: actors on one side of the market have much better information than those on the other. Borrowers know more than lenders about their repayment prospects, managers and boards know more than shareholders about the firm's profitability, and prospective clients know more than insurance companies about their accident risk."[2] The fact that the person with more information has an advantage seems like common sense, but a grasp of the impact of asymmetric information will lead to a better understanding of day-to-day economic activity.

Not only does **technology** change the way in which people communicate and work, but it also creates a new decision-making process that affects all aspects of industry and commerce. Informed decisions produce better outcomes. Competition has become a driving force in the pricing and marketing of health care. Payment methods that promote competition are encouraged by Medicare and Medicaid prospective payment systems (PPSs), health maintenance organizations (HMOs), preferred provider organizations (PPOs), and managed care. To offer a competitive and quality organization, information must be available to make decisions. More information is available to decision-makers with information technology.

> *The fact that the person with more information has an advantage seems like common sense, but a grasp of the impact of asymmetric information will lead to a better understanding of day-to-day economic activity.*

The application of the increased information available through technology to decision making in health care gives technologically driven organizations a competitive edge. To stay competitive in national and international health care, the health-care delivery system, and specifically nursing, must open itself to new information and ideas.

The health-care information revolution is progressing at the speed of light. Computers will be involved in almost every area of client care; the assessment of the quality of care; and the enhancement of decision making, management, planning, and medical research.[3]

Definition of Informatics

Two definitions of informatics are used in the health-care field. The term *medical informatics* was coined in the mid-1970s. Borrowed from the French expression *informatique medicale*, it described "those collected informational technologies which concern themselves with the client care, medical, decision-making process."[4] Mandil[5] uses the term *health informatics*, which is defined as the use of information technology with information management concepts and methods to support the delivery of health care. Mandil's definition encompasses medical, nursing, dental, and pharmacy informatics as well as all other health-care disciplines. The definition for health informatics focuses attention on the recipient of care rather than on the discipline of the caregiver.

The nursing community, however, is developing a discipline of informatics that is specific to the delivery of nursing care and is based on the science of nursing. Nursing has distinct and discrete information needs. The "data, information and knowledge of nursing are symbolic representations of phenomena of peculiar interest to nursing. The structure of this nursing information is substantively different from that of other disciplines. These information structures pose discipline-specific problems for the management and processing of nursing information."[6]

In 1989, Graves and Corcoran suggested a model for nursing informatics. In this model, nursing informatics is identified as "a combination of computer science, information science, and nursing science designed to assist in the management and processing of nursing data, information and knowledge to support the practice of nursing and the delivery of nursing care."[6]

Computer science refers primarily to the configuration and architecture of the computer system. Information science refers to the computer software, including how data or tasks are processed, how problems are solved, and where products are produced. Nursing science refers to the practice of nursing.[7]

Turley[8] added a fourth element, cognitive science, to the model for nursing informatics. He defined cognitive science as an interdisciplinary field that results from the convergence of psychology, linguistics, computer science, philosophy, and neuroscience. It is concerned with perception, thinking, understanding, and remembering. Turley's model unites information science, computer science, and cognitive science into a framework of nursing science.

Nelson and Joos[9] theorized that in addition to data, information, and knowledge, wisdom should be added as the fourth component. They view wisdom as knowing how and when to apply knowledge to manage a patient problem or need.

Data, Information, and Knowledge

When Graves and Corcoran developed their classic definition of nursing informatics, they defined *data* as raw and unstructured facts. The numbers 102 and 104 are raw data. By themselves, these numbers have little meaning because they lack interpretation.

Information consists of data that have been given form and have been interpreted. If the number 102 is given additional data so that it becomes a 102°F oral temperature of a 25-year-old man taken at 9 A.M., it becomes information that has meaning.

What Do You Think?

Have you used any of the computerized health-care records? Describe your experience.

Knowledge takes the process one step further, because it is a synthesis of data and information. Combining the information that an oral temperature of 102°F is higher than normal for a 25-year-old man with an understanding of human physiology and pharmacology provides the practitioner with the knowledge that enables him or her to make a decision concerning a course of treatment. This process is the basis for critical thinking and decision making and can also be used in research to create new knowledge.

The Graves and Corcoran model of "data to information to knowledge" is linear, but the process of synthesizing data into information to create knowledge is actually circular. New knowledge creates new questions and areas of research, which in turn lead to more new knowledge. To answer the research questions, new data are required that must be processed into information to create more knowledge. The goal of this process is to provide the most accurate and current information so that nurses can make informed decisions in their daily practice.

Areas of Focus in Informatics

Turley[8] suggests that the specialty of nursing informatics has evolved through three levels of special interest: technology, concepts of nursing theory, and function.

Early in the evolution, definitions of nursing informatics focused strictly on the use of technology. For example, in 1985 Hannah[10] defined nursing informatics as "any use of information technology by nurses in relation to the care of patients or the educational preparation of individuals to practice in the discipline is considered nursing informatics." Similarly, Saba and McCormick[7] continued to define nursing informatics in terms of technology: The use of technology and/or a computer system to store, process, display, retrieve, and communicate timely data and information in and across health-care facilities that:

- Administer nursing services and resources
- Manage the delivery of client and nursing care
- Link research resources and findings to nursing practice
- Apply educational resources to nursing education

A further evolution in the focus of nursing informatics is seen in those experts who advocate the underlying concepts of nursing theory. They argue that without a well-articulated theoretical basis to guide the gathering of data, nursing will soon be overwhelmed with meaningless data and information. They point out the need for definitions, a standardized nursing language, and criteria for organization of the data.

Nursing informatics is now recognized as a nursing specialty for which one can receive certification.

Those who focus on the concept of function in nursing informatics take the process one step further. They focus on how the management and processing of information help nurses enter, organize, or retrieve information. They stress the usability of the applications to achieve specific purposes. Although technology and concept are important in forming the foundation of informatics, the nurse's ability to use the system and make it function is the real test of the system's effectiveness.

In reality, nursing informatics includes all three of these areas of focus. However, the field of informatics has become so large that it is difficult for any one person to be an expert in all three areas.

Broader Definition

From the earlier definitions given by Hannah and Saba, a broader definition has evolved. The American Nurses Association (ANA) defines nursing informatics as:

> *A specialty that integrates nursing science, computer science, and information science in identifying, collecting, processing, and managing data and information to support nursing practice, administration, education and research; and to expand nursing knowledge. The purpose of nursing informatics is to analyze information requirements; design, implement and evaluate information systems and data structures that support nursing; and identify and apply computer technologies for nursing.*[11]

Nursing informatics is now recognized as a nursing specialty for which one can receive certification. The catalog of the American Nurses Credentialing Center (ANCC) states that the nursing informatics practice:

> *. . . encompasses the full range of activities that focus on the methods and technologies of information handling in nursing. It includes the development, support, and evaluation of applications, tools, processes, and structures that assist the practice of nurses with the management of data in direct care of patients/clients. The work of an informatics nurse can involve any and all aspects of information systems, including theory formulation, design, development, marketing, selection, testing, implementation, training, maintenance, evaluation, and enhancement.*[12]

Nursing informatics supports all areas of nursing, including practice, education, administration, and research. It facilitates and guides the management of data.

Importance of Nursing Informatics

Informatics is no longer just an elective subject. In today's competitive and rapidly changing health-care delivery system, informatics is an essential. The importance of the role of informatics is apparent in the need for the articulation of nursing practice. Articulation is an important way for nursing to demonstrate its accountability and credibility so that nursing can remain an essential element of the health-care system.

Articulation

Historically, the nursing profession has had difficulty in locating relevant nursing information quickly, because there was no universally agreed upon nomenclature and taxonomy for either nursing clinical information or management data. This lack of access to information has presented several seemingly insurmountable challenges for nurse executives, including being able to identify what the nursing staff actually does, determining the impact nurses have on outcomes, and establishing appropriate reimbursement for nursing activities.[13]

For example, how does a nurse interpret the term *weak grasp* when it is seen in the chart of a client? The meaning of weak grasp differs widely depending on the client. If the client is a premature infant with a weak grasp, the term has an entirely different meaning than if it is applied to a 25-year-old professional football player with a head injury or even a 60-year-old client with a stroke. Imagine the difficulty that a researcher will have when he or she is investigating the phenomenon of weak grasp because of the lack of a standardized definition among the nursing community. Because of the need to standardize nursing language to name and communicate what nurses do, nursing classification schemes, taxonomies, and vocabularies have come to the forefront with the evolution of nursing informatics.

The American Nurses Association Database Steering Committee was formed in 1991 to develop a common nursing language called the Unified Nursing Language System (UNLS). UNLS maps concepts and identifies common terms from different vocabularies and acknowledges them as synonyms of the same concept.

Box 17–1 lists standards and scoring guidelines for nursing languages. Twelve classification systems are recognized by the ANA as uniquely developed to document nursing care. They are designed to record and track the clinical care process for an entire episode of care for patients in the acute, home, and/or ambulatory care settings. They are listed in Box 17–2.

What Do You Think?

Think of four terms, not defined actions, carried out by nurses that have multiple meanings. How could these terms be clarified?

Box 17–1

Standards and Scoring Guidelines for Nursing Languages

1. Terms in data dictionaries and tables are appropriate to the domain of nursing.
2. Terms from ANA-recognized languages for nursing are used as a core for the nursing vocabulary.
3. The system allows for the development and addition of new terms as needed, without duplicating existing terms or disrupting the integrity of existing languages.
4. When using a "local" language, those terms are mapped to appropriate ANA-recognized nursing languages, which may include using reference terminologies.
5. The system accommodates the use of reference terminologies to map nursing languages with other existing standardized data sets, classification systems, or nomenclatures.

Box 17–2

Recognized Languages for Nursing

Source	Recognition Date
1. North American Nursing Diagnosis Association (NANDA)	1992
2. Nursing Interventions Classification (NIC)	1992
3. Home Health Care Classification (HHCC)	1992
4. Omaha System	1992
5. Nursing Outcomes Classification (NOC)	1997
6. Nursing Management Minimum Data Set (NMMDS)	1998
7. Patient Care Data Set (PCDS)	1998
8. Perioperative Nursing Data Set (PNDS)	1999
9. Systematized Nomenclature of Medicine Reference Terminology (SNOMED RT)	1999
10. Nursing Minimum Data Set (NMDS)	1999
11. International Classification for Nursing Practice	2000
12. ABC codes developed by Alternative Link	2000

Source: American Nurses Association, 2002. Available at: http://www.ana.org/nidsec/class1st.htm.

Standardization of the data in a client's record is the first step toward unifying information. The second step has been the development of criteria to determine the necessary elements that must be included in every client record or encounter. The Nursing Minimum Data Set (NMDS) developed in 1985 and accepted by the ANA in 1998 is a list of the data elements necessary in any computerized client record system or national database. The NMDS is considered to be the umbrella for other nursing process schemes. The purpose of the NMDS is to:

1. Describe the nursing care of clients and their families in various settings, both institutional and noninstitutional
2. Establish comparability of nursing data across clinical populations, settings, geographical areas, and time
3. Demonstrate or project trends regarding nursing care provided and allocation of nursing resources to clients according to their health problems or nursing diagnoses
4. Stimulate **nursing research** through linkages of detailed data existing in nursing information systems and in other healthcare information systems
5. Provide data about nursing care to influence health policy and decision making[14]

The NMDS has 16 elements divided into three main categories: nursing care (e.g., nursing diagnosis, intervention, outcome, and degree of nursing care), client demographics (e.g., the client's personal identification, date of birth, sex), and service elements (e.g., the unique service agency number, the admission and discharge dates, client's condition, and expected payer).

Accountability

Intuitively, the nursing profession has long known that the increased use of nurses improves the quality of care and also client outcomes, while decreasing the cost of health care. However, nurses traditionally have not been very good at documenting their worth and effectiveness. According to the Congressional Office of Technology Assessment,[15] better use of nurse practitioners could result in savings for clients, employers, and society owing to the cost-effectiveness of both their training and their services. Nurses affect client outcomes positively and contribute measurably to the goals of a competitive health-care delivery system.

In order to measure effectiveness with accurate information about client care and outcomes, nurses must use standardized language in both practice and documentation. The ability to measure the resources used and the client outcome achieved will help distinguish one health-care provider from another. As nursing practice becomes more efficient and can demonstrate improved client outcomes, both the quality of care will increase and health-care organizations will become more financially stable.

> *The amount of health-care information contained in scientific journals has grown to a point where no single individual is able to read all of the material.*

Credibility

The credibility of the nursing profession rests on the state of its documentation. Nurses must be able to measure their effectiveness with accurate information about both the care given and the client outcomes achieved. Nursing professionals must have control over the process of care as well as the information and assessments of the quality of care. Improvements in quality do not occur in isolation. Quality improvements result from a continual process of assessing care and measuring outcomes that produces improvements in treatments, changes in care procedures, and an increased number of support services.[16]

A standardized language will facilitate the nursing profession's ability to delineate the cost and benefits of nursing care from the costs and benefits of other health-care providers. If the nursing profession cannot articulate and measure the unique contributions that nurses make to the client's health and well-being, then the profession will continue to have difficulty justifying its higher costs over less educated and less qualified health-care providers.

Access to Information

An information explosion continues to restructure the world of health-care journals and textbooks. The amount of health-care information contained in scientific journals has grown to a point where no single individual is able to read all of the material. In 1994, 34,000 references from 4000 journals were added each month to the National Library of Medicine Medline database from among the more than 100,000 scientific journals published.[17] In the past 20 years, the number of articles indexed annually in the Medline database has nearly doubled, the number of clinical trials in cardiology has increased five times, and the number of clinical trials in health services has increased 10 times. One new article is added to the medical literature every 26 seconds. Coping with the volume of biomedical and nursing literature is an enormous task. With just a nightly perusal of the latest journals, even the most conscientious practitioners will have difficulty in keeping up with all the current research and new developments in their specialty field.

Although a great amount of new information is available, it would seem that only a small portion is actually transferred into the minds and practice of many health-care professionals. The traditional paradigm that seems to guide the decision-making process for many nurses is to:

- Refer back to the knowledge learned in school
- Confer with a colleague
- Look up the problem in any textbook/reference book available in the work setting
- Use previous experiences and "gut" instincts

Although this process is useful and has some merit, it is questionable whether it is adequate for the delivery of high-quality care.

Consider a new paradigm for decision making that may be more appropriate for the information age. This process includes:

- Accessing current literature concerning the latest diagnostic techniques and treatment modalities
- Conferring with a knowledgeable colleague
- Evaluating the effectiveness of previous experiences

Research shows that nursing interventions based on research produce better client outcomes.[18] This process is called evidence-based practice.

Ironically, even though evidence-based practice produces higher quality care, the health-care culture has been slow to implement its use. With increasing client care responsibilities, nurses rarely have time to go to the library to research solutions to client care problems. Furthermore, nurses are not rewarded for taking the initiative to do so. However, leaving the practice site in order to access relevant information is no longer necessary in the information age. Literature searching can be available at the point of care using automated systems.[19]

Royle described a Canadian study in which literature searching via a personal computer was available on the nursing unit. Nurses had access to six databases, the Health Science Library's online catalog, user manuals, search aids, textbooks, and reference books on medical-surgical and oncology nursing. The study extended over a 6-month period, and the nurses received 6 hours of training in the use of the system. Even after the training sessions, the nurses found that they still had difficulty finding time to use the system. However, with practice, they became more familiar with information that was available. They also claimed that "having access to literature about clinical issues gave them confidence in dealing with clients and other health professionals and allowed them to contribute more fully to the multidisciplinary health care team."[19]

Nurses must continue to demand access to and time for information searches that promote improved client care (Box 17–3). In recognizing the need for access to information, the goal of health services development in the United Kingdom was to provide e-mail and Web access at all nursing stations by March 2002. The creation of workplaces in which nurses can easily access client information, including research information, is essential to high-quality nursing practice.

Human Factors That Affect Informatics

The human factors that influence informatics include knowledge about human abilities, limitations, and characteristics that are relevant to the design of tools, machines, systems, and jobs. The terms *human factors*, *human engineering*, *usability engineering*, and *ergonomics* are often used interchangeably. The study of human factors examines how to make the interaction of people and equipment safe, comfortable, and effective. Cognitive science, one of the components of informatics discussed earlier, forms part of the foundation for the study of human factors. Cognitive science includes the human acts of perception, thinking, understanding, and remembering. In order to manage and process information, especially with an automated system, the individual must be able to understand and remember a great deal of data. The more logically this information is arranged, the easier it is to use the system.

Every day in their client care, nurses use complex machinery, including many types of monitors, ventilators, intravenous (IV) pumps,

Box 17–3

Principles for Access to Library and Information Services

1. All nurses should have access to a free library service funded by their employer that contains appropriate literature and multimedia resources.
2. Library services should have flexible opening hours and be staffed by qualified librarians.
3. Nurses should have equal rights, similar to those of other health-care professionals, to paid study time to update their practice.
4. Every nurse should have access to training on the Internet and appropriate databases.
5. Every nurse should be educated in electronic systems and services to support evidence-based practice.

Source: Urquhart, C, and Davis, R: The impact of information. Nursing Standard 12(8):23–31, 1997.

feeding pumps, suction devices, electronic beds and scales, lift equipment, and assistive devices. The directions for use of many of these machines are not self-evident and may be highly complicated. Although hospital equipment producers are becoming better at incorporating the human factor in the design and use of this complicated equipment, it would seem that consulting with practicing nurses or "field testing" equipment in the workplace prior to its mass production would make it more user friendly.

Similarly, new computer systems present many learning difficulties for health-care providers. Many computer systems are not user friendly. Computer systems designers are notorious for supplying computers with numerous advanced but obscure functions, but these systems often lack the ability to make daily tasks easier to accomplish. Millions of dollars have been wasted on computer systems that are not used or are underused because the user needs were not assessed before the systems were designed.

Individuals encountering complicated computer systems for the first time commonly feel that they are stupid, incompetent, or too old to learn because they cannot quickly master the use of the new technology. However, the fault often lies not with the individual but rather with the design of the technology. Nurses, through their education and philosophical orientation, are generally more in tune with the human factor than equipment designers, particularly as it relates to client care. Nurses can use their human factor orientation in the process of evaluating new technology before it is purchased. Also, nurses may be able to make suggestions to medical equipment producers to help improve the equipment after it has been used for some time.

The 2000 publication of the Institute of Medicine's (IOM) report, *To Err is Human: Building a Safer Health System*,[20] brought the problem of health-care error to the attention of the general public. According to the report based on a study conducted in New York, as many as 98,000 people die annually in the United States as a result of medical error. Statistics gathered in Utah and Colorado imply that at least 44,000 Americans die each year as a result of medical error. Medical error is the eighth leading cause of death in the United States.

The most common type of health-care error was drug complication (19 percent), followed by wound infections (14 percent) and technical complications (13 percent). The proliferation of new drugs and the increasing complexity of drug therapy have dramatically increased the risk of medication errors and adverse drug events both inside and outside hospitals. The Institute for

Safe Medication Practices has shown that well-designed physician order entry systems reduce serious prescribing errors by more than 50 percent;[21] but according to Weinstein, just 4 to 7 percent of physicians currently use on-line prescribing.[22]

Poor user design is responsible for thousands of health-care "accidents" each year. Complex medical devices are often used under extremely stressful conditions in which the user's cognitive abilities are not as focused as they might be in a less stressful situation.

Often the users are not considered during the design phase, because the designers believe that they know what is needed. The inevitable result of poor design in all types of equipment, ranging from paper laboratory forms to life-support devices, is an increased error rate. Cognitive science studies have shown that the average person's memory can retain only six to eight pieces of information at the same time. A well-designed system will take these elements into account (Box 17–4).

In a Harvard Medical Practice Study,[23] 30,121 client records were randomly selected from 51 New York hospitals. Adverse events were documented in 3.7 percent of the hospitalizations. Of the adverse events, 27 percent were determined to be preventable. Of the preventable events, 10 to 20 percent were related to the system or to devices. The authors suggest that the use of computerization and system analysis (human factors) would reduce the number of incidents. Most agree, however, that computers can just as easily contribute to errors as help reduce them.

> *According to the report based on a study conducted in New York, as many as 98,000 people die annually in the United States as a result of medical error. Statistics gathered in Utah and Colorado imply that at least 44,000 Americans die each year as a result of medical error. Medical error is the eighth leading cause of death in the United States.*

Training employees how to use a system is a common methodology for reducing error. Although training is important, by itself, it may not be adequate. According to McDonald,[24] error frequency was not well correlated with level of training, but a computer-based reminder system helped clinicians reduce errors significantly. Even with more training, errors returned to the previous level when the computerized reminder system was removed.

When automated and computer systems are properly designed using human factors engineering techniques, they can be a valuable part of the monitoring and prevention of error in clinical practice. As nursing professionals, it is important to understand that human performance is not perfect and cannot be perfected through education and training. Professionals must look for well-designed systems that can reduce and even eliminate errors.

Electronic Health Record

A health record serves multiple purposes. It is used to document client care and provides communication among health-care team members. It is a financial and a legal record. It is used for research and continuous quality improvement (CQI). Although the health record can take many forms, the most common forms are either paper or electronic. Both forms have advantages and disadvantages (Box 17–5).

Electronic health records (EHRs) have many advantages. They are accessible from remote sites to multiple care providers at the same time. They can provide reminders about completing information or carrying through with protocols as well as providing warnings about incompatibilities of medications or variances from normal standards. Redundancy is reduced with the EHR. Rather than every health-care worker asking a client for his or her past health history, allergies, and

Box 17–4

Elements of a Good Technology Design

- Can be operated intuitively with minimal reliance on complicated manuals.
- Easy-to-read displays that are logically arranged.
- Easy to use and reach controls.
- Positive and safe electrical and mechanical connections.
- Alarms that sound only when there is a real problem so that they are not turned off because of annoyance.
- Long-life reliability with few malfunctions.
- Easy and quick to repair and maintain.

current medications, the information is captured once and then transmitted to every record requiring the information. EHRs require less storage space, are more difficult to lose, and are much easier to research. Improved communication, increased completeness of documentation, and reduction in error are the most important advantages of the EHR.

However, EHRs have some obvious disadvantages. There is a high front-end cost in buying and converting from a paper to an electronic system. Employees may have problems adapting to the new system because of the large learning curve involved in converting from a paper system to an electronic system. EHR systems are nonportable but are breakable. Decisions must be made about who can enter data into the system and when the entries should be made. Many legal and ethical issues involving privacy and also access to information still remain to be resolved.

The ideal EHR will be a lifelong continuous record of all the care that the client has received, rather than the episodic, piecemeal data that it now provides. This one record will reflect an individual's current health status and lifetime medical history. It will be unique to the person and not to the institution. This record will reside in multiple data sites and will accept multiple data types (e.g., graphs, pictures, x-rays, text) and be accessible worldwide.

The information on the EHR does not physically reside in one place. When viewed from a computer workstation, the EHR only appears to

Box 17–5

Advantages and Disadvantages of the Paper Record

Advantages

- People know how to use it.
- It is fast for current practice.
- It is portable.
- It is nonbreakable.
- It accepts multiple data types, such as graphs, photographs, drawings, and text.
- Legal issues and costs are understood.

Disadvantages

- It can be lost.
- It is often illegible and incomplete.
- It has no remote access.
- It can be accessed by only one person at a time.
- It is often disorganized.
- Information is duplicated.
- It is hard to store.
- It is difficult to research, and CQI is laborious.
- Same client has separate records at each facility (physician office, hospital, home care).
- Records are shared only through hard copy.

be in one place. In reality, the individual records are retrieved from many information systems, such as laboratory, radiology, document imaging, anatomic pathology, anesthesiology, bedside, accounting, and others.

With proper authorization, this record could be accessed from anywhere in the world, at any time. Many people around the world could look at the same record at the same time. If an individual became critically ill abroad, this would be a valuable tool to facilitate the diagnosis and treatment.

Many barriers must be overcome before the ideal EHR can be fully implemented. The issues of maintaining confidentiality and security must be resolved. The high cost of starting up the system is still a barrier. Bob Boysen, Chief Information Officer of Iowa Health System, believes the universal ID or a unique client identifier could become the biggest bombshell to hit health-care informatics this century.[25] Many organizations use either their own client numbering system or social security numbers to identify individual records. Neither of these systems is adequate for the global access of the future. Fingerprinting, iris and retinal imaging, face prints, and voiceprints all are identification methods under investigation for use as the universal ID.

"Confidentiality is now becoming a commodity to be traded in exchange for health care," experts warned at the eighth annual Conference on Computers, Freedom and Privacy.

Information can be entered through a bedside system, a point-of-care system, or a unit system. A bedside system, as the name implies, is a computer terminal installed in each client's room or next to each bed. A point-of-care system has a broader meaning and includes not only the bedside but also many other points of care in the health-care environment and community, including the laboratory, radiology department, outpatient clinics, and even the home for home-health-care providers. Many facilities currently have a unit system that can be accessed at only one terminal in the client care area (e.g., the nurses' station).

Taking a paper record and typing it into a computer does not, in itself, constitute a modern electronic record. Automating the paper record in its present form only automates inefficient practices based on outdated requirements. Modern systems go beyond merely computerizing current paper records. These new systems gain control over the generation of information and develop new techniques for using it creatively. One of the most important characteristics of a bedside or point-of-care system is that client information can be input directly from the terminal rather than keeping notes or charting from memory at the end of the shift. Documentation at the time of care is an important change in workflow for most health-care workers who are accustomed to documenting at the end of a shift in a workroom with other professionals.

The re-engineering and streamlining of departmental workflow is accomplished by the automatic and continual routing of electronic documents and medical images from one person or department to another throughout the shift. With this system, traditional manual tasks are now automated, thus increasing the efficiency of management decisions and improving the distribution and evaluation of complex client records and electronic documents by authorized staff. It is this radical redesign of the old manual processes that provides the real return on investment for implementing the electronic health record.

Ethics, Security, and Confidentiality

Most people assume that all doctor-client communications are confidential. However, "confidentiality is now becoming a commodity to be traded in exchange for health care," experts warned at the eighth annual Conference on Computers, Freedom and Privacy.[26]

Examples of violation of client confidentiality abound. In 1996, a convicted child rapist working as a technician in a Boston hospital rifled through 1000 computerized records looking for potential victims. He was caught when the father of a 9-year-old girl used caller ID to trace the call back to the hospital. A banker on Maryland's State Health Commission pulled up a list of cancer clients from the state's records, cross-checked it against the names of his bank's customers, and revoked the loans of those clients diagnosed with cancer. At least a third of all Fortune 500 companies regularly review health information before making hiring decisions. More than 200 subjects in a case study published in *Science and Engineering Ethics* reported that they had been discriminated against as a result of genetic testing.[27]

One of the key ethical questions is "Who owns the client's health-care data?" Does the individual's health-care information belong exclusively to him or her? Does it belong to the organization (e.g., insurance company, PPO) that paid for the care? Or should the information belong to the physician who directed and ordered the care? What about the facility in which the care occurred—can they claim some ownership to the information, particularly if it is stored there? Or do all these groups and individuals own a part of the information?

Those who argue on the "individual rights" end of the ethical spectrum believe that each individual should have total and exclusive control over the information concerning his or her health and the care rendered. Those on the utilitarian or "social good" end of the ethical spectrum believe that society as a whole benefits from shared information about disease occurrence and treatment. Therefore, the information should be available to all interested parties. As with most ethical dilemmas, a single definitive answer has not been proposed regarding who owns the data.

However, public policy debates concerning the collection of health-care information for use as aggregate databases to underpin health-care planning are increasing. Many consumers are concerned about the status of future physician-client relationships. Driving the development of data collection policy is the public's fears about the damages that may result from excessive and uncontrolled health-care information disclosures through automated information systems.[28]

What Do You Think?

Who do you think owns health-care information? How does your decision affect health-care policy in the future?

When clients enter the health-care system, they are generally asked to sign consent forms so that other organizations can obtain information about their health status and the care that they received (particularly insurance companies so that bills can be paid). They are usually unaware that this information can be supplied to many other organizations or institutions. For example, reports to the trauma registry are made about injuries resulting from accidents. The tumor registry collects information about benign and malignant tumors, and infectious disease reports are made to the Public Health Department. In the future, sharing of health-care information will be used to support the development of payment systems, examine access to care, identify cost differences of treatment modalities, research disease trends and epidemiologic implications, and expand consumer information. Policies guiding the collection, development, and use of these data must be created around the core issues of confidentiality and security.

Even today, there is an expanded use of client information that would have been unacceptable only a few years ago. Some current, commonly accepted uses for client records include quality assurance, institutional licensing and accreditation, biomedical research, third-party reimbursement, credentialing, litigation, regional and national databases, court-ordered release of information, and managed care comparisons. Although automated information systems did not cause these information uses, automation does make acquiring this information much easier.

Unauthorized sharing of health-care information is generally unethical but is not always illegal. The code of ethics for most health-care professionals prohibits the unauthorized or unnecessary access to client information. In addition, most health-care institutions have policies prohibiting unauthorized access to confidential information. Although individuals can lose their jobs because of unauthorized access or sharing of client information, it is not illegal to do so.

Unauthorized access or sharing of information is not a new problem. It is just as easy to gain unauthorized access to a manual paper record as it is to the automated electronic record. The professional codes of ethics that stress client confidentiality have always been the primary protector of client information. Access to the paper record is available to anyone who picks up the chart. In some ways, the automated electronic record provides greater privacy to an individual. Access to the automated record is generally restricted to employees who have been issued a password. Also, most organizations have periodic **audits** that can track each person who has accessed a record, and some systems can even detect unauthorized access at the time of entry into the system.

Unauthorized sharing of health-care information is generally unethical but is not always illegal.

In an attempt to address the problem of unregulated processing and use of health-care information, the federal government developed the Health Insurance Portability and Accountability Act (HIPAA) in 1996. According to Cassidy,[29] the primary objectives of HIPAA are:

- Ensure health insurance portability
- Reduce health-care fraud and abuse
- Guarantee security and privacy of health information
- Enforce standards for health information

In 2000, HIPAA enacted rules governing the exchange of electronic administrative health-care information. The object of these rules was to simplify and standardize the electronic forms required for claims for services rendered. Every organization must now use the same form.

In 2001, the rules addressed the use and disclosure of individually identifiable health information in any form. Treatment providers must obtain patient consent before using or disclosing patient information for treatment, payment, or health-care operations.

Treatment providers must obtain patient consent before using or disclosing patient information for treatment, payment, or health-care operations.

HIPAA rules will continue to evolve and affect the manner in which traditional health-care entities such as payers, providers, and employer groups conduct business. Initially, the expense of complying with HIPAA regulations will be large, but an eventual cost savings is the expected result of the new regulations.

Threats to the security of information can be either accidental or intentional and affect both paper and electronic systems. Accidental threats involve naturally occurring events such as floods, fires, earthquakes, electrical surges, and power outages. The paper record has little security against many natural events. Typically, paper records are secured in a locked file cabinet or medical records room. Although current safety regulations require fire detection and suppression systems in these areas, even small fires can destroy a large number of paper records very quickly. There is little that can be done to protect paper records against major flooding. Once the charts are destroyed, they cannot be reproduced.

Facilities with automated systems usually have well-developed natural disaster plans built into the system design. These plans include the automatic production and storage of a backup tape of the data at a protected location some distance from the health-care facility. The frequency of data backup varies with the organization's requirements. Most systems automatically save all the data in the system every 24 hours, although this time interval can be shortened or increased to meet the facility's needs. Although these measures provide a high degree of protection from major natural events such as floods and fires, power surges and outages create problems for electronic systems that leave paper systems unaffected. Anyone who works at all with computerized equipment recognizes the major disruptions in service and work that occur when the "system goes down." Again, some safeguards can be built into the system so that not all the most recent information is lost when the power goes out. Power surges can be controlled with surge protection devices.

Intentional threats to the security of information involve the actions of an individual or individuals who wish to damage, destroy, or alter the records. In most cases, it is difficult to protect paper records from intentional tampering. It is a rather simple task for a determined individual to gain access to paper records and either erase, add to, or rewrite sections of the chart. These changes are often very difficult to detect. In addition, a person could simply remove the chart and destroy it so that there would be no record left at all.

Today, consumers are more knowledgeable about health care through use of the Internet.

Although automated electronic records are vulnerable to several different intentional threats, they are, over all, more secure than the paper record. All current automated systems have computer virus-checking programs that protect the automated record from the introduction of both intentional and accidental computer viruses into the system that will destroy information. Once data have been entered into the automated system, the data are difficult to alter. Modern automated systems are now designed with the "write once, read many" (WORM) programs. If a legitimate change in the electronic record needs to be made, it must be added as an addendum. Any changes made in the electronic record are logged by the time and the person who made them and can always be tracked to the point of origin. Although it is true that a determined and gifted hacker can still obtain access to almost any electronic database, electronic security systems are becoming more and more difficult to breach.

Uses of the Internet

For nursing professionals, the Internet has become a valuable resource for communicating with colleagues and professional organizations, researching clinical information, and educating consumers about health resources and information. Because of the lack of standardization and regulation, it is important that the nurse evaluate each site for accuracy of information, authority, objectivity, currency or timeliness, and coverage.[30]

Most professional organizations maintain a Web site containing information about the organization. Many include policy statements and lists of publications. **Continuing education units (CEUs)** can be obtained via the World Wide Web to help nurses remain current and retain licensure. The Nursing Network (http://www.nursingnetwork.com), for example, is a site that lists nursing education courses, nursing position vacancies, nursing conferences, and other pertinent information. News groups, such as those listed at http://www.nursingworld.org provide professional information and access to experts in specific areas of interest.

Disease-specific Web sites publish clinical information for both the consumer and the professional. OncoLink is an example of a resource for information about cancer. Often the most recent information about a disease is found on the Internet. Publishing is quicker and easier on the World Wide Web than in a peer-reviewed journal. Web-based support groups disseminate information on both technical and consumer levels. Protocols and policies are shared through Web sites and news groups.

Today, consumers are more knowledgeable about health care through use of the Internet. Clients are better informed than they were in the past, because they now have easy access to a wide range of health-care information. Preventive and wellness services are available electronically through articles, chat groups, and health risk assessment surveys posted on consumer Web sites. Kaiser Permanente has started an ambitious on-line pilot project that offers members various services, including 30,000 pages of disease-specific information; participation in discussion groups; and the ability to ask questions of a nurse, pharmacist, or specialist. In the future, members will be able to schedule themselves for nonurgent appointments at various clinics, order prescription refills or over-the-counter medications from an "on-line drugstore," and send e-mail messages directly to their physicians.[31]

Healthfinder is a consumer health and human services information Web site created and maintained by the federal government. The site links the user with on-line government publications, clearinghouses, databases, Web sites, support and self-help groups, as well as the government agencies and not-for-profit organizations that produce reliable information for the public. The goal of this information source is to help consumers make better choices about their health and human services needs for both themselves and their families.

Telehealth

For more than 30 years, clinicians, health services researchers, and others have been investigating the use of advanced telecommunications and information technologies to improve health care. Physicians examine and treat clients from distant sites with video cameras, thus saving money by exchanging office visits for on-line appointments. Telehealth is becoming more common in emergency rooms across the United States. The University of Pittsburgh offers neurologic consults to physicians at seven linked hospitals. In Baltimore, providers are taking telehealth to the streets, using cellular telephone lines to transmit live video and client data back to home base.[32] With expenditures for home health services expected to double within the next 5 years, HMOs and home health agencies are investing in telemedicine and information technologies to control costs and meet increased service demands.[33]

The terms *telehealth* and *telemedicine* are often used interchangeably. As defined here, telehealth is the use of electronic information and communications technologies to provide and support health care when distance separates the physician and the client. Telehealth includes a wide range of services and technologies, ranging from the "plain old telephone service" (POTS) to highly sophisticated digitized cameras, telemetry, and voice systems. Telemedicine is just one of the services provided by the overall telehealth system that primarily involves consultation with a physician.

Some uses of telehealth, such as emergency calls to 911, are so common that they are often overlooked when considering telehealth systems. Other applications such as telesurgery involve exotic technologies and procedures that are still in the experimental stage.

Historically, consumer concerns about access to health care have been the driving force behind the development of many clinical telehealth systems. Early applications focused on remote populations scattered across mountainous areas, islands, open plains, and arctic regions where medical specialists, and sometimes even primary care practitioners, were not available. Many telehealth projects from the 1960s through the early 1980s failed because they were expensive, awkward to use, and often not guided by the strategic plans of the facilities using them.

Renewed interest in telehealth has been spurred by managed care initiatives seeking to reduce health-care costs while maintaining or increasing the quality and access to care. Overall costs have decreased for many of the information and communications technologies used by telehealth systems. In addition, the ever-developing National Information Infrastructure is making these technologies more accessible and user friendly. As of October 2001, Medicare expanded reimbursement to include some types of telehealth care, but other third-party payers may still have difficulty determining reimbursement for telehealth services.

Telehealth offers many advantages affecting the cost of and access to the health-care system of the future. The telehealth system allows access to centralized specialists who can support primary care providers in outlying areas. Outlying areas can be either rural or urban areas that lack access to the full range of health-care services. Outlying clinics staffed only with nurse practitioners or physician assistants have immediate access to physician referrals through the telehealth system. University medical centers can offer specialist consulting services to primary care physicians at distant locations, thus reducing unnecessary travel and increased cost to clients. Here is an actual example of how the telehealth system functions in an emergency situation:

> In 1996, a 72-year-old man with a collapsed lung walked into the emergency room (ER) in a small town in North Dakota. The general practitioner who usually saw routine emergency cases immediately called the trauma II medical center in Bismarck and arranged a teleconsult with an ER physician and a thoracic surgeon. The man would die without a thoracotomy. Following the surgeon's instructions, the physician was able to insert the chest tubes needed to safely transport the client by helicopter to Bismarck.[32]

Telehealth services often save lives and prevent permanent disability, especially when time is a factor in treatment. For example, health-care providers know that if thrombolytic medications are given within 3 hours after the onset of symptoms of a stroke, the likelihood of death or permanent disability is reduced by 50 percent. Using telehealth technology, neurology specialists can evaluate a client's condition while he or she is still in the ambulance en route to the hospital, thus saving valuable time in making the decision about using lifesaving medications. The ER is prepared to administer the medications as soon as the client enters the department rather than having to wait several hours for all the routine evaluations and consults to be completed.

> *Nurses who practice in rural and underserved urban areas will have more autonomy and provide higher quality care when linked electronically with the support services of a large medical center.*

In the future, home care may benefit the most from telehealth. By investing in telehealth technologies, home care providers should be able to balance cost reductions with increased quality of care. Clients can be monitored at home using a combination of telephone calls, home visits, video visits, and in-home monitoring via the telehealth system. In-home monitoring devices for conditions ranging from congestive heart failure and diabetes to cancer and cardiac conditions can send information from the client's home to a central base for assessment by professionals. A Kaiser Permanente study in California demonstrated that when instant access from home to health-care professional was provided by telehealth systems, it reduced the cost of care by one-third while increasing its quality. Furthermore, the study showed that client anxiety levels were reduced, as noted in the agency's client satisfaction surveys.[32]

Future challenges remain for telehealth applications. Many of the older technical systems are poorly designed and do not meet the needs of the user's environment. As discussed earlier, human factor design and user assessments must be carefully considered when developing any new technologies. Although the overall costs of electronic systems continue to gradually

ISSUES NOW

Tomorrow's Technology Today

Almost any health-care provider with even a passing familiarity with the Star Trek movies or television shows has been envious of the tricorder used by fictional medical personnel to diagnose and treat a variety of ills by just waving the device over the client in distress. Although present technology is not quite to that point, it certainly is a lot closer than even a few short years ago.

Wearable computers, initially developed for use in the military as a type of flak jacket/telemetry vest is currently being tested. The Massachusetts Institute of Technology has improved upon the technology by developing a heart brooch that sends heart sounds back to the health-care provider. It looks like an elegant piece of jewelry that anyone can wear. The Japanese are beginning production of "smart" toilets that can collect, process, and transmit data based on their contents.

A technology company named BodyMedia has developed an integrated program that combines principles of wellness with technology. People who wish to join the program are fitted with a BodyMedia SenseWear Armband, a personal body monitoring apparatus. It is a little smaller than the current arm radio, weighs about 3 ounces, and is worn on the back of the right triceps. The brain of the unit is a computer, memory chip, and sensors that continuously monitor body motion, skin temperature, heart rate, evaporation heat loss, and the amount of heat being dissipated by the body. The devices, when programmed with the wearer's sex, age, height, and weight, provide data on the expenditure of energy while involved in various activities. The armband can be used to treat clients with congestive heart failure, improve client compliance, and alter lifestyle habits.

Nurses will soon be exposed to these smart devices. They will provide more data for integration into the health-care record, allow comparison of client's progress not only from day to day, but hour to hour or even minute to minute, and provide highly accurate and detailed information.

Another technology that nurses will be experiencing sooner rather than later is voice-activated information systems. We are used to seeing sportscasters, singers, and others in the media with the headset/microphone devices. Nurses will soon be wearing something very similar, a voice-activated headset that will allow them to dictate their documentation as they go about their daily tasks. Nurses have long realized that most of their work is highly activity directed and performed on the run. Sitting behind a computer, or even standing in a room at a computer console, is not the reality of nursing. It will allow for more timely documentation and free up some down time with paperwork.

These are just two areas of many that are around the corner in health care. One important element in any developing health-care technology is input from the people who are going to be using it. Too often new technology is developed by people who are experts in computers but have very little experience with health care. Unless a technology is user friendly, it is not going to be effective. Nurses need to play an active role in designing and testing new systems.

decrease, initial expenditures are still a barrier to implementation, especially in smaller facilities. Lack of **third-party payment** for telehealth systems also limits their development and use. Several legal issues still need to be resolved, including health-care provider licensure when consults are given across state lines and the liability incurred by providers who examine a client by television rather than in a face-to-face, hands-on encounter. Federal and state policies protecting privacy and confidentiality need to be developed with specific provisions for telehealth systems.

The telehealth system also affects nursing practice. Nurses are the primary users of telephone triage systems that rely on computerized decision-making trees to suggest appropriate actions when given a set of client symptoms. Nurses who practice in rural and underserved urban areas will have more autonomy and provide higher quality care when linked electronically with the support services of a large medical center. The use of remote monitoring devices provides nurses with immediate information about changes in their clients' conditions, improves outcomes, reduces complications, and lowers the number of re-admissions to the hospital.

The same types of technology used for telehealth can be used for distance and **nontraditional education** applications. Widespread use of **continuing education** is achieved through distance technology. Courses are video-conferenced with two-way interaction. Continuing education credits can be earned through courses on the Internet. Even college credits can be earned via Internet access. Grand rounds are conducted at multiple sites with video conferencing equipment, and in-services are beamed to multiple locations.

Conclusion

The information revolution affects every aspect of health care, not only in the United States but also throughout the world. The advent of advanced communications technology and its increased availability worldwide promotes ties between people and nations, bridging the gap between isolated rural communities and major metropolitan areas. The nursing profession needs to be actively involved in developing clinical information systems and the electronic health record, establishing care standards, safeguarding client privacy, using the Internet, and researching better ways of improving access and the quality of care through technology. The nursing profession is transformed, enhanced, and enriched as nurses become active participants in the information revolution.

Critical Thinking Exercises

- Debate the ethical issues of personal privacy and the greater social good in relation to availability of health-care information.
- Discuss how the design of equipment increases or decreases error rate.
- Discuss uses of telehealth for patient teaching and monitoring of home health clients.
- Write a vision paper describing your view of technology in health care in the year 2030.
- List all the pieces of data you had to give at your last visit to the doctor or hospital.
- Was all of the information necessary to provide your care?
- Who needed the information?
- How was the information recorded or transmitted?

References

1. Swerdlow, JL: Information revolution. National Geographic, October 1995, pp. 5–11.
2. The 2001 Sveriges Riksbank prize in economic sciences in memory of Alfred Nobel @The Bank of Sweden Prize in Economic Sciences press release:. Retrieved March 20, 2002 from http://www.nobel.se/economics/laureates/2001/press.html.
3. van Bemmel, JH, and Musen, MA (eds): Handbook of Medical Informatics. Springer-Verlag, Heidelberg, 1998.
4. Greenburg, AB: Medical informatics: Science or science fiction. Unpublished material, 1975.
5. Mandil, S: Health informatics: New solutions to old challenges. World-Health, August–September 1989, pp. 2–5.
6. Graves, J, and Corcoran, S: The study of nursing informatics. Image J Nurs Sch 21:227–231, 1989.
7. Saba, VK, and McCormick, KA: Essentials of Computers for Nurses, ed. 2. McGraw-Hill, New York, 1995, p. 226.
8. Turley, RJ: Toward a model for nursing informatics. Image J Nurs Sch 28(4):309–313, 1996.
9. Nelson, R, and Joos, I: On language in nursing: From data to wisdom. PLN Visions, Fall 1989, pp. 6–7.
10. Hannah K: Current trends in nursing informatics: Implications for curriculum planning. In Hannah, K, et al (eds): Nursing Uses of Computer and Information Science: Proceedings of the IFIP-IMIA International Symposium on Nursing Uses of Computers and Information Science. Calgary, Alberta, Canada, 1–3 May 1985. Elsevier Science Publishers, Amsterdam, 1985.
11. American Nurses Association: Scope and Standards of Nursing Informatics Practice. American Nurses Publishing, Washington, DC, 2001.
12. American Nurses Credentialing Center Catalog. American Nurses Publishing, Washington, DC, 2001.
13. Simpson, RL: Information is power. Nursing Administration 20(3):86–89, 1996.
14. Prophet, CM: Nursing interventions classifications. In Grobe, SJ, and Pluyter-Wenting, ESP (eds): Nursing Informatics: An International Overview for Nursing in a Technological Era. Elsevier, Amsterdam, 1994, pp. 692–696.
15. Congressional Office of Technology Assessment, 1988. Available at: www.cota.gov.
16. Casey, A: Nursing, midwifery and health visiting teams project. In Grobe, SJ, and Pluyter-Wenting, ESP (eds): Nursing Informatics: An International Overview for Nursing in a Technological Era. Elsevier, Amsterdam, 1994, pp. 639–642.
17. Elliott, S: Information overload and medical progress: When is enough too much? Minimally Invasive Surgical Nursing 8(1):23–27, 1994.
18. Bostrum, J, and Suter, W: Research utilization: Making the link to practice. Journal of Nursing Staff Development 9(1):28–34, 1993.
19. Blythe, J, et al: Linking the professional literature to nursing practice: Challenges and opportunities. American Association of Occupational Health Nursing 43(6):342–345, 1995.
20. Institute of Medicine: To Err is Human: Building a Safer Health System. National Academy of Sciences, Washington, DC, 2000.
21. The Leapfrog Group: Patient Safety, 2000. Retrieved June 6, 2001, from http://www.leapfroggroup.org/safety1.htm.
22. Weinstein, A: The bandwagon is outside waiting. Health Management Technology, May 2001, pp. 187–189.
23. Brennan, TA, et al: Incidence of adverse events and negligence in hospitalized patients. Results of the Harvard Medical Practice Study I. N Engl J Med 324:370–376, 1991.
24. McDonald, CJ: Protocol-based computer reminders, the quality of care and the non-perfectability of man. N Engl J Med 295:1351–1355, 1976.
25. Childs, B: A quick look forward. Healthcare Informatics, January 1994, pp. 87–88.
26. Miller, L, and Weise, E: Database sharing eroding medical confidentiality. USA Today, 23 February 1998, p. 10D.
27. Quittner, J: Invasion of privacy. Time, 25 August 1997, pp. 29–35.
28. Mills, ME: Data privacy and confidentiality in the public arena. In Proceedings of the AMIA Annual Fall Symposium on the Emergence of Internetable Health Care. Systems That Really Work. Nashville, TN, 25–29 October 1997. Hanley & Belfus, National Commission on Nursing Implementation Project, 1997.
29. Cassidy, B: Using web technology. Journal of AHIMA, June 2000. Available at: http://www.ahima.org/journal/features/feature.0006.4.html.
30. Alexander, J, and Tate, M: The web as a research tool: Evaluation techniques. Available at: http://www.science.widener.edu/~withers/alaslides/pptfirst.htm.
31. Schneider, P: Patient informatics is growing. Healthcare Informatics, August 1997, p. 14.
32. Davies, P: Delivering emergency care—In a heart beat. Telemedicine and Telehealth Networks, October 1997, pp. 28–32.
33. Kincade, K: Growing home-care business benefits from telemedicine tlc. Telemedicine and Telehealth Networks, October 1997, pp. 23–27.

Bibliography

American Nurses Association: Scope and Standards of Nursing Informatics Practice. American Nurses Publishing, Washington, DC, 2001.

Carty, B: Nursing Informatics: Education for Practice. Springer, New York, 2000.

DeBourgh, GA: Using Web technology in a clinical nursing course. Nurse Educator 26(5):227–233, 2001.

Englebardt, S, and Nelson, R (eds): Health Care Informatics: An Interdisciplinary Approach. Mosby, St. Louis, 2002.

Nicoll, LH: Nurses' Guide to the Internet, ed. 3. Lippincott, Philadelphia, 2001.

O'Brien, BS, and Renner, A: Nurses on-line: Career mobility for registered nurses. J Prof Nurs 16(1):13–20, 2000.

Sackett, K, et al: Interactive connections: Technologies used in nursing education. JNYSNA 32(1):7–10, 2001.

Timmons, S: Use of the Internet by patients: Not a threat to nursing but an opportunity. Nurse Education Today 21(2):104–109, 2001.

Williams, CA, and Gossett, MT: Nursing communication: Advocacy for the patient or the physician. Clinical Nursing Research 10(3):332–334, 2001

Young, KM: Informatics for Healthcare Professionals. FA Davis, Philadelphia, 2000.

4

Issues in Delivering Care

18

The Politically Active Nurse

Donna Gentile O'Donnell

Learning Objectives

After completing this chapter, the reader will be able to:

- Explain why it is important for nurses to understand and become involved in the political process.
- Discuss how a bill becomes a law.
- Identify the major committees at the federal level that influence health policy.
- Identify four points at which nurses can influence a bill.
- Give examples of how nurses may become politically involved.
- List and describe four methods of lobbying.

The word politics conjures up various images—some positive and some negative. There are images of great statesmanship, like the inaugural speech of John F. Kennedy exhorting the nation, "Ask not what your country can do for you, but what you can do for your country." Or images of more ignoble moments, like the national tragedy of Watergate, the resignation of Richard Nixon, the impeachment proceedings against Bill Clinton, the dubious election practices that elected George W. Bush, or the numerous negative campaign commercials vilifying a political opponent. Politics touches people's lives at all levels, crossing national boundaries, affecting individual states, and permeating local governments.

The goal of this chapter is to provide a foundation for understanding the political basics by using a "nuts and bolts" approach and to motivate nurses to become active in the political world. Politics is examined both within the profession of nursing and within society at large. In addition, this chapter discusses the forces that drive politics and the three concepts it comprises—partisanship, self-interest, and ideology.

Almost everyone has something to say about politics, ranging from political candidates, academicians, and members of the press to regular citizens. People define politics in many ways. One of the most cynical definitions of politics is offered by Ambrose Bierce in *The Devil's Dictionary*, describing it as "a strife of interests masquerading as a contest of principles. The conduct of public affairs for private advantage." Other, more widely accepted definitions include "the art or science of government," "the art or science concerned with guiding or influencing government policy," or "the total complex of relations between men in society."[1]

The Nursing Shortage

The nursing shortage is a good example of where nurses' concerns intersect with the political process. In many areas of the United States, the nursing shortage has reached crisis levels, and there does not appear to be any permanent cures on the near horizon. Different areas of the country are attempting to deal with the shortage in the short term with quick, stopgap political measures that may have an adverse effect on the nursing profession in the long term.

Politics touches people's lives at all levels, crossing national boundaries, affecting individual states, and permeating local governments.

One quick and easy solution some hospitals are initiating is recruitment of nurses from outside the country. Hospitals in Louisville, Kentucky, have started a program to bring nurses from the Philippines to the United States. Representatives from the Norton and University of Louisville hospitals traveled to the Philippines and interviewed 150 nurses interested in coming to the United States. They eventually selected and signed contracts with 25 nurses from this group. The Filipino nurses will receive the same pay and benefits as the American registered nurses (RNs) when employed by one of the five hospitals involved in the recruitment. They will also receive permanent resident visas and housing if desired. The recruitment plan does not address obtaining U.S. licensure by the foreign nurses, an issue that affects the state board of nursing and the nurse practice act.

The importation of foreign nurses to meet nursing shortages is not a new idea. It has been a potential solution for nursing shortages stretching back as far as the World War I. Health-care facilities, especially hospitals, strongly favor this approach to solve the nursing shortage. It is also a very good deal for the nurses who come into this country. They can easily make up to five times the salary they receive in their own countries in addition to upgrading their living conditions and lifestyle. However, as a profession, nurses need to examine this practice very closely because it seems to be an end-run attempt around existing regulations in the nurse practice act.

The primary concern is not one of quality of care. Nursing programs in the Philippines are 5 years long and require considerable clinical practice for their students. Although they are based on a medical model rather than nursing models, the Filipino schools produce nurses whose technical nursing skills are at levels comparable to those of new graduates from the United States.

The issue American nurses should be concerned with by the importation of foreign nurses is legislative in nature, namely institutional licensure. The underlying premise of institutional licensure is that individual health-care institutions are permitted to determine which individuals are qualified to practice nursing within general guidelines established by an outside board. The practice of institutional licensure has been universally rejected by every major nursing organization; however, health-care facilities continue to attempt "back-door" institutional licensure as is demonstrated by the Norton and Louisville hospitals. When foreign nurses are allowed to practice in specific institutions without taking the American licensure examinations, de facto institutional licensure exists even if it is not called by name.

So what's so bad about institutional licensure? The primary problem is the lack of external standards to determine the level of competency. Obviously, when the representatives of the Louisville hospitals interviewed the 150 candidates, they were looking for certain characteristics or qualities. What were these qualities? Ability to speak English? Not having a family?

Knowledge in critical care, obstetrics, pediatrics? No one really knows how the final 25 were selected. Without external standards, the designations of RN or LPN/LVN (licensed practical nurse/licensed vocational nurse) become relatively meaningless. In addition, without an American nursing license, these foreign nurses would not be under the control of the state board of nursing. What if the foreign nurse was practicing unethically or made grievous negligent errors that caused harm to the client? Who would be responsible? Who would discipline the nurse?

Nurses who are practicing in states where the importation of foreign nurses is being planned or actually practiced need to contact their state board of nursing. It is highly probable that the practice violates a standard in the nurse practice act, and the facilities conducting the practice should be investigated.

Some nurses are attempting to deal with the consequences of the nursing shortage, such as understaffing, mandatory overtime, supervision of undertrained personnel, and erosion of the quality of care, by seeking employment in what has become known as "luxury health-care centers." Luxury health-care centers are for-profit facilities that specialize in specific, high-revenue health care. In addition to offering high-end perks for the clients, such as gourmet meals, well-decorated, "resort-like"comfortable rooms that are sometimes called "guest suites," and one-room stays rather than moving from the intensive care unit (ICU) to a medical/surgical unit, these facilities also attract nurses who are tired of the working conditions of a traditional hospital.

The luxury health-care centers are focused on providing specific services for particular procedures that generate high profits. Heart and orthopedic hospitals, cancer centers, and free-standing surgery facilities currently are the most common focus for this type of health care. The heart hospitals offer the services usually found in a general hospital, such as angioplasty, pacemaker insertion, and bypass surgery, but with a much higher level of care. These hospitals use the client-focused care model in which a client stays in one room throughout the stay and is provided care by the same nurses until discharge.

> **What Do You Think?**
>
> *What experiences have you encountered, either as a client or a health-care worker, related to the nursing shortage? How might the political system help solve the shortage?*

These facilities generate revenue by offering only certain high-end medical procedures that have a large profit margin and are covered by insurance. The luxury facilities save money by having a minimal number of administrators and allowing the nurses more input into the policy decisions and day-to-day provision of care. In many of these facilities, up to 60 percent of the nursing staff is involved in direct client care, whereas the average in general hospitals is about 40 percent. Nurses are also cross-trained so that they can function in multiple roles in the facility. In addition, the facilities reduce cost by shortening the length of client stays. Several limited research studies have shown that in luxury facilities where the client-centered model is used, client stays are routinely reduced by 25 to 50 percent.

Nurses find this type of work environment attractive for several reasons. They feel that they can provide a higher level of continuity of care because the same nurse admits the client, cares for him or her during the stay, and then handles the discharge when the client goes home. Nurses feel that the quality of care is much higher in the luxury facilities. They work primarily with adequate numbers of well-trained professionals. Cross-training allows nurses to practice in several different settings, reducing the monotony of practice sometimes experienced in general hospitals. Also, by having a bigger say in the work environment, policies, and care they provide, one of the primary elements of burnout (lack of control) is significantly reduced. Finally, nurses in the luxury care facilities earn on average \$5.00 to \$7.00 more per hour than nurses in traditional hospitals. Retirement and health insurance plans are often better, and some even offer stock options as part of the benefit package.

So what is the downside to luxury hospitals? One significant problem is the siphoning off of the highest revenue procedures from the general hospitals. Most general, not-for-profit hospitals do a continual financial juggling act in an attempt to balance services that lose money or make little money (trauma centers, burn units, obstetric units) with areas that have a high income (cardiac centers, orthopedic centers, one-day surgery). Some analysts believe that the competition from the luxury hospitals will force the general hospitals to improve the quality of their care so that they can draw in more clients, but the reality is that if the general hospitals run at a deficit for too long, they will be forced to closed.

Another concern is that the most experienced and most qualified nurses are being lured away from the general hospitals. The nursing shortage has made it an employees' market. The luxury hospitals, because of the higher pay, can pick and choose from the best of the best. Heart hospitals are particularly interested in hiring ICU and critical care unit (CCU) nurses, as well as nurses with surgical and recovery room experience. This group represents some of the best-educated and most skilled nurses in any facility. As a result, the staffing shortages in the general hospitals will increase, and the quality of care suffers more by the loss of experienced nurses.

The long-term solution is to increase the supply of nurses by encouraging more young men and women to enter schools of nursing; however, the trend since the early 1990s is decreased enrollment in nursing schools. National trends in nursing school enrollments have shown a gradual but steady decline in enrollments of about 35 percent during this period. For those who do choose to enter the nursing profession, the future looks bright. There are many opportunities, and health-care facilities are beginning to appreciate and reward nurses at the level they deserve.

A recent example of the power of an alliance occurred in California in relation to the nursing shortage. The California state legislature made the precedent-setting move to establish minimum nurse-to-client ratios by enacting legislation in late 1999. The regulations are to be phased in over several years and to take effect in July 2003. Nurses' unions and consumer advocacy groups, such as the American Association of Retired Persons (AARP), support the proposal as a step toward increasing client safety and reducing the nursing shortage. Other states are following the development of this legislation closely. A bill has already been introduced in the Florida state legislature that has even more strict nurse-to-client ratios than the California bill. As always, there is opposition to these bills, generally by the state hospital associations and often the physicians' association too. The nursing shortage and the various attempts to resolve it are health-care issues that have become political. They have the potential to affect the profession of nursing greatly, and nurses need to get out in front of the issues if they want to have a say in what is decided about their future.[2]

Government and Politics

Keep in mind that government is a very broad term that refers to almost any type of hierarchical structure that functions to organize and direct an organization. From this context, the governance structure of any health-care facility can be considered a type of government that has its own politics. At this level, nurses have the potential to have a considerable amount of political influence.

Historically, most nurses avoided becoming engaged in government, perhaps because they share definitions similar to the one presented by Bierce. However, nurses, both as individual citizens and as a professional group, need to recognize that their personal lives and professional practice are affected by the political world. Some recent trends in health care, particularly the nursing shortage, managed care, and cost containment, have made nurses increasingly susceptible to the "bottom line." In addition, because of politics, nurses are confronting major changes in health care on a daily basis. They have experienced the erosion of the profession through their replacement with less-educated personnel and have seen the quality of client care deteriorate. Nurses, if they decide to act, are not powerless against such trends.

As a large group of voters, nurses have the power, influence, and skill to take an active role in the political process. Senator Daniel Inouye of Hawaii referred to nurses as the "sleeping giant in health care." Nurses can gain much by using the tools of political action, and now more than ever their professional survival depends on it.

There are attainable, deliberate actions individual nurses can take that can create a powerful, political force. However, before nurses can realize their full potential, a basic knowledge and understanding of the political system is necessary. Henry Adams stated long ago that "Knowledge of human nature is the beginning and end of a political education." If he is correct, it is logical to conclude that nurses, who are among the most astute observers of human nature, are in many ways ideally suited to the art and science of politics.

Why Should Nurses Be Involved?

A widely accepted definition of politics is the process of influencing **public policy**, including all forms and levels of governmental regulations. The effects of politics are pervasive and related to almost every aspect of life. On a personal level, politics influence where children go to school, the quality of food eaten, the water that flows from your kitchen tap, what medications are prescribed, and the speed limit on roadways. On a professional level, politics influences where nurses work, what they do and how they do it, the ability to organize professionally, and even the nurse's professional status through licensure and certification. The effects of politics on a person's life would seem to have no limits.

Nurses experience the effects of governmental regulations both directly and indirectly. Examples of directly experienced government regulations include some recent reforms that many states have initiated. Some state delegations have considered nurse-to-patient ratios. All states now have granted advanced practice nurses prescriptive privileges, although the regulations governing their implementation vary widely from state to state. Earlier attempts at national health-care reform have resulted in massive restructuring of the health-care system that led to dramatic decreases in the number of nurses employed in acute care hospitals. These reforms, initiated to forestall proposed legislation, continue to influence health care even today. Many nurses respond to these changes with sad acceptance and believe that they are beyond their control.

Alinsky provides useful pointers regarding tactics that nurses can use. Box 18–1 summarizes and gives examples for Alinsky's rules for tactics.

Definitions of Politics, Political Action, and Related Concepts

As a dynamic process, politics plays a key role in all forms and levels of government, including federal, state, and local. It can be seen as the complex interaction between the public policy and various public and constituent interests. Politics is directly and indirectly influenced by the self-interest of political officials, both elected and appointed. The mass media also have both a direct and indirect impact on the political process through numerous political commentators, political commercials, and investigations into the backgrounds of selected political figures.

Political action is a set of activities, methods, tactics, and behaviors that affect or have the potential to affect governmental and legislative processes and outcomes.[3] Examples of political action include grassroots efforts to change policies, the activities of lobbyists to change elected officials' opinions or votes, the give and take of political compromise within legislative bodies, and even the power of veto by the chief executive of a governmental structure. Government is often thought of as a series of processes used to

Box 18–1

Alinsky's Rules for Tactics (With O'Donnell's Comments)

- *Power is not only what you have but what the enemy thinks you have.*

This is widely used in political organizing. Fundraising reports are a classic example. Candidates will work very hard to get their financial commitments before filing their candidacy, to inform people of their ammunition.

- *Never go outside the experience of your own people.*

This is the fundamental mistake that has been made in some efforts to organize nurses. The American Nurses Association (ANA) and the state associations too often reflect an elite group not connected to the real world. Their leadership tends not to be nurses from the bedside or those intimately connected with front-line nursing. Their issues, although legitimate, are not the experience of the nurses entrenched in patient care issues.

- *Wherever possible, go outside the experience of your enemy. Pick your battlefields.*

During a press conference around the March on Washington in 1996, nurses talked about their experiences that were foreign territory to the press. They presented a compelling picture. Most of the press were not accustomed to listening to nurses talk about high-tech procedures and gained a new level of respect for what nurses do. To the extent to which you can impress people with your knowledge and go outside their experience, it forces them to compete.

- *Make them live up to their own book of rules.*

An example of this rule happened many years ago. Bob O'Donnell, former speaker of the Pennsylvania House, tells a story about when he was first breaking into the political world. There was a party machine that was not interested in supporting the common interests of the neighborhoods. Undaunted, he learned the rules by which the next ward leader and committee person election would be held. Ward leaders and committee people are the smallest unit of the partisan political system. Usually committee people are responsible for districts. The districts add up to the ward. The ward leader oversees the committee people who manage those districts and register people to vote. Standing within the system is necessary in order to be successful in a political system. The way to do that in the ward structure is to either be ward leader or to have significant influence over the ward leader. Over a period of several years, O'Donnell assisted his allies in obtaining committee people positions. When there was an election for the ward leader, the committee people elected O'Donnell to the position of ward leader. The party machinery refused to seat the ward leader. O'Donnell used their own rule book to bring the issue to federal court and forced them to seat him as the new ward leader. He beat them at their own game.

- *Ridicule is man's and woman's most potent weapon.*

This is also known as the Dan Quayle phenomenon. Dan Quayle has been repeatedly characterized as a political buffoon. Dan Quayle is not as unintelligent as people assume him to be. Unfortunately for him, Vice President Quayle did some uninformed things while he happened to be standing in front of a magnifying glass with the national press behind it. More recently, Bill Clinton became the focus of many a political joke because of his involvement with Monica Lewinsky. His Republican enemies seized on the incident to the point where they made it an issue of impeachment.

Box 18–1

Alinsky's Rules for Tactics (With O'Donnell's Comments) (*Continued*)

- *A good tactic is one that your people enjoy.*

The 1996 March on Washington is a wonderful example. Laura Gasparis Vonfrolio did a wonderful job of tapping into the anger disseminated all over the country. Nurses enjoyed the national forum that permitted a massive demonstration for their voices to finally be heard.

- *A tactic that drags on too long, becomes a drag; use the concepts of reward and momentum.*

This is the most dangerous element for nurses attempting political organizing. The process is difficult and takes time to reach a successful conclusion. Nurses can become discouraged by the slow pace of the change process in the political arena. Rather than focusing only on long-range goals, it is important to concentrate on smaller objectives as, for instance, achieving a significant role in a city council race.

- *Keep the pressure on. Become the constant by which all other variables are defined.*

Currently, the ANA defines issues and concepts at the national level. The ANA has raised money in every state and has translated that money into a political power base in Washington. When a senator or congressman who has been a beneficiary of the ANA's largess takes a position, it is with the ANA in mind. Nurses need to become the standard by which all related variables are measured in their states. State legislators need to consider nurses' opinions the same way they do now with the teachers' association.

- *The threat is usually more terrifying than the thing itself. Threat is multiplied by the unknown and the imagination of someone under attack.*

This principle can be used very effectively over time. Imagine if someone opposed pro-nursing legislation and nurses threatened to demonstrate. The public image of thousands of nurses donning their uniforms would be a very powerful image for legislators to contend with.

- *The major premise for tactics is the development of operations that will maintain a constant pressure on the opposition. The pressure must be sustainable over time.*

This is the concept of "if what, then what." In a tactical plan, you have to be able to look beyond and determine what happens after you reach the end of this tactic.

- *Pick the target. Freeze it. Personalize it. Polarize it. And use a focused and strategic attack.*

Essentially, nurses need to be focused in their political activities. For example, imagine that nurses have considerable support from various legislative groups for objective standards and want to pass a law. A solid bill has been drafted. But a Democrat or Republican will not introduce your bill. The strategy is to target the one person who is slowing it down, whether it is the speaker, the senate pro tem president, or majority leader. Pick the target. Freeze it. Go after it with a vengeance. Personalize the attack and look at their constituencies. If they have a large senior citizen constituency, proclaim to the media that the prevention of the passage of your legislation is putting senior citizens in your legislative district in danger. The legislator will have to respond. Remember the one cardinal tenet of legislative action, never hurt "mon," "pop," or the "little guy." That is a focused and strategic attack.

maintain society. As both an element of and result of politics, government is also influenced by the forces that drive politics and the three concepts that constitute it:

- Partisanship
- Self-interest
- Ideology

Partisanship refers to membership in a political party. Because of the limited nature of this chapter, it focuses on Democrats, Republicans, and to a lesser extent, independents.

Self-interest is almost always the most important factor in politics. It dictates the kind of issues that legislators become involved in and present to their constituencies as the key issues. For instance, a congressman who resides in a blue-collar industrialized district that has a majority who support unionization will most likely be a pro-union congressman. The legislative structure in the United States was designed so that elected officials represent the people in their districts rather than having the whole population of the United States trying to make policy decisions. If a candidate does not represent the beliefs of the district, it is unlikely that he or she will succeed in that district.

In the larger world of electoral politics, the principle of self-interest often means that an elected official will not make legislative or political decisions that could lead to professional damage, namely loss of an election. Occasionally, there are exceptions to this rule. There have been a few cases in which elected officials were so ideologically committed to an issue that they defied conventional wisdom and made decisions that went against their self-interest. Generally, in order to be effective in politics, a person needs to understand and accept the self-interests of his or her constituents and use these self-interests as the driving force in their political decision making.

Ideology is a broad concept that embodies beliefs and principles of an individual or group. Conservatives, liberals, populists, libertarians, and radicals represent five examples of ideologies.

Conservatives

Traditional conservatives support less governmental regulation and involvement in everyday life, fewer taxes, and smaller social programs. The general characterization of the conservative belief system is "less government equals better government." Applied to the current range of issues, conservatives tend to be anti-abortion, anti–gun control, anti–socialized health care, and pro-choice on education.

Liberals

Traditional liberals believe that government has a moral responsibility to do good for society and that government intervention is necessary for the greater good of the citizens. This ideology traditionally translates into larger government structures, increased taxes, and larger spending for a wide range of social programs. Liberals are traditionally pro-choice, pro–gun control, pro–government-regulated health care, and anti-choice on education.

Populists

Populists are probably the most dominant political force in America at a grassroots level. Although populists in general do not like paying high taxes, ideologically they may represent a variety of positions on any particular issue. For instance, one group of populists may be anti-abortion, whereas another may be pro-choice. The common bond among all populists is that they have a sense of being burdened by a large, oppressive governmental structure. "The middle class is under siege" is a major theme that has resonated throughout several recent presidential campaigns.

Libertarians

Libertarianism is both a political party and an ideology. As a political partisan group, they represent an electoral fringe element. Ideologically, Libertarians differ from populists because they do not have the underlying middle-class anger that often drives the populists to take political action. Although they do believe in fiscal conservatism and dislike paying high taxes, Libertarians tend to be "laid back" in their approach to politics. Typically, they avoid ideological battles because they do not want to be burdened with decisions about choice on gun control, health care, schools, or abortion.

Radicals

Radicals exist at either end of the ideological spectrum in both of the major parties. It is important to recognize that although most voters tend toward the middle of the political spectrum between conservatism and liberalism, radicals attempt to force their parties to the extreme ends of the spectrum. For instance, Republicans are challenged by the radical right, which consists of the anti–big government and pro-life forces that make conspicuous demands on the party. To counteract the rhetoric of the radicals, the Republican party tries to find candidates who are ideologically near the middle of the spectrum because they know that most Republican voters have opinions near the middle of the spectrum.

Understanding the Playing Field

Structure

The three branches of the government are the executive, judiciary, and legislative branches. These branches exist simultaneously at the federal, state, and local government levels (Fig. 18–1; Box 18–2). At the federal level, the executive branch consists of the President, Vice President, Cabinet, and various executive administrative bodies. The executive of a state is the governor. Boards and commissions can also be construed as part of the executive branch because they are appointees of the chief executive. Locally, in county government, one or more county commissioners function as executives. Larger cities usually have a mayor. Smaller cities and townships sometimes also elect mayors.

The judicial branch is the court system. It is important to note that there is a distinction between state court and federal court; however, appeals and supreme courts are found at both levels. At the state level, there are supreme courts, appeals courts, and the lower courts. At the federal level, there is the Supreme Court, federal courts of appeal, and district or circuit courts. Additionally, many cities and counties have a local court system.

The judicial branch of government should not be discounted as unimportant to nurses. Over the years, several important issues have been decided by courts that have an effect on the practice of nursing. These include the Supreme Court's decision regarding the right of nurses to organize into collective bargaining units (see Chapter 15 for more discussion), the requirement of health-care providers to report potentially violent patients to the police, the obligation for nurses to refuse to carry out physician orders they deem dangerous, and criteria for when nurses can withdraw life support measures. New test cases that are continually being brought before the Supreme Court have the potential to dramatically change the way that nurses are perceived and what they are permitted to do in the workplace.

At the federal level, the legislative branch of government consists of the House of Representatives and the Senate. Each state also has a legislative branch of government, and, except for Nebraska, all states have a bicameral legislature with both a House of Representatives and a Senate. The primary function of the legislative branch of government is the formation of policy by the making of laws.

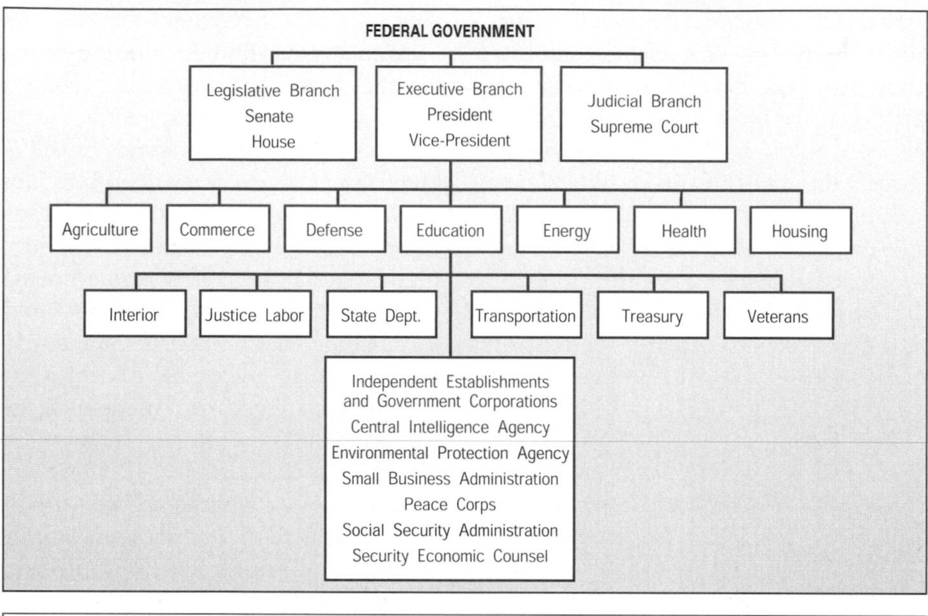

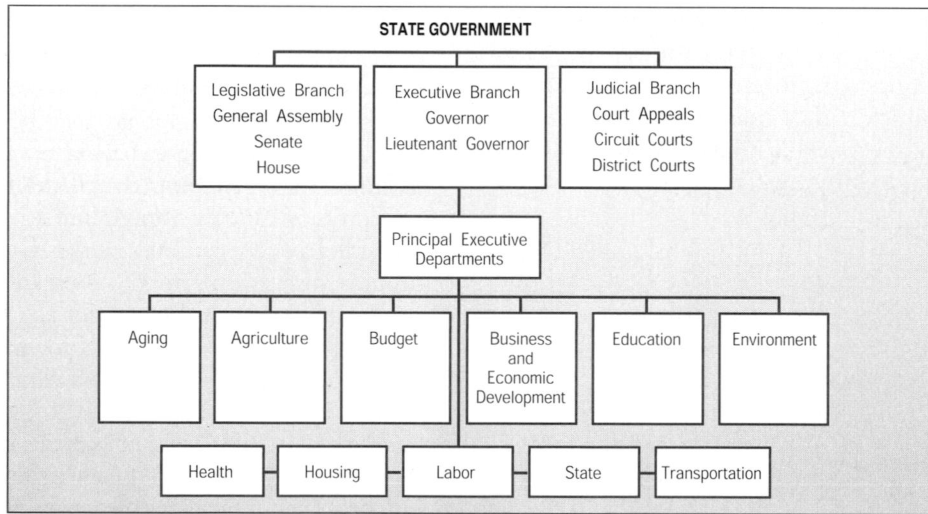

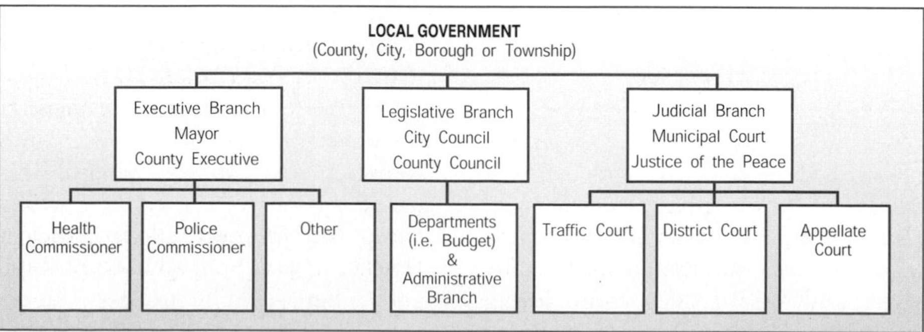

Figure 18–1. The organizational structure of the government.

Box 18–2

Know the Structure to Play the Game

One of the keys to creating power is understanding the organizational structure of the government. The Constitution of the United States establishes three separate branches of the federal government: legislative, judicial, and executive. The Constitution also ascribes certain auxiliary powers to the individual states. It is the role of the state governments to serve their citizens within these parameters and to delegate discrete areas of activity to local governments. Beneath the federal level of government in the United States, there exist state governments and five layers of local government identified by the U.S. Census Bureau: county, municipal, township, school district, and special district governments (which include various utility, construction, and facility authorities). The qualifications for the classification of these local government structures are generally determined by the parent state governments. State governments are governed by their individual state constitutions and in turn delineate responsibility for the local governments. It is important for nurses to understand that there are three levels in each governmental sector: federal, state, and local. These distinctions are important and are the most common source of confusion for nurses.

Key Players in the Formation of Policy (Agenda) and the Legislative Process

Members of the legislative branch of government have a wide range of ability and influence. It is important to remember that legislators are human, and they respond to the same forces that all people respond to, including interpersonal dynamics, peer pressure, and both internal and external factors.

The majority leader in the House is the person who generally supervises and directs the activities on the House floor. Some consider it to be the most powerful job in politics. The majority leader has control over the legislative calendar, which ultimately determines when many of the House session activities take place and even when bills are introduced for consideration. The majority leader is also the central figure in crafting the budget, which is the single most important activity the legislature performs on an annual basis.

The majority whip is responsible for collecting votes when legislators may be leaning toward voting against their party. At the same time the majority leader is supporting a bill, the whip is negotiating on the House floor for the votes necessary to successfully pass the bill. The whip is responsible for collecting support and votes for various issues both during the legislative session and when they are in recess.

The minority leader represents the party that does not have a numerical majority in the House and helps organize support against bills introduced by the majority leader. The minority leader presents an alternative point of view. There is an expression in the legislature: "The majority will have their way, and the minority will have their say." In most cases, the majority party

What Do You Think?

Who do you know in the legislature of your state government? Who is your representative or congressperson? Make a list of the things you would want that person to do for health care.

has the capacity to pass almost any bill they support over the objections of the minority. The minority leader usually only has the capacity to speak against it. However, there are some issues that legislators will almost never vote against—"mom," "pop," and the "little guy." When these issues are included in a bill, most legislators will support it even if they must vote against their party.

The conference committee attempts to reconcile differences in bills from the House and the Senate. The rules governing the structure, composition, and function of the conference committee vary from state to state. Generally, they consist of an equal number of appointed members from both the House and the Senate. Often a specified combination of votes, such as two votes from the House and two votes from the Senate, are necessary to approve a compromise bill and move it out of committee.

Caucuses are formed when the legislature divides into groups consisting of people with mutual interests. These groups operate as a unit, trading on their capacity to bring a block of votes for or against an issue or bill, rather than an individual vote. Examples are the Black Caucus, the Women's Caucus, the Hispanic Caucus, and the Business Community Caucus. Although caucuses may be bipartisan, many are partisan in nature. For example, the largest caucus groups are the Democratic Caucus and the Republican Caucus. Each caucus develops its own internal governance structure and version of leadership, including a speaker who leads the caucus and speaks for the group. After a group member achieves a leadership role, he or she must try to balance the wishes of the group against his or her own political survival in the caucus and the political pressures exerted by the larger world.

> *The media have become a tangible power in government, often driving and shaping public opinion that eventually evolves into a legislative agenda.*

The media and the voters are external forces that influence policy makers. The media have become a tangible power in government, often driving and shaping public opinion that eventually evolves into a legislative agenda. Although they claim to be objective, in reality the major news organizations decide what is and what is not news. The public often perceives media personalities as the people who know, write, and speak about the important public issues and matters of substance. One study performed at a large research university investigated how the media reported political campaigns for the years 1975 to 1995. The study compared the actual number of words recorded in writing or spoken on television by the candidates with the number of words spoken or written by the media about the candidate, which acted as a filter, translator, or commentator for the public. The results showed that the media consistently out-communicated the candidates at all levels.

Before media campaigns became the norm and millions of dollars were spent on television and radio advertising, the printed news media used to publish what the candidate said and often printed whole speeches. This approach allowed the public to read the speeches and make up their minds about which issues the candidate supported. Today, the trend is to give a 30-second sound bite of a speech, then have 10 minutes of political analysis by some well-known commentator who tells the public what the candidate is saying. Some of the printed media have adopted a similar approach to political issues. In newspapers, it is not unusual to see a lengthy editorial comment positioned right next to a statement made by a candidate. All elected officials have a great respect for the power of the media to influence public opinion. Those who learn to use the media to their advantage get elected.

Legislators, while recognizing and using the power of the media, have also become wary of it. They know that although they can use the media to proclaim their message, the media also pose a risk to their political survival, depending on the vulnerability of their position. Some legislators have a false sense of invulnerability because of the nature of their constituency base; for example, a legislator may have a large population of senior citizens in his district who have supported him for many years. The legislator publicly supports senior citizen issues and believes that the senior citizen support will always be there. However, during an election campaign, a political opponent's investigation uncovers information that the legislator actually voted against several bills that would have increased senior citizens' benefits. In addition, the opponent discovered that the legislator was having an affair with his married secretary. The opponent leaks this information to the media, which immediately put it on television and report it in the newspapers. If the story develops "legs," meaning it takes on a life of its own and continues to grow even without further information from the opponent, it will be on television news programs and in the newspapers every day. The major networks will do investigative reporting on the issues, and eventually the talk show and television tabloid programs will become interested and begin interviewing people who know or have heard about more "dirty little secrets" about the legislator. At this point, the legislator who is the subject of that story is in political jeopardy. There is little that a politician fears more than being the subject this type of negative story.

The Political Process

Who Introduces Legislation?

Laws serve to maintain order in a complicated society and regulate the interactions of its citizens. As society becomes more complex, more laws are needed to ensure the survival and smooth functioning of the population. For example, although computers and electronic communications have increased the quantity of information individuals can process and the speed at which it is transmitted, they have also added to the complexity of the world. Just a few years ago, there were no laws that dealt with "hacking," computer fraud, computer theft of bank funds, or on-line pornography. Today, there is an ever-growing body of law that deals with computers, and whole sections of police agencies have been dedicated to enforcing these laws, such as the Federal Bureau of Investigation's Computer Crime Unit. However, where do ideas for laws and policies come from? And how do these ideas become laws?

Any elected official, including governors, mayors, county commissioners, and city council members, can propose a program or initiative that requires passage by the legislature (i.e., a **bill**). The elected official will go to the legislative leadership in the parties and ask them either to submit the bill or to help move the bill through the legislative process.

Lobbyists, constituency groups, and advocates are a major source of proposed legislation. They represent various interests ranging from public interest groups to corporate lobbyists. Lobbyists frequently craft legislation and then pass it to a friendly legislator. Consumer groups are often visible at the legislature through demonstrations and lobbying.

Constituency groups can best be described by example, such as the AARP. These groups are made up of individuals interested in advancing an agenda that promotes a range of issues based on self-interests. Advocates, in contrast, can be described as groups who have a single issue or point of view that they are trying to advance, such as housing or abortion rights.

Legislation is also generated from governmental agencies. When agencies are seeking fee increases, or another type of policy reform, they can introduce legislation. For example, policy reforms in the Internal Revenue Service (IRS) are a type of agency-initiated legislation. Frequently the employees of the agency will draft the legislation and then direct it toward a supportive legislator.

What Issues Drive the Development of Legislation?

Funding. Because almost all government agencies depend on legislative funding to sustain their operations, they become actively engaged, overtly or covertly, in seeking the passage of a budget that will sustain their survival.

Public Demand. Legislators are very careful to listen to the demand of their voters and avoid voting against an issue to which the public is emotionally attached. A classic example of this process was seen in New Jersey, where a child was sexually molested and murdered by a known convicted sex offender who unknowingly moved into the child's neighborhood. The tragedy prompted a public outcry: How could this happen? Something needs to be done! Ultimately, the outcry produced the now famous Megan's Law, which requires public disclosure of a known sex offender's residence.

Program Issues. These issues recur periodically and require legislative attention. Requests for increases in television cable rates constitute an example of a programmatic issue. The cable industry will be very interested in the outcome of legislation that may affect what they can charge for their services. Both cable and consumer group lobbyists actively seek the ear of key legislators at these times.

Constituent-Specific Issues. Groups of voters may have specific interests that can lead to an introduction of a bill. For example, in legislative districts where a large population of senior citizens reside, the escalating cost of prescriptions may be an important issue. Legislation specific to that constituency will be introduced at a greater rate than in areas with fewer senior citizens in their populations.

What Do You Think?

Contact your state legislature's Web site and identify two bills that deal with health care. How do you feel about these bills? How should your representative vote on this issue?

What Is the Process of Introducing Bills?

Any legislator can introduce a bill from any source. Additional legislators can sign on as the bill's cosponsors. A bill is considered to be strong if it has strong sponsorship, including a number of powerful cosponsors, a high degree of bipartisanship, and the interest of powerful individuals, both political and nonpolitical. After the bill is introduced, it is taken to the chief clerk, who assigns it a number that permits it to be tracked throughout the process.

After the bill is assigned a number, it is referred to a **committee**. The House and Senate leaders make the decision on which committee considers the bill. This decision, greatly influenced by politics, is critical to the survival and ultimate passage of a bill. It is no coincidence that most bills die in committee. Invariably, the leadership discusses their expectation for the bill with the committee chairs, and if the leadership wants a bill to fail, it is referred to a committee where it will never be voted on or passed on to the House.

At the federal level, bills are referred to full committee and, generally, because of the enormous number of bills being introduced, to a subcommittee. It is within the committee structures that most of the work of Congress takes place. Committee action is perhaps the most important phase of the Congressional process, for this is where the most intensive consideration is given to proposed measures and where people are provided with an opportunity to be heard. The subcommittee studies the issue carefully, holds hearings, and reports the bill back to the full committee with recommendations. There are numerous standing committees in the House and Senate. In addition, there are several select committees and several standing joint committees. Each committee has jurisdiction over certain subjects, and often has two or more subcommittees. In the U.S. Congress, the committees with greatest jurisdiction over health matters and their subcommittees are:

- **House Ways and Means Committee**: Social Security and Medicare (health-care subcommittees)
- **House Commerce Committee**: Health legislation including Medicaid (Subcommittee on Health and the Environment)
- **Senate Finance Committee**: Medicare and Medicaid (health subcommittees)
- **Senate Labor and Human Resources Committee**: Health legislation in general; it also works cooperatively with the Senate Finance Committee in considering issues involving Medicare and Medicaid
- **House and Senate Appropriations Committee**: Authorizes all money necessary to implement action proposed in a bill (Subcommittees for Labor, Education, and Health and Human Services)

As a result of full committee hearings, several things may happen to a bill. It may be:

- Reported out of committee favorably and be scheduled for debate by the full House or Senate
- Reported out favorably, but with amendments
- Reported out unfavorably
- Killed outright

For example, a bill reforming the way that judges are elected ideally would go to the judiciary committee; however, there is no legal requirement that the Speaker or the Senate Pro Tem President send the bill to any particular committee. For political reasons, the speaker may refer the bill to the committee on intergovernmental affairs, where it will languish and die.

In order for a bill to survive, the bill's sponsor must have the knowledge and the political standing to move the bill out of committee. If sponsors are truly committed, they will trade on their political capital. *Political capital* is a term that generally refers to some type of favor or action that a politician can exchange for something he or she wants. It is an extremely important element in the legislative process and consists of, but is not limited to, votes, amendments to bills, appointments, and support from constituency groups. Political capital often consists of an "If you vote for my bill, I'll vote for your bill" type of exchange.

After a bill has been reported out of a House committee (with the exception of Ways and Means or Appropriations Committees), it goes to the Rules Committee, which schedules bills and determines how much time will be spent on debate and whether or not amendments will be allowed. In the Senate, bills go on the Senate calendar, after which the majority leadership determines when a bill will be debated. After a bill is debated, possibly amended, and passed by one chamber, it is sent to the other chamber, where it goes through the same procedure. If the bill passes both the House and the Senate without any changes, it is sent to the President for signature.

If the House and Senate pass different versions of a bill, however, the two bills are sent to a Conference Committee, which consists of members appointed by both the House and the Senate. This committee seeks to resolve differences between the two bills; if the differences cannot be resolved, the bill dies in committee. When the Conference Committee reaches agreement on a bill, it goes back to the House and Senate for passage. At this juncture, the bill must be voted up or down, because no further amendments are accepted.

If the bill is approved in both houses, it then goes to the chief executive—at the federal level, the President; or at the state level, the governor—who then makes determinations about bill. Governors can do one of two things: sign the bill into law or actively **veto** the bill. At the federal level, the President has the same options, with the addition of the pocket veto. Pocket vetoes, found only at the federal level, occur when the President, rather than actively vetoing a bill, simply does not sign it so that it does not become law. If vetoed, it is sent back to the House and Senate. In order to override the veto, a two-thirds vote by both chambers is required.

Clearly, the passage of a law can be a long and difficult process. This is often quite frustrating for "action-oriented" nurses who are used to seeing immediate outcomes, forming plans, and making things happen quickly.

All bills that are passed need a fiscal note attached to them. Therefore, the appropriations committee is operationally very powerful. A piece of legislation that is passed without a fiscal note attached will never become a reality. Over the years, many pieces of legislation have been passed by the legislature but have been starved to death financially. These are called unfunded mandates.

Major regulatory change occurs in laws in the form of housekeeping bills. Legislators can use this tactic to move a piece of legislation through the process, especially when the bill is more significant than the leadership acknowledges it to be. Although regulatory reform and change may seem tedious, they are important to the legislative process and have the capacity to do enormous public good or harm.

Executive Orders

Executive orders provide the chief executive, the governor, or the President with a means for moving an agenda item forward. Executive orders are in many cases a convenient way to formulate policy with minimal involvement from the legislature. They also allow the executive to make a statement about an issue that can be entered on the public record. The legislature can leave executive orders uncontested or challenge them, by characterizing them as beyond the scope of the executive branch. This may involve turning to the third branch of government, the judiciary.

Regulatory Agencies

Regulatory agencies are also arenas where policies are made and amended. For instance, the role of the Intergovernmental Regulatory Reform Commission (IRRC) is to examine regulatory issues across the state.

How to Be Politically Active

Why Organize or Be Politically Active?

The first step in becoming politically active is to identify the specific goals that nurses, as a group, want to accomplish. Nurses recognize many important issues in today's health-care system, including the increasing acuity of hospitalized clients who require higher levels of care and more complex levels of support than ever before, increasing responsibilities for nurses in supervision of rising numbers of unlicensed health-care personnel, loss of control of the work environment through managed care organizations, and ever-shortening hospitalizations resulting in clients being sent home "quicker and sicker." Any one of these issues can become a focal point at which nurses aim their considerable political power.

For example, most nurses are concerned that registered nurses who have traditionally been at clients' bedsides are being replaced by individuals who are less prepared and less able to deal with high-acuity clients. Nurses believe that when they are replaced in large numbers by unlicensed assistive personnel, including nursing assistants, as well as with personnel who provide specific services, such as monitor technicians who sit in front of cardiac monitors, the quality of client care decreases. Nurses know that these technicians are many times taking on responsibilities for which they have had little training. Rarely are there established national standards for these assistive personnel that require them to demonstrate their ability to provide a specific level of care or that even protect the public safety.

Nurses are usually employees at will and can be fired for any reason. Although some efforts have been made in this direction, whistle-blower protection is generally not available to protect nurses who wish to speak out against unsafe staffing levels or employment practices.[4] Nurses are, at times, torn between their obligations to maintain high standards of safe, ethical care and their obligations to their families. Although nurses often feel powerless against a giant monolithic health-care bureaucracy, in reality they have the potential to be a potent political force. Nationally, with almost 3 million nurses licensed to practice, the nursing profession constitutes the largest single body of health-care providers in the country.

Nurses in all health-care settings are saying "somebody's got to do something about this situation." The reality of the situation is that the "somebody" is nurses themselves. Once nurses identify exactly what it is that needs to be accomplished and understand what is possible within the political framework, then they can use their considerable political power to make changes that will benefit both the clients and the profession.

Nurses in all health-care settings are saying "somebody's got to do something about this situation." The reality of the situation is that the "somebody" is nurses themselves.

Rules for Radicals

Saul Alinsky, in *Rules for Radicals*, hypothesizes that human beings are divided into three groups: "the have's, the have nots, and the have a little and want mores." Nurses typically falls in the last group.

One problem nurses in this group encounter is the ongoing conflict between the status quo and progress. They want to obtain more power and control, gain more benefits, earn more money, and have more respect as professionals. However, the strong desire to advance is counterbalanced by fear of jeopardizing their current jobs and their professional standing. Their motivation to be something more, to do something new, or to believe in something bigger is held back and pulled in another direction by their fear of change. The result of this internal tug-of-war is an attitude of inertia and ambivalence that has prevented nurses from organizing politically and effectively using their numerical power.

Despite the inertia and ambivalence problems of individuals in the "have a little and want more" category, some of the most notable revolutionaries in history have come from this group, including Thomas Jefferson, Napoleon Bonaparte, Martin Luther King, Jr., and Vladimir Lenin. Each of these individuals came from the working middle class with a belief that it could be made better. Nurses can use their actions as examples of what individuals can accomplish to raise their own motivation levels to a point where it overwhelms the inertia of the status quo.

A fourth group of people, who seem to evolve from the inertia found among the "have a little, want more" group are the "do-nothings." These individuals can be heard saying things like, "I agree with what you are saying, I just don't agree with your means," "I'm not going to get involved in this," or "I'm too busy to belong to the organization." The do-nothings tend to watch the activities of others, and if their efforts are successful, then they will join in as a beneficiary because they feel they have supported the effort from an ideological standpoint. However, they avoid any active involvement in politics. The eighteenth century British politician Edmund Burke recognized the danger in the do-nothings. He said, "The only thing necessary for the triumph of evil, is for good men [and women] to do nothing."

What Can One Nurse Do?

It is important to remember that politics is a free market enterprise open to anyone who is willing to become involved and play the game. Success in the political arena is contingent on three elements: (1) knowledge and understanding of the process; (2) the ability to offer something of value to the political figure; and (3) the capacity to identify what will be necessary to accomplish the objective. Anyone who is interested in becoming politically active must recognize that all candidates and elected officials need three things: resources to run their political operation (money and volunteers), votes, and a means to shape public opinion.

Sufficient resources are essential to running a political campaign. The first and most necessary resource is always money. Would-be candidates soon discover that a lack of money to fund a campaign will inevitably lead to political failure. An unfunded candidate cannot travel, send mailings, produce radio and television commercials, post signs, or organize a telephone bank. Voters often fail to realize that political candidates are only as available as finances permit. Frequently, good candidates lose because they fail to garner the financial resources necessary to run an effective campaign. Nurses can gain a candidate's support for issues by donating to his or her campaign chest.

A second important resource in an election campaign is volunteers. Volunteers work in campaigns by manning telephone banks, making literature drops, placing signs, and conducting voter registration drives. Usually political candidates are very glad to have the free help for their campaigns. Although nurses may not be able to make large monetary contributions to a candidate's campaign, they can always volunteer some time. Working closely with a candidate on a volunteer basis allows individuals to discuss important issues on a personal basis and helps candidates win who support issues important to nurses. Most candidates need a considerable amount of education about health-related issues because of their lack of knowledge about medical and nursing concerns.

Obviously, votes are essential to any candidate. If a candidate does not have votes, he or she will not be elected. One of the most significant activities nurses can become involved in is to join and support a political party. The chosen party should reflect the nurse's value system and fundamental beliefs. Keep in mind that there is never a perfect fit with any political party. Almost everyone who belongs to a political party will disagree at some point with some element of the party, usually with the extremist views. However, differing opinions and beliefs should not serve as a barrier to membership in a political party. The only way to change a view or opinion is by active participation from within the party. The ultimate political power is the vote. Nurses need to be registered to vote and then actually go to the polls on election day to cast their ballots for the candidates who support legislation that empowers nurses and who recognize the needs for beneficial health-care reform.

Candidates need endorsements from their constituents so that they can build their support base. They generally consider endorsements from nurses as one of the most valuable assets to their campaign. By carefully selecting candidates who support legislation favorable to nursing and health care, endorsements can give nurses the capacity to shape public opinion. The periodic polls conducted by national news magazines asking readers to rank various professions on how much they are trusted have consistently shown that the public views nurses very highly, in the same category as police officers, firefighters, and teachers.

Nurses should use endorsements by choosing candidates in campaigns that have an impact on important issues. Often the campaigns for governor fall into this category, because governors, as chief executives, have a great deal of political power and can appoint people to a number of boards, committees, and positions. Nurses need to recognize that the members of the board of nursing in their state, as well as other important appointed positions in the health departments and other regulatory agencies, may be appointed by the governor and that this board has the final decision in the way that nurses practice. When nurses establish a working political relationship with the chief executive of the state, the governor is more likely to look favorably on those who have sustained him or her, provided financial supported, and given endorsements during the political campaign. They will be the people

ISSUES NOW

The Need for Organization at the State Level

Why do nurses need to organize at the state level? There is a debate that is just starting in nursing about the political activity the ANA is involved in at the federal level. The ANA over the last several years has successfully raised money through telemarketing in every state in the country. Many nurses do not realize that the ANA Political Action Committee (PAC) is now the second largest federal PAC in Washington. In the last election cycle, they raised $1.2 million, which was spent on political activities exclusively at the federal level. However, it is important to realize that many of the political battles that nurses have to fight are at the state level.

There is an ongoing discussion between the federal and state governments about what constitutes a legitimate course of action for the federal government and what constitutes a legitimate course of action for the state government. The 10th Amendment to the Constitution essentially says that any powers that are not expressly articulated to be part of the federal government mandate go to the states. This amendment underlies the current debate about Medicaid and Medicare and whether or not the states should be responsible for its administration.

The concept of unfunded mandates has come to the forefront in the past few years as a result of the states' rights push. There is an ongoing discussion among members of the National Governors' Association demanding that the federal government give more latitude to the way that governors are permitted to govern their states. They are saying: "Don't give us mandates. Give us the opportunity to set our own standards, to set our own regulatory actions, and to set our own legislative and governmental agenda." The nation is moving toward greater state control governmentally. It would be great if nurses could organize and just concentrate on issues at the federal level in Washington, but because most of nursing's issues are at the state level, this strategy is probably not going to work.

For nursing organizations to be effective, there has to be organized political action among nurses and by nurses in every state in this country. In those states where nurses are not active and organized politically, there is going to be in trouble, and the nurses in them will fare badly. Nurses need to be conscious of the fact that the trend is toward state nursing organizations becoming more active politically and determiners of their own fate. Consequently, nurses need to organize politically at the state level to increase their political power.

Another thing to keep in mind is that nurses' licensure, as well as the certification and regulation of hospitals, is a function of the state. Again, it does not make sense to concentrate all of nursing's resources at the national level. Of course, there are some issues and programs, particularly with respect to funding, in which federal action is necessary. But most of the issues that nurses are going to be dealing with occur at the state level, and that is where attention needs to be focused. The reality of the situation is that the states have the capacity to define and regulate objective standards for both nurses and hospitals. The mandate for nursing is to define how those standards are established and then develop an achievable agenda for political action by nurses at the state level.

Donna Gentile O'Donnell

that he or she is going to appoint to a board position.

Targeting endorsements will prevent nurses from making blind political decisions. Candidates should be assessed first on their willingness to be supportive to issues that nurses are interested in and then on their capacity to win the election.

A model for individual political development that encourages grassroots involvement in local issues is based on the belief that grassroots efforts may be more fulfilling than involvement in partisan politics.[5] This model is an activity-oriented ladder, including activities at four distinct levels:

- Rung 1—Civic involvement: Children's sports, parent-teacher association (PTA), neighborhood improvement group
- Rung 2—Advocacy: Writing letters to public officials and newspapers and making organized visits to officials on local issues
- Rung 3—Organizing: Independent organizing on local issues, incorporation of single-issue citizens' groups, and networking with similarly situated citizens' groups
- Rung 4—Long-term power wielding: Campaigning for oneself or another, local government planning, and agenda setting

Nurses usually shudder at the thought of running for political office. They tend to perceive political campaigns as something that is underhanded and tawdry, and they just do not want to be involved. However, it is not impossible for nurses to achieve high status in public office. Several nurses hold elected office in state and local government level, including Barbara Hafer, RN, State Treasurer of Pennsylvania, and Marilyn Goldwater, RN, who serves in the Maryland State Senate and has been a delegate to the national convention.

One way that nurses can direct their political activities is to develop a political relationship with a legislator or a political operative who can mentor and guide the nurse in finding a route through the political maze. As discussed earlier, the principle of self-interest is one of the most critical elements in politics, and in order to establish a relationship with a political figure, nurses must demonstrate that the issues they support have value to both themselves and to the politician.

There are several ways that a nurse can make decisions on whom to support when becoming involved in the political process. A first step is to begin identifying the issues particular legislators are interested in and will vote for. Editorial opinion pieces in the editorial section of newspapers can provide a sense of the issues of concern to legislators. It is a good idea to begin with local legislators and candidates, like the state representative, state senator, or the councilperson serving the neighborhood. Call their offices and find out when and where they are scheduled to speak, then go and listen to the speech to get a sense of who they are and what issues they support. Their speeches and the way that they answer questions will reveal their ideology and partisanship. Also, during question and answer periods, ask elected officials what they think about issues important to you.

Another way to become familiar with prominent political figures is by attending some of the many partisan events that occur during an election season. A good way to visualize the local political landscape is by observing who is talking to whom at the event. Nurses can make their own assessments of political candidates based on observations of the candidates in action, calling their offices for information, reading published literature, or talking to people who know the candidate. Beginning the process may seem difficult, but once a decision is made to become politically active, you'll become more confident.

Know the Issues

For nurses to be successful in the political process, they must know and understand the issues. At times an issue may be readily apparent in the nurses' community, for example, an increased number of homeless people. Other issues are easily identified by reading newspapers. Issues are generally presented in the editorial section; most newspapers also have a political watch section, which reports the results of any significant votes at the state and federal levels.

The American Nurses Association (ANA) newspaper, *American Nurse*, is an excellent source of information on issues of concern to the profession. In addition, the *American Journal of Nursing* Newsline feature and *Nursing and Health Care*'s Washington Focus serve as excellent, easily readable sources of information in journals. *Capitol Update*, the ANA legislative newsletter for nurses, reports on the activities of its nurse lobbyists and on significant issues in the Congress and regulatory agencies. This publication requires a subscription but is available in most nursing schools and hospital libraries.

State nurses' associations and many specialty-nursing groups also publish newsletters or legislative bulletins. Many of these are free to members but may be sent only when requested. When one is a member of a nursing organization, Action Alerts may also be sent to inform members of vital issues and the action needed by nurses. Most state legislatures now have on-line access to their proceedings so that bills of interest to nurses can be tracked as they progress through the legislative process.

Tactics

Tactics, essential tools for those who desire to be politically active, are the conscious and deliberate acts that people use to live and deal with each other and the world around them. In a political sense, tactics usually means using whatever resources are available to achieve a desired goal. Hannibal, one of the great tacticians in political history, said, "We will either find a way or we will make a way." Nurses, with their long history of accomplishing much with few resources, are natural tacticians. As nurses learn how to organize themselves for political purposes, they can use their well-developed tactical skills to achieve important political goals. Listed below are some easy-to-use tactics for political action.

Use the Resources That Have the Most Power (Money, Endorsements, Votes). For example, there are approximately 270,000 licensed nurses in Pennsylvania. By enlisting 25 percent of those nurses and collecting minimal dues, a powerful political force can be organized. If 25 percent of 270,000 nurses contribute $75 to a political action committee per year, approximately $5 million in annual revenue will be produced. In most states, $5 million would almost guarantee a win in any election.

Engage in Bipartisan Tactics. Both Republican and Democratic nurses need to be politically active to achieve unified goals. Political action across the spectrum of issues and across partisan lines is necessary to achieve the goal of bipartisanship. Nurses should understand that only by supporting candidates who favor nursing and its agenda, whether they are Democrat or Republican, can the profession make changes that will advance the agenda of the discipline. The most important thing, always, is the issue being addressed and not the personality or party of the candidate.

Sometimes communications with legislators take the form of lobbying. Lobbying may be defined as attempting to persuade someone (usually a legislator or legislative aide) of the significance of one's cause or as an attempt to influence legislation. Lobbying methods include letter writing; face-to-face communication or telephone calls; mailgrams, telegrams, or e-mail; letters to the editor; and providing testimony (verbal or written).

In order to lobby effectively, one should be both persuasive and able to negotiate. Lobbying is truly an art of communication, an area in which nurses can become skilled. Before beginning any lobbying effort, it is vital to gather all pertinent facts. In politics, getting the facts and laying the groundwork are analogous to developing a nursing care plan. Before visiting or writing a legislator, gather facts, delineate a problem or concern you wish to discuss, and develop a plan to articulate your concerns. Determine a method for evaluating your effectiveness.

If the plan is to visit the legislator's office, an appointment should be set up in advance. Most often the meeting may actually be with the legislative aide, particularly at the federal level. This should not be discouraging, because this is the individual who is often responsible for assisting in the development of position statements and offering committee amendments for the legislator.

To ensure that legislators listen to your concerns, it is important not only to be well prepared but also to show that others support your position. When one person speaks, legislators may listen, but when many people voice the same concern, legislators are much more likely to pay attention.

Benefit Through Collaboration. Nurses can increase their political power by making alliances with other powerful constituency groups who support similar issues, such as the AARP. The AARP is very interested in health-care issues, particularly managed care, national health insurance, and the decreased quality of care from the increased use of nonlicensed personnel. Nurses who are organized into collective bargaining units can use the alliance with powerful unions. Unions are traditionally concerned with issues such as working conditions, including staffing patterns in hospitals, wages, job security, and benefits. Nurses are concerned about the same issues.

How to Organize

"Know thine enemy" is one of the most fundamental rules that tacticians must follow, whether it is in war or politics. Napoleon was successful as a tactician and general because before he fought any battle, he walked the battlefield. He knew what the terrain was like, and he knew where the rocks and crevices were. He knew what to anticipate when he arrived on the battlefield. Nurses who want to be successful in a political battle must first learn the hills and valleys and rocks and crevices of the primary political battlefield, their own state demographics.

Important demographics for organizing nurses at the state level:

- Total population of the state. The total population of the state provides a demographic overview of the political arena.
- Total number of registered voters.
- Total number of registered voters by political party.
- Total number of likely voters in any given election cycle. To determine this number, the difference between an on-year election cycle and off-year election cycle should be understood. An on-year election cycle occurs when there is a major race in the state, usually during a presidential or gubernatorial race. An off-year cycle is when a major race is not being run. There may be city council races or even a state representative or senate race, but the majority of the population does not consider these major races, and fewer people tend to vote. Also, lower levels of political activity are seen in an off-year election cycle.
- Total number of registered nurses. The total number of registered nurses in a state

can be obtained from the state board of nursing. Comparing the number of actual voters with the number of registered nurses in a state provides an indication of the potential power of an RN voting block. For example, if there are 800,000 people who regularly vote in a state and there are a total of 100,000 nurses in the state who are organized into a voting block about a particular issue, then that group of nurses represents a significant percentage of voters, and candidates running for statewide office will be interested in having nurses' support. Nurses must be encouraged to register and vote to increase the power of the block.

- Comparing numbers helps define the political landscape of a state.

Important Characteristics of an Organizer

Many of the characteristics of an organizer listed in Box 18–3 are the same characteristics that are required of nurses on a daily basis in the practice of their profession. Although these characteristics may have varying degrees of value for the organizer, the one critical element a political organizer has to have is the capacity to communicate. Although nurses usually have a well-developed ability to communicate at the bedside, they may lack the confidence to communicate in the larger public and political arenas. Nurses need to recognize that the communication skills that they use on a daily basis, when explaining complicated medical jargon to clients, are the same skills they can use in translating health-care issues into language that the public and elected officials can understand. One way to gain the public's interest and elected officials' support is to personalize health-care issues by stressing the fact that nurses are the professionals who provide the bulk of direct care for their mothers, fathers, brothers, and children. Communication of issues that touch people personally is usually the most effective method.

Box 18–3

Characteristics of an Organizer

Curiosity
Motivation
Reverence
Realism
Flair for the dramatic
Sense of humor
Charisma
Self-confidence
Communication skills
Clear vision of the future
Capacity to change
Persistence
Ability to organize
Imagination

After Organization—What Then?

Drafting Legislation and Creating Change

The critical questions must be asked. The first question always must be, "Who is the decision-maker?" For example, if there is an issue that needs to be resolved in the state board of nursing, the first step is to identify who makes the decisions at the board. Although the board members make decisions, it is important to remember that the people who sit on the board are appointed. Who appoints them and what is the basis of those appointments? If they are political appointees, they usually have some sort of political benefactor or a political relationship with someone in power. By understanding these types of relationships, it becomes easier to determine their ideological and partisan positions on many issues. For example, if a nursing board is newly appointed by a recently elected Republican governor, it is probably safe to assume that most of the board members are Republicans who agree with the governor on many key issues.

The second question to address is: "How accessible is the appointee's benefactor?" Sometimes board members are appointed by the legislative leadership and not the governor. It is important to discover who appointed the board and whether or not individual voters have access to them. Generally, the access by individual voters to the power figures who make these types of appointments is very limited. Organized groups, like the ANA, provide the best avenue of access at the federal level. Other questions that need to be answered include:

> *Nurses need to recognize that the communication skills that they use on a daily basis, when explaining complicated medical jargon to clients, are the same skills they can use in translating health-care issues into language that the public and elected officials can understand.*

- How successful have nurses been in the past in achieving specific goals?
- What positions do nurses hold in government?
- What does the state board look like politically?
- Which legislators have supported nursing issues in the past?
- Which legislators traditionally oppose nursing and health-care issues?

Because of the failure to ask and answer these questions, numerous pieces of pro-nursing legislation that have been introduced have died in committee or lacked sponsors to move the bill through the process. In those states where nurses are in tune with the political issues and powers, nurses have more success moving bills through the legislative process so that they become law than in states where nurses are apathetic about the political process.

Even if a bill favorable for nurses or health care does not pass the first time, the fact that it was brought to a vote is important for several reasons. First, it has brought an issue to the attention of the whole legislature that they may otherwise have dismissed as unimportant. Second, the legislative process brings to light the proponents and opponents of the issue and allows nurses to specifically target those legislators who voted against the bill. One of two approaches can be used at this point. Nurses can either communicate with the legislators to explain why the bill is important in hopes of changing their minds, or they can organize as a voting block and attempt to vote the opposing legislators out of office. Third, after a bill has gone through the process the first time, it becomes much easier to identify the obstacles and sticking points in the language of the bill. Before the bill is re-introduced in a later session of the legislature, it can be modified and amended to eliminate those parts that may have caused ideological problems for specific legislators.

Other Factors That Have Potential Political Powers for Nurses

Historically, very few nurses have either sought or been elected to governmental positions. However, it is important to realize that not all nurses who hold elected positions are allies for nursing. Unless elected nurses identify themselves as nurses and support the profession, they may not be willing to support nursing issues politically. For example, a nurse currently elected to Congress from a Southern state refused to speak to the nurses who participated in the March on Washington Nurses. Although she is a nurse and has had a number of articles published in nursing journals in the past, she refused to support the nurses who marched. Elected officials must always be judged by what they do and what they deliver, and not by what they say, or look like, or think, or what people think they think.

ISSUES IN PRACTICE

How Do Politics Affect You and Your Family?

Why should nurses be involved in politics? Does it really make a difference who is elected and who makes the laws? Take a minute to go through the questions below and check the items that you think may be affected by politics.

Between the time you wake up and the time you leave the house several things usually happen to you. Do you think any of the following subjects are affected by politics?

- The water with which you wash your face and brush your teeth
- The electricity that lights the room
- The price and quality of food you have for breakfast
- The safety of the products you buy

As the average person's life span grows longer and the retirement age is lowered, these later years become more meaningful. Are any of the following decisions affected by our political systems?

- The age at which you can retire
- The income that you get during retirement
- The quality and cost of health care
- The life expectancy of each of us

We value our leisure time and the chance to get away from it all. Are any of the following areas affected by politics?

- The parks and lakes where vacationers fish and swim
- The air that you breathe
- The radio and television programs that entertain you

Conclusion

There is nothing magical about nurses becoming involved in politics. It is simply a matter of hard work and use of the critical thinking skills nurses already possess. It is clear, however, that nurses can and do make a difference in the political arena. Nurses must ask how and where they can make a difference and how they can become involved in the process. Not every nurse may choose to run for political office, but each nurse can and should make a contribution. Betts[6] believes that nursing's interest in public policy and politics is "the prescription for the power so necessary to our future." Carpe diem!

References

1. Webster's New Collegiate Dictionary, Simon & Schuster, New York, 2002.
2. Keating, SB, and Sechrist, KR: The nursing shortage in California: The public policy role of the California Strategic Planning Committee for Nursing. Online Journal of Issues in Nursing 6(1):14, 2001.
3. O'Donnell, DG: Unpublished material, 1996.
4. Cross, LL: Protected whistle-blowing or a legal firing? Oklahoma Nurse 47(1):14–16, 2002.
5. Chalich, T, and Smith, L: Nursing at the grassroots. Nurs Health Care 13:242–244, 1992.
6. Betts, AS: Nursing's agenda for health care reform policy, politics and power through professional leadership. Hospital Administration Quarterly 20(3):8, 1996.

Bibliography

Brewer, C, and Kovner, CT: Is there another nursing shortage? What the data tell us. Nurs Outlook 49(1):20–26, 2001.

Burke, RJ: The ripple effect: Staffing post restructuring. Nursing Management 33(2):41–43, 2002.

Carlson, ED: Welfare reform: Policy implications for health. Texas Journal of Rural Health 19(2):42–48, 2001.

Clemons, T: Highlights from the Hill: NIWI 2000: Issues and opportunities. ORL–Head and Neck Nursing 19(2):22–23, 2001.

Des Jardin, K: Political involvement in nursing—Politics, ethics, and strategic action. AORN J 74(5):614–618, 2001.

Frank, IC: Policy perspectives: The nursing shortage. Journal of Emergency Nursing 27(4):391–393, 2001.

Higgs, ZR, et al: Health care access: A consumer perspective. Public Health Nurs 18(1):3–12, 2001.

Malone, B: Making nursing's presence felt at the political party conferences. Nursing Standard 16(5):22, 2001.

O'Grady, ET: Health policy and politics. Access to health care: An issue central to nursing. Nursing Economics 18(2):88–90, 2001.

Rains, JW, and Barton-Kriese, P: Developing political competence. Public Health Nurs 18(4):219–224, 2001.

Roit, SM: When money talks, politicians listen. American Nurse 34(1):22, 2002.

19

Spirituality and Health Care

Nancy C. Sharts-Hopko

Learning Objectives

After completing this chapter, the reader will be able to:

- Develop a working definition of spirituality.
- Distinguish spirituality from religion.
- Describe what is meant by the nursing diagnosis Spiritual Distress.
- Describe research that supports the health benefit of spiritual practices.
- Describe the relationship between spirituality and one alternative healing modality used within nursing.

The emotional demands of working with people who are experiencing a crisis stimulate many health professionals to examine spiritual issues for themselves. Their interest may be sparked by the diverse spiritual practices that they witness in the course of their work or from a growing body of biomedical research that is showing that spiritual practices bring tangible benefits to health and well-being.

Spirituality refers to people's living with consciousness of a reality beyond that which is knowable through the five senses. This awareness of a transcendent reality may be experienced in terms of a divine creator, or it may be experienced in relation to the wonder of all creation or to fundamental values such as love, truth, or beauty. Health professionals have shown increased interest in spirituality since the early 1990s.

It is universally true that the human life cycle is marked by a rhythm of transitions: birth, the entry of a child into society, puberty, sexual awakening, entry into adulthood, marriage, parenthood, illness, loss, old age, and death. In all cultures there are other rhythms that people honor, such as the solar and lunar cycles, the agricultural cycle, and the reproductive cycles. These cycles constitute the rhythm of human life. All people recognize the importance of each of these transitions and in some way have ritualized them through their religions. People learn from their own cultural groups how to behave during each transition, and each cultural group has conceptualized an understanding of these human experiences; however, their importance is universal.

Nurses primarily have contact with clients in the health-care setting within the context of these transitions. Developmental crisis theory holds that these transitions are times of anxiety and vulnerability for families. Therefore, nurses are required to treat people who are going through these transitions with great tenderness and care. It is a sacred trust for nurses to be allowed into a family system in transition. During these transitions, clients and families may seek spiritual support or they may feel spiritual abandonment. Ideally, nurses can help people identify and find the spiritual support that they require.

Over a long period of time, from the enlightenment of the seventeenth century to the dawn of the twenty-first century, political leaders and educated people in Western cultures came to believe that all the answers to human suffering could be found in science and technology. For example, early in the twentieth century, antibiotics were thought of as "magic bullets" that cured diseases and reduced suffering. People were eager to take part in research studies to solve their health-care problems. It was in this context that the nursing profession embraced the Western scientific method as the measure for defining itself. Nurses believed, and some still do believe, that rigorous research involving testing of hypotheses would provide the theoretical base for the practice of professional nursing.

More recently, however, the horrors of terrorism, the harnessing of nuclear power, space exploration, and the mapping of the human genome are among new capabilities that have given urgency to reconsideration of the question: "What does it mean to be fully human in the universe as it is now understood?"

What Do You Think?

Make two lists—a list of the problems that science and technology have caused during the last 20 years, and a list of the problems that have been solved along with the benefits of technology and science. Which list is longer? Why?

More recently, however, the horrors of terrorism, the harnessing of nuclear power, space exploration, and the mapping of the human genome are among new capabilities that have given urgency to reconsideration of the question: "What does it mean to be fully human in the universe as it is now understood?" It is evident that science and technology cannot offer the solutions to all human problems; in fact, they have contributed to many of them.

Science, electronic communications, and the great social experiments of the last two centuries are among the influences directing humans to a consciousness of the individual's connectedness to the whole of creation and all peoples. One of the ways in which both consumers of health care and health professionals are responding to this realization is by reintegrating spirituality and spiritual modes of healing into health and illness practices. Another response is the growing inclination to examine and adopt the spiritual wisdom of traditions other than one's own.

A feature of postmodernism is the realization that the concept of truth is a relative one, allowing for an appreciation of diverse perspectives on what is true. Science, including nursing science since the mid-1980s, has expanded its ways of discerning truth, leaving behind traditional hypotheticodeductive, quantitative research. The emergence of **phenomenology** within the discipline of philosophy is one major influence that has led to an appreciation for qualitative methods of discovery within nursing. As a philosophical approach to understanding truth, phenomenology parallels and is closely related to existentialism, advocating the view that consciousness determines reality and truth in space and time. In the health-care setting, a phenomenologic approach appreciates the belief that the client's observations may be more objective than those of the nurse, because they are attached to the client's past experiences and knowledge, which includes rich descriptions of the person's experiences of life transitions. In nursing, intuition has emerged as a phenomenon worthy of further investigation. This change in viewpoint has coincided with increased interest in complementary and alternative therapies and with the importance of spirituality in healing and wellness.

The Nature of Spirituality

Spirituality is a broad and somewhat nebulous concept that has to do with people's search for answers to questions and issues such as those listed in Box 19–1. Similar concerns have been identified among children of various cultural backgrounds in research on the development of spirituality.

A rich heritage of spiritual practices, including systematic reflection for growth toward wholeness, is found in all the major religions of the world. The roots of the great traditions, including each religion's prayer practices, can be traced to the shift in human consciousness that occurred around 500 B.C. During this period, many great teachers and spiritual leaders emerged, including Confucius; Lao-tzu; Siddhartha Gautama, who became the Buddha; Zoroaster; the Greek philosophers Socrates, Plato, and Aristotle; and the Hebrew prophets Amos, Hosea, and Isaiah. St. Augustine, a Roman Catholic bishop who lived in North Africa during the fifth century, is credited with first identifying the relationships among contemplation, action, and wisdom within the Christian tradition. For Augustine, the contemplative life was properly focused on discernment of truth and was open to all people. However, Augustine equated truth, ultimately, with God.

Box 19–1

Spiritual Questions

- Why are we here?
- How do we fit into the cosmos?
- What power or intelligence created and orders the universe?
- What is the nature and meaning of divine or mystical experiences?
- How are we to make meaning of suffering?
- How are we to behave toward other people?
- How are we to deal with our own shortcomings and failures?
- What happens to us when we die, and where were we before we were born?

Spirituality is often defined as integrative energy, capable of producing internal human harmony or holism. Other definitions refer to spirituality as a sense of coherence. Spirituality also entails a sense of transcendent reality, which draws strength from inner resources, living fully for the present, and having a sense of inner knowing. Solitude, compassion, and empathy are important components of spirituality for many individuals.

The concept of hope is central to spirituality. Spirituality may be regarded as the driving force that pervades all aspects of and gives meaning to an individual's life. It creates a set of beliefs and values that influence the way that people conduct their lives. Spiritual activity involves introspection, reflection, and a sense of connectedness to others or to the universe. For many people, this connectedness focuses ultimately on a Supreme Being who is sometimes called God.

Traditionally, the term *spirituality* has been defined as a sense of meaning in life or associated with a sense of an inner spirit. However, it is difficult to identify what such a spirit is like and how it can be observed. In addition, spirituality can be defined from both religious and secular perspectives. A person with spiritual needs does not necessarily need to participate in religious rituals and practices.

The Religious Perspective

From the religious perspective, spirituality can be defined as encompassing the ideology of the *imago dei* (image of God), or soul, that exists in everyone. The soul makes the person a thinking, feeling, moral, creative being able to relate meaningfully to a Supreme Being and to others. This being or force may be called God, the divine creator and sustainer of the universe, the divine mystery, or other names that convey a profound sense of transcendence and awe. A religious perspective often entails a set of beliefs that help explain the meaning of life, suffering, health, and illness. These beliefs can be crucial to a believer's well-being.

Spirituality is often mistakenly understood to mean just religious practice; however, it should be considered in the broader sense of the term. Religion can be an approach to spirituality, and spirituality is often a component of religion, but the two concepts are different. It is quite possible for the members of a specific religion to be quite limited in their spirituality. Most people have known individuals who dutifully follow the rules of their religious tradition. They strongly believe that if they have adhered to the rules correctly, God will reward them with blessings such as health, success, affluence, social status, and power. For these individuals, adverse events like disease, death of a loved one, or loss of investments can be devastating, because they are perceived as a failure in religious practice or punishments from God. On the other hand, there are many deeply spiritual persons who do not belong to any organized religion but who may be profoundly reflective about the meaning of their life and experiences.

Huston Smith, a scholar of comparative religions at the University of California at Berkeley, has published books and coproduced several public television series with the intent of helping diverse nonacademic audiences appreciate religious traditions other than their own. For Smith,[1] all the world's religions seek to answer the same questions: "Why are we here?", "What does it all mean?", and "What, if anything, are we supposed to be doing with our lives?" All religions taken together can be perceived like a stained glass window that refracts the light in different colors and offers reflections of different shapes. Each of the world's religions is different because it has evolved to respond to unique histories and different cultural developments.

Definitions of religion usually identify a specific system of values and beliefs and a framework for ethical behavior that the members must follow. Religion can be thought of as a social construct that reflects its cultural context and specific philosophical influences. A religion evolves within a specific cultural group, situated in history, and attempts to discern what the group believes are God's commandments as the group has come to understand them. Religion, as an institutionally based, organized system of beliefs, represents only one specific means of spiritual expression. Participation in a specific religion generally entails formal education for membership, an initiation ceremony, participation in worship gatherings, adherence to a set of rules of behavior, the participation in prescribed rituals, a particular mode of prayer, and the study of that group's sacred texts. Religious groups vary widely in their tolerance of intragroup diversity of beliefs and behaviors as well as their respect for the belief systems of others. In addition, within a specific religious group there may be a wide range of understanding of what their practices represent.

Occasionally, health-care professionals may encounter individuals whose spiritual practices are highly questionable or discomforting to witness (e.g., worshipers of Satan or those who seek to invoke harm to others through their prayers and rituals).

The Secular Perspective

From a secular perspective, spirituality is seen as a set of positive values, such as love, honesty, or truth, chosen by the individual that ultimately become that person's supreme focus of life and organizing framework. These values have the capacity to motivate the individual toward fulfillment of personal needs, goals, and aspirations, leading ultimately to self-actualization.

What Do You Think?

How would you define your spirituality—is it religious or secular?

Manifestation of Spirituality

Both the religious and secular perspectives can exist at the same time in the totality of a person's life. A person's spirituality may be nourished by the ability to give and receive touch, caring, love, and trust. Spirituality may also entail an appreciation of physical experiences such as listening to music, enjoying art or literature, eating delicious food, laughing, venting emotional tension, or participating in sexual expression. A series of four developmental stages have been proposed for human spirituality:

- Stage 1: the chaotic (antisocial) stage, with its superficial belief system
- Stage 2: the formal (institutional) stage, with its adherence to the law
- Stage 3: the skeptic (individual) stage, with its emphasis on rationality, materialism, and humaneness
- Stage 4: the mystical (communal) stage, with its "unseen order of things"[2]

A Tradition of Spirituality in Nursing

Modern nursing has a rich legacy of the appreciation of spirituality in health and illness. Florence Nightingale's views of nursing practice were based on a spiritual philosophy that she set forth in *Suggestions for Thought*. She was the daughter of Unitarian and Anglican parents, and among her ancestors were famous dissenters against the Church of England. The skepticism fostered by her Unitarian upbringing may have influenced her to question and critique established religious doctrine. Her search for religious truth caused her to become familiar with the writings of Christian mystics (e.g., St. Francis of Assisi, St. John of the Cross) and also with various Eastern mystical writings, including the *Bhagavad-Gita*.

For Nightingale, spirituality involved a sense of a divine intelligence who creates and sustains the cosmos as well as an awareness of her own inner connection with this higher reality. The universe, for Nightingale, was the embodiment of a transcendent God. She came to believe that all aspects of creation are interconnected and share the same inner divinity. She believed that all humans have the capacity to realize and perceive this divinity. Nightingale's God can be described as perfection or as the "essence of benevolence."

Nightingale saw no conflict between science and mysticism. To her, the laws of nature and science were merely "the thoughts of God." Spirituality, for Nightingale, entailed the development of courage, compassion, inner peace, creative insight, and other "God-like" qualities. Based on this belief, Nightingale's convictions commanded her to lifelong service in the care of the sick and helpless. Nightingale endorsed the tradition of contemplative prayer, or attunement to the inner presence of God. All phenomena, Nightingale believed, are manifestations of God. A spiritual life entails wise stewardship of all the earth's resources, including human beings. Physical healing was seen by Nightingale as a natural process regulated by natural laws, and as she stated in her *Notes on Nursing*, "What nursing has to do . . . is to put the patient in the best condition for nature to act upon him."[3]

As nursing sought to establish itself as a profession with a legitimate knowledge base, the concern with human spirituality was downplayed and even consciously ignored until the early 1980s. Typically, the spiritual domain is assigned to the art rather than to the science of nursing, because of its seemingly subjective nature mistakenly equated with aesthetics and intuition.

Attention to the spiritual domain in providing holistic care depends on the beliefs and values of both the nurse and the client.

Spirituality and Religion in Nursing Theory

There are 26 major nursing theories and conceptual frameworks that have been developed since the 1960s. Although14 of them recognized the spiritual domain of health somewhere in their assumptions, only two theories mentioned it directly by name. Rogers' Science of Unitary Human Beings is an example of a profoundly spiritual view of humanity that does not directly name the concept of spirituality. Rogers' framework suggests that there are unbounded human energy fields in interaction with the environmental energy field. Rogers' spiritual definitions can apply as well to the concept of the soul (discussed later). Martha Rogers, who grew up in Tennessee amidst fundamentalist Christians, was loathe to be interpreted in that light; moreover, she had to establish her credibility at New York University during the 1950s, before nursing was accepted as a scientific discipline.

Neuman, in the later development of her theory, and Watson are the only theorists who clearly acknowledged the impact of spirituality in the development of their theories. But Watson alone defined and explained the spiritual terminology she used to discuss the spiritual aspect of holistic health.

Watson specifically identifies the awareness of the clients' and families' spiritual and religious beliefs as a responsibility of a nurse.[4] She advocates that nurses should appreciate and respect the spiritual meaning in a person's life, no matter how unusual that person's belief system may be. Watson states that nurses have an obligation to identify religious and spiritual influences in their clients' lives at home and to help clients meet their religious requirements in inpatient settings. For example, nurses can facilitate clients' use of measures such as the lighting of candles (real or electric), put flowers and personal objects in the room, ensure privacy, and play music to promote increased comfort and relieve anguish.

Spiritual Crisis

Since 1978, the North American Nursing Diagnosis Association (NANDA) has recognized the nursing diagnosis of Spiritual Distress.[5] It has most recently been defined as "disruption in the life principle that pervades a person's entire being and integrates and transcends one's biological and psychosocial nature." Defining characteristics of Spiritual Distress include concerns with the meaning of life and death, anger toward God, concerns about the meaning of suffering, concerns about the person's relationship to God, questions about the meaning of life, the inability to participate in preferred religious practices, seeking spiritual help, concerns about the ethics of prescribed medical regimens, black humor, expressing displaced anger toward clergy, sleep disturbances, and altered mood or behavior. Spiritual distress may occur in relation to separation from religious or cultural supports, challenges to beliefs and values, or intense suffering.

> *Spiritual distress may occur in relation to separation from religious or cultural supports, challenges to beliefs and values, or intense suffering.*

Nurses should be aware that some individuals have been seriously harmed by their religious communities. Examples of harm might include being shunned or excommunicated, being told that they are evil, being forced into a rigidly controlled lifestyle by a cult, or being physically or sexually assaulted by members of the religious community. For these people, illness may be seen as punishment for some sinful action, and they may perceive any offer of spiritual support from the religious community as profoundly threatening. They may believe that God has abandoned them or that the idea of God is foolish or even destructive. Given the rapid turnover of clients in most health systems, there may be little that the nurse can do other than to acknowledge their spiritual pain and accept them, with the assurance that "I am here for you now." If there is more time for contact, the nurse may be able to refer a client or family to appropriate support groups or clergy.

At times clients make health-care decisions that conflict with the beliefs of their religious communities. These often produce high levels of spiritual distress that may affect both the mental and physical well-being of the client. Consider the following case study:

> When I was a nursing student in the early 1970s, I cared for a woman who was undergoing a therapeutic abortion because of several medical complications of her pregnancy. She had her first child before RhoGAM was available, and she, an Rh-negative mother, had borne an Rh-positive baby. She had only one kidney, and her physicians were concerned that the immunologic complication of carrying a second Rh-positive baby would jeopardize that kidney's function. The decision was difficult for the woman and her husband to make, but they believed the first priority was to care for and raise their 7-year-old son. She needed to protect her kidney so that she could live and participate fully in the child's upbringing.
>
> The night before I cared for this woman, her clergyman came to the hospital and told her that she would go to hell for her decision. Being a devout church member, the woman was extremely distressed the next day. The primary nurse assigned to this woman recognized the spiritual distress caused by the clergyman and requested that a hospital chaplain spend time with her. The chaplain talked and prayed with the woman for several hours. These actions brought great comfort to the woman, who proceeded with the abortion.

Clients often make choices that are difficult for nurses to accept. For instance, based on religious beliefs, clients may refuse commonplace treatments, such as blood transfusions, medications, and even minor surgeries. End-of-life decisions are often based on family members' spiritual beliefs and can be controversial among the health-care personnel who are involved in the decision. In some acute care settings, regular group sessions are conducted with staff nurses by a chaplain or psychiatrist to assist them in understanding and accepting controversial client decisions.

The Human Energy System and the Soul

Most religious traditions include a concept called "the soul." Religious traditions usually offer explanations of what the soul is, how and when human beings acquire a soul, and what happens to the soul after death. But soul need not be a religious concept. Thomas Moore, a psychotherapist who has written extensively about spiritual development, describes the soul "not as a thing, but a quality or a dimension of experiencing life and ourselves. It has to do with depth, value, relatedness, heart, and personal substance . . . [not necessarily] an object of religious belief or . . . something to do with immortality."[6] Yet Moore observes that the soul must be nurtured, and religious practices can provide that nurturance. For Moore, spirituality is the effort a person makes to identify the soul's world view, values, and sense of relatedness to the whole of the person and of creation. The work of the soul is the quest for understanding or insight about major life questions.

Some people may depict the soul as an image of the person that extends several feet beyond the physical self, or the soul is characterized by color and energetic movement. The soul enters the body at some point during gestation and leaves the body at approximately the moment of death. Reincarnation, or the return of a soul for many earthly lifetimes, is a concept encountered in many religious frameworks, including certain mystical traditions within Judaism and Christianity, although not all denominations ascribe to it. The reason for the soul's return to earthly life is to learn, to develop, and to be purified. Some traditions express this process in terms of earning an improved position in the spiritual world to become closer to God after the final judgment.

The soul would seem to be an exquisitely precise and vast center for communication. Souls have the capacity to communicate with one another, with all living things, and with the divine source of all energy. Their capacity is not limited by the laws of physical matter. Some alternative modalities of healing rely on energy movement through the soul. Examples of therapies that capitalize on knowledge of the soul and the movement of a divinely generated energy, life force, or grace (*chi* in Chinese, *ki* in Japanese, or *prana* in Indian traditions) include therapeutic touch, Reiki, and shiatsu. Energy can move in many directions. When a person needs it, energy can be drawn from the divine source of energy into the person; excess energy can be moved from one person to another; and the flow of energy throughout the person's energy field can be balanced to achieve a state of health. Some alternative healing practices that use colors, herbs, aromas, and crystals can be regarded as consistent with a paradigm of repatterning the human energy field or altering the flow of energy throughout the person's body. The circulation of divine energy may be thought of as coming from God and circulating through all living things, the earth, and all the celestial bodies, thus interconnecting all creation.

Religious traditions of India and other Eastern cultures teach that the human energy system contains seven energy centers, or chakras. These might be considered as the primary openings in the human energy system through which energy flows. Each center has or controls a unique type of energy and spirituality that it allows to enter or leave the body. The root chakra is located at the base of the torso, or the perineum, and its energy has to do with the material world. The crown chakra, the highest level of energy at the top of the head, relates to spirituality.

Examining the religious art of many cultures, over many centuries, artists depict these areas of their subjects' bodies in similar ways. For instance, holy people are depicted with vivid, large, or colorful hearts, and their heads are surrounded by halos. At the very least, the chakras represent a paradigm for ordering the archetypal issues of human life.

Some individuals seem to be more aware of the nonphysical or spiritual realms than others. Many people have had a precognition or déjà vu experience during their lives. However, nurses may have more opportunities to glimpse a different reality than laypeople. Nurses have been involved in research on the near-death experience for more than 20 years. Across religious and cultural traditions, and throughout history, a common near-death experience has been documented, but it has been only since the early 1980s that it has gained credence among Western health professionals. Many clients describe the experience of near death as a sensation of floating in the air while visualizing their body lying below on a hospital bed, at the scene of an accident, or where the near death occurred. They often watch health-care personnel who are working to resuscitate the body. The person then experiences being drawn into a tunnel, perhaps accompanied by other forms or spiritual beings, and moving toward a bright light that emanates great energy or love. They also describe a communication with the light-being, generally identified as God, about whether they are to remain there or return to the earthly body. Obviously, in cases of near death, the decision is made to return. Individuals who have experienced near death often report that they have developed a great inner peace, they no longer fear death, and that their lives have been transformed by what they have experienced.

Nurses who spend much of their time working with clients who are near death, like hospice

What Do You Think?

What sources of religious energy do you have? When and how do you use them?

nurses, are most likely to have witnessed the experience of deathbed visions and gained a glimpse of a different realm of reality. Dying clients who are having a deathbed vision are often aware of multiple realities—the tangible here and now that family members and caretakers can observe, and "the other side," where they see loved ones who have previously died and are waiting for their arrival. The following personal experience is a good example of this phenomenon:

> At the time my maternal grandmother died in 1990 at the age of 98, she had been unable to communicate for many years as a result of a series of strokes. However, one afternoon in the nursing home, where she spent the last 14 years of her life, she rang for a nurse and asked for a glass of water. When the nurse returned 15 minutes later with the water, grandmother said, "Never mind—Frank is here for me." And within a few minutes she was dead. Frank, my grandfather, had died in 1937.

Some medical researchers attribute near death and deathbed experiences to progressive hypoxia in specific brain centers. However, others give the experiences a spiritual interpretation. Could it be that Frank had, indeed, come to meet his wife of many years past? There is a vast amount of literature on angels and spiritual guides emphasizing that people need not feel alone or frightened by future situations or crises. Angels and other spiritual guides are available to comfort them just for the asking.

Some authorities believe that children are more open to communication from the spiritual world than adults because they have not yet been contaminated with the laws of natural science that are generally accepted by Western society. For example, a young child related the following experience: When she was about 7 years old, she awoke in the middle of the night to find a beautiful lady in a gown of glowing white watching her. She had the experience at least one other time, but her mother, whom she called into the room at the time, was unable to see the lady.

Mystics are believed to be people who have a different relationship to time, space, matter, and energy than most of the population. It seems that they are able to understand the real nature and full capability of their souls and can apply that knowledge and ability to the physical world, producing changes that science has difficulty explaining and some call miracles. For example, the current-day Hindu holy man in India Sai Baba generates ash that has brought miraculous healing to some people who have touched it. Also, many healing miracles were documented by physicians and scientists during the lifetime of the Italian Franciscan priest Padre Pio before his death in 1968. The common message of mystics from around the world is that people are to live lives of love and compassion for all. The extraordinary love and compassion that most marks the early life of the Dalai Lama, a Buddhist holy man, is depicted in the historical films "Seven Years in Tibet" and "Kundun."

Spiritual Practices in Health and Illness

Jung, the Swiss psychoanalytic pioneer of the early twentieth century, was the first to directly propose that all human mental and even physical illnesses are the result of maladjustment between the physical and the spiritual being.[7] Although his father was a Protestant clergyman, Jung was a professed agnostic for most of his life. However, by the end of his life, Jung came to believe in the existence of God. But even before his conversion experience, Jung recognized that the truths contained within the world's religions and in ancient mythology convey knowledge about basic human nature. These truths are embedded in the human biologic being and manifest themselves in the unconscious mind. Jung is credited with explaining why ancient religious and secular stories survive over the centuries. These stories survive because they continue to resonate at the core of human nature.

During the last several decades, there has been growing realization that spiritual practices have an important role to play in modern health care.

Benson, a Harvard professor of psychiatry, published a ground-breaking book, *The Relaxation Response*, in 1975.[8] After reviewing numerous controlled studies of physiologic responses to transcendental meditation and other meditative techniques, Benson outlined a strategy of meditation for use by the general public. In 1975, Benson asserted that this practice required no spiritual underpinnings at all, and meditation on any word, even *potato*, would be beneficial. However, 20 years later, Benson was emphatically convinced of the health benefit of spiritual connectedness. He now teaches meditation on a spiritually meaningful word. Following this trend, in the mid-1990s the Harvard University Medical School initiated its conferences on Spirituality and Healing in Medicine.

Two phenomena that have unfolded since the mid-1970s support the trend toward spirituality in health care. First, in the tumultuous managed care environment now characterizing the health industry, clients and consumers increasingly feel that their health needs are not being addressed. More than one-third of American adults are seeking alternative solutions to health and illness problems from various nonmainstream sources, including spiritual practices. The second phenomenon is the growth of a body of well-designed and controlled research specifically examining relationships between spiritual practices and health outcomes of both clients and providers of care.

> *More than one-third of American adults are seeking alternative solutions to health and illness problems from various nonmainstream sources, including spiritual practices.*

In one study, 393 clients admitted to the coronary care unit at San Francisco General Hospital were randomly and blindly assigned to one of two groups.[9] In the first group, 192 clients were assigned anonymously to prayer groups throughout the San Francisco Bay area. The remaining 201 clients were assigned to a control group where no prayer was involved. Although some of the control group may have been prayed for by their own friends and family, the experimental group received from their assigned prayer groups regular and specific intercessory prayer that requested God's intervention for healing. In all other ways the two groups were similar. The group who received regular intercessory prayer had fewer episodes of cardiac arrest, congestive heart failure, and pneumonia, and they required less ventilatory assistance and fewer antibiotics and diuretics than the control group, who received no prayer interventions.

One of the more dramatic studies was conducted using a sample of 232 open-heart surgery clients at Dartmouth-Hitchcock Medical Center. Those clients who indicated that they had social support were one-third as likely to die as those who did not. Those who indicated that they had religious faith were one-third as likely to die as those who did not. And those who had both social support and religious faith were one-ninth as likely to die as those who had neither.

In another study, 203 family practice clients were interviewed regarding their views on the relationship between religion and health. They were very positive about their family practice physicians' involvement in spiritual issues; more than one-third of the group wanted their family practice providers to discuss religious issues related to their health with them more frequently, and half of the group wanted their physicians to pray with them. However, two-thirds of the group reported that their family practice physician had never discussed religious beliefs with them.[10]

Family practice physicians have, since the late 1980s, become more open to exploring the spiritual domain of health with their clients. In a 1989 study of 160 family practice physicians, most acknowledged the beneficial relationships among religious practice and both mental and physical health. Many thought that they should discuss these matters with their clients, and two-thirds of the physicians thought that prayer with their clients was appropriate at times. Yet only one-third of the group had prayed with clients. Praying with clients was more prevalent among younger physicians.[11] When a 1996 Yankelovich survey re-examined this issue among board-certified physicians in family medicine, 79 percent of that group agreed that prayer can actually effect healing—a substantial increase from previous surveys. There are a number of organizations and agencies that encourage the incorporation of spiritual practices into health care (Box 19–2 to Box 19–5).

Box 19–2

American Holistic Nurses' Association

The American Holistic Nurses' Association (AHNA) was founded in 1980 by a group of nurses dedicated to bringing the concepts of holism to every arena of nursing practice. They define holism as wellness, that state of harmony between body, mind, emotions, and spirit in an ever-changing environment.

AHNA offers certification in holistic nursing and has endorsed programs in Aroma Therapy, Interactive Imagery, and Healing Touch.

Visit the AHNA Web site at http://www.ahna.org.

Prayer

Surveys reveal that most Americans pray; and in response to recent world events, there has been a renewed interest in religion. Thoughts in general, and prayers in particular, should be regarded as powerful forces, and people need to learn how to direct and use them for positive ends. Individuals with a spiritual orientation have known for a long time that positive thoughts and affirmations influence events for the better, whereas negative thoughts and curses can bring about adversity. Thoughts and prayers should be viewed as exchanges of energy with creation. Prayer is sometimes defined as "communicating with God," or speaking with some type of divine entity. It is believed that all prayers are "heard" because they reverberate in the open system of the spiritual realm.

However, some prayers may appear to "backfire" because human wisdom is limited and it is impossible to know all the complexities of a given

Box 19–3

Parish (Congregational) Nursing

Parish (congregational) nursing is a movement of the last decade in which churches, synagogues, mosques, and other faith communities designate nurses to serve their membership. Parish nursing is viewed as a healing ministry, and parish nurses are attuned to spiritual issues raised by health transitions, as well as the healing nature of spiritual practice. They may function to assist people to remain in their own homes; they may connect them with other health services for which they are eligible; they may provide needed health teaching and support; and at times their role is to simply be present with them.

The International Parish Nurse Resource Center is now located in St. Louis, Missouri. They can be contacted at 314-918-2559, 314-918-2527, 877-627-5653, or on the World Wide Web at www.parishnurses.org.

Box 19–4

Office of Alternative Medicine

The Office of Alternative Medicine (OAM) was initiated at the National Institutes of Health in 1992 to evaluate the effectiveness of alternative medical treatment modalities. In addition to funding studies, they have developed a research database and a clearinghouse for disseminating information to the public.

The OAM's Web site is located at http://www.altmed.od.nih.gov/oam.

Box 19–5

International Center for the Integration of Health and Spirituality

The International Center for the Integration of Health and Spirituality (ICIHS) in Rockville, Maryland, disseminates research on the benefits of spiritual practices to health professionals and to the public through their publication, conferences, and speakers.

For further information about this resource, contact ICIHS at 310-984-7162, or visit their Web site at www.icihs.org.

situation nor what the long-term outcomes may be. Merely praying that a loved one may live does not address quality-of-life issues. Although the loved one may still be alive, he or she may be in great pain or exist in a vegetative state requiring complete and expensive care. Prayers of protection from the ill will or the mistaken, if well-intentioned, assistance of others may be preferred. Examples of protective prayer include the Lord's Prayer, the Prayer for Peace attributed to St. Francis, and the ancient Irish Prayer of St. Patrick's Breastplate. Rather than seeking a specific outcome to a problem, protective prayers ask for a protective shield of light and love in the time of need or simply that God's will be done.

Once a person believes that prayer can be an effective force in altering the world, he or she must then decide on what type of prayer is most effective. There are many and varying opinions about praying and types of prayer. A few simple principles need to be followed. First, pray with humility. Truly spiritual people are often characterized by humility. Prayers that express love and support or that seek forgiveness of self and others are powerful messages to their recipients. Consider the following case as an example of this principle:

> A man in the renal intensive care unit (ICU) at a large medical center many years ago was being cared for by a graduate nurse. He had experienced renal failure of unknown etiology. At that time, because of the primitive nature of dialysis and the very limited facilities, if a person did not regain renal function within 30 days, a committee would determine whether treatment should be continued or stopped. If it was stopped, obviously the person would die. Because this man was in his 60s and had seemingly already lived most of his life, he was not considered a priority case for dialysis. He owned a thriving hardware store in a small town in Indiana, where he was also the mayor. He was not known to be particularly religious, but after several weeks in the ICU, he began to ask that the Bible be read to him by the night shift nurses before he went to sleep. He also began to pray for the first time in many years. One night he talked with the graduate nurse about his realization that he had lived his life focused primarily on his work, rather than on the people he loved—his wife and his children. In his work he was a success, but in his relationships, he saw failure. He explained to the nurse that he told God that night that if he were allowed to recover, he would change the way that he lived his life. Near the end of the 30-day trial period, for no

reason that the doctors could determine, he began to produce urine. Eventually, he recovered full urinary function and was able to leave the ICU to go home. This man's prayers of repentance and for forgiveness seemed to have been answered.

Another interpretation for what was experienced by the man with renal failure is that disease, illness, or injury brings a message or a lesson to persons experiencing them that change their lives in some manner. This interpretation is based on the belief that all elements of creation are imbued with consciousness, and that pathogenesis, illness, or disease is but one manifestation of this consciousness. Contemplative, or meditative, prayer is a means by which people can become more sensitive to their internal environment so they can learn what the illness has to teach.

A belief in a universal consciousness is sometimes considered to be the underlying process causing psychosomatic illnesses. It is possible that healing and cure may be produced by therapeutic interventions at a subconscious level, even without the person's recognition or understanding of the message. Like the man with renal failure, however, the person may still need the illness and its message to become open to the healing process. When the person opens up to the message of the illness and understands why it happened, that message can then be absorbed into the whole of the person's life so that the illness is free to leave on its own. Although the recovery may seem to be most mysterious, in reality it is a result of a well-sequenced process.

Meditation and Healing

The relaxation response and prayer have been demonstrated to affect illnesses. The ability of people to participate in their own healing through prayer or meditation may use a source of healing power called "remembered wellness,"[12] sometimes called by others "the placebo effect." It is based on the belief that all people have the capacity to "remember" the calm and confidence associated with emotional and physical health and happiness. The benefit of remembered wellness is based on its acting as a source of energy to be tapped into and used for healing, not something to regard suspiciously. However, the effectiveness of remembered wellness depends on the individual's belief system.

Everyone involved in providing health care is in a position to make use of this energy as part of the healing process. One thing that health-care providers can do to promote healing is to speak positively of treatments and medications being used. For example, positive reinforcement occurs when the nurse refers to the clients' medication as the "drug your doctor prescribed to help your heart" or the food tray as "nutrition to help your body fight your infection." Remembered wellness depends on three components: belief and expectation of the client, belief and expectation of the caregiver, and belief and expectation generated by a caring relationship between the client and the caregiver. A warm and trusting relationship seems to enhance the effectiveness of the care that is provided.

In contrast, the "nocebo effect" is the fulfillment of an expectation of harm. It is also an effect that health professionals can cause. Examples of the nocebo effect include advising clients that a medicine will probably make them sick, telling them that chemotherapy will drain their energy and cause their hair to fall out, or informing them that a certain percentage of people die from a given procedure. Such warnings can actually bring about the warned against complications.

The relaxation response entails 20 minutes, twice each day, of quiet meditation on a word or image that is spiritually meaningful to the person. When an intrusive thought enters the person's consciousness, the person should lightly dismiss it, as if gently blowing a feather away, and return to the meditation word or image. Over time, individuals who use this method have lowered blood pressure, decreased incidents of dysmenorrhea, reduction in chronic pain, and improvement in a number of illnesses.

Relaxation, meditation, visualization, and hypnosis can help with seriously ill clients, including many with cancer. Meditation is a technique of listening. However, listening is not a passive process. Rather, it is a way of focusing the mind in a state of relaxed awareness to pay attention to deeper thoughts and feelings, to the products of the unconscious mind, to the peace of pure consciousness, and to deeper spiritual awareness. Some teachers of meditation suggest that the person select a spiritually symbolic word (e.g., God, love, beauty, peace, Mary, Jesus) on which to focus, whereas others suggest watching a candle flame. Still others teach practitioners to focus on their breathing. All these methods are intended to bring the person to a deeply restful state that frees the mind from its usual chatter. This is the experience of being centered. People may experience spiritual insights, but more often they experience a gradual enhancement of well-being.

Visualization is the practice of meditating with an image of a desired outcome or the process of attaining it. It is preferable that the image be selected by the person rather than someone else. For example, a person with a tumor might visualize miniature miners mining the unhealthy tissue and carting it away. Hypnosis is a process of suggesting an image of a desired reality to someone. Both these techniques have been demonstrated to stimulate the immune system. Siegel has also observed that some seriously ill people believe that they deserve their illness as a punishment for something they did in the past. Helping them forgive themselves often brings about dramatic improvements in their conditions. Releasing fear and hate has a similar effect. This process reflects back to Nightingale's belief that nurses need to help clients get out of the way of their own healing.

It might seem logical to conclude that clients who do not recover from illness, or who die, have failed to help themselves or did not adequately use their spiritual powers. However, that is not the case. Spiritual modes of healing do not always lead to cure. Spiritual healing takes a much broader view and includes enhanced comfort and an inner peace with disability or death.

Therapeutic Touch

Therapeutic touch (TT) is an active alternative healing modality that involves redirecting the human energy system. In recent years, TT has been retrieved from ancient traditions, studied, and refined. As a healing practice, TT is consistent with the Science of Unitary Human Beings developed by Martha Rogers. The Science of Unitary Human Beings defines persons as energy fields in interaction with the larger environmental energy field. The energy fields are characterized by patterns of waves. One way of altering the wave patterns of the human energy field is to use TT to move energy into and through it in deliberate ways. The practitioner of TT acts with the intent of relaxing the recipient, reducing pain and discomfort, and accelerating healing when appropriate. Early controlled studies of the effects of TT showed that the hemoglobin levels of a group of clients who received TT increased significantly more than the levels in a control group who did not receive TT.

Therapeutic touch (TT) is an active alternative healing modality that involves redirecting the human energy system.

The TT practitioner should approach the client with compassion and the intent to heal, and the recipient of care ideally approaches the healing encounter with receptivity and openness to change. The practitioner of TT first centers and then assesses the state of the recipient's energy field, noting energy levels and movement around the chakras. Cues may be determined through physical sensations in the practitioner's hands, direct visualization, inner awareness, or other intuitive modes of insight. After assessing the recipient, the TT practitioner, working from the center of the client's energy field to the periphery, directs energy from the environment into the client's field as needed, stimulates energy flow

ISSUES IN PRACTICE

Spiritual Care

Nancy C. Sharts-Hopko

My mother died 2 weeks after she had a stroke during coronary bypass surgery. My brother and I implemented her DNR (do not resuscitate) orders the Wednesday before the Monday that she died. During those days of terminal care, although she never had the same nurse 2 days in a row, we felt well cared for in a spiritual sense.

Some of the things that the staff did included making sure they made us aware that we were not restricted to visiting hours; staying with Mom when we left the room to get something to eat or go to the bathroom; offering to share their food and drinks with us; making sure that we had access to pastoral care—the hospital's or Mom's own; making sure that we had pillows, blankets, and even the other bed in Mom's room for our own use; allowing us as much privacy as we needed; coming in to talk with us; sharing their own stories of the loss of family members; explaining to us where in the physiologic process of dying she was; talking with Mom when they came into the room, both personally and in terms of explaining what they were going to do; handling Mom with great gentleness and respect; allowing us as much time alone with Mom after she died as we wanted; and after she died, calling the undertaker, and explaining clearly what steps we then had to take.

through the client's field, clears congested areas in the energy field, dampens excess energetic activity, and synchronizes the rhythmic waves of the energy flow depending on the client's needs. The practitioner is not diverting his or her own energy into the client because it would be detrimental to the practitioner. Rather, the TT practitioner redirects the client's energy field or directs energy from the environment outside the client.

Nursing Practice and Spiritual Wellness

Although the nursing profession is deeply rooted in religious traditions, modern nursing has spent considerable energy attempting to distance itself from this aspect of its history. Nursing as vocation has given way to nursing as profession. The current health-care system has required nurses to shift their identity from vocation to profession in order to achieve appropriate value in a system that is increasingly economically oriented.

People working in the helping professions, whose work is rooted in compassion and concern for others, are prone to depression and burnout.

Yet nursing is much more than the mere secular enterprise the modern world perceives it to be. Perhaps it is time that nurses re-evaluate the work they do and consider it a vocation, that is, a life calling in the spiritual sense of that word. The world's religions consistently allude to the symbolic and deep meaning of the work that nurses do. Nursing practice has the capacity to be richly imaginative and to speak to the soul on many levels. Nursing practice can be carried out mindfully and artistically, or it can be done routinely and unconsciously, like any other job. When nursing is practiced with deep consciousness and purpose, it nurtures the nurse as well as the client.

Some experts perceive that nursing is directly connected to the nurse's fantasy life, family myths, ideals, and traditions. The profession of nursing may be one way that nurses sort out their major life issues. Although the choice of nursing as a career may seem to have been serendipitous, in the spiritual context, it is reasonable to question whether anything really happens by accident. One's work can be viewed as an opus, or those undertakings that are central to the soul's lifetime work of self-definition and self-identification. As nurses practice nursing, they craft themselves.

As with most professions, at times it may become difficult, even impossible perhaps, to feel good about the work that is being done. Negative attitudes about work are detrimental to a person's self-development and tend to cause people to become overly invested in the surface trappings of work, such as money, power, and success. The phenomenon of burnout among nurses has been identified and studied for many years (see Chapter 11). Burnout can be viewed from a spiritual perspective, in which the well runs dry, energy fields become imbalanced, or the person experiences a prolonged "dark night of the soul," or even a finding that the nurse's life work is devoid of meaning.

People working in the helping professions, whose work is rooted in compassion and concern for others, are prone to depression and burnout. A concerted effort at spiritual development, or the nourishment of the soul, is essential to nurses' overall mental and physical well-being. Consider the following personal exchange:

> A nursing faculty colleague who is a psychotherapist recently confided in me that her burnout is caused precisely because she strives to live as Jesus would live in the same circumstances. I reminded her that Jesus also rested, partied enthusiastically with friends, and went on 40-day retreats when he needed to do so. I suggested to her that in her attempt to "live like Jesus," she might also consider caring for herself the way Jesus cared for himself.

In the attempt to maintain an internal state of balance, the first thing that nurses need to do is to take time to feed their spirit. Daily prayer or meditation is an important source of both insight and energy. Belonging to a group or community that actively pursues spiritual growth is also a powerful source of spiritual nourishment. Many individuals find that their spirit is nourished within the setting of a formal religion, although not necessarily the one in which they were reared. It is not uncommon for people to seek a faith community in midlife or later life, perhaps after being away from one for many years. The experience of trying various religions and modes of worship is, all by itself, a broadening, nurturing experience.

Periodic retreat from the hustle and bustle of modern living can be highly restorative of the spirit. A retreat may be for a few hours, a half-day, a weekend, a week, or longer. For some people, keeping a journal regularly is a retreat-like experience. For others, it may be a stroll through a beautiful park, a few hours watching waves on a beach, or a trip to the woods. Retreat is most effective when time is consistently set aside for introspection and reflection rather than for tasks.

Only when nurses begin to slow down and start centering their energy fields will they have the capacity to be fully present and be able to attend with complete consciousness to their loved ones, colleagues, and clients and focus completely on the present moment.

A sense of sacredness can infuse everyday life with meaning and zest if nurses would only open themselves to it. It is a part of normal human activity to celebrate seasonal and family holidays with specific rituals, music, decorations, group gatherings, and foods. These types of activities honor life cycles that are greater than the individual and nurture important relationships that serve as a **support system**.

Many people have routines for their weekends or days off that allow time for self-restoration. These special activities may include a large country breakfast while listening to favorite music; baking cookies, bread, or a pie; sitting for an extended period of time in a favorite easy chair; or even playing a physically demanding sport like basketball. Many people have favorite coffee mugs or dishes or special objects in their homes that are not only beautiful but may remind them of loved ones, wonderful trips, religious experiences, or other events that nourish them each time they view the object. One of the most spiritual aspects of a person's life is the enjoyment of beauty. It costs little or nothing to plant or cut flowers or listen to music. It is in these moments that a person's creativity and insight are most evident.

The hectic modern world continually urges people to enhance their capacity for dealing with multiple concerns at the same time. Some people even define success by looking at how many balls they can juggle simultaneously. *Multitasking* is the new buzzword for the health-care environment of the twenty-first century. Nurses must be able to talk on the telephone, send faxes and e-mail, surf the net, and use a word processor for entering client data at the same time that they are developing care plans, evaluating clients, answering call lights, supervising unlicensed assistive personnel, and providing physicians with information. Although this is highly productive, the more nurses multitask, the more disconnected they become from themselves. Multitasking can be thought of as the antithesis of spiritual nurturance. Spirituality is about personal wholeness, whereas multitasking is about fragmentation. Only when nurses begin to slow down and start centering their energy fields will they have the capacity to be fully present and be able to attend with complete consciousness to their loved ones, colleagues, and clients and focus completely on the present moment.

Critical Thinking Exercises

Mrs. Jan Steiner, 73 years old, has outlived two husbands. Ted, her second husband, died 20 years ago. Reared in the Roman Catholic faith, Mrs. Steiner converted to Judaism when she married Ted. Her two daughters by her first husband were also reared in the Roman Catholic tradition, one of whom, Kathy, continues to practice her religion. The other daughter, Judith, is Unitarian.

Mrs. Steiner experienced a stroke 2 years ago that left her moderately disabled. At that time she moved into a long-term care facility. Still, she was able to read and to enjoy visits with friends and family. But a second stroke 3 months ago left her incontinent and aphasic.

Mrs. Steiner has just had a major heart attack. Although bypass surgery could extend her life, she has never articulated any end-of-life desires. Her daughters are in conflict over how Mrs. Steiner's medical management should proceed. Kathy strongly believes that as long as Mrs. Steiner is alive, life should be actively supported. It would be morally wrong to do less than that. Judith, on the other hand, believes that what had been the "life" of Mrs. Steiner is essentially over and it is a waste of resources to merely delay the inevitable. The nursing staff, as they attempt to facilitate communication between the family and the medical staff, feel caught in the middle.

- What are your own spiritual beliefs about the proper approach to Mrs. Steiner's medical management?
- Analyze the positions of Kathy and Judith from both their ethical and spiritual contexts.
- What resources are likely to be available in the hospital or the community to help the daughters come to a decision?

Bypass surgery is not performed, and Mrs. Steiner returns to her long-term care facility. Her overall condition continues to deteriorate, and within 3 months she is very near death. She seems to have little awareness of her surroundings and she does not consistently recognize or respond to her daughters.

- Knowing the religious divergence within Mrs. Steiner's family, how might the nursing staff facilitate their preparation for the death of their mother and her funeral?
- What would happen within Mrs. Steiner's circle of family and friends if any "side"—Catholic, Jewish, or Unitarian—"won" in planning her end-of-life care?
- Have you seen blending of religious traditions in rituals such a marriage or burial? What are the advantages and disadvantages of such an approach?
- What might be the outcomes of handling their mother's death in a strictly secular or nonsectarian way and allowing all relatives and friends to mourn privately in accordance with their own spiritual traditions?

Conclusion

Spiritual development is not merely a task to be accomplished and checked off like an item on a checklist for personal improvement. Rather, spirituality is a way of life that involves a profound respect for self and for others and true living of the Golden Rule. Once individuals realize their self-goodness and the goodness of all creation, they have no choice but to live a spiritual life. Their ability to see their lives as abundantly blessed begets more goodness. Over time, they will feel more sustained, and the change will be recognized by the people for whom they are providing care. Spiritual development is a synergistic process. Some people may wonder whether there is a personal cost to spiritual development. Spiritual development does not cost the person anything, but it requires a shifting of priorities. What is regarded as abundant living may shift from a material focus to a focus on health, love, beauty, and a joy in life. It is never too late to begin to live in this way—but neither is it ever too soon.

References

1. Smith, H: The Illustrated World's Religions: A Guide to Our Wisdom Traditions. HarperCollins, New York, 1994.
2. Peck, MS: The Road Less Traveled and Beyond. Touchstone, New York, 1997.
3. Nightingale, F: Notes on Nursing. Dover, New York, 1969. (Originally published, 1860)
4. Watson, J: Nursing: Human Science and Human Theory of Care. Theory of Nursing. National League for Nursing, New York, 1988.
5. North American Nursing Diagnosis Association: Nursing Diagnosis: Definitions and Classification, 1997–1998. NANDA, Philadelphia, 1998.
6. Moore, T: Care of the Soul. HarperCollins, New York, 1992.
7. Bendit, LJ: The spirit in health and disease. In Kunz, D (ed): Spiritual Healing. Quest Books, Wheaton, IL, 1995, pp. 92–100.
8. Benson, H: The Relaxation Response. William Morrow, New York, 1975.
9. Byrd, RC: Positive therapeutic effects of intercessory prayer in a coronary care unit population. South Med J 81(7):826–829, 1988.
10. King, D, and Bushwick, B: Beliefs and attitudes of hospital inpatients about faith healing and prayer. J Fam Pract 39(4):349–352, 1994.
11. Koenig, H, et al: Physician perspectives on the role of religion in the physician–older patient relationship. J Fam Pract 28(4):441–448, 1989.
12. Dossey, L: Be Careful What You Pray For . . . You Just Might Get It. HarperSanFrancisco, New York, 1997.

Bibliography

Catanzaro, AM, and McMullen, KA: Increasing nursing students' spiritual sensitivity. Nurse Educator 26(5):221–226, 2001.

Kuuppelomki, M: Spiritual support of terminally ill patients. Journal of Clinical Nursing 10(5):660–670, 2001.

Lelis-Grice, D: Loving, human touch helps family cope with loss. AACN News 15(9):4–6, 1998.

Loscalzo, F: The essence of nursing is touching another soul. AACN News 15(10):3, 1998.

O'Mathna, DP, and Quiring-Emblen, JD: Making sense of complementary and alternative therapies. Journal of Christian Nursing 18(4):8–15, 2001.

Shelly, JA: Parish nursing: Firing the imagination. Journal of Christian Nursing 18(2):3, 2001.

Sutherland, K: Speak carefully. Journal of Christian Nursing 18(3):36, 2001.

Troussman, S: The human connection: Nurses and their patients. American Nurse 30(5):1–8, 1998.

Vandenbrink, RA: Spiritual assessment: Comparing the tools. Journal of Christian Nursing 18(3):24–26, 2001.

Wilson, J: Healing and curing. Oklahoma Nurse 43(1):4–5, 1998.

20

Cultural Diversity

Joseph T. Catalano

Learning Objectives

After completing this chapter, the reader will be able to:

- Define culture and identify its expression.
- Compare and contrast the "melting pot" and "salad bowl" theories of acculturation.
- Identify the components of an accurate cultural assessment.
- Distinguish between primary and secondary cultural characteristics.
- List and define the key aspects of effective intercultural communication.
- Name two sources for information about transcultural nursing.

Culture is a powerful influence on how nurses and clients interpret and respond to health care. Both nurses and clients expect to be treated with respect and understanding for their individuality no matter what their cultural origins. Nurses who understand the essential characteristics of transcultural nursing will be able to provide competent and culturally sensitive care for clients from all cultural backgrounds.

What Is Culture?

There are many definitions of culture and ways that culture is understood. Culture may be seen as a group's acceptance of a set of attitudes, ideologies, values, beliefs, and behaviors that influence the way that the members of the group express themselves. Cultural expression assumes many forms, including language; spirituality; works of art; group customs and traditions; food preferences; response to illness, stress, pain, **bereavement**, anger, and sorrow; decision making; and even world philosophy. An individual's cultural orientation is the result of a learning process that literally starts at birth and continues throughout the life span wherein behaviors, beliefs, and attitudes are transmitted from one generation to the next. Although expressions of culture are primarily unconscious, they have a profound effect on an individual's interactions and response to the health-care system.

Mrs. Sung Gwak, who is 74 years old, is brought into the emergency room (ER) by her family because of "very bad indigestion that won't go away." Three family members (a middle-aged man and woman and a younger woman) accompany the elderly lady. They are discussing her condition in a mixture of English and another language, which the nurse does not recognize. Because the client does not seem to understand any English, the nurse attempts to address the family. The younger woman speaks broken English but manages to explain that the client is her grandmother and she is accompanied by her mother and father, who speak even less English than she does.

By default, the granddaughter serves as the translator. After much prompting, she explains that her grandmother arrived in the United States for a visit only 2 days ago from a small mountain village in Korea where she had lived all her life. She had been having periodic episodes of "indigestion" for several weeks before the visit and used traditional herbal teas prescribed by the local healer to treat her condition. Based on further assessment and a diagnostic test, it is determined that Mrs. Gwak had an extensive myocardial infarction at least 1 week before her trip and is currently in a mild state of congestive heart failure (CHF).

She is given medications for the chest pain and CHF and is started on anticoagulant medications in the ER. She is then transferred to the coronary care unit (CCU), where she is scheduled to have coronary angiography the next day. The angiogram shows multiple blockages in her coronary arteries and extensive myocardial damage. Because of her age and also the extensive damage to her heart, the physician thinks that it would be too risky to attempt bypass surgery and decides to monitor her closely and treat her medically until she is stable enough to have a balloon angioplasty.

When the CCU nurse assigned to Mrs. Gwak enters the room at the beginning of her shift the day after the angiogram, she finds the client covered with four heavy blankets and a bedspread and sweating profusely. When the nurse attempts to remove the excessive bed covers, the client's daughter protests vehemently in Korean and puts the blankets back on as soon as the nurse leaves the room. The daughter seems to think that her mother is sick because she is too cold and gives the elderly woman hot herbal drinks from a thermos bottle that she had brought from home.

When the granddaughter arrives, the nurse explains to her why excessive heat is harmful to the client's cardiac status and the need to follow the diet restrictions prescribed by the physician. The ingredients of the herbal drinks were unknown, and there may be some serious interactions with the numerous medications that the client was receiving. The granddaughter translated this information to her mother, who seemed to become even angrier with the nurse. Although she outwardly seems to comply with the restrictions, she continues the traditional folk treatments in secret, believing that the Western hospital food is bad for her mother's health.

Mrs. Gwak is very quiet and hardly ever asks for help. When she does talk to her family, the conversation is usually about the airplane flight to the United States and the belief that the high altitude probably caused all Mrs. Gwak's problems.

Her condition gradually deteriorates during her hospitalization, despite all the medical treatment. The nurse and physician tell the family about the client's worsening condition and the likelihood that she will not survive the hospitalization, but they refuse to relay the information to the client.

Although this situation is fictitious, it demonstrates some of the potential problems that may be encountered when interacting with clients who come from a strong traditional cultural background. Culture, among other things, is a belief system that has been developed over a person's lifetime and, like all strongly held belief systems, is difficult to change. In the case of Mrs. Gwak, it is easy to see the futility of attempting to change her belief system in a short period of time with a limited number of interactions. Another important aspect of the situation is the effect of the **family**. Rather than being helpful to the care of this client or attempting to alter her belief systems to follow care recommendations, the family reinforced the client's beliefs.

Concepts of Culture

Culture is not a monolithic concept. Any individual probably belongs to several subcultures within his or her major culture. Subcultures develop when members of the group accept values in addition to those of their dominant culture. Even within a given culture, many variations may exist. For example, it is logical to conclude that people who live in the United States all belong to the American culture and would be very similar in most ways. However, teenagers living in the rural areas of Oklahoma may find it difficult to relate to the teenagers raised in the inner city of Philadelphia. Even though they speak the same language and share some similar interests, they have so many different past experiences that change their perspectives on life that it may be difficult for them to relate to each other.

Culture can be considered to be a type of flawed photocopy machine that makes duplicates of the original document with minor differences. A society attempts to preserve itself by passing down its values, beliefs, and customs to the next generation. Although some parts of the culture remain very similar, other parts change greatly owing to effects from both within and outside of the group.

Although some parts of the culture remain very similar, other parts change greatly owing to effects from both within and outside of the group.

Diversity

Diversity is a term that is used to explain the differences between cultures. The characteristics that define diversity can be divided into two groups: primary and secondary.

1. Primary characteristics are those that tend to be more obvious, including nationality, race, color, gender, age, and religious beliefs
2. Secondary characteristics, such as socioeconomic status, education, occupation, length of time away from the country of origin, gender issues, residential status, and sexual orientation, may be more difficult to identify, even though they may have an even more profound effect on the person's cultural identity than the primary characteristics.

When individuals make generalizations about others based on the obvious primary characteristics and do not take the time to consider the secondary characteristics, they are stereotyping the other person. Stereotyping is an oversimplified belief, conception, or opinion about another person (or group) based on a limited amount of information.

Melting Pot versus Salad Bowl

The United States has traditionally been considered a melting pot of world cultures. Early in the history of the United States, most people who came here from distant lands were eager to be assimilated into American culture. Many people Americanized their names; they shed their traditional dress; they learned American manners and customs as quickly as possible; and they made heroic attempts to learn English without the benefit of formal schooling—all so that they could "fit in" to their new homeland. Until recently, most people who immigrated to the new country were very willing to acculturate (i.e., to alter their own cultural practices in an attempt to become more like the new culture). The end result was a blending or melting pot of cultures.

However, since the early 1970s, the practice of intentional acculturation by immigrating cultures seems to have fallen by the wayside. Many individuals who migrate to the United States from other countries now cling tenaciously to their traditional cultural practices and languages, thus producing a phenomenon that is called multiculturalism. Rather than blending smoothly into the bigger pot as former immigrants had done, the modern immigrants maintain their own unique flavors and textures, much like the ingredients in a large tossed salad. As an ever-growing phenomenon, multiculturalism is something that health-care providers need to be aware of; they must learn ways of adapting their health practices to allow for these differences.

> *As an ever-growing phenomenon, multiculturalism is something that health-care providers need to be aware of; they must learn ways of adapting their health practices to allow for these differences.*

There are drawbacks and benefits in both approaches. In the era of the "melting pot," individuals who attempted to retain their native beliefs, customs, and languages were often ridiculed, scorned, and generally made to feel that they were outsiders to the mainstream culture. However, when they did become homogenized into the American culture, learned the language of the dominant society, and made an effort to be seen as belonging, they were more likely to be accepted as equals and quickly advanced up the socioeconomic ladder.

The current "salad bowl" trend in society has the advantage of allowing individuals in the dominant culture to gain an appreciation of other cultures for their unique contributions to society. The drawback of the salad bowl is that it tends to create pockets of culturally different individuals who live in, but only have minimal interaction with, mainstream American society. Because they do not speak the language or refuse to accept the customs of the dominant culture, it may be more difficult for them to advance their socioeconomic status.

The salad bowl process has also given rise to cultural relativism among some groups. Cultural relativism occurs when members of a strong cultural group understand their culture and group members only from their own viewpoint rather than from that of the larger culture. They do not try to understand its unique characteristics, values, and beliefs.

Some cultural groups manage to blend the melting pot and the salad bowl together through a rather complex process that is sometimes called heritage consistency. Outwardly, they may become acculturated to the point where they wear business suits, speak passable English, eat fast foods, and go to movies. However, when they are at home, or with groups from their traditional culture, they speak their native language, wear their traditional clothes, eat ethnically correct meals, and generally follow their native customs. This approach to acculturation has the advantages of allowing them to fit in and advance in the larger culture while retaining many of the elements of their traditional culture that provide a sense of stability to their lives. It does, however, create in some individuals a type of cultural confusion that may lead to increased tension and anxiety.

What Do You Think?

Identify and rank by priority at least five of your own health-care values (e.g., exercise, immunizations). Identify five health-care values of a culture with which you are familiar. How do these values compare with your own?

U.S. Ethnic Population Trends

Rapid population growth in ethnic groups has been the trend in the United States for many years. The last comprehensive national census was conducted in 2000. According to U.S. Bureau of Census statistics, in the year 2000 approximately 30 percent of the U.S. population was composed of minority groups. If current trends continue, it is projected that by the year 2080 the white population will actually be a minority group constituting 48.9 percent of the total population of the United States.

Contributing to the rapid growth in minority populations is the increasing number of immigrants coming to the United States. Between 1920 and 2000, the number of legal immigrants each year increased from 500,000 to more than 6 million. Currently the largest numbers of immigrants are from Asia, Mexico, and Central and South America. Fewer immigrants have come from Africa and Europe than in previous years.

"Despite the relatively low number of minority nurses, it is expected that nurses from one culture should be able to give culturally competent care to individuals from any other culture."

However, the percentage of minority nurses does not reflect the national population trends. Despite efforts on the part of the National League for Nursing (NLN), American Association of Colleges of Nursing (AACN), and other organizations concerned with nursing education, minority nurses have remained constant at approximately 10 percent of the RNs practicing in the United States. The latest reported statistics by the NLN demonstrate a leveling off of the number of minority students enrolled in basic nursing programs at about 15 percent. In a perfect world, the number and percentage of RNs from the various minority groups would mirror society as a whole to better meet the needs of a culturally diverse country.

Despite the relatively low number of minority nurses, it is expected that nurses from one culture should be able to give culturally competent care to individuals from any other culture. Being on the front lines of health care, nursing is the one profession that is continually confronted with cultural changes that result from ethnic shifts in population. Nurses now recognize that they can no longer use traditional ethnocentric models to guide their practice and protocols. Nurses are beginning to promote an understanding of individuals from other cultures and improve the overall quality of health care.

The Medicare and Medicaid laws that evolved out of the social programs of the 1960s have increased the number of culturally diverse clients with whom nurses come in contact. Historically, many minority groups tend to be among the poorest segments of the population. Before the Medicare and Medicaid legislation that expanded government-funded health care to cover all welfare recipients, some ethnic minorities were unable to afford health care and were seen in the health-care setting only when severely ill. Ethnic minorities are now covered by these laws and, by their increasing numbers in all levels and areas of health care, have prompted nurses to become more sensitive to the transcultural aspects of health care.

Since the 1970s, transcultural nursing has become an important subject in most nursing programs. However, nursing education has taken only the first unsteady steps on the path to seeking a true integration of cultural competence into daily practice. As technological and transportation advances bring more and more people from different cultures closer together, there will be an increased demand for nurses who can practice effectively in a culturally diverse society. Many challenges still lie ahead.

Developing Cultural Awareness

Developing a cultural awareness is the first step in becoming a culturally competent nurse. One of the main challenges for nurses who practice in a culturally diverse environment is to understand the client's perspective of what is happening in the health-care setting. From a cultural viewpoint, it may be very different from what the nurse believes is occurring.

A nurse develops cultural awareness only when he or she is able to recognize and value all

ISSUES NOW

Minority Nurses Needed for the Future of Nursing

Recruiting, retaining, and reshaping the role of minority nurses has been a primary concern of the health-care industry for almost a decade. Initiatives have been implemented by both the private sector and governmental agencies to increase the numbers of minority nurses and meet the needs of the ever-shifting client demographics.

Recent studies have shown that there has been a slight increase in the number of minority nurses 10%. The number of minority nurses increased at a faster rate than the overall number of RNs. Based on the estimated number of 2.5 million licensed RNs in the United States, the following percentages are found in each minority group:

- African American, 4.2% (107,500)
- Asian, 3.4% (86,000)
- Hispanic, 1.6% (40,600)
- Native American, 0.5% (12,000)

Hospitals have been the primary employer of minority nurses and recognize that their employment is a matter of survival. In the competition to attract clients, hospitals cannot afford to have clients feel uncomfortable because of cultural diversity issues. A recent survey showed that 88% of minority nurses are employed in nursing, whereas only 82% of non-minority nurses are. Also, 85% of minority nurses are working full-time, but that number drops to 70% for non-minority nurses.

Although hospitals and health care in general acknowledges the need for more minority nurses, some nurses are experiencing barriers to their career mobility. Although the core issues are not unlike those that all nurses experience—understaffing, frustration with paperwork and regulations, and unappreciative administration and physicians—they also feel that their ethnic background may be hindering their chance for promotion. Sometimes their capabilities are questioned because of their differences and that is a big deterrent.

The role of minority nurses continues to develop as an issue for the twenty-first century. Not only are they necessary because of the changing demographics of the population, many in the health-care system also believe that it is a sound economic policy to have more minority nurses. To help recruit nurses and retain those who are already practicing, several organizations have been established that nurses can contact. The national Coalition of Ethnic Minority Nurses Association and the Tenessee Hospital Association's Council on Diversity are available for assistance.

Source: Cooper, S: Diversity requires more from role of minority nurses. Oklahoma City Nursing Times, May 6, 2002, p. 17.

aspects of a client's culture, including beliefs, customs, responses, methods of expression, language, and social structure. However, merely learning about another person's culture does not guarantee that the nurse will have cultural awareness. Nurses must first understand their own cultural background and explore the origins of their own prejudiced and biased views of others. Several tools have been developed in recent years to measure a person's cultural awareness.

Box 20–1 contains a synthesis of several cultural assessment tools. Answer the questions honestly, then check how you rate in terms of cultural awareness. Keep in mind that there is always some degree of inaccuracy in all self-assessment tools and that the validity and reliability of tools vary widely. The specific score is not as important as gaining an insight into and understanding of what factors are important in developing cultural awareness. Cultural awareness begins with an understanding of one's own cultural health-care beliefs and cultural values.

To those unfamiliar with a particular culture's health-care beliefs, many of the health-care practices may appear meaningless, strange, or even dangerous. Beliefs about health care are based in part on knowledge and are often related to religious beliefs. For example, if a particular society has no knowledge of bacteria as a cause of infection, then the use of antibiotics may seem to them useless in achieving a cure for the disease. On the other hand, if a society believes that illness is caused by evil spirits entering the body from curses by witches or medicine men, then practices such as incantations, use of ritualistic objects like bones, feathers, or incense, and even bloodletting and purgatives to "release" the spirit from the body are a very logical approach to achieving a cure.

Cultural Belief Systems

Cultural belief system are highly complex. For example, some Native-American groups attributed twin births to witchcraft and believed that one of the twin infants had to die so that the other might live. These beliefs and practices are usually kept as closely guarded secrets among the group's members, and there may even be some type of sanction or punishment for members who reveal the belief.

Many cultural beliefs develop over time from a trial-and-error process that has both benefits and drawbacks. For instance, several Native-American tribes that live in the Western desert have developed the practice of keeping infants in cradle boards until they begin walking. This practice, from a safety viewpoint, protects the crawling infant from injury and bites from creatures that are commonly found in the desert, such as scorpions, rattlesnakes, and poisonous insects or lizards. However, the practice tends to delay the leg muscle development of the child and increases the incidence of hip dysplasia because of the child's position in the cradle board.

Some cultural beliefs have a primary purpose of explaining unusual or unpredictable events. For example, many traditional Vietnamese-Americans believe that mental illness results from some action that offended one or more of the gods. They also believe that a family member who is mentally ill brings disgrace upon the family, and thus knowledge of the illness must be kept secret, especially from strangers. As a result, traditional shamans or priest/doctors are sought to attempt to appease the offended deity through rituals and prayers. Only with great reluctance will a traditional Vietnamese-American family seek therapy or medication for a mental illness.

There are several sources for the development of cultural values, including religious beliefs, worldview and philosophy, and group customs. The values that underlie any particular culture serve as powerful forces that affect all aspects of a person's life, ranging from individual actions and decision making to health-care behaviors and life-goal setting. Values, which are discussed in Chapter 7, are the ideals or concepts that give meaning to an individual's life. They are deeply ingrained, and most individuals will strongly resist any attempt to change their value structure.

Box 20–1

Cultural Awareness Assessment Tool

Directions: Circle the number that best reflects your honest response to the statement. When you are finished, add up the total number of points and compare them to the Cultural Awareness Scale below.

Statement	Always	Sometimes	Never
I feel comfortable when discussing alternative lifestyles with clients.	3	2	1
I support the use of traditional cultural healing practices for hospitalized clients.	3	2	1
I know the limits of my communication skills with clients from different cultures.	3	2	1
Outside the work setting, I make an effort to be involved with people from different cultures.	3	2	1
When assessing clients, I recognize the biologic variations of different ethnic groups.	3	2	1
I accept that there is a strong relationship between culture and health.	3	2	1
I consider the race, gender, and age of my clients when administering medications.	3	2	1
When caring for clients from different cultures, I consider the specific diseases common among their group.	3	2	1
I openly acknowledge my own prejudices and biases when working with clients from different cultures.	3	2	1
I seek out and attend in-service classes that deal with cultural and ethnic diversity.	3	2	1
I remain calm when my health-care values or beliefs clash with those of a client.	3	2	1
I practice culturally competent nursing when dealing with all clients, not only those from different ethnic groups.	3	2	1
When assessing clients initially, I consider their geographic origins, religious affiliation, and occupation as important elements of the care plan.	3	2	1
I have a high level of knowledge about the beliefs and customs of at least two different cultures.	3	2	1
I use a standardized cultural assessment tool when performing admission assessments on clients from different cultures.	3	2	1
I take into consideration the policies of my institution that serve as barriers for the effective provision of culturally competent care.	3	2	1
I recognize the cultural differences between the members of the same culture.	3	2	1

Cultural Awareness Scale

40 to 51 points = High degree of cultural awareness
30 to 39 points = Average degree of cultural awareness
17 to 29 points = Low degree of cultural awareness

Cultural values are neither right nor wrong; they exist in a culture from a long-term process of development that can often be traced back to a need for group survival. However, when judged from the perspective of other cultures, they may seem strange or even harmful. Because it makes nurses feel secure and even superior, there is a tendency to transfer to clients health-care expectations based on the nurse's own cultural framework. However, this approach often leads the nurse to failure when trying to change health-care behaviors.

Recognizing Health-Care Practices

It is important to recognize that one of the primary functions of nurses is to change clients' values, particularly values about health care. It is not an easy task. The first step, always, is to recognize that the nurse comes from a particular culture that has its own set of health-care values. Like all values, these have developed over time and are dependent on the nurse's education, upbringing, religious beliefs, and cultural background.

The next step is to identify the culture of the client and recognize specific health-care practices that are both similar and different from those of the nurse. The nurse must then make a decision about whether it is desirable or possible to change the client's values, and if the end result is worth the effort.

For example, many cultures have strong values concerning pregnancy and the birth of children. In traditional Middle-Eastern families, the birth process is valued as an event strictly involving women, and the father is usually not present to either witness or assist in the delivery. However, midwives and obstetric nurses from the current American culture place a high value on the father's participation in the birth event as a way of promoting stronger family ties and starting the bonding process as soon as possible. The nurse who takes care of a Middle-Eastern family must decide whether or not to try to convince the father to stay in the delivery room during the delivery. In any event, the ultimate outcome remains relatively unchanged. Even without the father in the delivery room, the child is delivered safely, and only the bonding process with the father is delayed.

Some African cultures have discovered over time that a woman who delivers a small infant will have a much easier time during labor and delivery. Small infants usually have fewer traumatic birth defects; and there are fewer stillbirths and a higher maternal survival rate. In some traditional central African homeland settings where there is little skilled health care available, the value of having small infants helps in the survival of the group. The custom of feeding pregnant women only a corn-mush cereal throughout their pregnancies ensures small babies at birth. In the United States, where good prenatal nutrition is highly valued, this traditional practice is seen as dangerous to both the mother and the infant. Poor prenatal nutrition has been related to developmental delays, mental retardation, and skeletal deformities in infants as well as maternal malnutrition that can lead to infectious diseases and inability to breast-feed. In this situation, the benefits of a change in such practices of traditional African-American women would be rewarded by healthier babies and mothers.

Assessing Culture

Obtaining accurate cultural assessments can be time consuming and difficult. However, the only way that nurses can avoid imposing their cultural values and practices on others and develop plans of care based on knowledge about others' beliefs and customs is to make a concerted effort to obtain this information. Several different cultural assessment tools for clients have been developed—some short and directed, others lengthy and complicated. One of the most thorough cultural assessments developed to date is based on Purnell's Model of Cultural Competence (Box 20–2).

Although this tool is lengthy, it can provide a

Box 20–2

The 12 Domains of Cultural Assessment—Purnell's Model for Cultural Competence

I. Overview, Inhabited Localities, and Topography

Overview
Heritage and residence
Reasons for migration and associated economic factors
Educational status and occupation

II. Communications

Dominant language and dialects
Cultural communication patterns
Temporal relationships
Format for names

III. Family Roles and Organization

Head of household and gender roles
Prescriptive, restrictive, and taboo behaviors
Family roles and priorities
Alternative lifestyles

IV. Workforce Issues

Culture in the workplace
Issues related to autonomy

V. Biocultural Ecology

Skin color and biologic variations
Diseases and health conditions
Variations in drug metabolism

VI. High-Risk Behaviors

High-risk behaviors
Health-care practices

VII. Nutrition

Meaning of food
Dietary practices for health promotion

VIII. Pregnancy and Childbearing Practices

Fertility practices and views toward pregnancy

IX. Death Rituals

Death rituals and expectations
Responses to death and grief

X. Spirituality

Religious practices and use of prayer
Meaning of life and individual sources of strength
Spiritual beliefs and health-care practices

XI. Health-care Practices

Health-seeking beliefs and behaviors
Responsibility for health care
Folklore practices
Barriers to health care
Cultural responses to health and illness
Blood transfusions and organ donation

XII. Health-care Practitioners

Traditional versus biomedical care
Status of health-care providers

Source: Purnell, LD, and Paulanka, BJ: Transcultural Health Care. FA Davis, Philadelphia, 1998, with permission.

good overview of the client's culture. Nurses should not neglect completing an assessment of their own culture, as well.

True, most busy nurses do not have the time to complete this assessment on every client from a different culture. However, the following key questions can serve as a starting point for a cultural assessment:

- Why do you think you are ill? What was the cause of the illness?
- What was going on at the time the illness started?
- How does the illness affect your body and health?
- Do you consider this to be a serious illness?
- If you were at home, what type of treatments or medications would you use? How would these treatments help?
- What type of treatment do you expect from the health-care system?
- How has your illness affected your ability to live normally?
- If you do not get better, what do you think will happen?

Because clients from different cultures may feel uncomfortable revealing information about cultural beliefs, values, and practices to strangers, it is a good idea to begin your assessment by asking some general questions. A client is more likely to trust a nurse who demonstrates interest in that person as an individual. Only after a warm and trusting environment has been established will a client be willing to reveal the more hidden aspects of his or her culture to the nurse.

Physical assessments made on individuals from other cultures require a certain level of cultural awareness and competence. Although the assessment techniques used for different individuals may be identical, the nurse needs to possess knowledge of the basic biologic and physical variations among ethnic groups. The interpretation of assessment findings may be affected by ethnic variations in anatomic structure or characteristics (e.g., children from some Asian cultures may fall below the normal growth level on a standardized American growth chart because of their genetically smaller stature). Changes in skin color may also affect the interpretation of assessment findings (e.g., with regard to an assessment of cyanosis in people with a light versus a dark complexion). In order to determine whether the client's skin color is normal or abnormal, the nurse must know what constitutes the normal color for a particular ethnic group. In assessing for cyanosis, the nurse may need to examine the client's oral mucosa and may also need to measure capillary refill times to determine whether the client has cyanosis.

What Do You Think?

Using Purnell's cultural assessment tool, assess your own cultural background. In what areas of your own culture are you lacking knowledge?

The ultimate goal of cultural assessment, as with all assessments, is to provide the best care possible for the client. A fundamental belief that nurses hold to strongly is that all clients have a right to self-determination, including the customs, practices, and values that emanate from their culture. By considering both the cultural and ethnic variables of each client, nurses will avoid practice that is ethnocentric and conducted strictly from the nurse's cultural viewpoint.

Providing Culturally Competent Care

Cultural competence has become a buzzword for the twenty-first century. The term has several divergent definitions with little consensus among cultural experts. However, cultural competence as it relates to nursing can be regarded as the provision of effective care for clients who belong to diverse cultures, based on the nurse's knowledge and understanding of the values, customs, beliefs, and practices of the culture. Provision of culturally competent care requires the development of certain interpersonal skills that allow nurses to work with individuals and groups in the community. The primary skills required for cultural competence include communication, understanding, and sensitivity. Although the basic types of cultural skills are similar, their application within and between cultural groups may differ greatly. The development of cultural competence is not a one-time skill to check off on a skills checklist; rather, it is an ongoing process that continues throughout the nurse's career.

Transcultural Communication

The ability to communicate is the foundation on which culturally competent care is built. The most obvious barrier to culturally competent care for the non-English-speaking client is the lack of a common language (Box 20–3). Communication is a highly complex process that requires both verbal and nonverbal communication. Nonverbal communication includes (but is not limited to) body language, facial expressions, eye contact, personal space, touch and body contact, formality of names, and time awareness.

Other factors that affect communication are loudness of voice, tone, and acceptable greetings. Often clients communicate differently with family and friends than they do with health-care personnel. Nurses should also be aware that in some cultures (e.g., those with a strong caste system, which involves a class structure) communication between those in the upper and lower classes in that society may be affected. For example, different cultures may hold the role of women or of health-care personnel in more or less esteem.

Nurses must be cautious when interpreting the nonverbal responses from some cultural groups. Some cultures respond to all questions with the reply "yes," a nod, or a smile. This response, in the American culture, usually indicates understanding and **compliance**. However, particularly in Asian cultures, nodding and smiling can be signs of respect for the nurse's position or an attempt to avoid confrontation. The following is a classic example:

> An English-speaking nurse gave a non-English-speaking Asian client preoperative instructions about how to prepare an abdominal surgical site. She thought that she had shown the client how the bottle of povidone-iodine, a powerful skin disinfectant, was to be used in scrubbing the area. The client smiled and nodded throughout the instruction. When asked whether he had any questions, he did not respond. The nurse took the silence to mean that he had no questions. When the nurse left the room, the client promptly drank the whole bottle of povidone-iodine. Fortunately, the error was discovered immediately, and no long-term complications occurred from the accident.

Nurses who work with non-English-speaking clients need to develop other ways to measure how much a client understands rather than depending only on a verbal response. Return demonstrations provide more accurate information and better validation of the client's level of understanding in the absence of a common spoken language.

> *Nurses who work with non-English-speaking clients need to develop other ways to measure how much a client understands rather than depending only on a verbal response.*

The use of silence by some cultural groups has led to misunderstandings in communication in the health-care setting. For example, Asian-Americans consider silence to be a sign of respect, particularly for elders, whereas Arab-Americans and the English use silence to gain privacy. Among many people in Europe (e.g., the French, Russians, and Spanish), silence often indicates agreement.

Variations in communication style also account for misunderstandings and miscommunications. Factors such as loudness, intonation, rhythm, and speed of speech all are important in communication. Among certain cultural groups, American nurses have a reputation for speaking at a rapid rate and for using medical jargon. Some nurses also have a reputation for their tendency to increase the volume of their voices when communicating with clients who do not speak English, as if talking louder will increase understanding. On the other hand, groups such as Native-Americans and Asian-Americans speak more softly and may be difficult to hear even when the nurse is standing at the bedside. These groups may misinterpret the louder, more force-

Box 20–3

Guidelines for Communicating with Non-English-Speaking Clients

1. Use interpreters rather than translators. Translators just restate the words from one language to another. An interpreter decodes the words and provides the meaning behind the message.
2. Use dialect-specific interpreters whenever possible.
3. Use interpreters trained in the health-care field.
4. Give the interpreter time alone with the client.
5. Provide time for translation and interpretation.
6. Be aware that interpreters may affect the reporting of symptoms, insert their own ideas, or omit information.
7. Avoid the use of relatives who may distort information or not be objective.
8. Avoid using children as interpreters, especially with sensitive topics.
9. Use same-age and same-gender interpreters whenever possible. However, clients from cultures who have a high regard for the elderly may prefer an older interpreter.
10. Maintain eye contact with both the client and the interpreter to elicit feedback and read nonverbal clues.
11. Remember that clients can usually understand more than they express; thus, they need time to think in their own language. They are alert to the health-care provider's body language, and they may forget some or all of their English in times of stress.
12. Speak slowly without exaggerated mouthing, allow time for translation, use active rather than passive tense, wait for feedback, and restate the message. Do not rush; do not speak loudly. Use a reference book with common phrases, such as *Roget's International Thesaurus* or *Taber's Cyclopedic Medical Dictionary.*
13. Use as many words as possible in the client's language and nonverbal communication when unable to understand the language.
14. If an interpreter is unavailable, the use of a translator may be acceptable. The difficulty with translation is omission of parts of the message, distortion of the message, including transmission of information not given by the speaker, and messages not being fully understood.
15. Note that social class differences between the interpreter and the client may result in the interpreter's not reporting information that he or she perceives as superstitious or unimportant.

Source: Purnell, LD, and Paulanka, BJ: Transcultural Health Care. FA Davis, Philadelphia, 1998, pp. 16–17, with permission.

ful voice tone of the American nurse as an indication of anger. Arab-American groups are often noted for their dramatic communication styles. Nurses may misinterpret this behavior as hostility, when in reality they are merely trying to demonstrate a point using an emotional communication style. Nurses need to analyze their own speech patterns and consciously modify their tone and pace when working with different cultural groups to prevent misunderstandings.

Nurses also need to recognize that certain groups are much less willing to disclose private matters or personal feelings than others. In general, clients from American or European origins tend to be less secretive about almost all issues, because the practice of sharing has been encouraged from an early age. However, many Asian cultures, particularly the Japanese, are highly reluctant to discuss personal topics with either family or health-care providers. Other groups, such as Mexican-Americans, discuss personal issues openly with friends and family members but are reluctant to do so with health-care providers who they do not know well. However, even within these groups there are wide variations. American women probably constitute one of the most open groups when it comes to expressing personal feelings, whereas American men tend to have much more difficulty with this type of communication.

Nurses presume that all clients should trust them instantaneously just because they are nurses and should answer even the most personal questions immediately. As discussed earlier, it may be much more productive to start the communication process with small talk and general, nonthreatening questions to establish an atmosphere of trust. Often the use of open-ended questions and statements allows the client to express beliefs and opinions that would be difficult to discover through closed-end questions that the client can answer with a simple "yes" or "no." As the level of trust increases, the client will be more likely to reveal important information in the more sensitive areas of the assessment. In addition, sensitivity to the nonverbal aspects of the communication process allows nurses to use behaviors that increase trust and avoid gestures, facial expressions, or eye contact that may relay a message of superiority, hostility, anger, or disapproval.

The inappropriate touching of clients from different cultures is a leading cause of miscommunication. American nurses are taught early on in their first nursing classes, usually physical assessment or basic skill courses, that it is necessary to "lay on hands" in order to provide good care. Students who are reluctant to palpate the femoral pulses of their laboratory partner or remove a client's shirt to auscultate anterior heart and breath sounds may receive a failing grade for the course.

However, touching in other cultures conveys a number of alternative meanings, ranging from power, anger, and sexual arousal to affirmation, empathy, and cordiality. For example, it is generally not acceptable for men and women to touch in many Arab cultures, except in the privacy of the home and in the context of marriage. American female nurses who palpate pulses, listen to breath sounds, or palpate for tactile fremitus when assessing men from an Arab culture may be communicating a message that they never intended. Some groups, such as Mexican-Americans or Italian-Americans, who frequently touch and hug family members and friends, are much less receptive to touching by strangers during health-care examinations, particularly if the health-care provider is of the opposite sex. In these situations, it would be extremely important for the nurse to explain what he or she is going to do and why it is important before the particular physical contact occurs. The nurse should also avoid any unnecessary contact, such as palpation of femoral pulses when the client has pneumonia.

Closely related to the issue of touch is the concept of personal space. Personal space is a zone that individuals maintain around themselves in most casual social situations. When a person's personal space is violated, it often creates a generalized feeling of discomfort or threat, which causes the person to move away from the offending individual. Nurses routinely violate clients' personal space when performing physical assessments or providing basic care.

The actual distance required to maintain a comfortable personal space varies widely from one culture to another. People who belong to the European, Canadian, or American cultures usually require between 18 and 22 inches of distance for a comfortable personal space when communicating with strangers or casual acquaintances. In contrast, individuals from the Jewish,

Arab, Turkish, and Middle-Eastern cultures may require as little as 3 to 5 inches of personal space when talking with another person and often interpret physical closeness as a sign of acceptance. In addition, they prefer to stand face to face and maintain eye contact when they are talking. It is easy to understand why misinterpretations in communication might arise. A client from a Middle-Eastern culture might judge an American nurse to be cold and aloof, although she is merely maintaining a comfortable personal space from the client. Likewise, an American nurse may feel physically threatened by the close communication style of a Turkish-American client and find himself or herself continually backing away from the client in an attempt to re-establish his or her personal space.

Similarly, eye contact communicates different messages to different cultures. Among American and many European cultures, making periodic eye contact during conversations indicates that the person is attentive to the communication as well as acting as a means of measuring the person's sincerity. Common sayings such as, "Look me in the eye and say that," or admonitions for public speakers to "make eye contact" with the audience emphasize the underlying positive value these cultures place on eye contact. Lack of eye contact may be interpreted as inattention, insincerity, or disregard.

In contrast, some Native-American cultures believe that the eyes are the windows of the soul and that direct eye contact by another may be interpreted as an attempt to "steal the soul" from the body. Between Native-American men, direct eye contact is a sign of challenge and aggression and may precipitate a violent, physical confrontation. Among some South-American cultures, sustained eye contact is a sign of disrespect, whereas in other cultural groups, particularly Mexican-Americans, eye contact with a child is believed to convey the *mal de ojo*, or "evil eye." Many childhood and adult illnesses among these cultures are attributed to the effects of the evil eye, and practices such as tying red cloths or strings around the children's wrists are used to ward off the illnesses. Eye contact, a routine part of America culture, has diverse and powerful meanings to clients from other cultures.

The complexity and importance of communication should never be underestimated when working with clients from diverse cultures. Merely speaking a language does not encompass the entirety of communication. Awareness of the meanings of gestures, body positions, facial expressions, and eye movements is essential in culturally competent communications.

Looking Deeper

There are several other elements to be considered for effective transcultural nursing, including passive obedience, cultural synergy, building on similarities, and conflict resolution. The term *passive obedience* refers to a type of behavior that develops when clients from a different culture believe that the nurse is an authority figure or expert in health-care matters. Although many cultures may display this type of behavior to some extent, it is most commonly seen among Asian-American groups. These cultures try to cope with the uncertainty of their health status and the threat of an authority figure by becoming passively obedient. Rather than asking questions that they think will reveal their lack of knowledge or confusion about some health-care issue or that they believe may challenge the authority of the nurse, they become passively obedient and compliant.

Cultural Conflicts

It is inevitable that conflicts will arise from time to time when caring for clients of different cultures.

What Do You Think?

Think of the last client for whom you've provided care. What were the cultural differences that affected the care you gave? What measures did you use to overcome these? What might you have done differently to improve care?

It is important to recognize that the origins of many conflicts reside within the individual. Nurses may label clients from other cultures as noncompliant, when in reality the nurse has an incomplete understanding of the client's culture or unrealistic expectations for behavior.

Other common reasons for noncompliance among culturally diverse clients include the lack of external symptoms of disease, inconvenient or painful treatments, and lack of external support from family members or close friends. As discussed earlier, the nurse first needs to ask the client what traditional treatments are used in dealing with this disease. In some cases, where the traditional treatments are similar to the ones used by the health-care facility, the nurse may be able to demonstrate to the client that they are really very similar. In other cases, the treatments may be very different. However, if the traditional treatment does not disrupt the facility's treatment plan or threaten the client's health, they can be used simultaneously with the standard medical treatments. Nurses who work in the Native-American health-care system and hospitals have become accustomed to finding bone fragments, feathers, and leather medicine pouches in the beds of their clients.

> *Being on the front lines of health care, nursing is the one profession that is continually confronted with cultural changes that result from ethnic shifts in population.*

Cultural Synergy

Nurses who work actively to develop cultural synergy tend to be more successful in the delivery of competent transcultural care. *Cultural synergy* is a term that implies that health-care providers make a commitment not only to learn about other cultures but also to immerse themselves in those cultures. Nurses achieve cultural synergy when they begin to selectively include values, customs, and beliefs of other cultures into their own worldviews. The first step in cultural synergy is the desire to know everything there is about another culture and to purposely establish relationships with individuals from other cultures.

Closely related to cultural synergy is the recognition that cultures are really very much alike in many aspects. It would seem that most books and publications written about cultural diversity present only the diversity of cultures and not the similarities. Although recognition of cultural differences is important, it should be just one step toward the ultimate realization that there are more similarities than differences among cultures. Many colleges offer courses in comparative religions that identify the many similarities of the fundamental beliefs that underlie the major religions. However, many college courses on cultural diversity have not evolved past the point of identifying cultural differences. Perhaps this is due in part to the "salad bowl" approach to cultural communication that exists in current society. It would almost appear that a new approach to acculturation, based on similarities between cultures rather than on the differences, needs to be developed.

Information Sources for Transcultural Nursing

The recent explosion of interest in cultural diversity and transcultural nursing has led to a proliferation of literature on the topic. The origins of the current transcultural movement can be traced back to 1974, when a transcultural conference on communication and culture was held at the University of Hawaii School of Nursing. Following the success of this conference, a series of transcultural conferences were planned over the next year to bring together nurses, sociologists, anthropologists, and other social scientists to discuss issues that would eventually form the basis for transcultural nursing. Not long after this conference, the Transcultural Nursing Society was organized. It was incorporated in 1981 and began publishing its semiannual official journal, *Journal of Transcultural Nursing*, in 1989. It is now being published four times a year. In 1976, the American Nurses Association (ANA) recommended that multicultural content be included in nursing curricula. Since then, the ANA has organized the Council on Intercultural Nursing, which publishes the *Intercultural Nursing Newsletter*.

Since the 1980s, more and more universities and colleges have started offering graduate degrees in transcultural, cross-cultural, and international nursing. Graduates are now able to become certified transcultural nurses (CTNs) by completing oral and written examinations offered by the Transcultural Nursing Society. Nurses do not need to be from minority groups to obtain the CTN.

Society has not remained stagnant during this period of development and organization. Growing numbers of immigrants, changing governmental regulations, and grassroots movements all have contributed to the pressure placed on nursing to recognize and effectively care for clients from different cultures.

Conclusion

The major changes in U.S. demographics that began in the 1980s—and are accelerating as we enter the twenty-first century—require nurses to provide culturally sensitive care. Based on the fundamental belief of professional nursing that all individuals are to be cared for with respect and dignity regardless of culture, beliefs, or disease process, nurses must actively seek multicultural education. However, nurses need to keep in mind that cultural assessments and decisions about care are relative to the nurse's personal experiences, beliefs, and culture. There is a natural tendency to stereotype individuals from other cultures unconsciously on the basis of one's internal value system. There is also a tendency to batch all individuals from one culture into a single group, when in reality, there may be wide variations within the group.

It is a well-accepted belief that nurses who value cultural diversity will deliver higher quality care. Nurses who have a high level of cultural knowledge and sensitivity maximize their nursing interventions when they become coparticipants and client advocates for individuals who might otherwise be lost in an impersonal health-care system. Only when nurses can understand the client's perspective, develop an open style of communication, become receptive to learning from clients of other cultures, and accept and work with the ambiguities inherent in the care of multicultural clients will they become truly culturally competent health-care providers.

ISSUES IN PRACTICE

Consider the following case study:

In 1990, Jose Bisigan, aged 87 years, and his wife Carmen, aged 85, sold their small restaurant and immigrated to Los Angeles from a small town in the Visayan region of the Philippines. They came to join their first-born daughter, nurse Felicia, aged 54, her husband, and their three children aged 10 to 18. Mr. Bisigan speaks limited English and is in a poststroke rehabilitation unit. Since the stroke, he has had mild aphasia, mild confusion, and bladder and bowel continence problems. His hypertension and long-standing diabetes are controlled with medication and diet. His wife, daughter, and grandchildren have been supportive of him during this first hospitalization experience. Mr. Bisigan's family has cooperated with the health team, often agreeing with minimal resistance to the prescribed treatment management. The rehabilitation team recommended subacute rehabilitation treatment as part of the discharge plan.

As a businessman and the elder in the family household, Mr. Bisigan is looked to for counsel by the immediate and extended family. Mr. Bisigan's status, however, has caused friction between Felicia and her husband, Nestor, an American-born Filipino who works as a machinist. Nestor has accused Felicia of giving excessive attention to her mother and father. Felicia's worries about her parents' health have made Nestor very resentful. He increased his already daily "outings with the boys." Felicia maintains a full-time position in acute care and a part-time night shift position in a nursing home.

Mr. Bisigan's discharge is pending, and a decision must be made before Medicare coverage runs out. Felicia has to consider the possible choices available to her father and the family's circumstances and expectations. Mrs. Bisigan, who is being treated for hypertension, has always deferred decisions to her husband and is looking to Felicia to make the decisions. Because of her work schedule, the absence of a responsible person at home, her mother's health problems, and intergenerational friction, Felicia considers nursing home placement. She is, however, reluctant to broach the subject with her father, who expects to be cared for at home. Mrs. Bisigan disagrees with putting her husband in a nursing home and is adamant that she will care for her husband at home.

Felicia delayed talking to her father until the rehabilitation team requested a meeting. At the meeting, Felicia indicated that she could not bring herself to present her plan to put her father in a nursing home because of her mother's objection and her own fear that her father will feel rejected. Feeling very much alone in resolving the issue about nursing home placement, she requested the team to act as intermediary for her and her family.

- Identify cultural family values that contribute to the conflicts experienced by each family member.

- Identify a culturally competent approach that the team can use when discussing nursing home placement with the Bisigans.
- How might the rehabilitation program be presented to Mrs. Bisigan and still allow her to maintain her spousal role?
- Discuss at least three communication issues in the family that are culture-bound, and suggest possible interventions.
- Identify psychocultural assessments that should be done by the rehabilitation team to have a greater understanding of the dynamics specific to this family.
- Identify health promotion counseling that might be discussed with the Bisigans' grandchildren.
- Identify and explain major sources of stress for each member of this household.

Source: Purnell, LD, and Paulanka, BJ: Transcultural Health Care. FA Davis, Philadelphia, 1998, pp.269–270, with permission.

Bibliography

Brown, G: Culture and diversity in the nursing classroom: An impact on communication and learning. Journal of Cultural Diversity 8(1):16–20, 2001.

Child, R, et al: Managing diversity in the environment of care. Seminars for Nurse Managers 9(2):102–109, 2001.

DeSantis, L: Health-culture reorientation of registered nurse students. Journal of Transcultural Nursing 12(4):310–318, 2001.

Duffy, ME: A critique of cultural education in nursing. J Adv Nurs 36(4):487–495, 2001.

Esler, RO, and Nipp, DA: Worker designed culture change. Nursing Economics 19(4):161–163, 2001.

Lawrence, P, and Rozmus, C: Culturally sensitive care of the Muslim patient. Journal of Transcultural Nursing 12(3):228–233, 2001.

Marquand, B: Flying with the eagles. Minority Nurse 1(1):29–31, Spring 2002.

Nishimoto, PW, and Foley, J: Cultural beliefs of Asian Americans associated with terminal illness and death. Semin Oncol Nurs 17(3):179–189, 2001.

Orb, A, and Wynaden, D: Cross-cultural communication in heath care practices. Australian Journal of Holistic Nursing 8(2):31–38, 2001.

Purnell, LD, and Paulanka, BJ: Transcultural Health Care. FA Davis, Philadelphia, 1998.

21

Forensic Nursing: A Speciality for the Twenty-first Century

Anita G. Hufft and Cindy Peternelj-Taylor

Learning Objectives

After completing this chapter, the reader will be able to:

- Define forensic nursing.
- Discuss specialties in forensic nursing practice.
- Describe settings in which forensic nurses practice.
- Describe the populations for whom forensic nurses provide care.
- Identify resources for education and practice in forensic nursing.

Forensic nursing is an evolving specialty that has emerged as a dynamic and influential factor in the health care of individuals and communities. As society becomes more concerned about violence in its many forms, including acts of terrorism, and its impact on daily life, it becomes more likely that the health-care system will interface with the criminal justice system. With their orientation to holistic and comprehensive client care, their keen clinical skills, and an ability to collaborate with others, **forensic nurses** are ideally situated to provide quality care to both victims and perpetrators of crime. Trends in nursing education and nursing practice indicate that increased specialization and differentiation of practice will dominate career opportunities.

Definition of Forensic Nursing

Forensic nursing is still in an ongoing state of development. The American definition of this specialty is somewhat different from the definition found in the British literature. In order to provide for the broadest interpretation, a working definition of forensic nursing that bridges these two perspectives is presented.

Forensic nursing, which was first introduced in the United States as a term in 1991, was identified within the scope of four distinct nursing roles:

1. Clinical forensic nurse
2. Sexual assault nurse examiner
3. Forensic psychiatric nurse
4. Correctional/institutional nurse

A more succinct definition of forensic nursing is used in Great Britain. Based on an understanding of forensic psychiatry, forensic nursing is understood as nursing management of any client behavior that "links psychiatric symptomatology and offending behavior." Another related, but distinct definition of the forensic nurse states: "One who practices in a facility or program where the primary mission is the evaluation or treatment of mentally ill offenders."[1]

> *Forensic nursing is an evolving specialty that has emerged as a dynamic and influential factor in the health care of individuals and communities.*

> *Environments in which forensic nursing can be applied include secured settings, such as locked hospital units, jails, or correctional institutions.*

The American Nurses Association (ANA) recognized forensic nursing as a specialty in 1995 and further defined forensic nursing as the "application of forensic science combined with the biopsychosocial education of the registered nurse, in the scientific investigation, evidence collection and preservation, analysis, prevention and treatment of trauma, and/or death related to medical-legal issues."[2]

Although there are different classifications of nursing specialties within forensic nursing in the United States and abroad, the clarification of the role is dependent not only on what the nurse does (role expectations) but also on where the nurse works (role setting). The British approach emphasizes nursing relationships with perpetrators of crime, whereas the American approach emphasizes nursing relationships with the victims of crimes.

For the purposes of this discussion, forensic nursing is defined as a nursing specialty practice that integrates nursing science and forensic science to apply the nursing process to the health and well-being of individual clients, their families, and communities to help bridge the gap between the health-care system and the criminal justice system. This definition builds on the paradigm that emphasizes the "expanded role of the nurse in meeting the needs of victims and perpetrators of violent crime through enhanced quality of care and preventive services. Implementation of these roles occurs in many settings" (Box 21–1).

In order to make nurses visible and recognized for their contributions, any definition of forensic nursing should emphasize the uniqueness of nursing and clearly promote the idea that nurses do something different than other health-care providers or other members of a forensic team. The widest scope of practice within the forensic nursing specialty should be considered when defining forensic nursing. This consideration allows for the broadest possible application of forensic nursing knowledge in many settings and with as many populations as possible.

Forensic Nursing Knowledge

Nursing practice traditionally has been referred to as an art and a science. The knowledge that guides nursing actions is grounded in humanities, biology, physical sciences, and everyday experience. Nurses use knowledge from all these areas to understand human systems and the environments in which they practice.

Nursing science explains the relationships between the domain concepts of nursing: human

Box 21–1

Settings for Forensic Nursing Practice

Individuals practice forensic nursing in many settings, both in and out of formal institutions such as hospitals and correctional facilities. They work with both victims and perpetrators of crime and may focus their practice in various ways, including:

- Physical injury and violence
- Mental illness
- Dysfunctional family systems
- Community health promotion and accident prevention
- Policy making

Such a wide variety of clinical applications make forensic nursing an exciting opportunity for both new and experienced nurses.

systems, environment, and health. It is widely accepted that the scientific knowledge base of forensic nursing is derived from **forensic science**, criminal justice, police science, and legal studies. Forensic nursing uses forensic science as the context for nursing, incorporating knowledge of defining people and groups, understanding forensic communities and forensic environments, and identifying nursing therapeutics that differentiate forensic practice from other kinds of nursing. For example, people can be categorized as either victims or perpetrators of crime. Knowledge of theories that explain the behavior of victims and criminals is important information for the nurse. Environments in which forensic nursing can be applied include **secured settings**, such as locked hospital units, jails, or correctional institutions. Environments also include secured or special settings such as a medical examiner's office, a crime scene, or a shelter for women. Still other nurses may practice forensic nursing in emergency rooms or schools, adapting their nursing interventions to assess potential for violence or self-harm. The way in which nurses dispose of a contaminated dressing, how they touch a client, and how they set goals with a client can all be affected by whether or not the client is a victim of a crime or violence or an initiator of crime or violence. These are a few examples of how forensic nursing is different from other types of nursing and how knowledge of forensic nursing concepts can be valuable for any nurse. Forensic science is relevant to contemporary nursing, ensuring that clinicians are prepared to identify and report victims of crime, collect and preserve forensic evidence, evaluate issues of competence, and protect the rights and health of victims and perpetrators of crime.

Concepts Relevant to Forensic Nursing

Professional nursing practice is based, in part, on the use of theoretical knowledge and concepts in making decisions about client care. There are essential concepts that must be understood by nurses working in forensic settings and in forensic roles. The concepts of **victimization**, violence, manipulation, custody, and human rights serve to clarify the nursing profession's understanding of the client and his or her environment, to better guide the selection of therapeutic interventions, and to give meaning to nursing interactions with the client.

What Do You Think?

Do you know any nurses who are involved in forensic nursing? Is this a role that you might be interested in pursuing after graduation?

Box 21–2

Crime Victim's Bill of Rights

The right to be treated with fairness and with respect for the victim's dignity and privacy.
The right to be reasonably protected from the accused offender.
The right to be notified of court proceedings.
The right to be present at all public court proceedings related to the offense, unless the court determines that testimony by the victim would be materially affected if the victim hears other testimony at trial.
The right to confer with an attorney for the government in the case.
The right to restitution.
The right to information about the conviction, sentencing, imprisonment, and release of the offender.

Source: Evans, AM, and Wells, D: Scope of practice issues in forensic nursing. Psychosoc Nurs Ment Health Serv 39(1):38–45, 2001.

Victimization

In the 1970s, when the victim rights movement began, its primary goals were to help victims recover from the emotional trauma and physical injuries resulting from crime. Another goal included prevention of secondary victimization by ensuring that the criminal justice, health, and social services systems treat victims with dignity, respect, and compassion. Although significant advances in the care of victims has taken place in the since then, the belief that violence and victimization are caused only by criminals has proved to limit strategies for prevention of secondary victimization from the system. The current trend is to treat violence as a major criminal justice and health problem. Public health concepts have been used to provide a health-oriented model for understanding victims, treating victims, and preventing victimization. This approach focuses on public education, controlling the spread of violence (and the victim self-concept), and early detection of victimization.

Treatment of victims of violence and violence itself as a health issue, in addition to a criminal justice issue, opens the door to more health-care intervention. Early intervention and treatment by the health-care system, combined with criminal justice efforts, have the potential to decrease the experience of victimization. In response to the significance of this issue, a victim's bill of rights was developed (Box 21–2).

Violence

As a major example of antisocial behavior, violence is a concept integral to the understanding of forensic nursing. Although the mass violence of terrorism is very dramatic and has grabbed the imagination of the country, family violence (including abuse of children, spouses, and the elderly) is much more common, affects many more people, and represents a long-standing concern of health-care professionals. The American Medical Association (AMA) has linked violence in the family with the escalation of violence in the world at large.

Nurses use their knowledge of violence in the application of specific skills and interventions such as (1) increased awareness of family violence as a public health problem, (2) recognition of the risk factors and symptoms of abuse and neglect, (3) use of therapeutic communication techniques to ask questions nonjudgmentally, and (4) treatment and referral of clients for shelter and services when needed. The AMA has published guidelines for the diagnosis and treatment of abuse and neglect. Basic nursing diagnosis and care planning books contain chapters devoted to interventions with clients who are victims of abuse. Forensic nurses need to keep abreast of current research, which includes studies of the development of individual violent behavior, the effect of testosterone on aggression on children, the father's role in child/adolescent development and delinquency, effects of neighborhood characteristics on drug use and sales, peer social networks, and the relationship of child care arrangements to delinquency.

Manipulation

Manipulation is not necessarily a maladaptive or antisocial behavior. Its value is dependent on the context in which it occurs and the goals that are being achieved. Negative use of manipulation is a common characteristic of victims and perpetrators of crime, who often resort to maladaptive behaviors in order to have their needs met. For example, an inmate may tell prison authorities secrets or privately inform them of everyday illnesses to get special favors, such as release from work detail.

Providing health care in an environment where health-care delivery is not the primary goal leads to many complex challenges for the forensic nurse.

The following are characteristics of destructive or antisocial manipulation:

- It is the primary method used to have needs fulfilled.
- The needs and feelings of others are disregarded.
- People are treated as objects and dehumanized in order to fulfill the needs of the manipulator.

As one of the identifying characteristics of personality disorders, including sociopathic behavior, manipulation is also associated with maladaptive behavior patterns involving impulsiveness, aggression, and detachment. These behaviors are characteristics that define actions and relationships among both perpetrators and victims. Forensic nursing applications focus on the assessment of these characteristics and the assignment of meaning within the framework of criminal activity in which they occur.

Custody

Confinement of individuals who are accused of breaking the law or convicted of a crime involves sanctions that are unique, and these, in turn, influence nursing. These settings are referred to as "total institutions" and are characterized by their control over all aspects of an individual's life and daily routine, as is seen in the regimentation of scheduled activities and sequencing of events, the relinquishment of individual identity among those in custody, and the fact that the primary concern of all procedures and policies centers on what is best for the institution rather than the individual inmate. These characteristics are common to mental hospitals, prisons, and forensic psychiatric facilities.

Providing health care in an environment where health-care delivery is not the primary goal leads to many complex challenges for the forensic nurse. The priorities of the correctional system are built on confinement and security. As a result, nurses in this setting commonly face basic value conflicts, because the principles of security are often at odds with the principle of treatment. For example, if a prison has sick call only at 6:00 A.M., and an inmate becomes ill at 2:00 P.M., the inmate must wait until the following morning to obtain treatment. Unless the sickness is life-threatening, prison officials do not want to risk a lapse in security by altering the normal routine. Forensic nurses working with incarcerated perpetrators often struggle to find the balance between the security limitations of the institution and the health-care needs of the prison population. This contradiction, known as "custody and caring," can be immobilizing to nurses, who frequently find themselves caught between the proverbial "rock and a hard place." In other words, no matter how therapeutic a specific health-care program a nurse develops, a correctional institution will consistently sacrifice individual health needs to institutional needs.

Clinical forensic nursing is the management of crime victims from trauma to trial.

Human Rights

The basic human rights that are taken for granted in most nursing environments become an important issue of nurse advocacy in forensic nursing. There is little debate in the general health-care settings over the individual's right to self-determination, protection from discomfort and harm, maintenance of dignity, fair treatment, and respect for privacy. However, when viewed against the backdrop of the criminal justice system, these rights become controversial and complex issues. Take, for example, the case of the rape victim who wants to remain anonymous. She may fear the shame and retaliation if her identity is made public. The district attorney believes that public exposure of such cases will help destigmatize rape, encourage other women to testify, and increase the successful conviction of rapists, ultimately leading to a decrease of violence in society. When seen within a forensic context, the right of the individual rape victim to privacy comes into conflict with the right of society to be free from harm. Also, the issue of long-term best interests of the victim must be taken into consideration. Although public exposure of the rape victim may lead to immediate distress and possibly to further victimization, it may also increase the likelihood of successful resolution of the trauma through public dialogue and psychological processing of the event. The duty to do good for the client (beneficence) comes into conflict with the duty to protect from harm and to advocate for the patient's right to self-determination.

What Do You Think?

Have you or someone close to you ever been a victim of a crime? How did you deal with the experience? What experience did you have with the health-care and legal systems?

Forensic Nursing Specialties

Clinical Forensic Nursing Specialty

Clinical forensic nursing is the management of crime victims from trauma to trial. Nurses working in clinical forensics collect evidence through assessment of living victims, survivors of traumatic injury, or those whose death is pronounced in the clinical environment. Clinical forensic nursing involves making judgments related to client treatment associated with court-related issues. The **clinical forensic nurse** assesses victims of child and elder abuse and domestic violence. Forensic nurses are asked to differentiate between conditions that simulate accidental injury and those that are purposefully inflicted. An essential skill required by the forensic nurse is the ability to assess patterned injury by identifying marks such as defense wounds, grab marks, and fingernail marks. Clinical forensic nurses focus on observation of the communication and interaction patterns of suspected abuse victims and perpetrators. Many nurses come to forensic nursing from acute care settings of emergency room nursing, critical care nursing, and perioperative nursing.

In the coroner's office, death notification entails stabilization of the family situation and grief support, skills that are basic to nursing practice. Expert skills in physical assessment, clinical history taking and interviewing, and use of technology have helped advance this nursing role.

Because of their awareness of the effects of violence in society and their ability to assess situations in which potential for violence exists, clinical forensic nurses are often called upon for consultation. By identifying risk factors and cues for violence in health-care and workplace settings, these nurses can assist in the development of strategies, policies, and protocols to manage risk and reduce violence and injury. They will also assist in the debriefing or resolution of violent events in a workplace or community.

The **sexual assault nurse examiner (SANE)** is a registered nurse who has received specialized training to provide care to the sexual assault victim.[3] The SANE performs physical and psychosocial examination and collection of physical evidence, therapeutic interactions to minimize the trauma and initiate healing, coordination of referral and collaboration with community-based agencies involved in the rehabilitation of victims, and the judicial processing of sexual assault. The first programs training SANEs were developed in the United States in the late 1970s. The movement for national certification of SANE nurses continues to grow.

Forensic Psychiatric Nursing Specialty

Forensic psychiatric nurses integrate psychiatric/mental health nursing philosophy and practice with knowledge of the criminal justice system and assessment of the sociocultural influences on the individual client, the family, and the community to provide comprehensive psychiatric and mental health nursing. Forensic psychiatric nurses work with mentally ill offenders and with victims of crime. They help victims cope with their emotional wounds and assist in the assessment and care of perpetrators. They focus on identification and change of behaviors linking criminal offenses or reactions to them. These nurses assist perpetrators and victims of crime in dealing with the courts and other aspects of the criminal justice system, minimizing further victimization and promoting functional abilities.

Functional applications of forensic psychiatric nursing include assessment of inmates for mental and physical fitness, criminal responsibility, disposition, and early release. Forensic psychiatric nurses also provide mental health treatment for convicted offenders and those who are not found criminally responsible. In the criminal justice system, forensic psychiatric nurses deal with destructive, aggressive, and socially unacceptable behavior. These nurses provide interventions that encourage individuals to exercise self-control, foster individual change in behavior, and, in the process, protect other members of society and property.

There has been an increase in the involvement of forensic psychiatric nurses (especially those prepared for advanced practice) in the assessment and treatment of forensic psychiatric clients.

There has been an increase in the involvement of forensic psychiatric nurses (especially those prepared for advanced practice) in the assessment and treatment of forensic psychiatric clients. These practitioners are involved in the development and refining of clinical roles in forensic psychiatric nursing and are in a position to promote intervention strategies that increase the likelihood of rehabilitation and reintegration of the forensic client into society.

Correctional/Institutional Nursing Specialty

Correctional/institutional nurses work in secure settings, providing treatment, rehabilitation, and health promotion to clients who have been charged with or convicted of crimes. Settings include jails, state and federal prisons, and halfway houses. Before the 1960s, nurses in general gave little thought to working in the correctional system, even though jails and correctional facilities have always been a part of the community at large. There is a growing awareness of the potential for the correctional population as a target of successful health interventions. Some nurses have created private practices or consultation services in which they identify the health needs and arrange for the care of people detained in custody. This service is provided separate from acute care, which is located in a secured hospital or infirmary section of the institution. Such services are just emerging as health-care alternatives and will serve as the model from which community-based care, aimed at decreasing recidivism among those incarcerated, will develop. To guide professional nursing practice, the ANA first published Standards for Nursing Practice in Correctional Facilities in 1985; these standards were revised and updated in 1995 and 2001.[4]

In addition to the specialties of forensic nursing noted earlier, nurses are continuing to develop roles based on the integration of forensic knowledge into nursing practice (Box 21–3).

Box 21–3

Subspecialties of Clinical Practice Identified by the International Association of Forensic Nurses

- Forensic nurse educators/consultants
- Nurse coroners
- Death investigators
- Legal nurse consultants
- Nurse attorneys
- Clinical nurse specialists and those specializing in trauma
- Transplant and critical care nurses
- Forensic pediatric nurses
- Forensic gerontology nurses

Nurses in General Practice

In addition to nurses in specialty practice, nurses in general practice find forensic nursing knowledge of growing importance. Forensic applications in the acute care setting emphasize the use of forensic knowledge and awareness of criminal justice implications for the assessment, documentation of care, and reporting of information to police or other law enforcement agencies. Nurses who work in emergency rooms and in critical care units are often in positions to preserve evidence of what might be a criminal offense. Victims of automobile accidents or apparent accidental overdoses are not always what they appear to be. Knowledge of what to look for and how to collect evidence, in addition to knowing whom to call and when, can be valuable in finding out what really happened in such cases. Clients often come into acute care settings with what is first thought to be an injury that is the result of an accident. However, preservation of evidence such as stomach contents, clothing residue, or marks on the skin surface can provide a very different picture—one of injury caused by a self-inflicted wound or violence perpetrated by another person.

Clinical Applications

There are distinct advantages of using a sexual assault nurse examiner to care for victims of rape. Sexual assault victims are usually seen in a busy emergency room, and they are often not at the top of the triage list, where life-threatening cases are traditionally taken first. The wait for the rape victim can be agonizing. The victim has a long time to think about the rape, fear the worst, and worry about the pain and humiliation from the physical examination. The victim may feel alone and abandoned at a very stressful time in her life. Nurses are trained to listen, observe, support, and take care of the client. When the SANE intervenes, a multidisciplinary approach is used. The police officer is responsible for interviewing the victim about the sexual attack, whereas the nurse focuses on the forensic examination, collection of evidence with the use of a rape kit, and noting the presence of any injuries with written and photographic documentation.

Comprehensive nursing care includes an evaluation of immediate trauma as well as a referral to a rape crisis center, individual therapist, follow-up medical care, or other community health resources. In one case, the SANE noticed the presence of a dry, shiny substance on the victim's cheek. She sent a swab of the substance to the crime laboratory along with clothes and other body tissue evidence. None of the other evidence linked the victim to a perpetrator. However, the cheek swab did establish a DNA link to the accused rapist and was an important factor in the conviction of the assailant. The benefits of a community-based SANE team approach to sexual assault includes state-of-the-art evidence collection, compassionate care of victims, increased confidence among police and district attorneys that evidence collected is credible, and an increased likelihood that the process will yield convictions in court.

> *Sexual assault victims are usually seen in a busy emergency room, and they are often not at the top of the triage list, where life-threatening cases are traditionally taken first.*

Environments for Practice

The practice of forensic nursing can take place in several settings. The clinical forensic nurse may work in organizational settings under the control of local or state government, usually the office of the **coroner** or **medical examiner**. Similar to the emergence of nurse practitioners in the 1960s, the development of the role of nurse medical examiner appears to be related to the shortage of forensic pathologists. Nurses are adept at mastering the clinical skills required to assist in the investigation of death and violence. The need for forensic pathologists will continue to increase well into the future, reflecting the increased violence in society.

Clinical Forensic Nursing Settings

Clinical forensic nurses work in the laboratory, in the examination office, in the **autopsy** room, and in the field at crime scenes. Roles include field investigation, autopsy assistant, family liaison, and custodian of evidence. When investigating a death scene, the clinical forensic nurse interviews witnesses, takes charge of the body, examines the body, photographs the body, secures physical evidence, arranges body transport, and gathers records. When working with living victims, the tasks are similar, but they focus on injury assessment and the collection of evidence.

The coroner is usually in charge of death investigation. Nurses working in this capacity initiate or assist with death investigation under selected circumstances of homicide, violence, suicide, and suspicious circumstances that would indicate a violation of criminal law (e.g., the presence of illegal drugs, body found in water, fire, explosion).

Correctional Care Settings

Custody settings include jails, state and federal prisons, halfway houses, and other settings in which the individual who is accused of a crime or sentenced for a crime is held in confinement. In some states, private companies have been given contracts to manage either the entire secure setting or the health-care delivery system used by that setting. Prior to the 1970s, there was little in the way of systematic or planned health care for inmates of secured settings. Since the 1970s, the criminal justice system and the health-care system have worked both independently and in collaboration to develop systems of health care for those in custody.

Whatever the custody setting, the nurse is responsible for identifying and performing a role that is consistent with professional standards and state law in which he or she is licensed. Many health-care facilities in secure settings choose to be accredited, subjecting themselves to scrutiny of an outside agency that verifies the quality of the health care delivered in that setting. Most certified correctional health-care facilities in the United States affiliate with the National Commission on Correctional Health Care.

Administrators of correctional institutions find that, aside from overcrowding, the other major issue is providing health services for inmates. Limited resources constitute a persistent concern for health-care delivery in any setting. In correctional settings, the problem is compounded by political influences, legal issues, ethical concerns, special needs of some inmates, and emphasis on security. Nurses working in correctional settings must always frame their care planning within the limitations of the requirements of the institution and the characteristics of those for whom they provide care.

Prison and jail inmates are overwhelmingly from an impoverished environment and disproportionately represent minority groups. In the prison setting, many personal rights are lost, and individuals in confinement are subject to health care that is controlled by the confining agents, whether that is the local, state, or federal government. Inmates do not vote; they essentially have no power and few special interest groups to champion their welfare. In the prison setting, physical touch is discouraged; access to medication and comfort measures is limited; movement is restricted; and even talking is prevented at certain times. Inmates usually harbor strong negative attitudes and deep resentment toward authority figures or anyone identified with the correctional system, including nurses. In order to provide quality nursing care in correctional settings, nurses must excel in both clinical skills and interpersonal competencies (Box 21–4).

Box 21–4

The Skill Set of the Correctional Nurse

The skill set of the correctional nurse includes strategies to break barriers to nurse-client relationships, including mistrust, low self-esteem, chaotic and chronically unhealthy lifestyles, and poor communication abilities that characterize many inmates. Issues such as ethical standards, confidentiality, and informed consent have unique dimensions when considered within the correctional setting. Essential knowledge for the correctional nurse includes:

1. Understanding of the history of health care in corrections
2. Legal issues surrounding the provision of care in prisons
3. Ethical principles, including inmate participation in biomedical research
4. The organizational structure of prison health services
5. Staffing concerns related to custody rules and regulations
6. Inmates with special health needs, such as chronic illness and communicable diseases

Elements of the aforementioned content areas, along with an overview of a model health-care program that meets accreditation standards, should be part of any orientation program for new nurses working in correctional settings.

Education for Forensic Nursing

Nursing education for forensic nursing is developing rapidly in many areas. It is the responsibility of nursing educators to ensure the inclusion of forensic content in basic nursing curricula by teaching the basic skills for routine assessment, identification, treatment, and referral of victims of child, elder, and spouse abuse. Currently, there are growing numbers of schools of nursing that integrate forensic nursing into existing nursing courses, such as family nursing courses, comprehensive health and physical assessment courses, community health courses, and critical care or trauma courses. Elective nursing courses and programs of graduate nursing education in forensic nursing are slowly emerging. There is also an increase in the clinical placement of undergraduate and graduate students in forensic settings. These placements are found in research courses, nursing of adult courses, nurse practitioner courses, and psychosocial nursing courses.

Some hospitals and other health-care institutions are beginning to offer continuing education programs that integrate forensic science and nursing practice. Current programs include a wide range of academic offerings, such as the Utah Crime Scene Academy, the American Association of Legal Nurse Consultants' education program, and the College of Nursing, University of Massachusetts–Boston forensic nursing course. The Mercy College in New York incorporates prison sites into an RN program, as does the Indiana University Southeast baccalaureate program. The University of Virginia offers a forensic nursing major at the graduate level. Forensic nursing education has even come to the Internet via a comprehensive program of offerings from Mount Royal College, Alberta, Canada. Two courses of a seven-course series have already been developed and are currently available.

In general, most programs screen and carefully select students for experiences in a forensic setting (Box 21–5). Students must understand the logistical and behavioral restrictions that are inherent in forensic settings, whether they are in a correctional institution or a medical examiner's office.

What Do You Think?

Does your school offer any courses about forensic nursing? In what courses might this information best be included? Tell your instructors about your idea!

Characteristics of the Forensic Nurse

As with any other nursing specialty, forensic nursing is not for everyone. Who should be a forensic nurse? The same characteristics that predict a successful student learning experience in forensic settings (see Box 21–5) also apply to the practitioner. Social maturity, adaptability, analytical skills, and an optimistic disposition are critical to career management in any stressful setting. The nurse working in forensic settings should feel comfortable working in settings that

Box 21–5

Preferred Characteristics for Students in a Forensic Setting

Characteristics that promote optimal student experiences in forensic settings:

1. Social maturity—Skills interacting with diverse and unfamiliar groups of individuals
2. Objectivity—The ability to think critically, process information analytically, and be nonjudgmental
3. Adaptability—Constructive responsiveness to changing environmental demands
4. Sense of humor—Maintenance of idealism and optimism by not taking things personally and striving to see the positive aspects of situations

demand adherence to strict protocols and many rules. At the same time, the successful nurse will apply nursing knowledge to decisions about client care. Nurses who choose clinical forensic roles often have an acute care or emergency care background and enjoy working in situations that demand technological as well as organizational expertise and interpersonal skills.

Nurses working in custody or correctional settings need well-developed psychosocial assessment skills and must acquire a nonjudgmental attitude toward offenders. Studies have demonstrated that nurses who think of the criminal as someone who deserves respect and professional care, who believe in the ability of offenders to be rehabilitated, and who see their roles as caregivers experience increased work satisfaction, increased work productivity, and increased job longevity. Nurses who dislike working with offenders, see the role of prisons primarily as punishment, and consider their primary role as exerting control over offenders have low levels of job satisfaction with poor productivity and frequent job turnover.

Role conflict has been recognized as a major threat to job satisfaction and a source of stress for nurses working in forensic settings. An active involvement in professional organizations, combined with a well-defined program of career development that decreases isolation and places a strong emphasis on research-based clinical knowledge, reinforces the self-concept and the coping skills of the nurse in forensic practice. Networking with other forensic nurses can diminish the feelings of isolation that forensic nurses sometimes experience and can contribute further to the ongoing professional development of the forensic nurse.

Many opportunities are available for nurses to take an active role in forensic nursing. The practice of forensic nursing intersects with various professional and governmental groups that are traditionally viewed as being outside the domain of nursing, including forensic pathologists, law enforcement agents, and defense attorneys. However, the challenge is for nurses to adhere to the skills and practices that are unique to the nursing profession whenever they interface with the allied fields. Nurses need to cooperate with other disciplines but not be absorbed by them. Territoriality among health professionals can and does exist. As members of the nursing profession, forensic nurses must remain faithful to the principles of professional nursing.

Equipped with strategies to support independent and accountable nursing judgments, and with sensitivity to the roles and needs of others in the work setting, the forensic nurse is ideally situated in a position of power and influence in the criminal justice system. The ability to control aspects of the work environment and to achieve positive outcomes with clients results in increased job satisfaction and constructive, satisfying work relationships.

Applying Forensic Knowledge in General Practice Settings

The following case emphasizes the importance of applying forensic skills to preserve evidence:

> A nurse working in an emergency room cares for a client who eventually succumbs to cardiac arrest. Circumstances surrounding the death are confusing and troublesome to the nurse. The sisters of the deceased seemed unusually angry with the husband, who had refused to bring the sisters in to see the deceased the day before. An empty prescription bottle of medication, the contents of which were found in lethal doses at autopsy, was filled only a couple of days before. Stomach contents, which showed the medication, had been discarded at autopsy and were no longer available for analysis. At first the nurse was uncertain of her responsibility, of what all the circumstances meant, or whether they meant anything at all. By the time she reported the situation to the police, there was not enough evidence to conclude whether the death was an accident, an assisted

suicide, or an outright murder. If the medical examiner could have examined the gastric contents, he would have known how many pills had been ingested at once; however, the evidence was gone. No legal action was ever pursued. All that remained were accusations from the family and the nurse's feeling of frustration.

Conclusion

Forensic nursing is a developing nursing role that consists of two major practice specialties: clinical forensic nursing and correctional nursing. Clinical forensic nursing focuses on the application of forensic science to nursing interventions with victims of crime. Correctional nursing specialty practice involves the evaluation and treatment of those in custody. Forensic nursing takes place in various settings, including, but not limited to, medical examiner and coroner's offices, prisons and jails, and psychiatric facilities. Opportunities for nursing education in forensic nursing and for affiliations in professional organizations dedicated to forensic nursing are essential components of the growth of this role. Rewards for this area of practice include autonomous professional practice, challenges to expand repertoire of nursing skills to nontraditional settings, high demand for skills, diversity of clients and settings, and opportunities to work with peers in other disciplines.

Challenges often faced by the nurse in forensic practice include highly stressful work environments, threats to security and risk of physical violence, and risk of a confusing role with that of medical specialists, security officers, or other professionals. An exciting aspect of forensic nursing practice is involvement in a dynamic nursing specialty as it evolves within many settings. The opportunity to contribute to the increasing body of knowledge known as forensic nursing science provides the potential to make nursing for the twenty-first century relevant and responsive to the needs of society.

ISSUES IN PRACTICE

Application of Human Rights

What information do you need to make a decision? The reader is encouraged to explore applications of human rights from the point of view of the victim and the perpetrator of the crime. Think about how the issue of human rights would be defined and protected in the following examples. What is the nurse's role?

- A married father of two, an upstanding member of the community, is accused of child molestation and is admitted to the unit for psychiatric evaluation and submission of tissue samples.
- A female inmate becomes pregnant in prison and does not want anyone to know who the father is.
- A young man has a history of substance abuse and mental illness. He refuses medication to control psychotic behavior and is confined in a forensic psychiatric facility because of the claim that he is incompetent to stand trial for car theft.
- A mother of an infant is being interviewed in a suspected child abuse case. She admits that she was sexually and physically abused as a child and throughout her marriage. The priority is to establish her role in the current charges involving injury of her 3-month-old infant.

If You Were the Nurse on Duty, What Would You Do?

Below are scenarios that exemplify typical situations for the nurse in general practice. Identify your probable response. Critically analyze each situation in terms of what you know and do not know. What types of facts or skills are not part of your current knowledge base?

You are working on a maternity unit when a woman who is an inmate from a correctional institution is admitted in an advanced stage of labor. A correctional officer is in attendance; the woman is shackled at the feet and hands. As she is wheeled to the labor room, you note that the client has had 10 previous pregnancies and four live births.

- What factors make the care of this woman different from other pregnant women?
- Is she dangerous?
- How do you maintain confidentiality with this client?
- As an offender in custody, does she surrender any rights?

You work in a hospital setting that is experiencing an increase in violence in the workplace. Perpetrators of street, child, and domestic violence often follow their victims to the hospital setting and continue to pose a significant threat to the whole hospital community. It is important to assess the potential for violence.

- How will you contribute to the reduction of risk in the workplace?
- Identify risk factors and cues for violence.
- How would you implement strategies to assist violence management in the acute care setting?

A halfway house for paroled offenders is due to be constructed in your community. Residents are angry and afraid to have ex-convicts living in their neighborhood. A town meeting is scheduled in which the issue will be discussed. Does nursing have anything to contribute to the discussion?

- What do we know about mentally ill offenders, sex offenders, perpetrators of domestic violence, and others?
- What is the therapeutic outcome for those mentally ill offenders who have completed rehabilitation programs?
- What is the risk to the community?
- What stress management strategies are helpful to a community?

You work at a junior high school, providing sex education and health promotion programs for young teenagers. You notice that more and more young people are wearing gang colors and using gang-related language and hand signals.

- How does this affect your work?
- Does this change your priorities?
- Are there referrals or strategies that should be initiated because of the gang affiliations of your students?

References

1. Scales, CJ, et al: Survey report on forensic nursing. J Psychosoc Nurs 31(11):39–44, 1993.
2. International Association of Forensic Nurses and the American Nurses Association: Scope and Standards of Forensic Nursing Practice. American Nurses Association, Washington, DC, 1997.
3. Ledray, LE, et al: Sexual assault: Clinical issues, SANE advocate, forensic technician, nurse? Journal of Emergency Nursing 27(1):91–93, 2001.
4. Peternelj-Taylor, CA: Forensic psychiatric nursing: A work in progress. J Psychosoc Nurs Ment Health Serv 39(9):8–10, 2001.

Bibliography

Byrt, R, et al: Working with women in secure environments. J Psychosoc Nurs Ment Health Serv 39(9):42–50, 2001.

Drew, CS: Pediatric trauma. International Journal of Trauma Nursing 7(2):60–63, 2001.

Evans, AM, and Wells, D: Scope of practice issues in forensic nursing. J Psychosoc Nurs Ment Health Serv 39(1):38–45, 2001.

Faugno, D: Forensic coroner, DNA analysis, and SART programs integral to sexual assault cases. Journal of Legal Nurse Consulting 12(3):22–23, 2001.

Giardin, B: Is this forensic specialty for you? RN 64(12):37–41, 2001.

Maeve, MK, and Vaughn, MS: Nursing with prisoners: The practice of caring, forensic nursing or penal harm nursing? ANS Adv Nurs Sci 24(2):47–64, 2001.

McConkey, TE, et al: Assessing the female sexual assault survivor. Nurse Practitioner 26(7):28–30, 2001.

McCrone, S, and Shelton, D: An overview of forensic psychiatric care of the adolescent. Issues in Mental Health Nursing 22(2):301–305, 2001.

Moore, A: Pioneering practice . . . Nurse forensic examiners. Nursing Standard 15(27):20–21, 2001.

Sekula, K, et al: Forensic psychiatric nursing. J Psychosoc Nurs Ment Health Serv 39(9):51–59, 2001.

22

Alternative and Complementry Healing Practices

Lydia DeSantis

Learning Objectives

After completing this chapter, the reader will be able to:

- Compare the philosophy and objectives of alternative and complementary healing modalities with those of conventional Western medicine.
- List major reasons why a growing number of people are using alternative and complementary healing modalities.
- Describe major types of alternative and complementary healing modalities.
- Summarize methods by which nurses and clients can obtain information about alternative and complementary healing modalities.
- Evaluate a client for use of alternative and complementary healing modalities.
- Identify the strengths and weaknesses of alternative and complementary healing modalities.

In North America, alternative and complementary healing practices refer to those that are outside of conventional, science-based Western medicine and not sanctioned by the official health-care system. Alternative and complementary healing practices and products have grown and continue to grow dramatically in popularity with clients of all ages and backgrounds. Indeed, the range of practices and concepts included in alternative and complementary healing is considerable, as outlined in the accompanying glossary at the end of this chapter.

According to the World Health Organization (WHO), 80 percent of the world's population uses what Americans call "alternative" practices as their primary source of health care. Because of the widely accepted use of these practices, WHO has officially sanctioned the incorporation of "safe and effective [alternative] remedies and practices for use in public and private health services." Currently, between 34 and 42 percent of Americans (60 to 83 million people) use alternative and complementary healing practices, as do 20 to 70 percent of people in Western Europe, 33 percent in Finland, and 49 percent in Australia.

The trend toward alternative practices continues to grow. In the United States since the 1990s, studies show that 40 percent of people developed an increasingly positive attitude toward alternative prac-

---

Inclusion of particular ideas or practices in this chapter implies no endorsement of them. Health-care practitioners and their clients must carefully evaluate the claims and qualifications of alternative and complementary healing practices and practitioners before making conclusions about them.

tices, whereas only 2 percent had more negative opinions. Both the general public (72 percent) and health maintenance organizations (HMOs) (73 percent) expect consumer demand for this area of health care to remain moderate to strong. Few persons (4 to 11 percent) rely solely on alternative practices to treat illness, but the number relying only on conventional health care is declining.

Defining Alternative and Complementary Healing

There is no universally accepted definition for alternative and complementary healing practices. Many of the modalities originated long ago in other cultural belief systems and healing traditions. A commonly used definition in the United States for alternative and complementary modalities comes from the National Center for Complementary and Alternative Medicine (NCCAM), which is an agency of the National Institutes of Health: "those treatments and healthcare practices not taught widely in medicals schools, not generally used in hospitals, and not usually reimbursed by medical insurance companies."

> *Alternative health-care practices are most popular among women, people aged 35 to 49, people with higher educational levels (some graduate education), and those with annual incomes of more than $50,000.*

One concern with this definition is that courses on alternative and complementary modalities are being included in more and more medical, nursing, and other schools for Western health professionals. Also, the practice of alternative medicine is not limited to healers outside the conventional health-care system. Nurses, physicians, and other health-care professionals are responding to the growing public use of these practices by incorporating selected ones into their own client care. Physicians have begun referring clients to a variety of alternative healers. The use of alternative modalities by conventional health-care professionals for their own health is also increasing.

In this chapter alternative and complementary medicine is defined as the understanding and use of healing modalities not commonly considered to be part of Western biomedicine. The focus here is mainly on methods of self-care, wellness, self-healing, health promotion, and illness prevention. Modalities are called alternative when used alone or with other alternative therapies and complementary when used with conventional therapies.

The term *healing* is preferable to *medicine* because alternative and complementary modalities typically are based in holistic philosophies that go beyond treatment or cure of the physiologic and psychological dimensions of care commonly associated with modern, scientific biomedicine. Holism refers to treatment of the whole person (body-mind-spirit) in that person's environmental context (physical, biologic, social, cultural, and spiritual).

What Do You Think?

Do you use any alternative health-care practices? What are they? Why do you use them?

Who Uses Alternative Therapies

No single client characteristic or profile consistently predicts the use of alternative and complementary therapies. However, these practices are most popular among women, people aged 35 to 49, people with higher educational levels (some graduate education), and those with annual incomes of more than $50,000.

In most national studies of alternative therapy users, ethnic and racial minorities are underrepresented, particularly among persons who do

Box 22–1

Reasons for Use of Alternative and Complementary Modalities

People use alternative therapies alone or together with conventional health care for a variety of reasons. There is no single predictor of use, and the reasons for use may vary from context to context and situation to situation. Persons who seem to benefit the most from the alternative approach are those who:

- Prefer a personalistic relationship with healers
- Refuse to give up hope and hopefulness, regardless of the illness or life-state
- Desire to focus on wellness, health promotion and maintenance, and illness prevention
- Are concerned with gentle alleviation and management of suffering and illness rather than aggressive management of the end-stage of life through technology, medications, surgery, and other invasive procedures
- Wish to participate actively in decision making about their health care
- Believe in the holistic aspects of existence rather than in the primacy of biologic and physiologic aspects
- Are "culture creatives"—persons at the leading edge of innovation and culture change and who have been exposed to alternative lifestyles and worldviews compatible with those from which alternative and complementary modalities and theories have arisen
- Share cultural and philosophical views similar to those from which alternative and complementary modalities have developed

Sources: Aspen Reference Group: Holistic Health Promotion and Complementary Therapies: A Resource for Integrated Practice. Aspen, Gaithersberg, MD, 1998.

Austin, JA: Why patients use alternative medicine. JAMA 279:1548, 1998.

Cassidy, CM: Cultural context of complementary and alternative medicine systems. In Micozzi, MS (ed): Fundamentals of Complementary and Alternative Medicine. Churchill Livingstone, New York, 1996, p. 9.

Delbanco, T: Leaches, spiders, and astrology: Predilections and predictions. JAMA 280:1564, 1998.

Jonas, WB: Alternative medicine: Learning from the past, examining the present, advancing to the future. JAMA 280:1616, 1998.

not speak English. Such exclusions raise questions about whether the use rate of alternative therapies in the United States may exceed 42 percent, because the use of alternative therapies among immigrant populations and those with lower incomes tends to be high. Many such populations have grown up with these therapies as "folk" medicine, and they have worldviews that encompass different concepts of health, illness, and healing.

Why Use of Complementary and Alternative Medicine Has Grown

Three general theories have been advanced to explain the growing use of alternative and complementary healing: dissatisfaction with conventional health care, a desire for greater control over one's health, and a desire for cultural and philosophical congruence with personal beliefs about health and illness. Many other client-specific reasons have also been postulated, such as belief in the efficacy of alternative therapies and the individual's health status (Box 22–1). The rising cost of conventional health care may play a role as well.

Dissatisfaction

Disillusionment with the ability of conventional health care to deal with major health problems and improve general health contributes to the increasing use of alternative therapies. This feeling is especially strong among people who rely primarily on alternative therapies and have a general distrust of conventional health care. Lack of trust has begun to increase for a variety of reasons. They include:

- Contradictory and ever-changing information from epidemiologic studies and clinical trials about risk prevention and health promotion. For example, clients no longer know what to believe about salt intake, normal cholesterol levels, alcohol use, or hormone replacement therapy.
- Continuing emphasis of conventional health care on curative rather than preventive aspects of care. The lack of emphasis on illness prevention limits the ability of individuals to live long lives relatively free of disability from major chronic illnesses, such as arthritis, diabetes, cancer, and cardiovascular disease.
- Growing concern about the cost and safety of conventional health care. Concerns center on the prevalence of iatrogenic illnesses, adverse results of medications, progressively more invasive procedures, growing resistance to antibiotics, and reliance on technology.

Control

Some people who use alternative therapies express a growing intolerance of the authoritarianism and depersonalization of conventional care. They feel that health-care professionals are insensitive to the wishes of clients and their families when formulating treatment plans, depriving them of a partnership role in decision making about their care.

In the United States, the majority of people (61 percent) are reluctant to tell conventional health-care professionals that they use alternative therapies, and almost all (89 percent) who use them do so with supervision by an alternative healer. Nearly half (46 percent) of people who use alternative therapies do so without consulting a conventional health-care professional. Fourteen percent of persons see both conventional health-care professionals and alternative healers. Similar patterns of self-care and nondisclosure to conventional health-care professionals are found throughout the industrialized world.

What Do You Think?

Do you tell your physician or primary health-care provider that you use alternative therapies? What is their response?

Holistic Philosophy

Conventional health care is often faulted for its focus on the physiologic dimension of health and curing rather than on the holistic approach that espouses the unity of mind-body-spirit and healing. For some, another negative characteristic is its dependence on medicine, surgery, and technology rather than on the more natural and noninvasive alternative approach with its focus on self-care and self-healing.

Belief

Clients who use alternative therapies do so because they believe those therapies will work, either alone or combined with conventional treatments. Persons who consider their health to be poor or who have chronic illnesses report greater benefits from alternative than conventional health care and are more likely to try both at once. Referral from conventional health-care professionals, friends, or other users of alternative therapies is also a prominent reason for the simultaneous use of both systems. For many clients, alternative therapies simply make them feel better than conventional health care does.

Cost of Conventional Care

Most people (58 percent) in the United States pay out-of-pocket for alternative therapies.

Payments to alternative healers rose from $23 billion in 1990 to $33 billion 1997. However, this is slightly less than the total out-of-pocket expenses paid for physician services ($29 billion) and hospitalizations ($9 billion). Estimated costs of alternative medicines (herbs and nutritional supplements), diet products, equipment, and books/courses totaled another $14 billion.

Sixty-seven percent of HMOs cover one or more alternative and complementary healing (ACH) modalities, but coverage is uneven and varies regionally. Chiropractic (65 percent) is the most common covered service, followed by acupuncture (31 percent), massage therapy (11 percent), and vitamin therapy (6 percent). By 2005, HMOs expect to increase coverage for acupuncture to 36 percent, acupressure to 31 percent, massage therapy to 30 percent, and vitamin therapy to 27 percent. The most important reasons for adding coverage for these services are public demand (38 percent), legislative mandate (38 percent), and demonstrated clinical effectiveness (8 percent).

Classifying Alternative Methods

Basic to all healing systems are the goals of preventing illness, promoting and maintaining health, and caring for people while alleviating the suffering caused by illness. However, despite their underlying commonality, healing systems vary profoundly in their modalities (technologies); types, preparation, and monitoring of practitioners; concepts (models) of health and illness; delivery of care; and social and legal mandates to provide care. Such variation gives rise to a large number of health-care systems, practitioners, and healing modalities that are part of different worldviews and explanatory models. Two systems that can be used to help define and classify the alternative and complementary approach are the Healing Matrix, by Engebretson and Wardell, and the NCCAM classification.

Healing Matrix

The Healing Matrix (Table 22–1) contrasts conventional and alternative modalities and practitioners. The alternative modalities shown are (1) representative of those most commonly known by the general public; (2) sought in the United States and industrialized world; and (3) practiced most often by conventional health-care professionals, including nurses.

Modalities in column 1 are technologies that cross various healing systems. The technologies are arranged vertically from the most concrete to the most abstract. The remaining columns include various healing modalities from conventional, marginal, and alternative healing systems.

Physical Manipulation Technologies. These are often termed bodywork therapies done by a therapist or as part of self-care and include rituals and breathing exercises to bring about the union of body-mind-spirit.

Ingested or Applied Substances. Technologies included are herbs, vitamins and other nutritional supplements, and dietary regimens that are taken to help the body heal itself, rid itself of toxins, and promote health and wellness.

Energy. These technologies maintain and restore health through the balancing of energy flow of vital forces, life essences, or other such vitalities.

Mental (Psychic) and Spiritual. Included are group or individual counseling technologies that promote and attain spiritual and personal growth. Examples are intuiting, revelations, visualization, astrological and other readings, and invoking the spirit world.

Modalities in column 2 (orthodox [conventional]) are part of the official health-care system in the United States and elsewhere. Their explanatory model is derived from knowledge rooted in scientific and biomedical principles.

Modalities in column 3 (marginal) are generally learned through the study of formal curricula in institutions of higher education. Alternative healers practicing such modalities are usually

Table 22–1

The Healing Matrix

TECHNOLOGIES	ORTHODOX	MARGINAL	ALTERNATIVE	
Physical manipulation	Surgery Physical therapy	Chiropractic	Rolfing Feldenkrais	Craniosacral alignments Massage therapy Yoga, Akido, Tai Chi Reflexology
Ingested or applied substances	Pharmacology	Homeopathy Vitamin therapy	Naturopathic remedies Herbs Flower remedies	Aromatherapy Diet alternatives
Uses of energy	Laser surgery	Acupuncture Acupressure	Reiki Magnetic or polarity healing Therapeutic touch	Chakra balancing Radionics Use of color, gems and crystals
Mental Spiritual	Psychiatry	Secular or spiritual counseling Established support groups (e.g., 12-step programs)	Self-help groups Visualizations Affirmations	Psychic, spiritual or intuitive healing

Source: Adapted from Engebretson, J, and Wardell, D: A contemporary view of alternative healing modalities. Nurse Pract 18:51, 1993.

licensed by one or more states, and most have credentialing and professional bodies. They are not considered conventional therapies in the United States but may be part of conventional health-care systems in other nations. For example, acupuncture is a prominent healing modality of traditional Chinese medicine, which along with biomedicine forms the conventional health-care system in the People's Republic of China. In 1997, The National Institutes of Health Consensus Panel on Acupuncture reviewed research studies and other information on its safety, efficacy, and effectiveness. The panel concluded that there is sufficient evidence to support acupuncture as a therapeutic intervention for adult general and dental postoperative pain and nausea and vomiting from chemotherapy.

Modalities in column 4 (alternative) are derived from progressively more intuitive types of knowledge. Most alternative healers practicing such modalities are self-taught, have learned through working with other, more experienced practitioners, and/or have had courses or workshops on particular modalities. Alternative modalities in the bottom cell on the far right have the most intuitive knowledge base, that is, insights about the spiritual or physical self are gained through direct revelations or as interpreted by another, such as readers (e.g., astrologers or seers) or spiritual healers in touch with divine forces.

NCCAM Classification

In 1992, Congress mandated the establishment of an Office of Alternative Medicine in the National Institutes of Health to enhance the study of ACH modalities to determine their effectiveness. In 1998, the Office became the National Center for Complementary and Alternative Medicine (NCCAM). Its mission is to conduct and support both basic and applied research and training and the dissemination of ACH information to conventional health-care professionals, alternative healers, and the public.

Complementary and alternative medicine (CAM) is defined by the NCCAM as those practices not commonly included in or used by conventional medicine. Seven major categories of CAM are defined and subdivided into practices that (1) fall under CAM; (2) are found in conventional health care but are classified as behavioral medicine; and (3) are overlapping, that is, they can fall in the domain of either CAM or behavioral medicine. Table 22–2 summarizes the NCCAM classification.

Category I

Category I includes alternative systems of theory and practice developed outside of Western biomedicine. For example, acupuncture and Oriental medicine are grounded in traditional Chinese medicine or its derivatives. Also included in this category are traditional indigenous systems, which are all medical systems other than acupuncture and Oriental medicine developed outside of Western biomedicine. It also includes unconventional Western systems not classified elsewhere that were developed in the West but are not considered part of biomedicine, such as homeopathy. Finally, this category includes naturopathy, which is an unconventional medical system that has gained prominence in the United States. This eclectic approach consists of a variety of natural systems, such as herbalism, lifestyle therapies, and diet as therapy.

Category II

Category II includes mind-body practices, religion and spirituality, and social and contextual areas. Mind-body medicine involves a variety of approaches to health care and contains three subcategories. Mind-body systems are seldom practiced alone, are usually combined with lifestyle interventions, and may be part of a traditional medical system. Mind-body methods include individual approaches and are often considered as conventional practice. They are characterized as CAM when used for health conditions for which they are not normally prescribed. Religion and spirituality include nonbehavioral characteristics of spirituality and religion that are examined in relation to biologic functions or clinical conditions. Social and contextual areas are modalities not included in other categories. They are approaches that are considered cultural, symbolic, social, and contextual interventions.

Category III

Biologically-based therapies include products, interventions, and practices that are natural and biologically based and may or may not overlap with conventional medicine and its use of dietary supplements. Phytotherapy or herbalism is use of plant-derived products for purposes of prevention and treatment. Special diet therapies are therapeutic dietary approaches and special diets applied to risk factors or chronic disease. Orthomolecular medicine is use of nutritional products and food supplements that are not included in other categories for prevention and treatment of disease. Pharmacologic, biologic, and instrumental interventions are products and interventions not covered in other categories that are administered in an unconventional manner.

Category IV

Manipulative and body-based methods include body manipulation and/or body movement.

Category V

Energy therapies include biofield and bioelectromagnetic-based therapies. Biofields include energy systems and energy fields internal and external to the body that are used for medical purposes. Bioelectromagnetics is the use of electromagnetic fields in an unconventional manner for medical reasons.

Table 22–2

NCCAM Categories of Alternative Practice

I. ALTERNATIVE MEDICAL SYSTEMS

Traditional Oriental Medicine

Acupuncture
Diet
External and internal qi gong
Herbal formulas
Massage and manipulation (Tui Na)
Tai Chi

Traditional Indigenous Systems

Ayurvedic medicine
Curanderismo
Central and South American
Kampo medicine
Native-American medicine
Traditional African medicine
Traditional Aboriginal medicine
Unani-tibbi
SIDDHI

Alternative Western Systems

CAM	Overlapping
Homeopathy	Anthroposophically extended medicine
Naturopathy	
Orthomolecular medicine	

II. MIND-BODY INTERVENTIONS

Mind-Body Methods

CAM	Behavioral Medicine	Overlapping
Yoga	Hypnosis	Art, music, and dance therapies
Tai Chi	Meditation	Humor
Internal qi gong	Biofeedback	Journaling
	Imagery	

Religion and Spirituality

CAM

Confession
Nonlocality
Nontemporality
Soul retrieval
"Special" healers
Spiritual healing

Social and Contextual Areas

CAM	Overlapping
Caring-based approaches (e.g., holistic nursing, pastoral care)	Community-based approaches (e.g., Native-American "sweat" rituals)
Intuitive diagnosis	Explanatory models
	Placebo

III. BIOLOGICALLY BASED THERAPIES

Phytotherapy or Herbalism

Aloe vera	Echinacea	Ginseng	Mistletoe
Bee pollen	Evening primrose	Green tea	Peppermint oil
Biloba	Garlic	Hawthorne	Saw palmetto
Cat's claw	Ginger	Kava Kava	Witch hazel
Dong Quai	Ginkgo	Licorice root	Valerian

Special Diet Therapies

Atkins	McDougall	Fasting	Paleolithic
Diamond	Ornish	High fiber	Vegetarian
Kelly-Gonzalez	Pritikin	Macrobiotic	
Gerson	Wigmore	Mediterranean	
Livingston-Wheeler	Asian	Natural hygiene	

Table 22–2

NCCAM Categories of Alternative Practice (*Continued*)

Orthomolecular Therapies

Single Nutrients (Partial Listing)

Amino acids	Folic acid	Lysine	Niacinamide	Thiamine
Ascorbic acid	Glutamine	Manganese	Potassium	Tyrosine
Boron	Glucosamine sulfate	Magnesium	Selenium	Vanadium
Calcium	Iodine	Medium-chain triglycerides	Silicon	Vitamin A
Carotenes	Inositol		Glandular products	Vitamin D
Choline	Iron	Melatonin	Riboflavin	Vitamin K
Fatty acids	Lipoic acid	Niacin	Taurine	

Pharmacologic, Biologic, and Instrumental Interventions

Products

Antineoplastons	Cone therapy	Hyperbaric oxygen
Bee pollen	Enderlin products	Induced remission therapy
Cartilage	Enzyme therapies	Ozone
Cell therapy	Gallo immunotherapy	Revici system
Coley's toxins	H_2O_2	

Procedures/Devices

Apitherapy	Electrodiagnostics	Neural therapy
Bioresonance	Iridology	
Chirography	MORA device	

IV. MANIPULATIVE AND BODY-BASED METHODS

Chiropractic Medicine

Massage and Bodywork

Acupressure	Feldenkrais technique	Reflexology
Alexander technique	Osteopathic manipulative therapy (OMT)	Rolfing
Applied kinesiology		Swedish massage
Chinese Tui Na massage	Pilates method	Trager bodywork
Craniosacral OMT	Polarity	

Unconventional Physical Therapies

Colonics	Heat and electrotherapies	Light and color therapies
Diathermy	Hydrotherapy	

V. ENERGY THERAPIES

Biofield Therapies

External qi gong	Healing touch	Reiki
Healing science	Huna	Therapeutic touch

Bioelectromagnetic-Based Therapies

(Unconventional Use of Electromagnetic Fields)

Alternating and direct current fields	Magnetic fields	Pulsed fields

Source: Adapted from National Center for Complementary and Alternative Medicine: Classification of Alternative Medicine Practices. April 26, 2000 [On-line]. Available at: wysiwyg://14/http://ccam.nih.gov/fcp/classify/index.html.

Comparing Conventional and Alternative Practices

Many similarities and differences exist between alternative and conventional health care. As they attempt to achieve similar goals, they may overlap in method, even though the methods are derived from different concepts of reality and theoretical models. Table 22–3 summarizes characteristics often cited as common to alternative healing and contrasts them with those usually associated with conventional health care.

In general, conventional medicine focuses on the physical or materialistic part of the person-body, that is, the structure, function, and connections or communications between material elements that compose the body, such as bones, muscles, and nerves. Human beings are generally viewed as biologically similar, and disease is seen as a deviation from measurable biologic or somatic variables. Conventional medicine is sometimes considered reductionistic because it tends to reduce very complex entities (humans) to seemingly equal and more simple beings who are all anatomically and physiologically similar. From this perspective, it is believed that all individuals will respond in more or less the same ways to causative agents and common treatments. In other words, a person with measles, cirrhosis of the liver, or breast cancer will have a similar course of illness as other persons with those illnesses and will respond to treatments in basically the same manner. Extensive disease categories have been developed, and great emphasis is placed on diagnosis and cure based on the evaluation of physical signs and symptoms. Most newly developed medications, when they are in the human-testing phase, are tested on men between the ages of 25 and 35 years old, with the presumption that they will work similarly in women, the elderly, and children. That presumption is not always accurate.

The physical body is the primary site of conventional therapeutic intervention. The almost exclusive focus on the physical body limits consideration and incorporation of nonmaterialistic aspects of health and illness in diagnosis and treatment decisions. Thus, spiritual, psychologi-

Table 22–3

Contrasts Between Conventional and Alternative Health Care

CONVENTIONAL	ALTERNATIVE/COMPLEMENTARY
Chemotherapy	Plants and other natural products
Curing/treating	Healing/ministering care
Disease category	Unique individual
End-stage	Hope/hopefulness
Focus is on disease and illness	Focus is on health and wellness
Illness treatment	Health promotion and illness prevention
Individual is viewed as disease category	Individual is viewed as unique being
Nutrition is adjunct and supportive to treatment	Nutrition is the basis of health, wellness, and treatment
Objectivism: Person is separate from disease	Subjectivism: Person is integral to the illness
Client	Person
Practitioner as authority	Practitioner as facilitator
Practitioner paternalism/client dependency	Practitioner as partner/person empowerment
Positivism/materialism: Data is physically measurable	Metaphysical: Entity is energy system or vital force
Reductionistic	Holistic
Specialist care	Self-care
Symptom relief	Alleviation of causative factors
Somatic (body biologic and physiologic) model	Behavioral-psycho-social-spiritual model
Science is only source of knowledge and truth	Multiple sources of knowledge and truth
Technology/invasive	Natural/noninvasive

cal, sociocultural, behavioral, and energy system aspects commonly play little, if any, role in conventional medical treatment. The human body is not seen as an integrated person-body that incorporates and responds simultaneously to both materialistic and nonmaterialistic dimensions in everyday functioning. That integration is not seen as basic to the person's state of wellness or illness, nor is it seen as essential that therapies be based on the concept of holism. The concept of a psychosocial body has been given additional attention in Western practice, but it has not been effectively incorporated into conventional care. The energetic and spiritual bodies are largely denied.

Most newly developed medications, when they are in the human-testing phase, are tested on men between the ages of 25 and 35 years old, with the presumption that they will work similarly in women, the elderly, and children. That presumption is not always accurate.

In contrast, the alternative approach conceives of the person-body as multiple, integrated bodies that incorporate both the materialistic and nonmaterialistic aspects of existence, including physical (materialistic), spiritual, energetic, and social bodies. Such a concept allows for a variety of interpretations of how the various components of the person-body are structured and how they function, affect health and illness, and direct and respond to therapeutic interventions.

The integration of multiple bodies into a unified but distinctly individual person-body results in the concept that the person-body responds as a whole to factors that affect its state of well-being. Similar signs and symptoms of illness may indicate different underlying internal and external causal and risk factors based in a variety of materialistic and nonmaterialistic components of the overall individual. Diagnostic measures and interventions cannot be based on only one aspect of the person's being, but must be tailored to the person-body of each individual.

A variety of alternative modalities are needed to diagnose and treat each individual holistically because it may not be apparent when the functioning of the physical body merges into the dynamics of the energetic body, the energetic body merges with the spiritual body, and how all are mediated and integrated into the psychosocial body. The mediating role of the psychosocial body in the alternative approach emphasizes each person's capacity for self-healing, the importance of the mind-body effect in the form of the placebo response, and the need for people to have an integral role in the monitoring and maintenance of their health and well-being and in the diagnosis and treatment of their illness.

The multiple body concept of the alternative approach requires a rather eclectic approach to health promotion and maintenance and the diagnosis and treatment of illness rather than dependence on a single healing tradition that centers on a one-body concept or on a particular type of diagnostic criteria. The alternative approach requires active participation of well and ill persons in their health promotive, diagnostic, and treatment processes rather than on their passive acceptance of a diagnosis and treatment prescription of external authorities such as conventional health-care professionals. The alternative philosophy includes both the materialistic and nonmaterialistic aspects of the individual's being, stimulation of the self-healing forces of each individual, and the determination of a person's unique needs. It simultaneously uses the concepts and treatment modalities of a variety of healing traditions based on different worldviews or concepts of reality to address the healing needs of each person. From this perspective, acupunc-

What Do You Think?

Name someone you know or know of who has gotten better after an illness although not expected to? Why do you think this happened?

turists may also use massage and a variety of other types of bodywork and energy-system methods; chiropractors may incorporate diet, herbs, and other kinds of naturopathic methodologies into chiropractic spinal manipulations; and massage therapists may include mind-body techniques such as meditation, imagery, and visualization.

Central and constant to alternative and complementary healing is the concept of a multiple-body individual, with healers functioning as facilitators in the promotion of health and healing (Box 22–2). Central and constant to conventional therapy is the physical-body individual, with conventional health-care professionals functioning as experts in determining the meaning of physical signs and symptoms of health or illness and prescribing interventions to promote health or cure illness.

Certain specific concepts can be used to compare and contrast alternative and conventional methods of healing. They include wellness and holism, self-healing, energy systems, nutrition, and using plants as medicine.

Wellness and Holism

Wellness, from the perspective of conventional health care, tends to focus on individuals deemed at risk for illness. Prevention often begins when signs or symptoms arise and is directed at alleviating them rather than treating or removing their underlying cause. Individuals can continue to engage in risky behaviors as long as conventional health care can find treatments or palliative measures for diseases it cannot prevent. From this perspective, health is often defined as the absence of disease and is considered synonymous with wellness.

The focus of conventional health care is

Box 22–2

Defining Alternative Healers

Alternative healers are those persons who practice one or more alternative or complementary modalities and who are not also licensed as conventional health-care professionals. Conventional health-care professionals who incorporate hands-on alternative and complementary modalities into their conventionalpatient care are termed *integrative practitioners.* They should undergo the same educational, certification, and licensing processes of both conventional and alternative healers for the modalities they use.

Keep in mind that creating a universally applicable definition of alternative healers is extremely difficult because of the wide variety of healing traditions in use and the number of specialized healing techniques contained within them. The difficulty is compounded by the fact that many alternative healers incorporate various modalities from different healing traditions into their practices. For example, chiropractors commonly use therapeutic touch, acupuncture, acupressure, massage therapy, and naturopathic or homeopathic therapies. Massage therapists may combine multiple types of massage (such as Alexander, Swedish, Trager, and sports) with therapeutic touch, aromatheraphy, reflexology, nutritional supplements, and electromagnetic therapies. The growing use of alternative practices by conventional health-care professionals further complicates the task of defining and classifying alternative healers and their practices.

reductionistic rather than holistic because treatment and diagnosis are frequently centered on the cellular, organ, or system levels of the body. Emphasis is mainly on the biologic-physiologic (body) dimension of the client and the disease entity that may occur or for which signs and symptoms are already evident. Illness is commonly regarded as being primarily caused by external forces or risk factors that "invade" the body from the surrounding physical, social, or biologic environments.

Treatment endeavors for the biomedical model usually center on identifying potentially dangerous or invading agents and destroying, immobilizing, or extracting them from the person-body. Interventions consist mainly of chemotherapeutic agents (medications), surgery, or other externally imposed activities or technologies to prevent those at risk from becoming ill or to prevent signs and symptoms from becoming full-blown diseases.

In contrast to conventional health care, wellness in the alternative model is a state in which individuals are in harmony or balance with their internal and external worlds. This approach is often seen in nursing models or theories (see Chapter 4). Usually, wellness cannot be conferred by an outside entity or agency but is achieved mainly by individuals through the process of self-care, that is, assuming responsibility for their own state of health or wellness and for returning themselves to a state of wellness when signs and symptoms of illness (imbalance or disharmony) occur in themselves or some disruption (imbalance or disharmony) occurs in their external world. External disruptions—such as work stress, personal tragedy, a troublesome interpersonal relationship, or illness of a parent, spouse, or child—are seen as capable of affecting internal harmony and producing signs and symptoms of physical, emotional, or spiritual illness. Thus, individuals are seen as one with their internal and external environments, and their care must be holistic in nature. Treatment must address the whole individual (body-mind-spirit) in an environmental (physical, biologic, social, cultural, and spiritual) context. Integral to holistic treatment is the concept of spirituality. The human spirit incorporates the values, perception of meaning, and purpose in life that can positively or negatively affect the ability to heal and achieve wellness. From this perspective, health (balance or harmony), or the absence of illness, is but one aspect of wellness.

The human spirit incorporates the values, perception of meaning, and purpose in life that can positively or negatively affect the ability to heal and achieve wellness.

Self-Care

In the alternative system, self-care measures for wellness that a person may undertake range from those performed purely by the individual to those that require a high degree of specialist assistance. Examples of the former are exercising, eating a well-balanced diet, praying, getting enough sleep, cleaning the house, using defensive driving measures, doing breast or testicular self-examinations, applying sunscreen at the beach, and practicing good hygiene.

The next level of self-care requires seeking the assistance of others to achieve balance in self and the environment. This level includes getting help to find satisfying employment, seeking prenatal care or taking parenting classes when pregnant, going to community meetings to address environmental safety and citizen quality-of-life issues, undergoing routine health screening examinations (such as mammography and dental checkups), obtaining glasses to correct myopia, and getting and keeping vaccinations up to date.

The third level of self-care requires a high degree of specialist assistance from alternative healers and others to deal with major disruptions in internal or external well-being. Measures focus on the spiritual dimension and include searching for personal awakening, enlightenment, and self-actualization through modalities rooted in other systems of health care such as traditional Chinese medicine, Ayurveda, or spiritualism. Others may require use of alternative modalities to deal with illnesses when conventional health care has been deemed no longer effective or needs to be enhanced.

Self-Healing

Both alternative and conventional health care believe that the body heals itself. The alternative system considers self-healing a central principle of its explanatory model and sees it as the basis of all healing. Thus, alternative healers focus on helping people determine why the cells of their body are sick and search for imbalances from a holistic perspective.

Conventional health care views the ability of the body to heal primarily through its normal routine of replacing cells and the physiologic and biologic processes involved in wound healing. It approaches the concept of body self-healing by questioning why the cells of the body are not replacing themselves and attempts to facilitate body healing through external means, such as surgery, medications, or invasive measures.

Placebo Response

Conventional health care tends to dismiss the effects of healing measured after the application of alternative modalities by citing the placebo response or placebo effect (healing takes place because the patient assumes or believes that a treatment is effective). In conventional medicine, the term *placebo* has come to signify a type of sham treatment instituted to please difficult or anxious clients or a sugar pill given when conventional health-care professionals have nothing more to offer the healing process than "sugar-pill promises." In biomedical clinical research, a placebo is a nontreatment given to participants because it is assumed that its inactivity will not cause the structural or physiologic responses that result from active treatments.

The concept of the placebo response is integral to the testing of new drugs in double-blind studies, where neither investigators nor study participants know which participants receive the study drug and which receive an inert substance (the control group). At the conclusion of the study, scientists compare whether a higher percentage of the experimental group experienced the hoped-for results from the active medication than the control group received from the placebo.

However, clinical studies have shown that participants respond positively to placebo medications and interventions 30 to 70 percent of the time. It seems especially effective in clients with:

- Pain from chronic disease, such as cancer pain, arthritis, back pain, angina pectoris, and gastrointestinal tract discomfort
- Autonomic nervous system disorders, such as phobias, psychoneuroses, depression, and nausea
- Neurohormonal disorders, such as asthma, other bronchial airflow conditions, and hypertension

The mechanism by which the placebo response operates is not understood. The placebo effect is believed to be at work in every therapeutic intervention regardless of whether the intervention is an alternative or a conventional modality. It has been attributed to four variables:

- An endorphin-mediated response
- Belief of the client
- Belief of the healer
- The client-healer relationship

What Do You Think?

What are the ethical issues involved in using placebos? If you were being given a placebo and you found out, how would you feel? What if you improved with the placebo, would you still feel the same way?

Endorphins are the body's natural painkillers that, when released, reduce pain and bring about a degree of euphoria. Relaxation therapies and other types of stress-reducing and stress-controlling techniques are believed to promote the release of endorphins and enhance the relief of pain. Medications that block the release of endorphins have been shown to inhibit or reverse the placebo treatment effects in the reduction of postoperative dental pain.

A person's belief in the effectiveness of the therapy is seen as an active ingredient to the success of the therapy and may be just as important as the therapy itself. The placebo response acts to change the perception of the client but not the underlying disease process. Studies of client compliance in taking prescribed beta blocker heart medications in the first year after myocardial infarction showed that mortality rates were almost equal for those failing to take either the beta blocker or placebo. Mortality rates for both groups were higher than the rates for those who faithfully took their prescribed medications or placebos.

> *A person's belief in the effectiveness of the therapy is seen as an active ingredient to the success of the therapy and may be just as important as the therapy itself.*

Healers who believe in the therapeutic effectiveness of interventions and have the ability to convey that belief to their clients achieve more positive placebo responses in clients than healers who remain skeptical about the interventions they are prescribing. An attitude of caring and being in control tends to alleviate client anxieties and fears while increasing their hope and positive expectations.

A trusting and close relationship between the client and healer has a positive psychological effect on clients and can become their mental catalyst for recovery. The ability of healers to communicate in an empathetic manner increases client satisfaction with care, compliance with mutually set goals, and feelings of empowerment, self-confidence, and self-worth, and decreases depression and anxiety.

Although conventional health care considers many of these approaches as speculative, incomplete, or insufficient to explain the placebo response, alternative healers see the placebo response as measurable and reproducible evidence that the mind and body are intertwined. The placebo response is viewed as proof that feelings, thoughts, and beliefs can change the physiologic and structural functioning of individuals.

Remembered Wellness

The term *remembered wellness* is sometimes used in place of placebo effect to describe the physiologic response that occurs after active or passive therapeutic interventions. Remembered wellness includes the person's prior learning, experiences and environment, beliefs and perceptions, and biologic factors or genetic interactions. It is triggered by memories of past events or times when good health and feelings of confidence, strength, hope, and peace were part of the person's life. Memories are accessed through alternative modalities that stimulate relaxation, such as the quieting of the body and mind to promote healing. Clinical research has demonstrated relaxation to be effective in treating anxiety, pain, high blood pressure, and tachycardia, as well as showing the effectiveness of stress management on disease prevention. Research studies have also found a relationship between the central nervous system and the immune system and shown that communication exists between two mind-body pathways: the autonomic and neuroendocrine.

A scientific explanation of the psychophysiologic interaction of mind and body, its relationship to the placebo response and remembered wellness, and the method by which the placebo response operates will depend on multidisciplinary research, especially by the sciences of psychology and neurobiology. The placebo response remains an enigma to conventional health care and seems to imply an element of deceitfulness when used deliberately in client treatments. For alternative medicine, the placebo response and remembered wellness are forces that can be harnessed to bring about healing.

Energy Systems

It has long been known scientifically that the human body is regulated by its own internal electrical energy system and that humans could not survive without the low levels of electricity that sustain and regulate life at the cellular and molecular levels. Electrical-chemical stimuli from the nervous system regulate other body systems; electrical impulses trigger heartbeats; and minute electrical and magnetic forces exist in each body molecule.

Conventional health care has long utilized various types of energy systems (e.g., electrical, magnetic, microwave, and infrared) for screening, diagnosis, and treatment through the use of electrocardiograms, magnetic resonance imaging, electroencephalograms, electomyelogram, x-rays, radiation treatments for cancer, low-frequency electric current to stimulate growth of bone cells (osteoblasts) to accelerate healing of fractures, and types of electric shock therapy for cardiac arrest, cardioversions for cardiac arrhythmia, and pacemakers. Conventional health care has also used bioenergy (body energy) to determine the degree of pathology and estimate prognosis through the study of cells as they decompose, die, reproduce, and respond to pathogens and traumas. The majority of conventional treatments for many diseases are chemical (medications), surgical, and/or immobilization or manipulation of the affected body part. They are used primarily *after* the disease has been diagnosed.

Although conventional medicine does not use the energy of the body for purposes of healing, alternative modalities conceptualize energy systems in such terms as fields, vital essences, balance, and flow that are used by individuals to heal themselves, prevent illness, and promote health. The basic concept is that external forces are not able to cause harm if the person is in the well state. Alternative healers may be needed to assist individuals to manipulate the energy system primarily for self-protection or healing. Major alternative and complementary modalities using bioenergy and other energy fields are energy medicine, vital essences and balance, and external energy forces.

Energy Medicine

This modality includes a broad range of therapies that use external energy sources to stimulate tissue regeneration or improve the immune system response. Relaxation of muscles through electrical stimulation is thought to promote relaxation, increase circulation, enhance waste removal, improve nutrition and oxygenation, and restore energy balance. Examples of energy medicine include electroacupuncture, biofeedback, magnet therapy, and sound and light therapy.

Vital Essences and Balance

In many alternative models, illness reflects blockage, loss, or imbalance of body energy or vital essence. Disturbance of internal body energy can result from external or internal factors. Treatment may be directed at removing the blockage of energy flow through such measures as acupuncture, acupressure, chiropractic adjustment, craniosacral therapy, or reflexology. It may also be directed at increasing the amount of energy and vital essence to restore balance in the body. Ways that these changes are brought about include diet, herbs, exercises, and spiritual techniques, such as yoga, meditation, and internal qi gong. Therapies related to the creative arts, such as music, drawing, singing, chanting, and dancing are also used to restore balance and vital essences.

External Energy Forces

The central belief is that application of a variety of disparate external energy forces has the capacity for healing. Some of these external energy forces are actual energy treatments. Other forces include mobilizing the healing energy of faith, spirituality, prayer, shamanism, crystals, and hand-mediated energetic healing techniques, such as therapeutic touch and healing touch (Box 22–3).

Nutrition

Nutrition and diet have long been recognized by both alternative and conventional healing systems as important in health promotion and illness treatment, as well as being causative or risk factors for illness. In conventional health care, nutrition and diet are usually considered as adjuncts to biomedical treatment. In alternative systems, nutrition is commonly seen as a way of life and as a method of preventing illness.

Natural Benefits

Conventional health care commonly focuses on the need for food and a well-balanced diet without close regard to food production or processing. The safety of food sources in the contemporary diet has been called into question by both alternative healers and conventional health-care professionals because of increasing evidence of toxins in the food chain. These include:

- Pesticides used in agricultural production, lawn care, and pest control
- Industrial pollutants discharged into the air and water in which plants and animals live and obtain nutrients

Box 22–3

Therapeutic Touch

Therapeutic touch (TT) and healing touch (HT) are two forms of hand-mediated energetic healing. TT refers to the Krieger-Kunz method, and HT to the techniques taught to health-care professionals and certified by the American Holistic Nurses' Association. HT relies on the ability of practitioners to choose appropriate energy healing techniques based on their interpretation of the patent's energy flow, whereas TT follows a set of rules and protocols based in traditional or ancient healing concepts of energy, such as aura (electromagnetic field), chakras, and prana (life-force or vital essence in Ayurvedic medicine).

No actual physical contact takes place between practitioner and client in either technique. The practitioner's hands are held, palms-down, 2 to 6 inches away from the client. Slow, rhythmic motions are made over the client from head to toe to detect blockage in the normal energy flow in the body. When energy blockages or imbalances are detected or sensed, they are rectified by transference of energy from the practitioner's hands to the client's energy field, replenishing the client's energy flow, removing energy obstructions, and releasing energy congestion. The transference of energy stimulates the healing powers of the body through the reduction of stress and anxiety, promotion of relaxation, and relief of pain. TT is also believed to relax crying babies, relieve asthmatic breathing, increase wound healing, and reduce fever, inflammation, headache, and postoperative pain.

- Chemicals added to food for preservation, to increase shelf life, or make food more aesthetically appealing and pleasing in texture and taste
- Irradiation used to kill organisms, retard sprouting, and preserve shelf life
- Antibiotics, hormones, and other drugs given to animals to improve their health and increase their size, weight, and speed of growth
- Alteration of nutrients during food processing

Alternative modalities typically advocate consumption of foods produced in a natural manner in their natural environment. Emphasis on natural products stems, in part, from (1) concerns about food production and processing; (2) the concept of the person-body as both an energy system and a physical entity that exist in a natural environment and an ecological context; (3) beliefs that what we eat directly affects our health; and (4) growing scientific evidence that shifting to a more sedentary lifestyle and greater affluence has increased consumption of nutrient-poor and energy-rich foods, leading to conditions such as obesity, coronary artery and arteriosclerotic disease, micronutrient deficiencies, congenital abnormalities, and cancer. Most alternative systems advocate consumption of plant-based, whole foods and carbohydrates and eating food lower on the food chain to decrease overall intake of meat, saturated fats, and processed foods. Examples of natural food diets include the macrobiotic and vegetarian diets.

Dietary Supplements

The Food and Drug Administration (FDA) defines dietary supplements as "any product intended for ingestion as a supplement to the diet. This includes vitamins; minerals; herbs, botanical, and other plant-derived substances; and amino acids . . . and concentrates, metabolites, constituents and extracts of theses substances." Conventional health-care professionals typically view nutritional supplements (vitamins and minerals) as replacement or preventive therapy for nutrition-deficient conditions, such as rickets and osteoporosis from inadequate vitamin D, scurvy from inadequate ascorbic acid (vitamin C), neural tube defects in newborns from insufficient maternal intake of folic acid (vitamin B_9) during the prenatal period, pellagra-induced mental illness from niacin (vitamin B_3) deficiency, hair loss from lack of zinc intake, and heart disease from insufficient quantities of essential fatty acids that the body cannot manufacture for itself. To prevent deficiency diseases or conditions from overabundant intake of vitamin and minerals, the FDA, based on research by the National Academy of Sciences, has established maximum recommended daily allowances (RDAs) for vitamin and mineral intake. RDAs are usually well above the amount at which deficiency diseases would occur but below the level at which toxicities would develop.

Studies suggest that approximately two-thirds of adults fail to consume the RDAs of fruits and vegetables and that RDA levels may be too low for certain vitamins, minerals, and micronutrients to prevent the onset of chronic diseases in persons whose diets do not meet the recommended daily nutrient requirements. Especially susceptible are growing children, alcoholics, people with conditions preventing normal nutrient absorption, and pregnant, lactating, and postmenopausal women. Conventional health-care professionals consider general daily supplements, such as vitamin pills, sufficient to prevent deficiency diseases in persons with special dietary needs.

Alternative systems, like conventional health care, consider nutritional supplements as both necessary to promote health through assurance of adequate dietary intake and as replacement therapy for conditions caused by nutrition defi-

What Do You Think?

Should dietary supplements be considered medications? What are the advantages and disadvantages of classifying supplements as medications?

ciency. Alternative systems also postulate that orthomolecular therapy or megavitamin therapy (the administration of "megadoses" far in excess of RDAs for vitamins and minerals) is effective in curing diseases, increasing vitality, and enhancing overall well-being.

Concern about nutritional supplements also exists because, unlike drugs and most food additives, they are not regulated by the FDA and are not tested for safety and effectiveness before marketing if manufacturers make no claims that they are effective against a disease. However, the 1994 Dietary Supplement and Health Education Act (DSHEA) created a special category of 20,000 protected substances previously sold as supplements. The DSHEA defined supplements as including vitamins, minerals, amino acids, herbs, botanicals and other plant-derived products, and the extracts, metabolites, constituents, and concentrates of supplements. The FDA can remove supplements from the market if it receives numerous reports of their adverse effects and then proves they are dangerous to consumers' health. The FDA issues public warnings when supplements are linked to safety concerns. The DSHEA also gave the FDA authority to improve and enforce product labeling, package inserts, and accompanying literature. To enhance product comparison, guidelines instituted in 1999 require a panel of "Supplemental Facts" or "Nutrition Facts Box" on labels, which include ingredients.

The U.S. Postal Service and the Federal Trade Commission (FTC) also regulate nutritional supplements and herbal products. The U.S. Postal Inspection Service monitors products purchased by mail and may intercept supplements shipped through the mail for false claims, such as stating that they can cure AIDS or cancer. The Office of Criminal Investigation can be contacted at (202) 268-2000.

The FTC has issued guidelines to ensure that advertising claims are substantiated by reliable scientific evidence. No longer acceptable are claims of effectiveness and safety based on testimonials and other anecdotal evidence. Also outlawed are vague disclaimers, such as "results may vary," traditional use (e.g., folk remedy) that implies product efficacy without scientific evidence, and failure to give risks or qualifying information that is prominently displayed and easily understood.

Plants as Medicine

Both alternative and conventional health care use plants as medicines. Herbalism or "botanical medicine," also known a phytotherapy or phytomedicine in Europe and England, is the study and use of herbs or crude-based plant products for food, medicine, or prophylaxis to heal, treat, or prevent illness and improve the spiritual and physical quality of life. Herbs may be angiosperms (flowering plants, trees, or shrubs), algae, moss, fungus, seaweed, lichen, or ferns. Herbs for medicinal purposes consist of some part of the plant (leaf, root, flower, fruit, stem, bark, or seed), its syrup-like exudates, or some combination of them. In some herbal traditions, nonplant products are used alone or in combination, with or without plants. They may include animal secretions and parts (such as bones, organs, or tissues), stones and gemstones, minerals and metals, shells, and insects and insect products.

Botanical healing in the form of herbal medicines had been widely used in the United States until the early nineteenth century, when it was gradually displaced by the increasing prominence of the scientific method and labeled quackery. Phytomedicine continues to be a prominent branch of conventional health care in Europe. Botanicals are used by 40 percent of German and French physicians in their daily practices.

Herbal Traditions

Herbal paradigms vary by cultural tradition. Three major herbology systems utilized worldwide are from Western medicine, traditional Chinese medicine, and Ayurvedic medicine.

The Western herbal tradition relies primarily on the pharmacologic action of herbs, most of which are derived from the plant kingdom. There are presently 119 plant-derived pharmaceutical medicines. Plant chemicals constitute about 25 percent of prescriptions by conventional health-care professionals, and another 30 percent are for medicines from plant products.

Herbology is used in traditional Chinese medicine to enhance the flow and amount of chi and to restore the harmonious balance of the complementary forces of yin and yang and the five elements (fire, earth, metal, water, and wood). Medicinal plants are prescribed and evaluated based on their effects on the five elements and their corresponding organs, tissues, emotions, temperatures (climates), and other qualities. The five elements give rise to the five tastes that produce particular medicinal actions. Bitter-tasting herbs (fire) act to dry and drain. Sweet tasting herbs (earth) reduce pain and increase tone. Acrid herbs (metal) serve to disperse. Salty herbs (water) nourish the kidney. Sour herbs (wood) astringe to preserve chi and to nourish yin. Herbs are also symbolically classified according to temperature changes they are said to bring about in the body in the treatment of conditions: cold, cool, neutral, warm, and hot. The temperatures correspond to the symbolic climate qualities of the organs and the five elements.

> *The pharmaceutical qualities of most plants have yet to be documented, so their toxicities are relatively unknown. The world supports an estimated 250,000 to 500,000 flowering plant species, but only 5000 have been researched for their pharmacologic attributes.*

The taste or "essence" of the herb is also integral to the herbology of Ayurvedic medicine. Ayurveda recognizes six essences (sweet, sour, salty, pungent, bitter, and astringent) and five elements (ether, water, fire, air, and earth). The elements are manifested as three doshas or humors (vata, pitta, and kapha) that govern body functioning and that must be kept in balance to maintain or restore a healthy state. Vata, the principle of air, wind, or movement, is decreased by herbs that are sweet, sour, and salty, which exert a symbolic heating effect on the body. Vata is increased by herbs that are pungent, bitter, astringent, and cooling. Pitta, the principle of fire, is decreased by herbs that are sweet, bitter, astringent, and cooling and increased by those that are pungent, sour, salty, and heating. Kapha, the principle of water, is decreased by herbs that are pungent, bitter, astringent, and heating and increased by those that are sweet, sour, salty, and cooling.

Concerns About Alternative Therapies

There is growing concern in the United States about the use of herbal preparations by the general public without consultation with either conventional health-care professionals or alternative healers. In 1999, herbal sales exceeded $1.5 billion and are expected to exceed $5 billion in 2000. Another concern is the lack of licensing and standards for herbalists. Except for naturopaths, most herbalists have no foundation in phytochemistry or botanical medicine. Also, in other cultural traditions, herbs are not prescribed based on the biologic effects of their chemical ingredients. They are commonly prescribed based on the "doctrine of signatures" or their physical and taste characteristics. For example, herbs with heart shaped leaves may be used to treat heart problems; those with red flowers or leaves may be used to control bleeding or blood disorders; and those with a sour taste may be given to decrease swelling or counteract the effects of "sugar" (diabetes mellitus).

Additional problems may arise because the public views most herbal remedies as natural products and therefore considers them to be pure, safe, relatively harmless, and more healthy than manufactured medicines. The pharmaceutical qualities of most plants have yet to be documented, so their toxicities are relatively unknown. The world supports an estimated 250,000 to 500,000 flowering plant species, but only 5000 have been researched for their pharmacologic attributes.

The Paradox of Alternative Healing Practices

Variation in definitions and concepts of alternative and complementary healing modalities, their widespread use, and the lack of regulation of alternative healers present nurses with a paradox. It arises because most nursing knowledge comes from the biomedical sciences, but most alternative modalities (1) have not yet been scientifically validated or proven safe based on the scientific method and (2) are based in concepts of holism, self-care, and theoretical constructs that emanate from worldviews different from that of biomedicine and the scientific perspective.

In other words, for most alternative modalities, little is known about if or how they work, their side effects, or their interactions with conventional or other alternative modalities. Claims regarding their effectiveness come largely from testimonials of users or alternative healers rather than from evidence in scientific studies. Equally limited is valid knowledge about which conditions the various alternative modalities are effective against and about their short- and long-term effects.

Central to the credibility of the nursing profession is decision-making based on knowledge derived primarily from the scientific method, as well as thinking critically, being culture competent, and promoting self-care by clients able to make informed choices about their health-care options.

The technical competence and knowledge of alternative healers are of considerable importance for nurses caring for patients who pursue alternative and complementary practices. Nurses and the general public are accustomed to determining the qualifications, assumed competency, and scope of practice of conventional health-care practitioners through externally regulated mechanisms, such as graduation from an accredited school of the health professions, a state-regulated licensing process, credentialing, and attainment of specialty certifications from professional organizations or institutions of higher education. No such external processes or criteria exist to validate the competence and knowledge of most alternative practitioners.

The relative lack of regulatory standards makes selection of competent alternative practitioners exceedingly difficult. It is a major concern of the public, conventional health-care practitioners, and insurers, because patients may be subject to financial exploitation, ineffective therapies, and psychological and physical abuse.

The challenge presented to nurses by alternative healing modalities relates to professional accountability. Nurses must learn about alternative modalities, their general safety and efficacy, and their use in specific health and illness conditions. Human caring and cultural competence also require that nurses are able to develop therapeutic partnerships with culturally diverse patients, empower them to take charge of their lives and health care, and preserve their right to self-determination, to practice alternative lifestyles, and to pursue a variety of conventional or alternative modalities with or without consulting alternative healers or conventional health-care professionals. As a nurse, you are charged with both keeping an open mind and relying on sound evidence for your recommendations about alternative practices and practitioners.

Ask Questions

Box 22–4 lists questions that you should ask when attempting to determine the quality and validity of information about an alternative modality when scientific research is limited or nonexistent. Teach your clients to ask similar questions as they ponder their potential use of an alternative therapy and the often conflicting advice they receive

Box 22–4

Questions to Ask About Alternative Modalities

1. What evidence exists that the therapy is effective/harmful?
   - Is there experimental evidence? How effective is the alternative modality when examined experimentally?
   - Is there clinical practice evidence? How effective is the alternative modality when applied clinically?
   - Is there comparative evidence? How effective is the modality when compared with other treatments?
   - Is there summary evidence? Has the modality been evaluated and a consensus reached regarding its use and effectiveness for various health conditions?
   - Is there demand evidence? Is the modality wanted by clients and/or practitioners?
   - Is there satisfaction evidence? Does the alternative modality meet the expectations of clients and/or practitioners?
   - Is there cost evidence? Is the modality covered by health insurance? Is it cost effective?
   - Is the meaning evident? Is the modality the best and right one for the client?
2. How strong is the evidence? Is it based on testimonials, clinical observations, or scientific research?
3. Can the results be attributed to the placebo effect? Is the benefit from the placebo effect adequate to alleviate the client's needs?
4. Does evidence exist that the benefits of the therapy outweigh the risks?
   - Is the alternative modality potentially useful?
   - Is the modality essentially without value except for the potential placebo effect?
   - Is the modality potentially harmful?
5. Is there another way to obtain the same hoped-for results?
6. Who else has tried this alternative modality, and what was their experience?
7. Are there reputable (licensed and certified) alternative healers available? What has been their experience with this alternative modality?
8. What information do regulatory agencies have about the modality or the alternative healers?
9. What information is available in the popular media about the modality or alternative healers? Has it/can be verified by clinical observations or research studies?

Sources: Barrocas, A: Complementary and alternative medicine: Friend, foe or OWA (other weird arrangements). J Am Diet Assoc 97:1373, 1997.

Kurtzweil, P: An FDA Guide to Dietary Supplements. January 1999 [On-line]. Available at: http://vm.cfsan.fda.gov/~dms/fdsupp.html.

Micozzi, MS (ed): Fundamentals of Complementary and Alternative Medicine. Churchill Livingstone, New York, 1996.

National Center for Complementary and Alternative Medicine: Considering CAM? March 1, 2000 [On-line]. Available at: wysiwyg://22/http://nccam.nih.gov/nccam/fcp/faq/considercam.html.

National Center for Complementary and Alternative Medicine: NCCAM Clearinghouse. April 6, 2000 [On-line]. Available at: wysiwyg://3/http://nccam.nih.gov/nccam/faq/clearinghouse/index.html.

Spencer, JC, and Jacobs, JJ: Complementary/Alternative Medicine: An Evidence-Based Approach. Mosby, St. Louis, 1999.

from family, friends, conventional health-care professionals, alternative healers, and the media.

Many clients use alternative healing modalities without ever talking to a conventional health professional about it. They may fear a negative reaction. Others are not aware of the potential harm that may occur, especially when combining alternative therapies or alternative and conventional therapies. Some may consider the scientific evidence and conclude that most noninvasive and nondrug alternative therapies are harmless. Others may mistakenly assume that alternative modalities are regulated by the government and would not be available if they were dangerous.

Find Information

Lack of scientific information about alternative healing modalities is of concern to alternative healers, conventional health-care professionals, and clients. For yourself and your clients, you will need to know where and how to find up-to-date, reliable information on alternative modalities. The NCCAM offers one of the best general governmental resources for information on alternative modalities. You can find the NCCAM Web site at http://nccam.nih.gov.

Several authoritative sources on herbal medicines are available for practitioners and clients. The FDA maintains a site for reporting and obtaining information about adverse effects and interactions of herbals through MedWatch (800-FDA-1088 or http://www.fda.gov/medwatch). FA Davis maintains a Web site on herbal medicines (http://www.DrugGuide. com) as does the United States Pharmacopeia (http://www.usp.org/information/index.html). The American Botanical Society (512- 926-4900) has a Web site (http://www. herbal gram.org) and publishes the *Herbalgram*, a newsletter on herbal medications. MICROMEDEX has an evidence-based series on herbal medicines and dietary supplements, toxicologies, clinical protocols, and client education (800-643-8116 or http://www.micomedex.com). It also links to the electronic database on herbal medicines from the Royal Pharmaceutical Society of Great Britain. Tyler's *The Honest Herbal* is one of the most reputable guides for the use of herbs. *The Physician's Desk Reference for Herbal Medicine* contains scientific findings on the efficacy, potential interactions, clinical trials, and case reports of herbs, as well as indexes on Asian, Ayurvedic, and homeopathic herbs.

An English translation of *The Complete German Commission E Monographs: Therapeutic Guide to Herbal Medicine* is a compendium of monographs published by Commission E, a panel of experts responsible for regulating herbal products in Germany, much as is done by the FDA in the United States. It contains information about the therapeutics of individual herbs, dosages, adverse effects, and pharmacology. The lack of regulatory standards for herbal products in the United States poses problems in applying findings from Commission E to herbal products manufactured in this country.

What Do You Think?

Does the facility where you do your clinical practice ask about alternative therapies during the admission assessment? Are you taught to assess for this information in your nursing program?

A growing number of clients and even professionals are turning to the Internet for information about alternative products and local practitioners of alternative therapies. Because information posted to the Internet is not regulated, this avenue of inquiry requires caution. Only one Web site is available with reputable information about ACH and specific modalities.

- Quackwatch (http://www.quackwatch. com/) offers fact sheets and reviews of specific alternative modalities, as well as those associated with certain illnesses. It also has sections on how to determine whether a Web site devoted to alternative modalities is trustworthy.

Above all, do not neglect to ask your clients about their use of alternative therapies. Not doing so may place clients at risk for adverse health outcomes. When and how to actually assess for the use of ACH during the client-assessment process is a matter of judgment and should be guided by your knowledge of individual clients. An appropriate time is often after the chief complaint has been documented, because this is the time when you explore clients' reasons for seeking health care and investigate what they have already done for their problem. Discuss the use of alternative therapies tactfully and supportively. Keep complete and accurate documentation of your interactions with patients about alternative therapies and healers. And as much as possible, help direct clients toward the safest therapies and the most qualified practitioners.

Critical Thinking Exercises

1. Contact three of the Web sites on alternative practices listed in the chapter. Evaluate them according to their quality, content, and usefulness to your practice.

2. Identify a nurse practitioner or physician or other health-care provider in your area who uses alternative practices. Interview that person and arrange for a presentation to the class about alternative health-care practices.

3. Select a client from your clinical experiences who is having pain. How might alternative practices help this client? Develop a care plan using both traditional and alternative methods for pain control.

4. Identify and discuss three advantages of and three problems with alternative health-care practices.

5. Select three nursing theories from Chapter 4 that use a holistic approach to nursing. Identify how and what alternative practices would work well with each one of these theories.

Conclusion

Alternative and nontraditional health-care practices are a growing part of health care in the United States. It is essential that nurses become aware of what these practices entail and how they may affect or interact with conventional therapies that the client is already receiving. Admission assessments for these practices, when clients enter the health-care system for whatever reason, should become a routine part of client evaluation. Nurses traditionally have approached health care from a holistic viewpoint that addresses all of the client's needs—mind, body, and spirit. As health care moves more toward alternative practices, nurses would be the logical choice to coordinate a comprehensive approach to health care that includes both traditional and alternative practices. Without this coordination, an already fragmented health-care system will become even more fragmented.

Glossary of Terms for Alternative and Complementary Healing

Acupressure From traditional Chinese medicine. Practitioner uses fingers or hands to apply pressure over acupuncture points on meridians to restore or enhance the flow of chi to maintain or restore balance.

Acupressure massage Practitioner uses massage techniques such as rubbing, kneading, percussion, and vibration over acupuncture points to improve circulation of chi.

Acupuncture From traditional Chinese medicine. Now commonly considered a complete treatment system on its own. The object of acupuncture is to re-establish the balance of energy in the body by inserting needles along meridian channels to alleviate blockage of chi. The points of insertion are believed to be linked to internal body organs.

Alexander technique A type of bodywork developed by Frederick Matthias Alexander to decrease muscle tension and fatigue, stress, and back and neck pain. Based on the belief that poor posture during daily activities contributes to physical and emotional problems. Use of body posture realignment through imaging and relaxation.

Allopathic medicine From Greek words *allos* (other) and *pathos* (suffering). A synonym for conventional medicine. Practitioner uses medicines to counteract symptoms or heal by producing different effects or a second condition different from the one being treated.

Applied kinesiology Study of muscle activity and strength and heath effects via the muscle-gland-organ link. Muscle dysfunction may be counteracted by nutrition, manual procedures (such as massage), applying pressure over muscle attachment points, and realignment.

Aromatherapy A type of herbal medicine. Uses odors of essential oils extracted from plants to treat various conditions, such as headaches, tension, and anxiety. Chemical composition of the oils provides pharmacologic effects that include antibacterial, antiviral, antispasmodic, diuretic, vasodilatation, and mood-harmonizing actions. The oils may be applied via massage, inhaled, placed in baths and other forms of hydrotherapy, or taken internally.

Art therapy Use of artistic self-expression through drawing, sculpture, and painting to diagnose and treat behavioral or emotional problems.

Aura Magnetic field said to surround every person, plant, and animal. Adjustment of the field is said to affect health, emotions, spirit, and mind.

Auriculotherapy Also known as ear acupuncture and developed in France. Points on the external ear are believed to have neurologic connection to other body areas. The points can be stimulated with acupuncture needles, massage, electronic stimulation, or infrared treatment.

Ayurvedic medicine From East Indian medicine. A personalistic, holistic, and naturalistic approach to health maintenance and treatment of illness. Maintains balance of the three doshas (bioenergies) of the body through diet and herbs, meditation, breathing exercises (pranayama), massage with medicated oils, yoga and other forms of vigorous exercise, and exposure to the sun for higher consciousness.

Bach flower essences Originated by Edward Bach, an English physician. Homeopathic preparations of oil concentrates extracted from flowers are administered to remedy emotional states rather than treating the signs and symptoms of physical illness. Specific concentrates or combinations of concentrates are associated with various emotional states. Each client is diagnosed individually because there is no corresponding psychological equivalent for every physical state.

Biofeedback Form of training that helps a person to consciously control or change normally unconscious body functions to improve overall health. Also refers to the method of immediately reporting back to the person information about a biologic process that is being measured so the person can consciously alter or influence the process.

Bodywork General term used to describe various forms of massage therapy, energy balancing, deep-tissue manipulation, and movement awareness.

Botanical medicine Use of the entire plant or herb for treating illness or maintaining health.

Chakras Circles found along the midline of the body, in alignment with the spinal cord, that distribute energy throughout the body. If blocked, energy flow is inhibited.

Chelation therapy From the Greek word *chele* (to bind or to claw). Chelation uses minerals combined with amino acids, given intravenously or orally, to help cleanse the body of unnecessary or toxic minerals that block blood circulation.

Chi (Qi, Shi) From traditional Chinese medicine. Chi is the invisible life-force that circulates through the body along meridians, or channels. Maintaining or restoring the flow of chi restores and promotes health.

Chiropractic A Western medical system that postulates that partial joint dislocations (subluxations) cause the body to be misaligned. Removal or adjustment of subluxations balances the spinal-nervous system and restores and maintains health.

Craniosacral therapy *Cranio* refers to the cranium and *sacral* to the sacrum. In this therapy, bones of the skull are manipulated to treat craniosacral dysfunctions caused by restriction in the flow of cerebrospinal fluid and misalignment of bones.

Crystal therapy Also called *gem therapy*. Quartz and other gemstones are believed to emit electromagnetic energy. Used frequently with light and color therapy.

Cupping From traditional Chinese and Ayurvedic medicines. Practitioner places a heated cup over the skin to draw out impurities, decrease blood pressure, increase circulation, and relieve muscle pain.

Curanderismo From the Spanish verb *to heal*. Healing tradition found in Mexican-American communities. Based in concepts of supernaturalism, balance, holism, and natural world illnesses.

Dance therapy Use of dance movement to enhance wellness and aid healing. Sharpens levels of awareness, enhances self-confidence, helps with motor coordination and physical skills, and assists with communication, especially with severely disturbed psychiatric clients.

Doshas Three (*vata*, *pitta*, and *kapha*) basic metabolic types, life-forces, or bioenergies in Ayurvedic medicine. Each has certain characteristics and tendencies that combine to determine a person's constitution. When in balance, mind and body are coordinated, resulting in vibrant health and energy. When out of balance, the body is susceptible to outside stressors, such as microorganisms, poor nutrition, and work overload.

Energy medicine Measurement of electromagnetic frequencies emitted by the body. The object is to diagnose energy imbalances that may cause or contribute to present or future illnesses and to use electromagnetic forces to counteract imbalances and restore the body's energy balance.

Environmental medicine Explores the role of environmental and dietary allergens in health and illness.

Feldenkrais method A type of bodywork or physical movement developed by Moshe Feldenkrais that stresses awareness through movement and helps the body to work with gravity. Incorporates imaging, active moving, and forms of directed attention designed to re-educate the nervous system, teach subjects how to learn from their own kinesic feedback, and avoid movements that strain joints and muscles.

Gerson therapy Metabolic therapy developed by Max Gerson, a German physician. It is based on the belief that cancer results from metabolic dysfunctions in cells that can be countered by detoxification, a vegetarian diet, coffee enemas to stimulate excretion of liver bile, and the exclusion of sodium and an abundance of potassium.

Guided imagery A facilitated flow of thoughts that helps a person see, feel, taste, smell, hear, and touch something in the imagination. The power of the mind or imagination is used to stimulate positive physical responses and provide insight into health and an understanding of emotions as a cause of ill health.

Healing touch Healing tradition based in the belief of a universal energy system. Humans are seen as interpenetrating layers of energy systems just above and outside the body that are integrated with energy fields in the environment. Manipulation of such energy fields through touch can help restore a person's energy balance and health.

Hellerwork A type of bodywork developed by Joseph Heller as an outgrowth of Rolfing. It combines dialog, body movement education, and deep touch to achieve greater mind-body awareness and structural body alignment with gravitational forces. Therapy is individualized to different body types.

Herbal medicine The most ancient known form of health care. Also known as botanical medicine, phytotherapy, and phytomedicine. It uses the chemical makeup of herbs in much the same manner as conventional medicine uses pharmaceuticals. Herbal medicine is basic to traditional Chinese, Ayurvedic, and American Indian medical systems.

Homeopathy A Western medical system based on the principle "like cures like." Natural substances are prescribed in minute dilutions to cause the symptoms of the disease they are intended to cure, helping the body cure itself.

Humor therapy Deliberate use of laughter to improve quality of life by encouraging relaxation and stress reduction, distracting individuals from awareness of constant pain, and providing symptom relief.

Hydrotherapy Also known as "water cure." Use of hot, cold, or contrasting temperatures to maintain or restore health. Water, steam, or ice may be used in combination with baths, compresses, hot and cold packs, showers, and enemas or colonic irrigations. Minerals, herbs, and oils may be added to enhance the therapeutic effects.

Hypnotherapy Use of hypnosis, power of suggestion, and trance-like states to access the deepest levels of the mind to bring about changes in behavior, treat health conditions, and manage medical and psychological problems.

Integrative medicine *Integrative* is synonymous with *complementary*. This is practiced by conventional health-care professionals who prescribe a combination of therapies from both systems.

Iridiology Iris diagnosis. In this belief system, each area of the body has a corresponding point on the iris of the eye. Thus, the state of health (balance) or disease (imbalance) can be diagnosed from the color, texture, or location of pigments in the eye.

Jin Shin Jyutsu A Japanese form of massage in which combinations of healing points on the body are held for a minute or more with the fingertips. The purpose is to enhance or restore the flow of chi.

Light and color therapy A method by which light is converted into electrical impulses, travels along the optic nerve to the brain, and stimulates the hypothalamus to send neurotransmitters to regulate the autonomic nervous system. Various colors of light are believed to stimulate different parts of the body.

Magnet therapy A type of electromagnetic therapy or energy medicine in which magnets are used to stimulate circulation, increase oxygen to cells, and facilitate healing by correcting disturbed or malfunctioning electromagnetic frequencies that the body emits.

Mantra A technique of Ayurvedic medicine used to reach a higher level of spiritual and mental functioning. It is a type of sound therapy used to change the "vibratory patterns of the mind" to release unconscious negative thoughts, psychological stress, and emotional distress. Often achieved by uttering a mystical word or phrase and associated with meditation.

Meditation Known as "mind-cure" or the use of contemplation to exercise the mind, which is an unseen force of healing. Thoughts and deep feelings are believed to be the primary arbiters of health through relaxation. Also known as a form of mental cleansing that enhances self-awareness and awareness of one's environment.

Megavitamin therapy A type of orthomolecular medicine in which diseases are prevented and cured by taking doses of vitamins larger than the normal or recommended amounts needed for general good health or prevention of deficiencies. The disease to be treated or prevented determines the type, dosage, and mode of administration of vitamins, minerals, and nutrient supplements.

Meridians From traditional Chinese medicine. Meridians are invisible channels by which chi flows through the body. Blockage along a meridian causes illness.

Mind-body medicine Healing based on the interconnectedness of the mind and body, individual responsibility for self-care, and the self-healing capabilities of the body. Uses a wide range of modalities, such as imaging, massage, hypnotherapy, meditation, yoga, concepts of balance, herbs, and diet.

Moxibustion From traditional Chinese medicine. Burning of *moxa* (dried or powered herbs) on or close to acupuncture points on the meridians to restore or improve the flow of chi.

Music therapy Use of music to enhance well-being and promote healing. Helps improve physical and mental functioning, alleviate pain, ease the psychological discomfort of illness, and improve quality of life, especially of terminally ill persons. Aids ability of mentally handicapped, autistic, and elderly persons with dementia to interact with others, learn, and relate to their environments.

Naturopathy A Western healing system. Heals through holism, use of natural substances, treating cause rather than symptoms (effects), empowering and motivating individuals to take responsibility for their own health, preventing disease through lifestyle and education, and doing no harm beyond using safe, natural therapies.

Neurolinguistic programming Focuses on how individuals learn, communicate, and change. *Neuro* refers to how the brain works and the consistent and observable patterns that emanate from human thinking. *Linguistic* refers to the expression (verbal and nonverbal) of those patterns of thinking. *Programming* refers to how such patterns of thinking are interpreted and how they can be changed. Changing the patterns gives people the ability to make better choices for healthy behavior.

Orthodox Used as a synonym for conventional, Western, scientific, biomedicine, or official health-care system.

Orthomolecular medicine *Ortho* means normal or correct. This system treats physiologic and psychological disorders by re-establishing, normalizing, or creating the optimal nutritional balance in the body by administering vitamins, minerals, amino acids, and other types of nutritional substances.

Osteopathy A Western system of medicine that considers the structural integrity of the body the most important factor in maintaining and restoring the person to health. The structural integrity or balance of the musculoskeletal system is maintained through physical therapy, joint manipulation, and postural re-education.

Oxygen therapy Use of various forms of oxygen to destroy pathogens and promote body healing. Includes hyperbaric, ozone, and hydrogen peroxide therapies.

Pharmacognosy Scientific study of the chemical properties of plants and natural products. A goal is to standardize herbal products to make sure they are free of harmful components and contain the identical amount of active ingredients.

Phytomedicine/phytotherapy A branch of botanical medicine especially prominent in Europe that includes the pharmaceutical study and therapeutic use of herbs, herbal derivatives, and herbal synthetics. Merges ancient herbal traditions with contemporary scientific investigation to standardize the active ingredients of herbal products.

Polarity therapy A combination of bodywork therapies and other hands-on techniques to restore the natural flow of energy through the body. Other therapies may include reflexology, hydrotherapy, and breathing techniques.

Prana From Ayurvedic medicine. Vital energy or life-force that runs through the body.

Qi Gong (Chi Kung, Chi Gong) From traditional Chinese medicine. Combines movement, meditation and deep relaxation, and regulation of breathing to enhance the flow of chi throughout the body to nourish vital organs.

Reflexology In this belief system, every part of the body has a corresponding area on the hands and feet. Thus, body parts can be stimulated by applying pressure to the appropriate sites on the hands or feet. Reflexology is applied to relieve tension, improve circulation, promote relaxation, and restore energy balance by unblocking nerve impulses.

Reiki An ancient Buddhist version of healing touch practiced in Tibet and Japan. The word also means universal life-force. Energy is transferred to the person through the hands of the healer to restore energy balance in the body.

Relaxation response Physiologic mechanism described by Herbert Benson in which body stress is reduced through regulation of internal activity, such as reduced metabolism and slowing of other physiologic reactions.

Relaxation therapy Use of the relaxation response to reduce stress through release of physical and emotional tension. Various therapies are commonly included in other types of therapeutic programs. Examples are mind-body therapies such as biofeedback, hydrotherapy, imaging/visualization, meditation, qi gong, Tai Chi, and yoga.

Rolfing Developed by Ida Rolf. Technique of deep massage using the knuckles that is designed to counteract the effects of gravity on body balance. Fascia, connective tissue, and muscle are loosened and lengthened to help them return to their correct position.

Rosen technique A type of bodywork in which muscle tension is seen as repressed emotional conflicts. Deep and gentle pressure is applied as persons are questioned about what they are experiencing.

Shamanism Ancient healing approach found in most cultural systems. Shamans communicate with the spirit world via trances and other altered states of consciousness. They attempt to control spirits and effect change in the physical world. The belief is that the soul of the shaman separates from the body and explores the cosmos in search of cures for ill patients.

Sound therapy Elements of sound affect different parts of the brain, regulate corticosteroid hormone levels, and can affect the body's own rhythmic patterns.

Shiatsu Japanese form of massage whose literal meaning is *finger pressure*. Consists of firm pressure in a sequential and rhythmic manner. Pressure is exerted for 3 to 10 seconds on points along the body that correspond to acupuncture meridians. It is designed to "awaken the meridian."

Spiritual healing Cosmic healing energy is transferred or channeled from practitioner to client via laying on of the hands.

Swedish massage The most common form of massage, it focuses on superficial muscle layers. Practitioner uses kneading, friction, and long, gliding strokes to relieve muscle tension and promote relaxation.

Tai Chi From traditional Chinese medicine. Derived from qi gong but practiced at a much slower pace. Also one of the body-mind therapies. Combines contemplation (meditation) with movement or "moving meditation" and coordinated breathing.

Therapeutic massage Manipulation of soft tissues through a variety of techniques to affect the circulatory, lymphatic, and nervous systems.

Therapeutic touch A healing touch modality that does not involve actual touching of the patient's body. The therapist's hands are used to sense and interact with the client's energy field to redirect it, alleviate energy blockage, and restore balance.

Traditional Chinese medicine A complete system of healing based on the concept of the uninterrupted flow of chi or vital essence and the concept of balance (yin and yang), representing corresponding and interrelated elements in the internal world of the body and the external world. All illness is attributed ultimately to a disturbance of chi.

Trager therapy A method of bodywork developed by Milton Trager. Use of gentle, rhythmic touch and movement exercises to assist in the release of accumulated tensions. Uses sensory-motor feedback or mental gymnastics (Mentastics) to learn how body moves. Purpose is to develop the ability to move more effortlessly.

Vibration medicine Healing systems that treat the body on an energy level. Cure is effected by ingestion of substances that adjust energy or rate of energy field vibration. Homeopathy is an example.

Visualization Also called guided imagery, centering, focusing, meditation, or distraction. Use of the imagination or power of the mind to get in touch with one's inner self. Involves all, several, or one of the senses to bridge the mind, body, and spirit.

Yin/yang Complementary but opposing phenomena or correspondents in Taoist philosophical thought that form the underpinning of traditional Chinese medicine. Yin and yang represent the interdependence of all elements of nature and body and mind. Yin represents the female force and passive, still, reflective aspects. Yang represents the male force and active, warm, moving aspects. For health to be maintained and wellness achieved, yin and yang must be in balance.

Yoga Means *union* or the integration of mental, physical, and spiritual energies. Part of Ayurvedic medicine. The integration is accomplished through exercise in the form of assuming different body postures, meditation, and breathing.

Bibliography

Barrocas, A: Complementary and alternative medicine: Friend, foe or OWA (other weird arrangements). J Am Diet Assoc 97:1373, 1997.

Bodeker, GC: Global health traditions. In Micozzi, M (ed): Fundamentals of Complementary and Alternative Medicine. Churchill Livingstone, New York, 1996, p. 279.

Eisenberg, DM, et al: Trends in alternative medicine use in the United States, 1990–1997. JAMA 280:1569, 1998.

Fisher, P, and Ward, A: Complementary medicine in Europe. BMJ 309:107, 1994.

Glisson, J, et al: Review, critique, and guidelines for the use of herbs and homeopathy. Nurse Practitioner 24:44, 1999.

Jonas, WB: Alternative medicine: An overview. CARING Magazine, December 1996, p. 16.

The mainstreaming of alternative medicine. Consumer Reports, May 2000, p. 17.

National Center for Complementary and Alternative Medicine: Frequently Asked Questions. March 1, 2000 [On-line]. Available at: wysiwyg://18/http://nccam.nih.gov/nccam/fcp/faq/index.html.

Spencer, JC, and Jacobs, JJ: Complementary/Alternative Medicine: An Evidence-Based Approach. Mosby, St. Louis, 1999.

World Health Organization: WHO's Policy and Activities on the Traditional Medicine. 1999 [On-line]. Available at: http://www.who.int/dap/trm0.html.

Glossary

abandonment Leaving a client without the client's permission; terminating the professional relationship without providing for appropriate continued or follow-up care by another equally qualified professional.

accountability Concept that each individual is responsible for his or her own actions and the consequence of those actions; professional accountability implies a responsibility to perform the activities and duties of the profession according to established standards.

accreditation Approval of a program or institution by a voluntary professional organization to provide specific education or service programs.

act Legislation that has become law.

active euthanasia Acts performed to help end a sick person's life.

acute-severe condition Health problem of sudden onset; a serious illness or condition.

adaptation Process of exchange between a person and the environment to maintain or regain personal integrity; the key principle in the Roy Model of Nursing.

administrative A governmental agency that implements legislation agency.

administrative rule or regulation An operating procedure that describes how a government agency implements the intent of a statute; state boards of nursing implement the nurse practice act.

advanced nursing education Master's or doctoral level education that provides knowledge and skills in areas such as research, education, administration, or clinical specialties.

advanced placement A process by which a student is given credit for a required course through transfer or examination rather than by enrolling in and completing the course.

advanced practice Extended role; increased responsibilities and actions undertaken by an individual because of additional education and experience; nurse practitioners are advanced practice nurses.

advocate One who pleads for a cause or proposal; one who acts on behalf of another.

affidavit Written sworn statement.

affiliation agreement A formal agreement between an educational institution and another agency that agrees to provide clinical areas for student practice.

aggressiveness Harsh behavior that may result in physical or emotional harm to others.

ambulatory care center Type of primary care facility that provides treatment on an outpatient basis.

answer Document filed in the court by the defendant in response to the complaint.

anxiety Uneasiness or apprehension caused by an impending threat or fear of the unknown.

apathy Lack of interest.

appeal Request to a higher court to review a decision in the hopes of changing the ruling of a lower court.

appellant Person who seeks an appeal.

arbitrator Neutral third party who assesses facts independently of the judicial system.

articulation Type of education program that allows easy entry from one level to another; for example, many BSN programs have articulation for nurses with an associate degree.

artificial insemination Insertion of sperm into the uterus with a syringe.

assault Attempt or threat to touch.

assertiveness Ability to express thoughts, feelings, and ideas openly and directly without fear.

assessment Process of collecting information about a client, to help plan care.

associate degree nursing program Type of nursing education program that leads to an associate degree with a major in nursing; usually located in a community or junior college, these programs nominally last 2 years.

audit Close review of records or documents to detect the presence or absence of specific information.

auscultation Assessment technique that requires listening with a stethoscope to various parts of the body to detect sounds produced by organs.

authoritarian A type of leadership style in which the leader gives orders, makes decisions for the group as a whole, and bears most of the responsibility for the outcomes. Also called autocratic, directive, or controlling.

autonomy State of being self-directed or independent; the ability to make decisions about one's future.

autopsy Examination of a body after death to determine the cause of death.

baccalaureate degree nursing program Type of nursing education program that leads to the bachelor's degree with a major in nursing; usually located in a college or university, the length of the program is 4 years.

bargaining agent Organization certified by a governmental agency to represent a group of employees for the purpose of collective bargaining.

baseline data Initial information obtained about a client that establishes the norms for comparison as the client's condition changes.

basic human rights Those considerations society deems reasonably expected for all people; right to self-determination, protection from discomfort and harm, dignity, fair treatment, and privacy.

battery Nonconsensual touching of another person that does not necessarily cause harm or injury.

behaviorism Psychological theory based on the belief that all behavior is learned over time through conditioning.

behavior modification Method to change behavior through rewards for positive behavior.

belief Expectations or judgments based on attitude verified by experiences.

beneficence Ethical principle based on the beliefs that the health-care provider should do no harm, prevent harm, remove existing harm, and promote the good and well-being of the client.

bereavement State of sadness brought on by the loss or death of a significant other.

bill Proposed law that is moving through the legislative process.

bill of rights List of statements that outline the claims and privileges of a particular group, such as the Client's Bill of Rights.

bioethical issues Issues that deal with the health, safety, life, and death of human beings, often arising from advances in medical science and technology.

biofeedback Ability to control autonomic response in the body through conscious effort.

body substance isolation (BSI) Universal precautions; guidelines established by the Centers for Disease Control and Prevention (CDC) and the Occupational Safety and Health Administration (OSHA) to protect health-care professionals and the client from diseases carried in the blood and body fluids, such as HIV and hepatitis B; involves the use of gloves whenever one is in contact with blood or body fluids and the use of masks, gowns, and eye covers if a chance of aerosol contact with fluids exists.

brain death Irreversible destruction of the cerebral cortex and brain stem manifested by absence of all reflexes; absence of brain waves on an electroencephalogram.

breach of contract Failure by one of the parties in a contract to fulfill all the terms of the agreement.

burden of proof Requirement that the plaintiff submit sufficient evidence to prove a defendant's guilt.

burnout syndrome A state of emotional exhaustion that results from the accumulative stress of an individual's life, including work, personal, and family responsibilities.

cadaver donor Clinically or brain-dead individual who previously agreed to allow organs to be taken for transplantation.

capitated payment system System of reimbursement in which a flat fee is paid for health-care services for a prescribed period of time. Expenses incurred in excess of this fee are provider losses.

capricious Unpredictable; arbitrary.

career ladder Articulation of educational programs that permit advancement from a lower level to a higher level without loss of credit or repetition of coursework.

career mobility Opportunity for individuals in one occupational area to move to another without restrictions.

case management Health-care delivery in which a client advocate/health-care coordinator helps the client through the hospitalization to obtain the most appropriate care.

case manager Health-care provider who coordinates cost-effective quality care for individuals who are generally at high risk and require long-term complex services.

certification Official recognition of a degree of education and skills in a profession by a national specialty organization; recognition that an institution has met standards that allow it to deliver certain services.

challenge examination Examination that assesses levels of knowledge or skill to grant credit for previous learning and experience; passing a challenge examination gives the individual credit for a course not actually taken.

chart Legal document that contains all the pertinent information about a client who is in a hospital or clinic; usually includes medical and nursing history, medical and nursing diagnosis, laboratory test results, notes about the client's progress, physician's orders, and personal data.

charting Process of recording (written or computer-generated) specific information about the client in the chart or medical record.

civil law Law concerned with the violation of the rights of one individual by another; it includes contract law, treaty law, tax law, and tort law.

claims-made policy A type of malpractice insurance that protects only against claims made during the time the policy is in effect.

client More modern term for patient; an individual seeking or receiving health-related services.

client goal Statement about a desired change, outcome, or activity that a client should achieve by a specific time.

clinical education Hands-on part of a nursing program that allows the student to practice skills on actual clients under the supervision of a nursing instructor.

clinical forensic nurse Professional nurse who specializes in management of crime victims from trauma to trial through collection of evidence, assessment of victims or making judgments related to client treatment associated with court-related issues.

clinical ladder Type of performance evaluation and career advancement in which nursing positions for direct client care have two or more progressive levels of required skill leading to advancement in salary and responsibility; it allows nurses to remain in direct client care while making career advancements rather than having to move into administration.

clinical pathways Case-management protocols used to enhance quality care, encourage cost-effectiveness, and promote efficiency.

closed system System that does not exchange energy, matter, or information with the environment or with other systems.

code of ethics Written values of a profession that act as guidelines for professional behavior.

collective bargaining Negotiations for wages, hours, benefits, and working conditions for a group of employees.

collective bargaining unit Group of employees, recognized as representatives of the majority, with the right to bargain collectively with their employer and to reach an agreement on the terms of a contract.

committee Group of legislators, in the House or Senate, assigned to analyze bills on a particular subject.

common law Law based on past judicial judgments made in similar cases.

comparable worth Method for determining employees' salaries within an organization so that the same salary is paid for all jobs that have equivalent educational requirements, responsibilities, and complexity regardless of external market factors.

competencies Behaviors, skills, attitudes, and knowledge that an individual or professional has or is expected to have.

competency-based education Courses or programs based on anticipated student outcomes.

complaint Legal document filed by a plaintiff to initiate a lawsuit, claiming that the plaintiff's legal rights have been violated.

compliance Voluntary following of a prescribed plan of care or treatment regimen.

computer technology Use of highly advanced technological equipment to store, process, and access a vast amount of information.

concept Abstract idea or image.

conceptual framework Concept, theory, or basic idea around which an educational program is organized and developed.

conceptual model Group of concepts, ideas, or theories that are interrelated but in which the relationship is not clearly defined.

confidentiality Right of the client to expect the communication with a professional to remain unshared with any other person unless a medical reason exists or unless the safety of the public is threatened.

consensus General agreement between two or more individuals or groups regarding beliefs or positions on an issue or finding.

consent Voluntary permission given by a competent person.

consortium Two or more agencies that share sponsorship of a program or an institution.

constitutional law Law contained within a federal or state constitution.

continuing care Nursing care generally provided in geriatric day care centers or in the homes of elderly clients.

continuing education Formal education programs and informal learning experiences that maintain and increase the nurse's knowledge and skills in specific areas.

continuing education unit (CEU) Specific unit of credit earned by participating in an approved continuing education program.

continuous quality improvement (CQI) A type of total quality management whose primary goal is the improvement of the quality of health care.

contract Legally binding agreement between two or more parties.

contractual obligation Duty to perform a service identified by a contract.

copayment Percentage of the cost of a medical expense that is not covered by insurance and must be paid by the client.

core curriculum Curriculum design that enables a student to leave a career program at various levels, with a career attained and with the option to continue at another higher level or career; it is organized around a central or core body of knowledge common to the profession.

coroner Elected public official, usually a physician, who investigates deaths from unnatural causes, including homicide, violence, suicide, and other suspicious circumstances.

correctional/institutional nurse Registered nurse who specializes in the health care of those in custody in secure settings such as jails or prisons.

credentialing Process whereby individuals, programs, or institutions are designated as having met minimal standards for the safety and welfare of the public.

crime Violation of criminal law.

criminal action Process by which a person charged with a crime is accused, tried, and punished.

criminal law Law concerned with violation of criminal statutes or laws.

criterion-referenced examination Test that compares an individual's knowledge with predetermined standard rather than to the performance of others who take the same test.

critical thinking The intellectual process of rationally examining ideas, inferences, assumptions, principles, arguments, conclusions, issues, statements, beliefs and actions for which all the relevant information may not be available. This process involves the ability to use the five types of reasoning (scientific, deductive, inductive, informal, practical) in application of the nursing process, decision making, and resolution of ambiguous issues.

curriculum Group of courses that prepare an individual for a specific degree or profession.

customary, prevailing, and reasonable charges The typical rate in a specific locale that payers traditionally reimburse physicians.

damages Money awarded to a plaintiff by a court in a lawsuit that covers the actual costs incurred by the plaintiff.

database Information collected by a computer program on a specific topic in a specified format.

defamation of character Communication of information that is false or detrimental to a person's reputation.

defendant Person accused of criminal or civil wrongdoing. A party to a lawsuit against whom the complaint is served.

delegation Assignment of specific duties by one individual to another individual.

democratic A type of leadership style in which the leader shares in the planning, decision making, and responsibilities for outcomes with the other members of the group. Also called participative leadership.

deontology An ethical system based on the principle that the right action is guided by a set of unchanging rules.

dependent practitioner Provider of care who delivers health care under the supervision of another health-care practitioner; for example, a physician assistant is supervised by a physician, or an LPN is supervised by an RN.

deposition Sworn statement by a witness that is made outside the courtroom; sworn depositions may be admitted as evidence in court when the individual is unable to be present.

diagnosis Statement that describes or identifies a client problem and is based on a thorough assessment.

diagnosis-related groups (DRGs) Prospective payment method used by the U.S. government and many insurance companies that pay a flat fee for treatment of a person with a particular diagnosis.

differentiated practice Organizational process of defining nursing roles based on education, experience, and training.

dilemma Predicament in which a choice must be made between two or more equally balanced alternatives; it often occurs when attempting to make ethical decisions.

directed services Health-care activities that require contact between a health-care professional and a client.

discharge planning Assessment of anticipated client needs after discharge from the hospital and development of a plan to meet those needs before the client is discharged.

disease Illness; a functional disturbance resulting from an individual organism's inability to adapt to certain stressors; an abnormal physiologic state caused by microorganisms, cancer, or other conditions.

distributive justice Ethical principle based on the belief that the right action is determined by that which will provide an outcome equal for all persons and will also benefit the least fortunate.

due process Right to have specific procedures or processes followed before the deprivation of life, liberty, or property; the guarantee of privileges under the Fifth and Fourteenth Amendments to the U.S. Constitution.

duty Obligation to act created by a statute, contract, or voluntary agreement.

emerging health occupations Health-care occupations that are not yet officially recognized by government or professional organizations.

employee Individual hired for pay by another.

Employee Retirement Income Security Act (ERISA) Federal law that grants incentives to employers to offer self-funded health insurance plans to their employees.

employer Individual or organization that hires other individuals for pay to carry out specific duties during certain hours of employment.

empowerment Process in which the individual assumes more autonomy and responsibility for his or her actions.

endorsement Reciprocity; a state's acceptance of a license issued by another state.

end product Output of a system not reusable as input.

energy Capacity to do work.

entry into practice Minimal educational requirements to obtain a license for a profession.

environment Internal and external physical and social boundaries of humans; all those things that are outside a system.

essentials for accreditation The minimal standards that a program must meet to be accredited.

ethical dilemma An ethical situation that requires an individual to make a choice between two equally unfavorable alternatives.

ethical rights (moral rights) Rights that are based on moral or ethical principles but have no legal mechanism of enforcement.

ethical system System of moral judgments based on the beliefs and values of a profession.

ethics Principles or standards of conduct that govern an individual or group.

ethnic group Individuals who share similar physical characteristics, religion, language, or customs.

euthanasia Mercy killing; the act or practice of killing, for reasons of mercy, individuals who have little or no chance of recovery by withholding or discontinuing life support or by administering a lethal agent.

evaluation Fifth step in the nursing process used to determine whether goals set for a client have been attained.

evaluation criteria Outcome criteria; desired behaviors or standards.

expanded role Extended role; increased responsibilities and actions undertaken by an individual because of additional education and experience.

expert witness Individual with knowledge beyond the ordinary person because of special education or training who testifies during a trial.

external degree Academic degree granted when all the requirements have been met by the student; a type of outcomes-based education in which credit is given when the individual demonstrates a certain level of knowledge and skill, regardless of how or when these skills are attained; challenge examinations are often used.

false imprisonment Intentional tort committed by illegally confining or restricting a client against his or her will.

family Two or more related individuals living together.

Federal Tort Claims Act Statute that allows the government to be sued for negligence of its employees in the performance of their duties; many states have similar laws.

feedback Reentry of output into a system as input that helps maintain the internal balance of the system.

fee for service Payment is expected each time a service is rendered. Includes physician office visits, diagnostic procedures (laboratory tests, x-rays) and minor surgical procedures.

fellowship Scholarship or grant that provides money to individuals who are highly qualified or highly intelligent.

felony Serious crime that may be punished by a fine of more than $1000, more than 1 year in jail or prison, death, or a combination thereof.

fidelity The obligation of an individual to be faithful to commitments made to self and others.

for-profit Health-care agencies in which profits can be used to raise capital to pay stock holders dividends on their investments. Also called proprietary agencies.

foreign graduate nurse Individual graduated from a school of nursing outside the United States. This individual is required to pass the U.S. NCLEX-RN CAT to become a registered nurse in the United States.

forensic nurse A registered nurse who specializes in the integration of forensic science and nursing science to apply the nursing process to individual clients, their families, and the community, bridging the gap between the health-care system and the criminal justice system.

forensic psychiatric nurse A registered nurse who specializes in application of psychosocial nursing knowledge linking offending behavior to client characteristics; nurse specializing in forensic psychological evaluation and care of offender populations with mental disorder.

forensic science Body of empirical knowledge used for legal investigation and evidence-based judgment in police or criminal cases.

fraud Deliberate deception in provision of goods or services; lying.

functional nursing Nursing care in which each nurse provides a different aspect of care; nurses are assigned a set of specific tasks to perform for all clients, such as passing medications.

general systems theory Set of interrelated concepts, definitions, and propositions that describes a system.

genetics Scientific study of heredity and related variations.

gerontology Study of the process of aging and of the effects of aging on individuals.

goal Desired outcome.

Good Samaritan Act Law that protects health-care providers from being charged with contributory negligence when they provide emergency care to persons in need of immediate treatment.

grievance Complaint or dispute about the terms or conditions of employment.

group practice Three or more physicians or nurse practitioners in business together to provide health care.

health Complete physical, mental, and social well-being; a relative state along a continuum ranging from severe illness to ideal state of being; the ability to adapt to illness and to reach the highest level of functioning.

health-care consumer Client or patient; an individual who uses health-care service or products.

health-care team Group of individuals of different levels of education who work together to provide help to clients.

health insurance purchasing cooperative (HIPCs) Large groups of people or employers who band together to buy insurance at reduced costs. HIPCs may be organized by private groups or the government.

health maintenance organization (HMO) Prototype of the managed health-care system; method of payment for a full range of primary, secondary, and tertiary health-care services; members pay a fixed annual fee for services and a small deductible when care is actually given.

health policy Goals and directions that guide activities to safeguard and promote the health of citizens.

health practitioner Individual, usually licensed, who provides health-care services to individuals with health-care needs.

health promotion Interventions and behaviors that increase and maintain the level of well-being of persons, families, groups, communities, and society.

health systems agency (HSA) Local voluntary organization of providers and consumers that plans for the health-care services of its geographic region.

hearsay Evidence not based on personal knowledge of the witness and usually not allowed in courts.

holistic Treatment of the total individual,

including physical, psychological, sociologic, and spiritual elements, with emphasis on the interrelatedness of parts and wholes.

home health care Health care services provided in the client's home.

hospice care Alternative way of providing care to terminally ill clients in which palliative care is used; the major goals of hospice care are control of pain, provision of emotional support, promotion of social interaction, and preparation for death; family support measures and anticipatory grieving counseling are also used if appropriate.

hospital privileges Authority granted by a hospital, usually through its medical board, for a health-care practitioner to admit and supervise the treatment of clients within that hospital.

hypothesis Prediction or proposition related to a problem, usually found in research.

ideal role image A projection of society's expectations for nurses that clearly delineates the obligations and responsibilities, as well as the rights and privileges those in the role can lay claim to. Is often unrealistic.

illness Disease; a functional disturbance resulting from an individual organism's inability to adapt to certain stressors; an abnormal physiologic state caused by microorganisms, cancer, or other conditions.

implementation Fourth step in the nursing process, in which the plan of care is carried out.

incidence Number of occurrences of a specific condition or event.

incident report Document that describes an accident or error involving a client or family member that may or may not have resulted in injury; the purpose of the incident report is to track incidents and to make changes in the situations that caused them; the incident report is not part of the chart.

incompetency Inability of an individual to manage personal affairs because of mental or physical conditions; the inability of a professional to carry out professional activities at the expected level of functioning because of lack of knowledge or skill or because of drug or alcohol abuse.

indemnity insurance Health insurance in which the contractual agreement is between the consumer and the insurance company. Providers are not involved in these arrangements, and rates are not pre-established.

independent nurse practitioner Nurse who has a private practice in one of the expanded roles of nursing.

independent practice association (IPA) Type of HMO usually organized by physicians that requires fee-for-service payment.

independent practice organization (IPO) Type of IPA in which a group of providers deals with more than one insurer at a time.

independent practitioner Health-care provider who delivers health care independently with or without supervision by another health-care practitioner.

indirect services Health-care actions that do not require direct client contact but that still facilitate care, such as the supply and distribution department of a hospital.

informed consent Permission granted by a person based on full knowledge of the risks and benefits of participation in a procedure or surgery for which the consent has been given.

injunction Court order specifying actions that must or must not be taken.

input Matter, energy, or information entering a system from the environment.

inquest Formal inquiry about the course or manner of death.

institutional licensure Authority for an individual health-care provider to practice that is granted by the individual's employing institution; the institution determines the educational preparation, training, and functions of each category of provider it employs; no longer legally permitted, UAPs act under a form of de facto institutional licensure.

intentional tort A willful act that violates another person's rights or property and may or may not cause physical injury.

interrogatories Written questions directed to a party in a lawsuit by the opposing side as part of the discovery process.

intervention Nursing action taken to meet specific client goals.

invasion of privacy A type of quasi-intentional tort that involves (1) an act that intrudes into the seclusion of the client; (2) intrusion that is objectionable to a reasonable person; (3) an act that intrudes into private facts or published as facts or pictures of a private nature; and (4) public disclosure of private information.

Joint Commission on Accreditation of Healthcare Organizations (JCAHO) Organization that performs accreditation reviews for health-care agencies.

judgment Decision of the court regarding a case.

jurisdiction Authority of a court to hear and decide lawsuits.

justice Fairness; giving people their due.

Kardex Portable card file that contains important client information and a care plan.

laisseze-faire A type of leadership style in which the leader does little planning, sets few goals, avoids decision making, and fails to encourage group members to participate. Also called permissive or nondirective leadership.

law Formal statement of a society's beliefs about interactions among and between its citizens; a formal rule enforced by society.

legal complaint Document filed by a plaintiff against a defendant claiming infringement of the plaintiff's legal rights.

legal obligations Obligations that have become formal statements of law and are enforceable under the law.

legal rights (welfare rights) Rights that are based on a legal entitlement to some good or benefits and are enforceable under the legal system with punishment for violations.

legislator Elected member of either the House of Representatives or the Senate.

legislature Body of elected individuals invested with constitutional power to make, alter, or repeal laws.

liable Obligated or held accountable by law.

libel Written defamation of character.

license Permission to practice granted to an individual by the state after he or she has met the requirements for that particular position; licensing protects the safety of the public.

licensed practical nurse (LPN) Licensed vocational nurse; technical nurse licensed by any state, after completing a practical nursing program, to provide technical bedside care to clients.

licensing board Government agency that implements the statutes of a particular profession in accordance with the Professions Practice Act.

licensure Process by which an agency or government grants an individual permission to practice; it establishes a minimal level of competency for practice.

licensure by endorsement Method of obtaining a license to practice by having a state acknowledge the individual's existing comparable license in another state.

licensure by examination Method of obtaining a license to practice by successfully passing a state board examination.

living will Signed legal document in which individuals make known their wishes about the care they are to receive if they should become incompetent at a future date; it usually specifies what types of treatments are permitted and what types are to be withheld.

lobbyist Person who attempts to influence political decisions as an official representative of an organization, group, or institution.

locality rule standard of care Legal process that holds an individual nurse accountable to both what is an acceptable standard within his or her local community and to national standards as developed by nurses throughout the nation through ANA, national practice groups, and health-care agencies.

malfeasance Performance of an illegal act.

malpractice Negligent acts by a licensed professional based on either omission of an expected action or commission of an inappropriate action resulting in damages to another party; not doing what a reasonable and prudent professional of the same rank would have done in the same situation.

managed care System of organized health-care delivery systems linked by provider networks; health maintenance organizations are the primary example of managed care.

mandatory licensure Law that requires all who practice a particular profession to have and to maintain a license in that profession.

manslaughter Killing of an individual without premeditated intent; different degrees of manslaughter exist, and most are felonies.

mediation A legal process that allows each party to present their case to a mediator, who is an independent third party trained in dispute resolution.

medical examiner Coroner; a physician who investigates deaths that appear to be from other than natural causes.

Medicaid State health-care insurance program, supported in part by federal funds, for health-care services for certain groups unable to pay for their own health care; amount and type of coverage vary from state to state.

medically indigent Individuals who cannot personally pay for health-care services without incurring financial hardship.

Medicare A federally run program that is financed primarily through employee payroll taxes and covers any individual who is 65 years of age or older as well as blind and disabled individuals of any age.

Medicare Utilization and Quality Peer Review Organization (PRO) Organization that reviews the quality and cost of Medicare services.

Medigap policies Health insurance policies that are purchased to cover expenses not paid by Medicare.

midwife Individual experienced in assisting women during labor and delivery; they may be lay midwives, who have no official education, or certified nurse midwives, who are RNs in an expanded role, having received additional education and passed a national certification examination.

misdemeanor Less serious crime than felony punishable by a fine of less than $1000 or a jail term of less than 1 year.

model A hypothetical representation of something that exists in reality. The purpose of a model is to attempt to explain a complex reality in a systematic and organized manner.

morality Concept of right and wrong.

moral obligations Obligations based on moral or ethical principles but are *not* enforceable under the law.

morals Fundamental standards of right and wrong that an individual learns and internalizes during the early stages of childhood development, based primarily on religious beliefs and societal norms.

mores Values and customs of a society.

mortality Property or capacity to die; death.

motivation Internal drive that causes individuals to seek achievement of higher goals; desire.

multicompetency technician Allied health care provider who has skills in two or more areas of practice through the process of cross-training.

multiskilled practitioner Health-care professional who has skills in more than one area of health care, such as an RN who has training in physical therapy.

national health insurance Proposed system of payment for health-care services whereby the government pays for the costs of the health care.

negative entropy Tendency toward increased order in a system.

negligence Failure to perform at an expected level of functioning or the performance of an inappropriate function resulting in damages to another party; not doing what a reasonable and prudent person would do in a similar situation.

no-code order Do not resuscitate (DNR) order; an order by a physician to withhold cardiopulmonary resuscitation and other resuscitative efforts from a client.

nonfeasance Failure to perform a legally required duty.

nonmaleficence Ethical principle that requires the professional to do no harm to the client.

nontraditional education Methods of education that do not follow the traditional lecture and clinical practice methods of learning; may include computer-simulated learning, self-education techniques, or other creative methods.

nonverbal A type of communication that uses any methods except written and spoken messages and constitutes 93 percent of the communication between individuals. It includes body language, gestures, facial expression, tone, pace, personal space, etc.

normative ethics Questions and dilemmas requiring a choice of actions where there is a conflict of rights or obligations between the nurse and the client, the nurse and the client's family, or the nurse and the physician.

norm-referenced examination Examination scored by comparison with standards established on the performance of all others who took the same examination during a specific time; the NLN achievement examinations are norm referenced.

not-for-profit (nonprofit) agencies Agencies in which all profits must be used in the operation of the organization.

nurse clinician Registered nurse with advanced skills in a particular area of nursing practice; if certified by a professional organization, a nurse clinician may also be a nurse practitioner, but more often this designation refers to nurses in advanced practice roles such as nurse specialists.

nurse practice act Part of state law that establishes the scope of practice for professional nurses, as well as educational levels and standards, professional conduct, and reasons for revocation of licensure.

nurse practitioner Nurse specialist with advanced education in a primary care specialty, such as community health, pediatrics, or mental health, who is prepared independently to manage health promotion and maintenance and illness prevention of a specific group of clients.

nurse specialist (clinical nurse specialist) Nurse who is an expert in providing care focused on a specialized field drawn from the range of general practice, such as cardiac nurse specialist.

nurse theorist Nurse who analyzes and attempts to describe what the profession of nursing is and what nurses do through nursing models or nursing theories.

nursing assessment Systematic collection and recording of client data, both objective and subjective, from primary and secondary sources using the nursing history, physical examination, and laboratory data, for example.

nursing diagnosis Statements of a client's actual or potential health-care problems or deficits.

nursing order Statement of a nursing action selected by a nurse to achieve a client's goal; may be stated as either the nurse's or the client's expected behavior.

nursing process Systematic, comprehensive decision-making process used by nurses to identify and treat actual and potential health problems.

nursing research Formal study of problems of nursing practice, the role of the nurse in health care, and the value of nursing.

nursing standards Desired nursing behaviors established by the profession and used to evaluate nurses' performance.

obligations Demands made on individuals, professions, society, or government to fulfill and honor the rights of others. Obligations are often divided into two categories—moral and legal (welfare).

occurrence policy A type of malpractice insurance that protects against all claims that occurred during the policy period regardless of when the claim is made.

omission Failure to fulfill a duty or carry out a procedure recognized as a standard of care; often forms the basis for claims of malpractice.

oncology Area of health care that deals with the treatment of cancer.

open curriculum Educational system that allows a student to enter and leave the system freely; often uses past education and experiences.

open system System that can exchange energy, matter, and information with the environment and with other systems.

ordinance Local or municipal law.

outcome criteria Standards that measure changes or improvements in clients' conditions.

out-of-pocket expenses Amount the client is responsible for paying for a health-care service.

output Matter, energy, or information released from a system into the environment or transmitted to another system.

palliative Type of treatment directed toward minimizing the severity of a disease or illness rather than curing it; for example, for a client with terminal cancer, relief of pain is the main goal (palliative), rather than cure.

panel of approved providers A list of physicians, nurse practitioners, pharmacies, and other health-care providers that are approved by an insurance plan and to whom reimbursement will be made by the insurer.

patient Client; an individual seeking or receiving health-care services.

patient day Client day; the 24-hour period during which hospital services are provided that forms the basis for charging the patient, usually from midnight to midnight.

pediatrics Study and care of problems and diseases of children younger than the age of 18.

peer review Evaluation against professional standards of the performance of individuals with the same basic education and qualifications; formal process of review or evaluation by coworkers of an equal rank.

perceived role image The individual's own definition of the role, which is usually more realistic than the ideal role, involving rejection or modification of some of the norms and expectations of society.

percussion Physical examination involving the tapping of various parts of the body to determine density by eliciting different sounds.

performed role image The actual duties performed by the practitioner of a role. Often produces reality shock in new graduate nurses.

perjury Crime committed by giving false testimony while under oath.

permissive licensure Law that allows individuals to practice a profession as long as they do not use the title of the profession; no states now have permissive licensure.

phenomenology Philosophical approach that holds that consciousness determines reality in space and time.

plaintiff Individual who charges another individual in a court of law with a violation of the individual's rights; the party who files the complaint in a lawsuit.

point-of-service plans Insurance plans in which consumers can select providers outside of a prescribed provider panel if they are willing to pay an additional fee.

political action Activities on the part of individuals that influence the actions of government officials in establishing policy.

political involvement Group of activities that, individually or collectively, increase the voice of nursing in the political or health-care policy process.

politics Process of influencing the decisions of others and exerting control over situations or events, includes influencing the allocation of scarce resources.

practical nursing program Vocational nursing program; a program of study leading to a certificate in practical nursing, usually 12 to 18 months in length; these programs are located in a vocational or technical school or in a community or junior college; after passing the NCLEX-LPN CAT examination, students become licensed practical nurses (LPNs).

precedent Decision previously issued by a court that is used as the basis for a decision in another case with similar circumstances.

preceptor Educated or skilled practitioner who agrees to work with a less educated or trained individual to increase the individual's knowledge and skills; often staff nurses who work with student nurses during their senior year.

precertification Approval for reimbursement of services prior to their being rendered.

preferred provider organization (PPO) Method of payment for employee health-care benefits in which employers contract with a specific group of health-care providers for a lower cost for their employees' health-care services but require the employee to use the providers listed.

premium Amount paid on a periodic basis for health insurance or HMO membership.

prescriptive authority Legal right to write prescriptions for medications, granted to physicians, veterinarians, dentists, and advanced practice nurses.

preventive care Well care; nursing care provided for the purpose of maintaining health and preventing disease or injury, often through community health clinics, school nursing services, and storefront clinics.

primary care Type of health care for individuals and families in which maintenance of health is emphasized; first-line health care in hospitals, physicians offices, or community health clinics that deal with acute conditions.

primary care nurse Hospital staff RN assigned to a primary care unit to provide nursing care to a limited number of clients, who are followed by the same nurse from admission to discharge.

primary intervention Health promotion, illness prevention, early diagnosis, and treatment of common health problems.

private-duty nurse Nurse in private practice; nurse self-employed for providing direct client care services either in the home or the hospital setting.

privileged communication Information imparted by a client to a physician, lawyer, or clergyman that is protected from disclosure in a court of law. Communication between a client and a nurse is not legally protected, but nurses can participate in privileged communication when they overhear information imparted by the client to the physician.

profession Nursing; an occupation that meets the criteria for a profession, including education, altruism, code of ethics, public service, and dedication.

professional review organization Multilevel program to oversee the quality and cost of federally funded medical care programs.

professionalism Behaviors and attitudes exhibited by an individual that are recognized by others as the traits of a professional.

prospective payment system (PPS) System of reimbursement for health-care services that establishes the payment rates before hospitalization based on certain criteria, such as diagnostic-related groups (DRGs).

protocol Written plan of action based on previously identified situations; standing orders are a type of protocol often used in specialty units that have clients with similar problems.

provider Person or organization who delivers health care including health promotion and maintenance and illness prevention and treatment.

provider panel Health-care providers selected to render services to a group of consumers within a managed-care plan.

proximate cause Nearest cause; the element in a direct cause-and-effect relationship between what is done by the professional and what happens to the client. As, for instance, when a nurse fails to raise the side rails on the bed of a client who has received a narcotic medication, and the client falls out of bed and breaks a hip as a result.

public policy Decision made by a society or its elected representatives that has a material effect on citizens other than on the decision makers.

quality Level of excellence based on pre-established criteria.

quality assurance Activity conducted in health-care facilities that evaluates the quality of care provided to ensure that it meets pre-established quality standards.

quasi-intentional tort A violation of a person's reputation or personal privacy.

reality shock (transition shock) A sudden and sometimes traumatic realization on the part of the new graduate that the ideal or perceived roles do not match the actual performed role.

recertification Periodic renewal of certification by examination, continuing education, or other criteria established by the accrediting agency.

reciprocity Endorsement; a state's acceptance of a license issued by another state.

registration Listing of a license with a state for a fee.

registry Published list of those who are registered; the agency that publishes the list of individuals who are registered.

regulations Rules or orders issued by various regulatory agencies, such as a state board of nursing, which have the force of law.

rehabilitation Restoration to the highest possible level of performance or health of an individual who has suffered an injury or illness.

relative intensity measures (RIMs) Method for calculating nursing resources needed to provide nursing care for various types of clients; helps determine the number and type of staff required based on client acuity and needs.

respondent superior Legal doctrine that holds the employer or supervisor responsible for the actions of the employees or of those supervised; for example, under this doctrine, RNs are held responsible for the actions of unlicensed assistive personnel under their supervision.

responsibility Accountability; the concept that all individuals are accountable for their own actions and for the consequences of those actions.

restorative care Curative care; nursing care that has as its goal cure and recovery from disease.

resume Curriculum vitae; a summary of an individual's education, work experience, and qualifications.

retrospective payment system Payment system for health care in which reimbursement is based on the actual care rendered rather than on preset rates.

right Just claim or expectation that may or may not be protected by law; legal rights are protected by law, whereas moral rights are not.

risk management Evaluating the risk of clients and staff for injuries and for potential liabilities and implementing corrective and preventive measures.

secondary care Nursing care usually provided in short-term and long-term care facilities to clients with commonly occurring conditions.

secondary intervention Acute care designed to prevent complications or resolve health problems.

secured settings Any institutional setting imposing restriction of movement, confinement, and limitations to activity and access; jails, locked units or locked mental institutions, prisons.

service insurance Health insurance in which services are provided for a prescribed fee that is established between the providers and the insurance company.

sexual assault nurse examiner (SANE) A registered nurse specializing in care of victims of sexual assault, performing physical and psychosocial examination, collection of physical evidence, and therapeutic interventions to minimize trauma.

significant other Individual who is not a family member but is emotionally or symbolically important to an individual.

slander Oral defamation of character.

sliding-scale fees Fees for services that are based on the client's ability to pay.

slow-code order Physician's order that the efforts for resuscitation of a client who is terminally ill should be initiated and conducted at a leisurely pace; the goal of a slow-code order is to allow the client to die during an apparent resuscitation. Slow-code orders are not acceptable practice and do not meet standards of care.

staff nurse Nurse generalist who works as an employee of a hospital, nursing home, community health agency, or some other organization providing primary and direct nursing care to clients.

standards Norms; criteria for expected behaviors or conduct.

standard of best interest A type of decision made about an individual's health care when he or she is unable to make the informed decision for his or her own care, based on what the health-care providers and/or the family decide is best for that individual.

standards of care Written or established criteria for nursing care that all nurses are expected to meet.

standards of practice Written or established criteria for nursing practice that all professional nurses are expected to meet.

standing order Written order by physician for certain actions or medication administration to be initiated or given in certain expected circumstances; similar to protocols.

statute Law passed by a government's legislature and signed by its chief executive.

statute of limitations Specific time period in which a lawsuit must be filed or a crime must be prosecuted; most nursing or medical lawsuits have a 2-year statute of limitations from the time of discovery of the incident.

statutory law Law passed by a legislature.

stereotype Fixed or predetermined image of or attitude toward an individual or group.

stress Crisis situation that causes increased anxiety and initiation of the flight-or-fight mechanism.

stressor Internal or external force to which a person responds.

structure criteria Physical environmental framework for client care.

subpoena Court document that requires an individual to appear in court and provide testimony; individuals who do not honor the subpoena can be held in contempt of court and jailed or fined.

subsystem Smaller system within a large system.

summary judgment Decision by a judge in cases in which no facts are in dispute.

sunset law Law that automatically terminates a program after a pre-established period of time unless that program can justify its need for existence.

support system Environmental factors and individuals who can help an individual in a crisis cope with the situation.

systems theory Theory that stresses the interrelatedness of parts in any system in which a change in one part affects all other parts; often, the system is greater than the sum of its parts.

taxonomy Classification system.

team nursing Method of organizing nursing care in which each client is assigned a team consisting of RNs, LPNs, and nursing assistants to deliver nursing care.

technician Individual who carries out technical tasks.

technology Use of science and the application of scientific principles to any situation; often involves the use of complicated machines and computers.

teleology Utilitarianism; an ethical system that identifies the right action by determining what will provide the greatest good for the greatest number of persons. This system has no set, unchanging rules; rather, it varies as the situation changes.

tertiary care Nursing care usually provided in long-term care and rehabilitation facilities for chronic diseases or injuries requiring long recovery.

tertiary intervention The provision of advanced and long-term health care services to acutely ill clients, including the use of advanced technology, complicated surgical procedures, rehabilitation services and care of the terminally ill.

testimony Oral statement of a witness under oath.

theory Set of interrelated constructs (concepts, definitions, or propositions) that presents a systematic view of phenomena by specifying relations among variables with the purpose of explaining and predicting phenomena.

third-party payment Payment for health-care services by an insurance company or a government agency rather than directly by the client.

third-party reimburser An organization other than the client, such as an employer, insurance company or governmental agency that assumes responsibility for payment of health care charges for services rendered to the client.

throughput Matter, energy, or information as it passes through a system.

tort Violation of the civil law that violates a person's rights and causes injury or harm to the individual. Civil wrong independent of an action in contract that results from a breach of a legal duty; a tort can be classified as unintentional, intentional, or quasi-intentional.

tort-feasor Person who commits a tort.

total quality management (TQM) A method for monitoring and maintaining the quality of health care being delivered by a particular institution or health-care industry.

trial Legal proceedings during which all relevant facts are presented to a jury or judge for legal decision.

Tri-Council Nursing group composed of the American Nurses Association (ANA), National League for Nursing (NLN), American Association of Colleges of Nursing (AACN), and American Organization of Nurse Executives (AONE).

two plus two (2+2) program Nursing education program that starts with an associate (2-year) degree and then moves the individual to a baccalaureate degree with an additional 2 years of education.

Uniform Anatomical Gift Act Legislation providing for a legal document signed by an individual indicating the desire to donate specific body organs or the entire body after death.

unintentional tort A wrong occurring to a person or that person's property even though it was not intended; negligence.

universal health-care coverage Health-care reimbursement benefits for all United States citizens and legal residents.

universal precautions Body substance isolation; guidelines established by the Centers for Disease Control and Prevention (CDC) and the Occupational Safety and Health Administration (OSHA) to protect health-care professionals and clients from diseases carried in the blood and body fluids, such as HIV and hepatitis B; involves the use of gloves whenever in contact with blood or body fluids and masks, gowns, and eye covers if a chance exists of contact with aerosol fluids.

upward mobility Movement toward increased status and power in an organization through promotion.

utilitarianism Teleology; an ethical system that identifies the right action by determining what will provide the greatest good for the greatest number of persons. This system has no set, unchanging rules; rather, it varies as the situation changes.

utilization guidelines Guidelines that stipulate the amount of services that can be delivered by a health-care provider.

value Judgment of worth, quality, or desirability based on attitude formed from need or experience; a strong belief held by individuals about something important to them.

values clarification Process by which individuals list and prioritize the values they hold most important.

veracity The principle of truthfulness. It requires the health-care provider to tell the truth and not intentionally deceive or mislead clients.

verbal A type of communication based on written or spoken messages that constitutes approximately 7 percent of the total communication between individuals.

veto Signed refusal by the President or a governor to enact a bill into law. If the President vetoes a bill, the veto may be overridden by a two-thirds vote of the membership of both the House and Senate.

vicarious liability Imputation of blame on a person for the actions of the other.

victimization Experience of physical, emotional or psychological trauma in which the individual suffers injury, fear, self-blame and/or other dysfunction.

vocational nursing program Licensed practical nursing program in Texas and California; a program of study leading to a certificate in vocational nursing, usually 12 to 18 months in length; these programs are located in a vocational or technical school or a community or junior college; after passing the NCLEX-LPN CAT examination, students become licensed vocational nurses (LVNs).

Appendix A

Boards of Nursing

Alabama Board of Nursing
770 Washington Avenue
RSA Plaza, Suite 250
Montgomery, AL 36130-3900
Phone: (334) 242-4060
Fax: (334) 242-4360
www.abn.state.al.us
Contact Person: N. Genell Lee, MSN, JD, RN, Executive Officer

Alaska Board of Nursing
550 West Seventh Avenue, Suite 1500
Anchorage, AK 99501-3567
Phone: (907) 269-8161
Fax: (907) 269-8196
www.dced.state.ak.us/occ/pnur.htm
Contact Person: Dorothy Fulton, MA, RN, Executive Director

American Samoa Health Services Regulatory Board
LBJ Tropical Medical Center
Pago Pago, AS 96799
Phone: (684) 633-1222
Fax: (684) 633-1869
Contact Person: Etenauga Lutu, RN, Executive Secretary

Arizona State Board of Nursing
1651 E. Morten Avenue, Suite 210
Phoenix, AZ 85020
Phone: (602) 331-8111
Fax: (602) 906-9365
www.azboardofnursing.org
Contact Person: Joey Ridenour, MN, RN, Executive Director

Arkansas State Board of Nursing
University Tower Building
1123 S. University, Suite 800
Little Rock, AR 72204-1619
Phone: (501) 686-2700
Fax: (501) 686-2714
www.state.ar.us/nurse
Contact Person: Faith Fields, MSN, RN, Executive Director

California Board of Registered Nursing
400 R Street, Suite 4030
Sacramento, CA 95814-6239
Phone: (916) 322-3350
Fax: (916) 327-4402
www.rn.ca.gov
Contact Person: Ruth Ann Terry, MPH, RN, Executive Officer

California Board of Vocational Nurse and Psychiatric Technician Examiners
2535 Capitol Oaks Drive, Suite 205
Sacramento, CA 95833
Phone: (916) 263-7800
Fax: (916) 263-7859
www.bvnpt.ca.gov
Contact Person: Teresa Bello-Jones, JD, MSN, RN, Executive Officer

Colorado Board of Nursing
1560 Broadway, Suite 880
Denver, CO 80202
Phone: (303) 894-2430
Fax: (303) 894-2821
www.dora.state.co.us/nursing
Contact Person: Patricia Uris, PhD, RN, Program Administrator

Connecticut Board of Examiners for Nursing
Department of Public Health
410 Capitol Avenue, MS# 13PHO
P.O. Box 340308
Hartford, CT 06134-0328
Phone: (860) 509-7624
Fax: (860) 509-7553
www.state.ct.us/dph
Contact Person: Jan Wojick, Board Liaison

Delaware Board of Nursing
861 Silver Lake Boulevard
Cannon Building, Suite 203
Dover, DE 19904
Phone: (302) 739-4522
Fax: (302) 739-2711
www.professionallicensing.state.de.us/boards/nursing/index.shtml
Contact Person: Iva Boardman, MSN, RN, Executive Director

District of Columbia Board of Nursing
Department of Health
825 N. Capitol Street, N.E., 2nd Floor
Room 2224
Washington, DC 20002
Phone: (202) 442-4778
Fax: (202) 442-9431
www.dchealth.dc.gov
Contact Person: Karen Scipio-Skinner, MSN, RNC, Executive Director

Florida Board of Nursing
Capital Circle Officer Center
4052 Bald Cypress Way
Room 120
Tallahassee, FL 32399-3252
Phone: (850) 488–0595
www.doh.state.fl.us/mqa
Contact Person: Dan Coble, RN, PhD, Executive Director

Georgia State Board of Licensed Practical Nurses
237 Coliseum Drive
Macon, GA 31217-3858
Phone: (478) 207-1300
Fax: (478) 207-1633
www.sos.state.ga.us/plb/Ipn
Contact Person: Jacqueline Hightower, JD, Executive Director

Georgia Board of Nursing
237 Coliseum Drive
Macon, GA 31217-3858
Phone: (478) 207-1640
Fax: (478) 207-1660
www.sos.state.ga.us/plb/rn

Guam Board of Nurse Examiners
P.O. Box 2816
1304 East Sunset Boulevard
Barrgada, GU 96913
Phone: (671) 475-0251
Fax: (671) 477-4733
Contact Person: Lucy Cruz Iona, RN, FNP, Active Executive Officer

Hawaii Board of Nursing
Professional and Vocational Licensing Division
P.O. Box 3469
Honolulu, HI 96801
Phone: (808) 586-3000
Fax: (808) 586-2689
www.state.hi.us/dcca/pvl/areas_nurse.html

Contact Person: Kathleen Yokouchi, MBA, BBA, BA, Executive Officer

Idaho Board of Nursing
280 N. 8th Street, Suite 210
P.O. Box 83720
Boise, ID 83720
Phone: (208) 334-3110
Fax: (208) 334-3262
www.state.id.us/ibn/ibnhome.htm
Contact Person: Sandra Evans, MA, Ed, RN, Executive Director

Illinois Department of Professional Regulation
James R. Thompson Center
100 West Randolph, Suite 9-300
Chicago, IL 60601
Phone: (312) 814-2715
Fax: (312) 814-3145
www.dpr.state.il.us
Contact Person: Deborah Taylor, RN, EdD, Nursing Act Assistant Coordinator

Illinois Department of Professional Regulation
320 W. Washington Street
3rd Floor
Springfield, IL 62786
Phone: (217) 782-8556
Fax: (217) 782-7645

Indiana State Board of Nursing
Health Professions Bureau
402 W. Washington Street, Room W041
Indianapolis, IN 46204
Phone: (317) 232-2960
Fax: (317) 233-4236
www.statc.in.us/hpb/boards/isbn
Contact Person: Kristen Kelley, Director of Nursing of IN BON

Iowa Board of Nursing
RiverPoint Business Park
400 S.W. 8th Street
Suite B
Des Moines, IA 50309-4685
Phone: (515) 281-3255
Fax: (515) 281-4825
www.state.ia.us/government/nursing
Contact Person: Lorinda Inman, MSN, RN, Executive Director

Kansas State Board of Nursing
Landon State Office Building
900 S.W. Jackson, Suite 551-S
Topeka, KS 66612
Phone: (785) 296-4929
Fax: (785) 296-3929
www.ksbn.org
Contact Person: Mary Blubaugh, MSN, RN, Executive Administrator

Kentucky Board of Nursing
312 Whittington Parkway, Suite 300
Louisville, KY 40222
Phone: (502) 329-7000
Fax: (502) 329-7011
www.kbn.state.ky.us
Contact Person: Sharon Weisenbeck, MS, RN, Executive Director

Louisiana State Board of Practical Nurse Examiners
3421 N. Causeway Boulevard, Suite 203
Metairie, LA 70002
Phone: (504) 838-5791
Fax: (504) 838-5279
www.Isbpne.com
Contact Person: Claire Glaviano, BSN, MN, RN, Executive Director

Louisiana State Board of Nursing
3510 N. Causeway Boulevard, Suite 501
Metairie, LA 70002
Phone: (504) 838-5332
Fax: (504) 838-5349
www.Isbn.state.la.us
Contact Person: Barbara Morvant, MN, RN, Executive Director

Maine State Board of Nursing
158 State House Station
Augusta, ME 04333
Phone: (207) 287-1133
Fax: (207) 287-1149
www.state.me.us/boardofnursing

Contact Person: Myra Broadway, JD, MS, RN, Executive Director

Maryland Board of Nursing
4140 Patterson Avenue
Baltimore, MD 21215
Phone: (410) 585-1900
Fax: (410) 358-3530
www.mbon.org
Contact Person: Donna Dorsey, MS, RN, Executive Director

Massachusetts Board of Registration in Nursing
Commonwealth of Massachusetts
239 Causeway Street
Boston, MA 02114
Phone: (617) 727-9961
Fax: (617) 727-1630
www.state.ma.us/reg/boards/rn
Contact Person: Theresa Bonanno, MSN, RN, Executive Director

Michigan CIS/Bureau of Health Services
Ottawa Towers North
611 W. Ottawa, 4th Floor
Lansing, MI 48933
Phone: (517) 373-9102
Fax: (517) 373-2179
www.cis.state.mi.us/bhser/genover.htm
Contact Person: Diane Lewis, Policy Manager for Licensing Division

Minnesota Board of Nursing
2829 University Avenue, S.E.
Suite 500
Minneapolis, MN 55414
Phone: (612) 617-2270
Fax: (612) 617-2190
www.nursingboard.state.mn.us
Contact Person: Shirley Brekken, MS, RN, Executive Director

Mississippi Board of Nursing
1935 Lakeland Drive, Suite B
Jackson, MS 39216-5014
Phone: (601) 987-4188
Fax: (601) 364-2352
www.msbn.state.ms.us
Contact Person: Delia Owens, RN, JD, Executive Director

Missouri State Board of Nursing
3605 Missouri Boulevard
P.O. Box 656
Jefferson City, MO 65102-0656
Phone: (573) 751-0681
Fax: (573) 751-0075
www.ecodev.state.mo.us/pr/nursing
Contact Person: Lori Scheidt, BS, Acting Executive Director

Montana State Board of Nursing
301 South Park
P.O. Box 200513
Helena, MT 59620-0513
Phone: (406) 841-2340
Fax: (406) 841-2343
www.discoveringmontana.com/dli/bsd/license/bsd_boards/nur_board/board_page.htm
Contact Person: Barbara Swehla, MN, RN, Executive Director

Commonwealth Board of Nurse Examiners
P.O. Box 501458
Saipan, MP 96950
Phone: (670) 664-4812
Fax: (670) 664-4813
Contact Person: Rosa M. Tudela, Associate Director for Public Health and Nursing

Nebraska Health and Human Services System
Department of Regulation and Licensure, Nursing Section
301 Centennial Mall South
Lincoln, NE 68509-4986
Phone: (402) 471-4376
Fax: (402) 471-3577
www.hhs.state.ne.us/crl/nursing/nursingindex.htm
Contact Person: Charlene Kelly, PhD, RN, Executive Director

Nevada State Board of Nursing
Administration, Discipline and Investigations

1755 East Plumb Lane
Suite 260
Reno, NV 89502
Phone: (775) 688-2620
Fax: (775) 688-2628
www.nursingboard.state.nv.us
Contact Person: Debra Scott, MS, RN,
Executive Director

Nevada State Board of Nursing
License Certification and Education
4330 S. Valley View Boulevard
Suite 106
Las Vegas, NV 89103
Phone: (702) 486-5800
Fax: (702) 486-5803
www.nursingboard.state.nv.us
Contact Person: Don Rennie MS, RN,
Associate Executive Director for Licensure and Certification

New Hampshire Board of Nursing
P.O. Box 3898
78 Regional Drive, Building B
Concord, NH 03302
Phone: (603) 271-2323
Fax: (603) 271-6605
www.state.nh.us/nursing
Contact Person: Cynthia Gray, MBA, BS, RN,
CPN, Executive Director

New Jersey Board of Nursing
P.O. Box 45010
124 Halsey Street, 6th Floor
Newark, NJ 07101
Phone: (973) 504-6586
Fax: (973) 648-3481
www.state.nj.us/lps/ca/medical.htm
Contact Person: Patricia Lynch Polansky, MS,
RN, Executive Director

New Mexico Board of Nursing
4206 Louisiana Boulevard, N.E.
Suite A
Albuquerque, NM 87109
Phone: (505) 841-8340
Fax: (505) 841-8347
www.state.nm.us/clients/nursing
Contact Person: Debra Brady, PhD, RN,
Executive Director

New York State Board of Nursing
Education Building
89 Washington Avenue
2nd Floor West Wing
Albany, NY 12234
Phone: (518) 474-3817, Ext. 120
Fax: (518) 474-3706
www.nysed.gov/prof/nurse.htm
Contact Person: Barbara Zittel, PhD, RN,
Executive Secretary

North Carolina Board of Nursing
3724 National Drive, Suite 201
Raleigh, NC 27612
Phone: (919) 782-3211
Fax: (919) 781-9461
www.ncbon.com
Contact Person: Polly Johnson, MSN, RN,
Executive Director

North Dakota Board of Nursing
919 South 7th Street, Suite 504
Bismarck, ND 58504
Phone: (701) 328-9777
Fax: (701) 328-9785
www.ndbon.org
Contact Person: Constance Kalanek, PhD, RN,
Executive Director

Ohio Board of Nursing
17 South High Street, Suite 400
Columbus, OH 43215-3413
Phone: (614) 466-3947
Fax: (614) 466-0388
www.state.oh.us/nur
Contact Person: John Brion, RN, MS,
Executive Director

Oklahoma Board of Nursing
2915 N. Classen Boulevard, Suite 524
Oklahoma City, OK 73106
Phone: (405) 962-1800
Fax: (405) 962-1821

www.youroklahoma.com/nursing
Contact Person: Kimberly Glazier, MEd, RN, Executive Director

Oregon State Board of Nursing
800 N.E. Oregon Street, Box 25
Suite 465
Portland, OR 97232
Phone: (503) 731-4745
Fax: (503) 731-4755
www.osbn.state.or.us
Contact Person: Joan Bouchard, MN, RN, Executive Director

Pennsylvania State Board of Nursing
P.O. 2649
124 Pine Street
Harrisburg, PA 17101
Phone: (717) 783-7142
Fax: (717) 783-0822
www.dos.state.pa.us/bpoa/cwp/view.asp?a=1104&q=432869
Contact Person: Miriam Limo, MS, MSN, RN, Executive Secretary

Commonwealth of Puerto Rico Board of Nurse Examiners
800 Roberto H. Todd Avenue
Room 202, Stop 18
Santurce, PR 00908
Phone: (787) 725-7506
Fax: (787) 725-7903
Contact Person: Magda Bouet, Executive Director of the Office of Regulations and Certifications of Health Care Professions

Rhode Island Board of Nurse Registration and Nursing Education
105 Cannon Building
Three Capitol Hill
Providence, RI 02908
Phone: (401) 222-5700
Fax: (401) 222-3352
www.healthri.org/hsr/professions/nurses.htm
Contact Person: Charles Alexandre, MSN, RN, Executive Officer

South Carolina State Board of Nursing
110 Centerview Drive
Suite 202
Columbia, SC 29210
Phone: (803) 896-4550
Fax: (803) 896-4525
www.llr.state.sc.us/pol/nursing
Contact Person: Martha Bursinger, RN, MSN, Executive Director

South Dakota Board of Nursing
4300 South Louise Avenue, Suite C-1
Sioux Falls, SD 57106-3124
Phone: (605) 362-2760
Fax: (605) 362-2768
www.state.sd.us/dcr/nursing
Contact Person: Diana Vander Woude, MS, RN, Executive Secretary

Tennessee State Board of Nursing
426 Fifth Avenue North
Cordell Hull Building, 1st Floor
Nashville, TN 37247
Phone: (615) 532-5166
Fax: (615) 741-7899
www.state.tn.us/health
Contact Person: Elizabeth Lund, MSN, RN, Executive Director

Texas Board of Nurse Examiners
333 Guadalupe, Suite 3-460
Austin, TX 78701
Phone: (512) 305-7400
Fax: (512) 305-7401
www.bne.state.tx.us
Contact Person: Katherine Thomas, MN, RN, Executive Director

Texas Board of Vocational Nurse Examiners
William P. Hobby Building, Tower 3
333 Guadalupe Street, Suite 3-400
Austin, TX 78701
Phone: (512) 305-8100
Fax: (512) 305-8101
www.bvne.state.tx.us
Contact Person: Terrie Hairston, RN, CHE, Executive Director

Utah State Board of Nursing
Heber M. Wells Building, 4th Floor
160 East 300 South
Salt Lake City, UT 84111
Phone: (801) 530-6628
Fax: (801) 530-6511
www.commerce.state.ut.us
Contact Person: Laura Poe, MS, RN, Executive Administrator

Vermont State Board of Nursing
109 State Street
Montpelier, VT 05609-1106
Phone: (802) 828-2396
Fax: (802) 828-2484
www.vtprofessionals.org/opr1/nurses
Contact Person: Anita Ristau, MS, RN, Executive Director

Virgin Islands Board of Nurse Licensure
Veterans Drive Station
St. Thomas, VI 00803
Phone: (340) 776-7397
Fax: (340) 777-4003
Contact Person: Winifred Garfield, CRNA, RN, Executive Secretary

Virginia Board of Nursing
6606 W. Board Street, 4th Floor
Richmond, VA 23230
Phone: (804) 662-9909
Fax: (804) 662-9512
www.dhp.state.va.us
Contact Person: Nancy Durrett, MSN, RN, Executive Director

Washington State Nursing Care Quality Assurance Commission
Department of Health
1300 Quince Street, S.E.
Olympia, WA 98504-7864
Phone: (360) 236-4700
Fax: (360) 236-4738
www.doh.wa.gov/nursing
Contact Person: Paula Meyer, MSN, RN, Executive Director

West Virginia State Board of Examiners for Licensed Practical Nurses
101 Dee Drive
Charleston, WV 25311
Phone: (304) 558-3572
Fax: (304) 558-4367
www.lpnboard.state.wv.us
Contact Person: Lanette Anderson, RN, BSN, JD, Executive Secretary

West Virginia Board of Examiners for Registered Professional Nurses
101 Dee Drive
Charleston, WV 25311
Phone: (304) 558-3596
Fax: (304) 558-3666
www.state.wv.us/nurses/rn
Contact Person: Laura Rhodes, MSN, RN, Executive Director

Wisconsin Department of Regulation and Licensing
1400 E. Washington Avenue
P.O. Box 8935
Madison, WI 53708
Phone: (608) 266-0145
Fax: (608) 261-7083
www.drl.state.wi.us
Contact Person: Kimberly Nania, Director, Bureau of Health Service Professions

Wyoming State Board of Nursing
2020 Carey Avenue, Suite 110
Cheyenne, WY 82002
Phone: (307) 777-7601
Fax: (307) 777-3519
www.nursing.state.wy.us
Contact Person: Cheryl Lynn Koski, MS, RN, CS, Executive Director

Source: National Council of State Boards of Nursing, Inc.

Appendix B

Specialty Nursing Organizations

Academy of Medical-Surgical Nurses (AMSN)
North Woodbury Road, Box 56
Pitman, NJ 08071
Phone: (609) 589-6677
Fax: (609) 589-7463
www.medsurgnurse.org

American Academy of Ambulatory Care Nursing (AAACN)
North Woodbury Road, Box 56
Pitman, NJ 08071
Phone: (609) 582-9617
Fax: (609) 589-7463
www.aaacn.org

American Association of Critical-Care Nurses (AACN)
101 Columbia
Aliso Viejo, CA 92656-1491
Phone: (800) 899-2226/(949) 362-2000
Fax: (949) 362-2020
www.aacn.org

American Association of Diabetes Educators (AADE)
444 N. Michigan Avenue
Suite 1240
Chicago, IL 60611-3901
Phone: (312) 664-2233/(800) 644-2233
Fax: (312) 644-4411
www.aadenet.org

American Association of Neuroscience Nurses (AANN)
224 N. Des Plaines #601
Chicago, IL 60661
Phone: (312) 993-0043
www.aann.org

American Association of Nurse Anesthetists (AANA)
222 South Prospect Avenue
Park Ridge, IL 60068-4001
Phone: (847) 692-7050
Fax: (847) 692-6968
www.aana.com

American Association of Occupational Health Nurses (AAOHN)
50 Lenox Pointe
Atlanta, GA 30324
Phone: (404) 262-1162
Fax: (404) 262-1165
www.aaohn.org

American Association of Spinal Cord Injury Nurses (AASCIN)
75-20 Astoria Boulevard
Jackson Heights, NY 11370-1177

Phone: (718) 803-3782
Fax: (718) 803-0414
www.aascin.org

American College of Nurse-Midwives (ACNM)
1522 K Street, N.W., Suite 1000
Washington, DC 20005
Phone: (202) 289-0171
Fax: (202) 289-4395
www.acnm.org

American Nephrology Nurses Association (ANNA)
North Woodbury Road, Box 56
Pitman, NJ 08071
Phone: (609) 589-2187
Fax: (609) 589-7463
www.inurse.com/anna

American Psychiatric Nurses' Association (APNA)
6900 Grove Road
Thorofare, NJ 08086
Phone: (609) 848-7990
Fax: (609) 848-5274
www.apna.org

American Society of Anesthesiologists (ASA)
520 North Northwest Highway
Park Ridge, IL 60068
Phone: (847) 825-5586
Fax: (847) 825-1692
www.asahq.org

American Society of Ophthalmic Registered Nurses, Inc. (ASORN)
655 Beach Street
P.O. Box 193030
San Francisco, CA 94119
Phone: (415) 561-8513
Fax: (415) 561-8575
http://webeye.ophth.uiowa.edu/asorn

American Society of Pain Management Nurses (ASPMN)
7794 Grow Drive
Pensacola, FL 32514-7072
Phone: (888) 34-ASPMN
Fax: (850) 484-8762
www.aspmn.org

American Society of Plastic and Reconstructive Surgical Nurses, Inc. (ASPRSN)
North Woodbury Road, Box 56
Pitman, NJ 08071
Phone: (609) 589-6247
Fax: (609) 589-7463

American Society of Post Anesthesia Nurses (ASPAN)
11512 Allecingie Parkway
Richmond, VA 23235
Phone: (804) 379-5516
Fax: (804) 379-1386
www.aspan.org

American Urological Association Allied, Inc. (AUAA)
11512 Allecingie Parkway
Richmond, VA 23235
Phone: (804) 379-1306
Fax: (804) 379-1386

Association for Practitioners in Infection Control (APIC)
505 E. Hawley Street
Mundelein, IL 60060
Phone: (708) 949-6052
Fax: (708) 566-7282

Association of Perioperative Registered Nurses (AORN)
2170 S. Parker Road, Suite 300
Denver, CO 80231-5711
Phone: (303) 755-6300/(800) 755-2676
Fax: (303) 750-2927
www.aorn.org

Association of Pediatric Oncology Nurses (APON)
11512 Allecingie Parkway
Richmond, VA 23235
Phone: (804) 379-9150
Fax: (804) 379-1386
www.apon.org

Association of Rehabilitation Nurses (ARN)
5700 Old Orchard Road, First Floor
Skokie, IL 60077-1057
Phone: (708) 966-3433
Fax: (708) 966-9418
www.rehabnurse.org

Association of Women's Health, Obstetric and Neonatal Nurses (AWHONN)
2000 L Street, N.W., Suite 740
Washington, DC 20036
Phone: (800) 673-8499
Fax: (202) 728-0575
www.awhonn.org

Dermatology Nurses' Association (DNA)
North Woodbury Road, Box 56
Pitman, NJ 08071
Phone: (609) 582-1915
Fax: (609) 589-7463
www.dna.inurse.com

Emergency Nurses Association (ENA)
915 Lee Street
Des Plaines, IL 60016-6569
Phone: (800) 243-8362
Fax: (847) 460-4001
www.ena.org

Federated Ambulatory Surgery Association (FASA)
700 N. Fairfax Street, #306
Alexandria, VA 22314
Phone: (703) 836-8808
Fax: (703) 549-0976
www.fasa.org

International Society of Nurses in Genetics, Inc. (ISONG)
University of North Dakota
Department of Pediatrics/Genetics
501 Columbia Road
Grand Forks, ND 58203
Phone: (701) 777-4243

Intravenous Nurses Society, Inc. (INS)
Two Brighton Street
Belmont, MA 02178
Phone: (617) 489-5205
Fax: (617) 484-6992

National Association of Nurse Massage Therapists (NANMT)
6851 Yumuri Street, #8
Coral Gables, FL 33146
Phone: (305) 667-6821
www.nanmt.org

National Association of Nurse Practitioners in Reproductive Health (NANPRH)
2401 Pennsylvania Avenue, N.W., #350
Washington, DC 20037-1718
Phone: (202) 466-4825
Fax: (202) 466-3826

National Association of Orthopaedic Nurses (NAON)
North Woodbury Road, Box 56
Pitman, NJ 08071
Phone: (609) 582-0111
Fax: (609) 589-7463

National Association of Pediatric Nurse Associates and Practitioners (NAPNAP)
1101 Kings Highway North, Suite 206
Cherry Hill, NJ 08034
Phone: (609) 667-1773
Fax: (609) 667-7187
www.napnap.org

National Association of School Nurses, Inc. (NASN)
P.O. Box 1300
Scarborough, ME 04070-1300
Phone: (207) 883-2117
Fax: (207) 883-2683
www.nasn.org

National Federation for Specialty Nursing Organizations (NFSNO)
East Hully Avenue, Box 56
Pitman, NJ 08071
Phone: (856) 256-2333
Fax: (856) 589-7463
www.inurse.com/nfsno

National Flight Nurses Association (NFNA)
6900 Grove Road
Thorofare, NJ 08086-9447

Phone: (609) 384-6725
Fax: (609) 848-5274
www.astna.org

National Nurses Society on Addictions (NNSA)
5700 Old Orchard Road, First Floor
Skokie, IL 60077-1057
Phone: (708) 966-5010
Fax: (708) 966-9418

Oncology Nursing Society (ONS)
501 Holiday Drive
Pittsburgh, PA 15220-2749
Phone: (412) 921-7373
Fax: (412) 921-6565
www.ons.org

Society of Ambulatory Anesthesiologists (SAMBA)
520 N. Northwest Highway
Park Ridge, IL 60068-2573
Phone: (847) 825-5586
www.sambahq.org

Society of Critical Care Medicine (SCCM)
701 Lee Street, Suite 200
Des Plaines, IL 60016
Phone: (847) 827-6869
Fax: (847) 827-6886
www.sccm.org

Society of Gastroenterology Nurses and Associates, Inc. (SGNA)
1070 Sibley Tower
Rochester, New York 14604
Phone: (716) 546-7241
Fax: (716) 546-5141
www.sgna.org

Society of Otorhinolaryngology and Head-Neck Nurses, Inc. (SOHN)
116 Canal Street, Suite A
New Smyrna Beach, FL 32168-7004
Phone: (904) 428-1695
Fax: (904) 423-7566
www.sohnnurse.com

Affiliate Members

American Association of Nurse Attorneys (TAANA)
720 Light Street
Baltimore, MD 21230
Phone: (410) 752-3318
Fax: (410) 752-8295
www.taana.org

American Holistic Nurses Association (AHNA)
4101 Lake Boone Trail, Suite 201
Raleigh, NC 27607
Phone: (919) 787-5181
Fax: (919) 787-4916
www.ahna.org

National Association of GCRC Nurse Managers (NAGCRCNM)
Clinical Research Center
The Center for Health Sciences
27-066 CHS 169747
10833 Le Conte Avenue
Los Angeles, CA 90024-169747
Phone: (310) 825-5225
Fax: (310) 206-9440

National Association for Health Care Recruitment (NAHCR)
P.O. Box 5769
Akron, OH 44372
Phone: (216) 867-3088
Fax: (216) 867-1630
www.nahcr.com

National Student Nurses' Association, Inc. (NSNA)
555 West 57th Street
New York, NY 10019
Phone: (212) 581-2211
Fax: (212) 581-2368
www.nsna.org

Nursing Organization Liaison Forum (NOLF)
600 Maryland Avenue, S.W.
Suite 100 West
Washington, DC 20024
Phone: (202) 554-4444

Index

Page numbers followed by *b* indicate boxes; page numbers followed by *f* indicate figures; page numbers followed by *t* indicate tables.

A

D

E

F

G

J

K

L

O

P

Q

R

S

Y